Seltzer and Bender's Dental Pulp

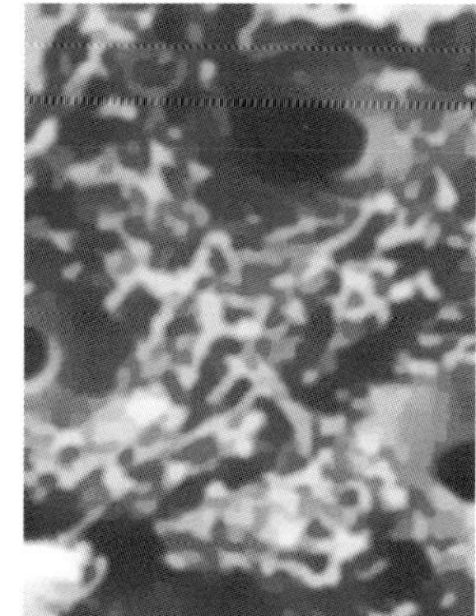

Seltzer and Bender's Dental Pulp

With great expectations
IB Bender 4-31-03

Edited by

KENNETH M. HARGREAVES, DDS, PHD
Professor
Departments of Endodontics and Pharmacology
University of Texas Health Science Center at San Antonio
San Antonio, Texas

HAROLD E. GOODIS, DDS
Professor
Department of Restorative Dentistry
University of California at San Francisco
San Francisco, California

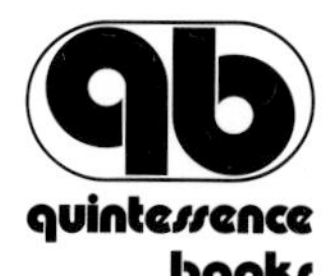

Quintessence Publishing Co, Inc
Chicago, Berlin, Tokyo, London, Paris, Milan, Barcelona,
Istanbul, São Paulo, New Delhi, Moscow, Prague, and Warsaw

Library of Congress Cataloging-in-Publication Data

Seltzer and Bender's dental pulp / edited by Kenneth M. Hargreaves,
Harold E. Goodis.
p. ; cm.
Rev. ed. of: The dental pulp / Samuel Seltzer, I.B. Bender. 3rd ed.
c1984.
Includes bibliographical references and index.
ISBN 0-86715-415-2 (hardcover)
1. Dental pulp. 2. Endodontics.
[DNLM: 1. Dental Pulp. 2. Dental Pulp--physiology. 3. Dental Pulp
Diseases. 4. Endodontics--methods. WU 230 S4675 2002] I. Title:
Dental pulp. II. Hargreaves, Kenneth M. III. Goodis, Harold E. IV.
Seltzer, Samuel, 1914- Dental pulp.
RK351 .S4 2002
617.6'342--dc21
2002000198

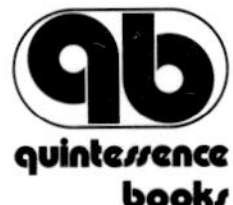

© 2002 by Quintessence Publishing Co, Inc

Published by Quintessence Publishing Co, Inc
551 Kimberly Drive
Carol Stream, IL 60188
www.quintpub.com

All rights reserved. This book or any part thereof may not be reproduced, stored in a retrieval system, or transmitted in any form or by any means, electronic, mechanical, photocopying, recording, or otherwise, without prior written permission of the publisher.

Editor: Lisa C. Bywaters
Assistant Editor: Kathryn O'Malley
Design and Production: Dawn Hartman
Printed in China

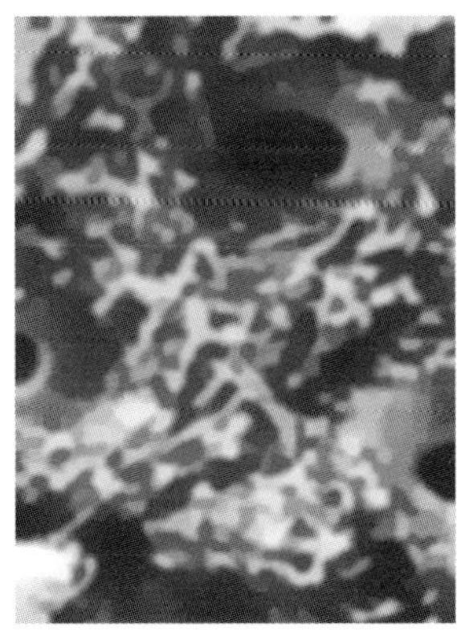

Dedication

To my wife, Holly, and our children, Nick and Mike, for their love, support, and remarkable patience.
To my colleagues at San Antonio, for their advice, support, and friendship. Mange tusen tak.

—KMH

To my dear wife Joan and our children and grandchildren. I couldn't have done it without your support, understanding, and love. I love you all.
To my colleagues at UCSF for your patience, understanding, and most of all, your friendship. You have made this book possible.

—HEG

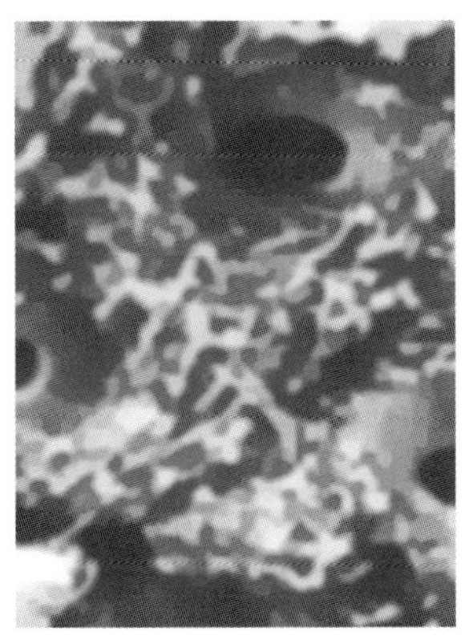

Table of Contents

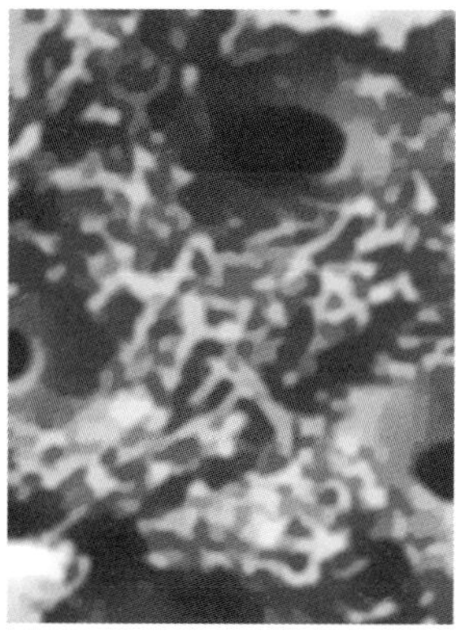

Contributors

J. Craig Baumgartner, DDS, PhD
Professor and Chair
Department of Endodontology
Oregon Health Sciences University
Portland, Oregon

I. B. Bender, DDS
Chairman Emeritus
Department of Dentistry
Albert Einstein Medical Center
Philadelphia, Pennsylvania

George Bogen, DDS
Private Practice
Los Angeles, California

Margaret R. Byers, PhD
Research Professor
Departments of Anesthesiology, Biological Structure, and Endodontics
University of Washington
Seattle, Washington

Charles F. Cox, DMD, PhD
Professor
Department of Restorative Dentistry
University of California at Los Angeles
Los Angeles, California

Rena D'Souza, DDS, MS, PhD
Professor and Director of Research
Department of Orthodontics
University of Texas Health Science Center
Houston, Texas

Ashraf F. Fouad, DDS, MS
Associate Professor
Department of Endodontology
University of Connecticut Health Center
Farmington, Connecticut

Harold E. Goodis, DDS
Professor
Department of Restorative Dentistry
University of California at San Francisco
San Francisco, California

Kenneth M. Hargreaves, DDS, PhD
Professor
Departments of Endodontics and Pharmacology
University of Texas Health Science Center at San Antonio
San Antonio, Texas

Hideharu Ikeda, DDS, PhD
Department of Restorative Sciences
Tokyo Medical and Dental University
Tokyo, Japan

Hugh M. Kopel, DDS, MS
Professor Emeritus
University of Southern California
Los Angeles, California

Lecturer
Section of Pediatric Dentistry
University of California at Los Angeles
Los Angeles, California

Linda Levin, DDS, PhD
Associate Professor
Department of Endodontics
University of North Carolina
Chapel Hill, North Carolina

Harold H. Messer, DDS, PhD
Professor of Restorative Dentistry
The University of Melbourne
Melbourne, Australia

Matti V. O. Närhi, DDS, PhD
Professor of Pain Physiology
University of Turku
Turku, Finland

Professor
Department of Physiology
University of Kuopio
Kuopio, Finland

Takashi Okiji, DDS, PhD
Professor
General Dentistry and Clinical Education Unit
Niigata University Dental Hospital
Niigata, Japan

David Pashley, DMD, PhD
Professor
Department of Oral Biology
Medical College of Georgia
Augusta, Georgia

John D. Ruby, DMD, PhD
Postgraduate Fellow and Assistant Professor
Department of Pediatric Dentistry and Specialized Caries Research Center
University of Alabama
Birmingham, Alabama

R. Bruce Rutherford, DDS, PhD
Department of Cariology and General Dentistry
University of Michigan
Ann Arbor, Michigan

Samuel Seltzer, DDS
Professor Emeritus
Department of Endodontology
Temple University
Philadelphia, Pennsylvania

Anthony J. Smith, BSC, PhD
Professor
Department of Oral Biology
University of Birmingham
Birmingham, United Kingdom

Adam Stabholtz, DDS
Professor
Department of Endodontics
The Hebrew University
Jerusalem, Israel

Harold Stanley, BS, MS, DDS
Professor Emeritus
Department of Oral and Maxillofacial Surgery and Oral Diagnostic Sciences
University of Florida
Gainesville, Florida

Philip Stashenko, DMD, PhD
Senior Member of Staff and Head
Cytokine Biology Unit
Forsyth Dental Institute
Norfolk, Massachusetts

Hideaki Suda, DDS, PhD
Department of Endodontics
Tokyo Medical and Dental University
Tokyo, Japan

Martin Trope, BDS, DMD
Jake Freedland Professor and Chair
Department of Endodontics
University of North Carolina
Chapel Hill, North Carolina

Henry O. Trowbridge, DDS, PhD
Professor Emeritus
Department of Pathology
University of Pennsylvania
Philadelphia, Pennsylvania

Attending Staff
Division of Endodontics
Albert Einstein Medical Center
Philadelphia, Pennsylvania

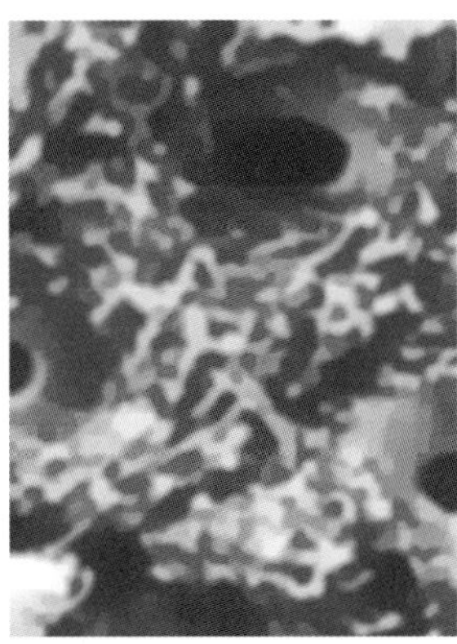

Preface

This book is about the dental pulp and its interaction with other tissues during health and disease; it is intended for practicing dentists as well as for residents and dental students. Each chapter provides an introduction to its major themes, allowing the busy clinician an opportunity to become reacquainted with the subject matter. It then presents the latest research on that topic for the dental pulp. Importantly, this research is interpreted in terms of biologically based recommendations for restorative and endodontic dental procedures. Thus, the goal of this book is to provide a biologic framework for the practice of dentistry.

We have named this book in honor of Sam Seltzer and I. B. Bender, two dental pioneers who were instrumental in developing biologically based recommendations for endodontics and restorative dentistry. Indeed, the philosophical basis for the present book has evolved from a similar work published by Sam and I. B. nearly three decades ago. They have actively participated in several chapters of the current book.

Sam and I. B. long ago said that the dental pulp is a "big issue about a little tissue." And, in a way, they are correct. The big issue is simply the central role that pulp tissue plays in dental health. Both local (eg, caries, periodontitis) and systemic (eg, AIDS, hyperparathyroidism) disease can contribute to pulpal pathosis. In turn, pulpal pathosis can contribute to both local (eg, root resorption, periodontitis) and systemic (eg, referred pain) conditions. The astute clinician needs this information to provide accurate diagnoses and effective treatments. Accordingly, we have focused on the biology of dental pulp and its interaction with other tissues during health and disease in order to provide comprehensive, biologically based clinical recommendations for practicing dentists.

During the final preparation of this book, we were greatly saddened to learn of the passing of Professor Harold Stanley. Dr Stanley made numerous important contributions during his long and productive career, and his chapter represents a summary of many of his important findings.

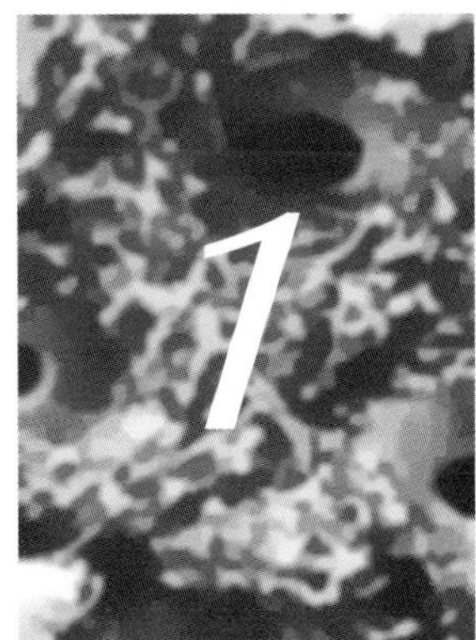

History of Pulp Biology

Harold E. Goodis, DDS

Why Study Dental Pulp?

From many perspectives, dental health is directly related to the health of a unique tissue—that is, dental pulp. However, the study of dental pulp is not restricted to this tissue alone, but extends to its interactions with many other tissues in health and disease. For example, since dentin and pulp are anatomically and functionally integrated, they are often referred to as the *pulpodentin complex*.[1]

The pulp also interacts with other tissues such as the periodontium (chapters 17 and 18) and even the central nervous system (chapters 7 and 8). Indeed, the interrelationship between dental pulp and other tissues is a major theme in the field of dentistry, in pulp biology research, and of course, in this textbook. It also serves as a rationale for the specialty of endodontics. According to one recent endodontics text, the purpose of endodontic treatment is not to preserve the pulp but to eliminate it, so as to remove those factors found in necrotic and infected pulp that stimulate apical periodontitis.[2] Thus, the biologic rationale for nonsurgical endodontic treatment is to manage the apical periodontitis that results from the functional relationship between infected dental pulp and apical tissue.

The importance of the relationship between dental pulp and other tissues has also been recognized in other clinical fields. For example, restorative dental procedures are closely linked to the biology of the pulpodentin complex. Indeed, the focus on prevention and treatment of noncavitated caries lesions is based on the premise that the potential for subsequent pulpal pathosis will be minimized.[3] Moreover, cavitated lesions often are now treated by adhesive restorations that take advantage of the exposed collagen fibers, expressed by odontoblasts, that are unmasked in demineralized dentin.[4] A recent series of articles in *Quintessence International* on pulpal responses to restorative materials was introduced by the statement that "reactions in dentin and pulp should be at the center of attention in restorative dentistry."[5] Contemporary periodontics textbooks emphasize the importance of recognizing the interrelationship of dental pulp with the periodontium when evaluating potential pulpal-periodontal pathoses.[6] It is clear that clinical dentistry is built on a foundation of knowledge of the dental pulp and its interrelationships with other tissues.

In addition to its clinical implications, dental pulp is worthy of study from a scientific perspective. Basic science research on dental pulp has recognized several unique features of this tissue. Its location within relatively hard, unyielding walls and its particular vascular supply and dynamic cellular content have led to an increasing interest in its responses to injury and bacterial infection. Scientists have used this unique tissue to study ectodermal-mesodermal interactions during development (chapter 2), growth factors embedded in dentin (chapter 3), phenotype plasticity of nociceptors ("pain neurons") (chapters 7 and 8), bacterial-host interactions (chapters 5, 11, 12, and 17), and a number of other topics. To close the circle, many of these topics have important implications in the diagnosis and management of diseases related to the dental pulp.

History of Dental Pulp and Related Dental Procedures

The history of pulp biology and related dental procedures is, surprisingly, long and varied. Several excellent reviews of dental history offer considerable information about the dental pulp and dental procedures designed to treat pulpal infections.[7,8] The following review summarizes these contributions in three broad historical eras.

Early recognition of the role of dental pulp in oral health

Early writings from around the world indicate a recognition of the relationship between caries, pulpal inflammation, and pain. Fu Hsi (2953 BC) is credited with one of the earliest surviving descriptions of several types of toothache, including pain caused by cold and mastication. Later, Pliny the Elder (23–79 AD) advised that a toothache could be relieved by chewing the root of the hyocyamus soaked in vinegar, or the roots of the plantain. Interestingly, extracts of plantain are now known to possess antimicrobial and anti-inflammatory properties.[9] He also stated that a mixture of plant extracts with opium was effective for treating tooth pain. Scribonius Largus (physician to the Emperor Claudius) reported the application of "certain" medicaments, or the mechanical removal of caries, were alternatives to tooth extraction due to pain. Root canal treatments were performed in the European and Mediterranean Basin in antiquity,[10] and the ancient Greeks attempted to hermetically seal root canal systems.[11] At the time, caries was thought to be caused by small worms that existed in the tooth and consumed enamel. An early reference to worms causing caries, or the "legend of the tooth worm," is found in Mesopotamia in the sixth century BC.

Archigenes of Syria (98–117 AD) treated pain due to traumatic injuries to teeth by cauterizing them with a red-hot iron. He also reported that drilling small trephines directly into the pulp chamber was effective for relieving pulpal pain. Galen (130–201 AD) believed that teeth were bones and were innervated by sensory neurons originating from a pair of cranial nerves. Galen also described two types of toothache, one originating from pulpal inflammation and the second originating from the periodontal tissues. When all remedies failed to cure pulpal pain, he too suggested trephination of teeth in order to expose the dental pulp. The casual reader will observe only the gross nature of the observations and treatment. However, upon reflection, the insightful nature of these observations reveals a dedication to the well-being of patients.

A great Persian clinician, Rhazes (865–925), published a comprehensive text on pathology and therapeutics. He and others treated toothache as a result of caries by applying arsenic and opium. If pain was not relieved, red-hot needles were placed through the caries into the root canal system. The "second Galen," Avicenna (980–1037), also believed in the tooth worm theory of caries. To treat pain due to pulpitis, he drilled into the tooth to relieve pressure and to release the "morbid humors." Abulcasis (1013) used cauterization (hot butter applied on a probe) to remove the "worm" causing dental pain. Although the methods are not representative of contemporary techniques (thankfully), it should be appreciated that these clinicians based their treatments on the prevailing beliefs of the pathologic process (eg, tooth worm) involved and that the treatments were designed to remove this pathology.

Development of dental therapeutics

These observations and remedies continued for several hundred years until the time of Vesalius in the middle of the sixteenth century, who corrected the proposition by Galen that teeth were bones. Pierre Fauchard, the father of modern dentistry (1678–1761), rejecting the theory of worms in the teeth, used a lead-filled root canal space to hold a pivot crown. Bourdet (1757) treated infected dental pulp by intentional reimplantation, in which teeth were luxated with a forceps and the pulp extirpated by means of an instrument with a three-sided point. Teeth were instrumented and then replaned once the root canal space was packed, reportedly with some degree of success. The treatment of diseased teeth and study of the dental pulp begun by these practitioners reached its zenith in the nineteenth century.

During this time, similar observations were made by clinicians in England. Though most treated toothache with Galen's remedies, others, more observant, attempted to understand the cause of the pain. John Baumster in the latter part of the sixteenth century described the presence of nerves and arteries and veins that had been dissected out of the tooth. Peter Lowe (1654), having discovered that worms in the teeth were not the cause of toothaches, used some of the same remedies, such as cautery, as had the other advanced French dentists.

At the beginning of the eighteenth century, a few studied teeth more thoroughly. John Hunter's work established a sound foundation for scientific procedures in dental treatment. He understood the profound necessity of reaching the end of the root when performing pulp debridement procedures. James Snell, in the early nineteenth century, employed acetate of morphia, silver nitrate, and cautery for the destruction of inflamed and sensitive pulp tissue. He devised a steel instrument with a bulb at the end of a platinum wire, which retained heat long enough to cauterize the pulp tissue. Similar discoveries followed in the United States, in the work of Horace Hayden (1769–1844) and Chapin Harris (1806–1860), who lectured extensively on diseases of the dental pulp.

Discoveries of asepsis by Pasteur and Lister were incorporated into dental practice. The advent of rubber dam in the late 1800s allowed for a practical method of aseptic root canal procedures. Advances in root canal treatment appeared rapidly from 1890 to 1920, guided by an ever-growing understanding of the histopathology of the pulp and periradicular tissues and their reactions to treatment.

The development of vital treatment for diseased pulpal tissue without removing that tissue has been reviewed by Francke.[12] Philip Pfaff is credited with some of the first attempts to treat vital pulp. He cut small pieces of gold or lead so that they fitted over the pulpal exposure. A unique feature of the cap was the presence of a concavity to prevent contact with dental pulpal tissue. At about the same time, James Snell described applying silver nitrate to the "ulcerated surface" of the pulp that was then protected by a temporary filling of mastic. The apparent purpose of this type of treatment was pulp capping, a common practice of the time.

Others have described responses of the pulpodentin complex to various dental treatments. Frederick Hirsh recommended that a diseased tooth should be treated by cauterizing the pulp with a red-hot probe and filling the opening with lead. There are no records of patient responses to this treatment. Leonard Koecker of Philadelphia (1828) performed similar pulpal cauterizations. Jacob Linderer and his son Joseph (1837) recommended that the pulp be made insensitive by placing essential or narcotic oils on it and then a

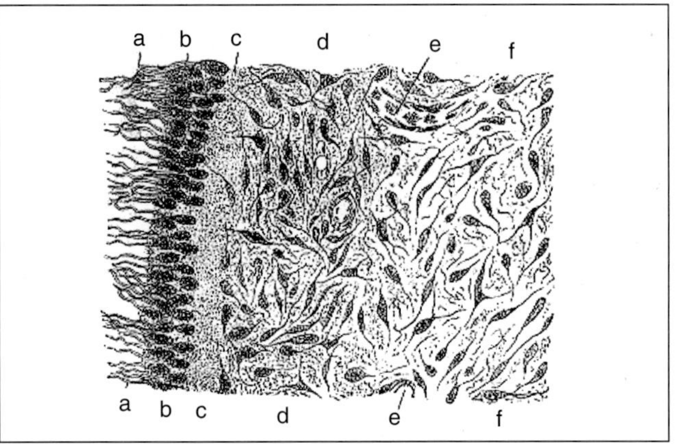

Fig 1-1 Margin of the dental pulp: a, dentinal fibrils; b, membrana aboris or odontoblast layer; c, transparent zone between odontoblasts and pulp cells; d, densely packed cell layer; e, blood vessels; f, cells less closely packed (1/10 inch objective). (Reprinted from Black.[13])

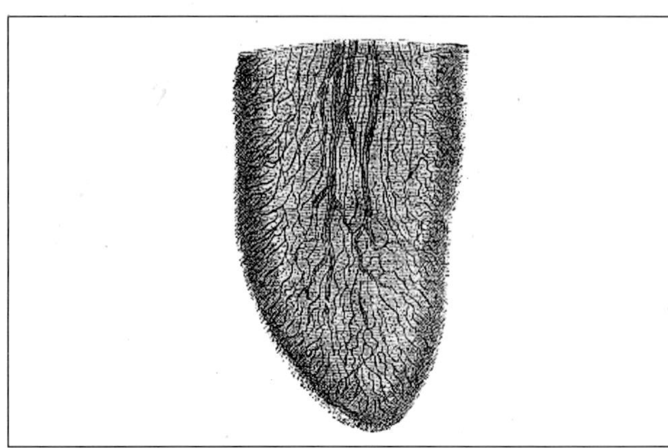

Fig 1-2 Visualization of the apex of an incisor injected with Beale's blue to show the blood vessels (original magnification ×25). (Reprinted from Black.[13])

covering of wax or stopping. A permanent filling was to be placed, cautiously, several days later. Also recommended was a thin gold plate to be placed over pulpal exposures. Gold was believed to have unique healing capabilities and to be necessary to produce a suitable barrier.

Jonathan Taft (1858) continued this theme by introducing a new therapeutic concept to the dental community. He proposed that the vital pulpodentin complex was valuable in providing greater resistance to caries. Taft stated that therapy directed at maintaining pulpal vitality could lead to the formation of a "boney deposit," ie, secondary dentin. This was an incredibly insightful observation for the period. The development of secondary dentin was not generally recognized until the 1960s.

Others of that era developed new methods of diagnosis. Adolph Witzel (1879) recommended that, after caries removal and pulpal exposure, cold water should be placed into the cavity: if that caused acute but transitory pain, then the pulp was viewed to be reversibly inflamed and could be capped; if the pain lingered, other treatments were recommended.

Leber and Rottenstein (1867), finding a microorganism on the surface of a tooth and in the decaying cavity and dental tubules, concluded that caries could cause pulpal necrosis. At about this time, Joseph Lister (1867) reported using carbolic acid for the aseptic treatment of wounds. This led to use of antiseptic substances in pulp-capping treatments. Julius Parreidt (1879) recommended "Carbolgypse," a 5% water solution of carbolic acid mixed with plaster. W. E. Harding (1883), in England, is said to have believed that dental surgeons should ask first not "Can I save the root?" but "Can I save the tooth?" John Wessler, a Swede, found metal caps too difficult to apply. In 1894, he proposed the use of "Pulpol," a cement of oil of cloves containing 80% to 90% eugenol mixed with zinc oxide. It relieved pain and could easily be placed over exposures.

The following illustrations (Figs 1-1 to 1-15) define the thinking of those involved in the treatment of pulpal diseases at the end of the nine-

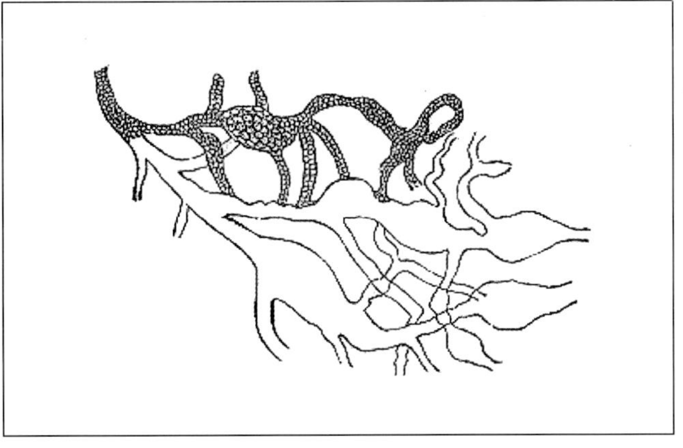

Fig 1-3 Related blood vessels in pulpal hyperemia from a tooth extracted during a paroxysm of intense pain. (Reprinted from Black.[13])

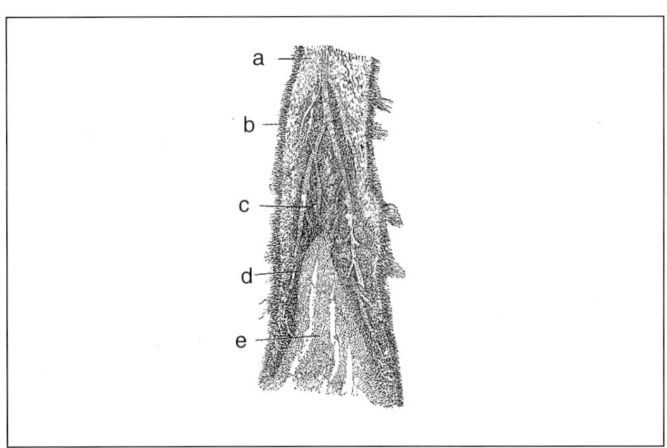

Fig 1-4 Progressive suppuration of the pulp of an incisor: a, healthy tissue; b, odontoblast layer or membrane eboris; c, inflamed tissue in which veins are seen to be dilated; d, line of demarcation of the suppurative process; e, abscess. (Reprinted from Black.[13])

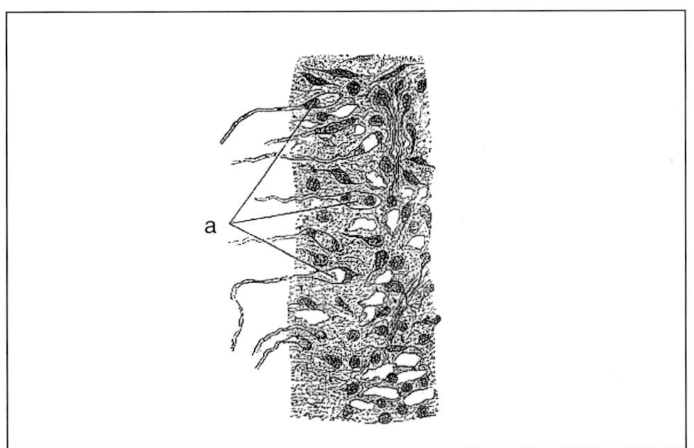

Fig 1-5 Atrophy of the odontoblasts: a, odontoblasts that have taken the stain in an irregular manner (1⁄10 inch immersion). (Reprinted from Black.[13])

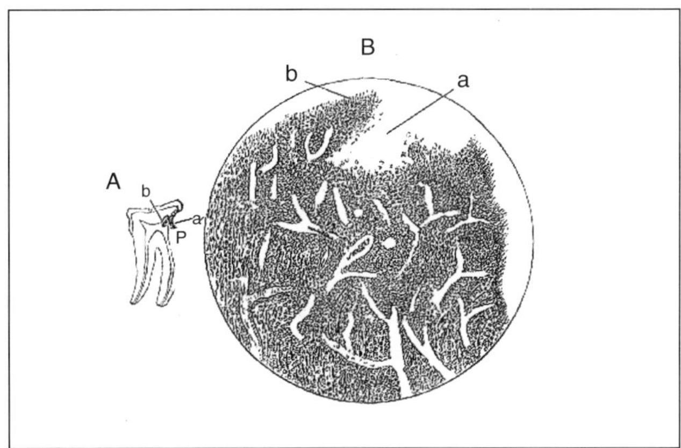

Fig 1-6 *(A)* Diagram of mandibular molar, with caries (a), which exposed the pulp (P). The darkened portion (b) shows the extent of the inflammation. *(B)* Illustration of the inflamed tissue of the abscess (a). The odontoblasts are undermined (b). The blood vessels that were filled with blood clot in the section are left blank to make them more apparent. (Reprinted from Black.[13])

teenth century. They point to an era of enlightenment and discovery about pathoses most pulp biologists and endodontists now take for granted. More than pioneers, they were thinkers, and no history of the evolution of information would be complete without their findings. The illustrations taken from textbooks published in the 1880s and 1890s include both photographs and drawings of what was seen microscopically. Where possible, the persons responsible for them are credited.

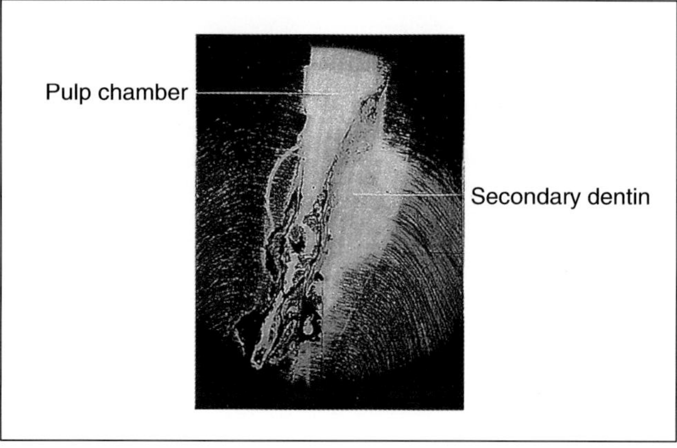

Fig 1-7 Secondary dentin on wall of pulp chamber (original magnification ×100). (Reprinted from Marshall.[14])

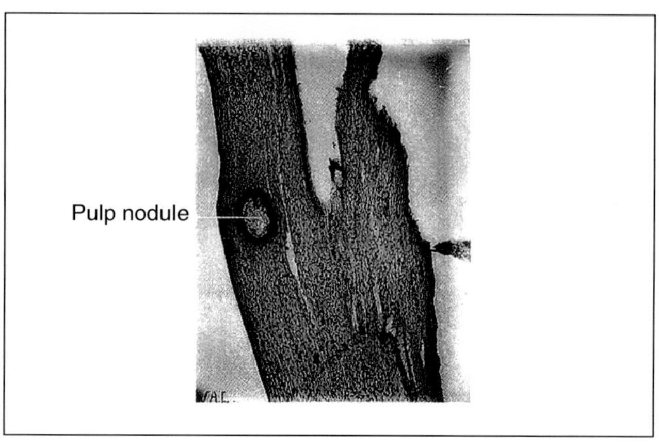

Fig 1-8 Section of dental pulp with secondary dentin in chamber (original magnification ×100). (Reprinted from Marshall.[14])

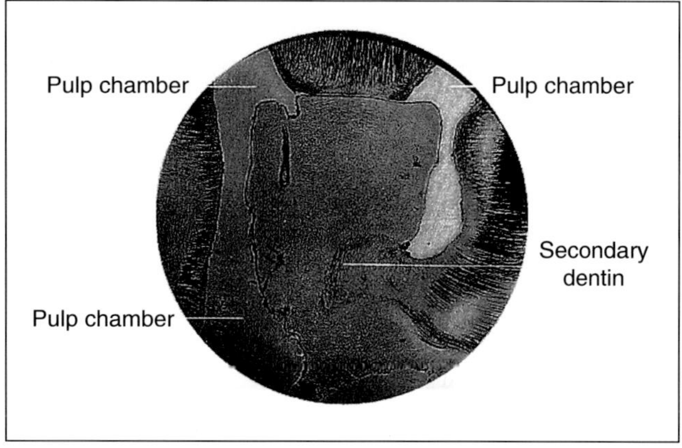

Fig 1-9 Section of tooth pulp undergoing fibroid degeneration (original magnification ×110). (Reprinted from Marshall.[14])

TABLE OF INFLAMMATORY PHENOMENA

1. Irritants.
   - a. Traumatic.
   - b. Chemic.
   - c. Bartoric or septic.
   - d. Electric.
   - e. Thermic.
2. Irritation.
3. Determination or active hyperaemia.
4. Disturbance of circulation.
5. Increased motion and retardation or oscillation.
6. Stasis (partial).
7. Vascular dilatation.
8. Exudation, —diapedesis, rhexis.
9. Swelling, —ocdema.
10. Terminations
    - a. Resolution, or absorption or organization.
      - a. Vascularization
      - b. Granulation
      - c. Scar-tissue
    - b. Fibroid thickening or chronic inflammation
      - Hyperplasia
      - New formations.
    - c. Suppuration.
    - d. Abscess,—necrosis.
    - e. Ulceration.
    - f. Gangrene.

Fig 1-10 Inflammatory phenomena. (Reprinted from Marshall.[14])

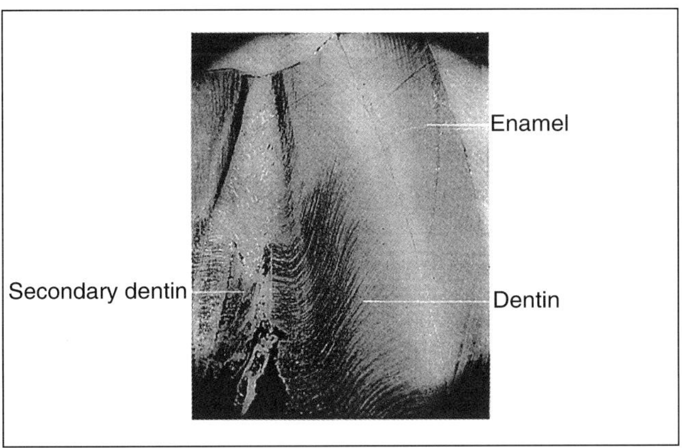

Fig 1-11 Vertical section of human canine, showing formation of secondary dentin in the coronal portion of the pulp chamber as a result of loss of tissue at the dorsal edge (original magnification ×100). (Reprinted from Marshall.[14])

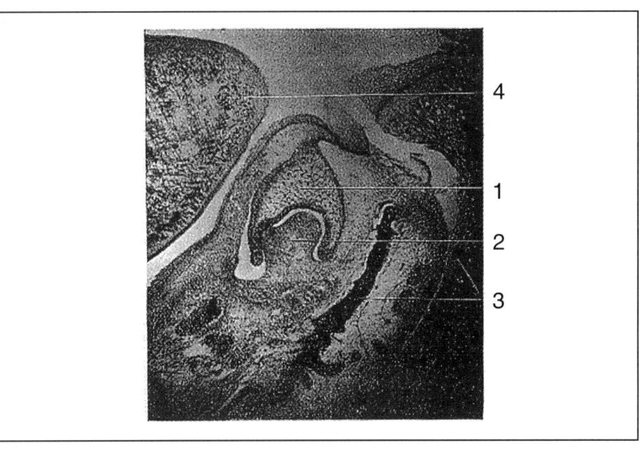

Fig 1-12 Growth of enamel organ and dental germ (ie, dental papilla) in section of pig jaw embryo: 1, enamel organ; 2, dental germ; 3, growth of jaw; 4, tongue. (Reprinted from Kirk.[15])

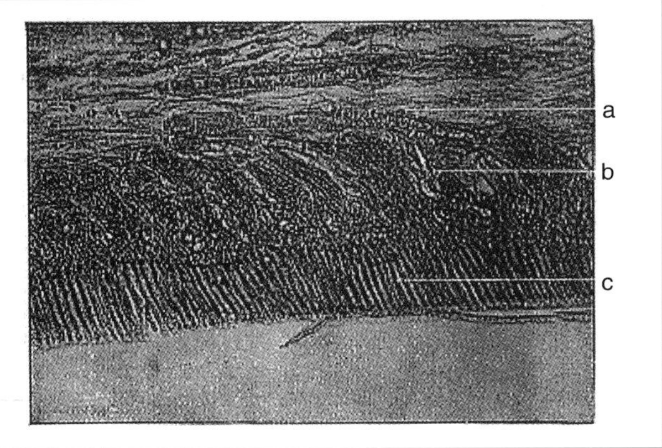

Fig 1-13 Section of rat incisor: a, blood vessels with erythrocytes in situ; b, branch of blood vessels descending to supply capillary loops around secreting papillae; c, ameloblasts (original magnification ×175). (Reprinted from Bourchard.[16])

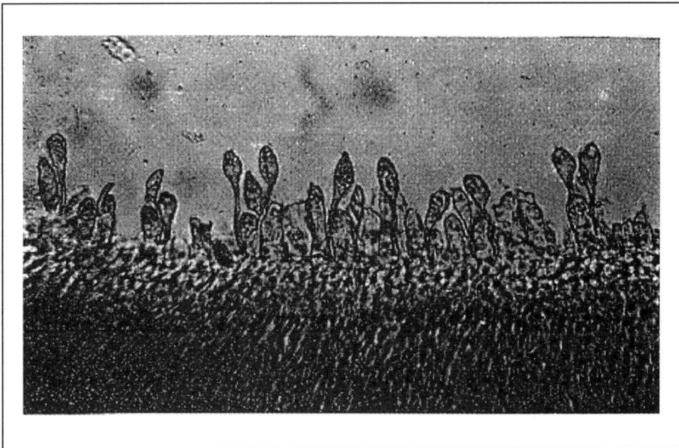

Fig 1-14 Layer of odontoblasts and fibril cells attached to the forming dentin in section of growing tooth of calf at birth. (Reprinted from Kirk.[15])

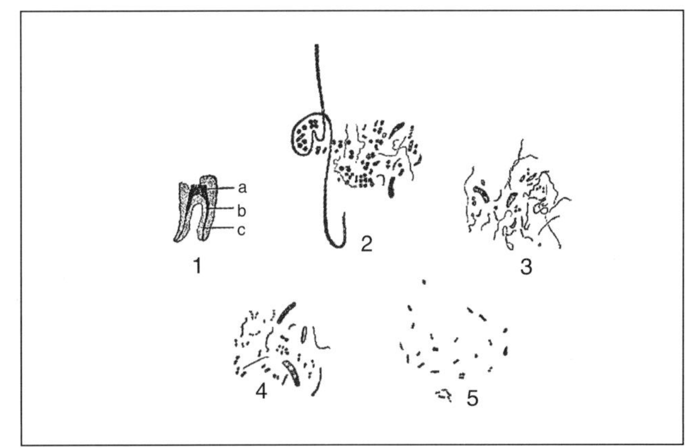

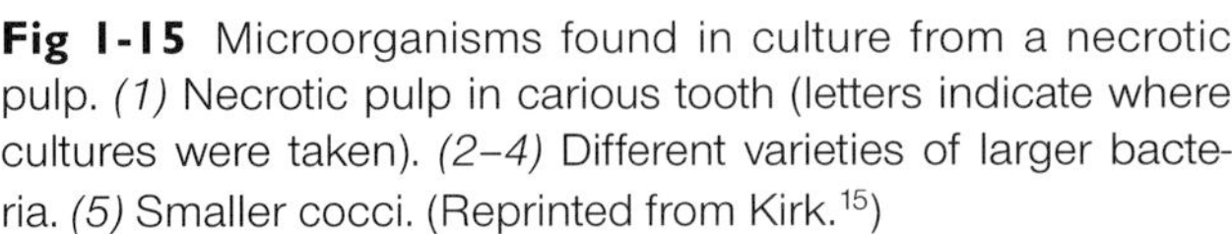

Fig 1-15 Microorganisms found in culture from a necrotic pulp. *(1)* Necrotic pulp in carious tooth (letters indicate where cultures were taken). *(2–4)* Different varieties of larger bacteria. *(5)* Smaller cocci. (Reprinted from Kirk.[15])

Development of endodontic techniques and the impact of the focal infection theory

The sequence of events in the above history of the protection of the dental pulp allows us to better understand the evolution of the study of the biology of the dental pulp. Despite their limited facilities and instrumentation, the dentists of the seventeenth and eighteenth centuries laid the foundation for those following in the nineteenth and early twentieth, whose work has in turn led in the late twentieth century to the publication of studies of pulp biology too numerous to quote in this brief history. Suffice it to say that our forefathers were bright, observant men who laid the groundwork for today's investigations into the biology of the dental pulp. Despite this overall progress, some events, such as the focal infection theory, still lead to the loss of millions of teeth.

In their book *Clinical Endodontics*,[17] Sommer, Ostrander, and Crowley reviewed previous histologic studies of pulpal tissue thought to be infected. At the time (early twentieth century) many physicians and dentists believed that teeth with infected pulps were foci of infection for systemic disease.[18] The focal infection theory was based on culture results from extracted teeth, with little regard to the possibility that the bacteria recovered may have been part of the normal flora of the oral cavity. Interestingly, a supporter of the focal theory did not find any proof that the organisms found played a role in focal infection.[19] Although the theory of focal infection had little experimental support, it resulted in the needless extraction of countless teeth. When reviewing this period of dental history, we must remember that the majority of contemporary dental pulp research has been conducted only in the last 40 years. For example, only in the 1970s did clinical studies demonstrate that flossing and tooth brushing reliably produce transient bacteremias without the risk of a systemic infection.[20,21] These and numerous other studies (see chapter 12) have refuted the theory of focal infection due to bacteria in necrotic teeth.

A variant of this concept has appeared in recent studies advancing the theory that periodontal disease is associated with systemic health. Many of these studies are based on cross-sectional correlations of one factor (eg, periodontitis) with another factor (eg, the systemic disease of interest). However, since a correlation of factor A with factor B could imply that factor A causes B, or that factor B causes A, or that both A and B are caused by some underlying common disorder (ie, A and B caused by factor C), correlation does not equal causation. Moreover, large-scale prospective studies (N = 8,032) and meta-analyses of published studies (N = 74,103) have failed to detect a significant substantial correlation between periodontal disease and systemic health.[22,23] Thus, there is little evidence in support of a causative relationship between chronic oral infections such as infected pulps or periodontitis and systemic disease. Other risk factors, however, may eventually lead to determinations of a causative relationship between systemic disease entities and oral diseases. For example, a recent study[24] of upper body obesity suggested that this may be a common disorder linking both cardiovascular disease and periodontitis.

It was not until the mid- to late 1930s that the "presence" of organisms (ie, colonization) and "infection" were considered not to be synonymous.[25] This distinction between colonization and infection continues to be a topic for contemporary reviews (see also chapter 12).[26] Histologic examination of pulp tissue from extracted teeth has demonstrated the presence of microorganisms where there is no evidence of inflammatory changes.[27] This may have been due to an experimental confound, since the same investigators showed that it was impossible to sterilize tooth surfaces and that bacteria from the oral cavity could be forced into the pulp canal space during tooth extraction.

Several advances in endodontic treatment were made during this period. A focus on new aseptic techniques offered the opportunity to disrupt and significantly reduce the presence of oral flora during root canal treatment.[27-29] Aseptic techniques made it possible, therefore, to control and prevent infection. More recent papers describe the history of other types of endodontic treatment. A history of formocresol pulpotomy[30] and a historical review of the management of tooth hypersensitivity[31] have been published. G.V. Black prepared 88 handmade microscope slides, staining or double staining different sections of the same material to describe the histopathologic features of the dental pulp. The slides were reviewed by Loevy and Kowitz.[32]

Others have examined the history of endodontics from its origins to the beginning of, and into, the twentieth century.[33-38] A recent president of the American Association of Endodontists explained the use of immediate root fillings in the latter part of the nineteenth century, the use of arsenic in the treatment of dentin and the dental pulp,[39] and the Herbst method of treating the dental pulp.[40,41] A three-part review of the history of endodontics from 1889 to 1963 was presented by Cruse and Bellizzi.[42-44] They surveyed the evolution of root canal treatment from the time of Fauchard to that of the recognition of endodontics as a dental specialty. A history of the use of gutta percha in endodontics described its use beginning in the 1500s and its evolution over the next several hundred years.[45] Rosenberg and Schilder[46] summed up the specialty of endodontics by reviewing its past, present and future.

The foregoing review is essentially a prelude to treatment modalities and instrumentation from the 1920s to the present. However, coincident with the development of the study of the diseased pulp has been the exploration of the pathophysiology of the pulpal tissue itself.

Development of Pulp Biology As a Scientific Discipline

The events described above coincided with an evolution of "experimental" science. The Renaissance in Europe (fifteenth and sixteenth centuries) included fundamental new research on dental pulp. Its morphology was first described by Coiter in the mid-sixteenth century, and developmental changes occurring in teeth were described by Ingrassia. Anthony van Leeuwenhoek (1632–1723) used an early microscope to describe dentinal tubules. Bichat described dentin as bone and noted the presence of secondary dentin. Later, Bertin described pulp anatomy, and concluded that secondary dentin was formed by cells in dental pulp. Retzius (1837) predicted that dentinal tubules would be found to contain a peculiar kind of vessel functioning by elaborating a nourishing and supporting fluid.

Additional studies laid the groundwork for understanding the pulpodentin complex.[47-49] In 1881, Baume reviewed the status of pulpodentin biology at the time of the Dental School of Geneva's establishment in 1881.[50] Later, Sigron reviewed the anatomic contributions of Walter Hess, an early dental pulp researcher.[51] The studies of Professor Hess revealed the complexity of root canal systems—their branching and their multiple portals of exit.

Interest grew when, in 1963, a group led by Dr Sidney B. Finn applied to the National Institute of Dental Research (now named the National Institute of Dental and Craniofacial Research) for financial aid for a symposium on the basic science of the dental pulp organ and related fields. The meeting in 1964 at Lake Martin, Alabama, helped to establish a formal network of pulp biology scientists. This led to the formation of the Pulp Biology Group in 1975 under the leadership of Dr William Cotton, the group's first president. The Pulp Biology Group is a component of the International Association for Dental Research. Research in pulp biology has truly become international in scope.

The Pulp Biology Group has organized and sponsored symposia at various venues throughout the world. These include the Charlotte conferences in 1984 and 1991 in Charlotte, North Carolina; the conference on Hypersensitive Dentin at Callaway Gardens, Georgia in 1993; the Symposium on Dental Innervation in Seattle in

1994; and the Pulp/Dentin Complex Conference in Chiba, Japan, in 1995 and 2001. The published proceedings of these conferences have proven an incredible source of scientific studies on the dental pulp. Several of the more interesting books include *Biology of the Dental Pulp Organ*[52] in 1967, *Dynamics Aspects of the Dental Pulp* in 1990,[53] the *Proceedings of the Finnish Dental Society*[54] in 1992, and the *Dentin/Pulp Complex* in 1996[55] and 2002.[56]

Conclusions

A review of dental history illustrates the pivotal role of dental pulp in oral health. Moreover, we now recognize many and important interactions between dental pulp and other tissues in health and disease. This has led to the recognition that a clinician cannot select the most appropriate and effective dental procedures without a fundamental knowledge of dental pulp biology. Drs Samuel Seltzer and I. B. Bender were among the first to incorporate contemporary research findings emphasizing these important links between pulp biology and clinical dentistry. In 1974, Seltzer and Bender published *The Dental Pulp*, the first textbook to devote its entire content to this tissue and its relationship to clinical dentistry. With characteristic humor, they succinctly encapsulated this concept by stating that the study of dental pulp was "a big issue over a small tissue." In the following chapters, our coauthors have used this philosophy to review current knowledge of pulpal biology for the purpose of improving our care of our patients.

References

1. Pashley DH. Dynamics of the pulpodentin complex. Crit Rev Oral Biol Med 1996;7:104–133.
2. Ørstavik D, Pitt Ford TR. Prevention and treatment of apical periodontitis. In: Ørstavik D, Pitt Ford TR (eds). Essential Endodontology. Oxford: Blackwell Science, 1998:1–8.
3. National Institutes of Health Consensus Development Conference Statement. Diagnosis and Management of Dental Caries Throughout Life. March 26–28, 2001. http://odp.od.nih.gov/consensus/cons/115/115_statement.htm
4. Dietschi D, Spreafico R. Adhesive Metal-Free Restorations. Chicago: Quintessence, 1997.
5. Wathen WF. The biological approach to restorative dentistry. Quintessence Int 2001;32:425.
6. Carranza F, Takei H. Treatment of furcation involvement and combined periodontal-endodontic therapy. In: Carranza F, Newman M (eds). Clinical Periodontology. Saunders: Philadelphia, 1997:chapter 58.
7. Lufkin AW. A History of Dentistry. Philadelphia: Lea & Febiger, 1947.
8. Asbell MB. Dentistry: A Historical Perspective. Bryn Mawr: Dorrancet Comp, 1988.
9. Gomez-Flores R, Calderon CL, Scheibel LW, Tamez-Guerra P, Rodriguez-Padilla C, Tamez-Guerra R, Weber RJ. Immunoenhancing properties of Plantago major leaf extract. Phytother Res 2000;14:617–622.
10. Nardoux M. Endodontics of the European of the Mediterranean basin in antiquity. Ligament 1978;16:61–69.
11. Ramsey WO. Hermetic sealing of root canals. The Greeks had a name for it. J Endod 1982;8:100.
12. Francke OC. Capping the living pulp: From Philip Pfaff to John Wessler. Bull Hist Dent 1971;19:17–32.
13. Black GV. Pathology of the dental pulp. Part IV. In: Litch WF (ed). The American System of Dentistry, vol 1. Philadelphia: Lea Brothers, 1886:829–887.
14. Marshall JS. Principles and Practice of Operative Dentistry. Philadelphia: Lippincott, 1901.
15. Kirk EC (ed). The American Text-Book of Operative Dentistry. Philadelphia: Lea Brothers, 1897.
16. Bourchard HH. Dento-alveolar abscess. In: Kirk EC (ed). The American Text-Book of Operative Dentistry. Philadelphia: Lea Brothers, 1897.
17. Sommer RF, Ostrander FD, Crowley MC. Clinical Endodontics, ed 3. Philadelphia: Saunders, 1966.
18. Billings F. Chronic focal infections and their etiologic relations to arthritis and nephritis. Arch Intern Med 1918;9:484.
19. Meyers FK. The present status of dental bacteriology. N.D.A.J. 1917;4:966.
20. Baumgartner C, Heggers J, Harrison J. The incidence of bacteremia related to endodonic procedures. I. Nonsurgical endodontics. J Endod 1976;2:135–140.
21. Hockett R, Loesche W, Soderman T. Bacteremia in asymptomatic human subjects. Arch Oral Biol 1977;22:91–98.
22. Hujoel P, Drangsholt M, Spiekerman C, DeRouen T. Periodontal disease and coronary health risk. J Am Med Assoc 2000;284:1406–1410.
23. Hujoel P, Drangsholt M, Spiekerman C, DeRouen T. In Reply. J Am Med Assoc 2001;285:40–41.

24. Saito T, Shimazaki Y, Koga T, Tsuzuki M, Ohshima A. Relationship between upper body obesity and periodontitis. J Dent Res 2001;80:1631-1636.
25. Logan WHG. Are pulps and investing tissues of completely imbedded teeth infected? J Am Dent Assoc and Dent Cosmos 1937;24:853.
26. Henderson B, Wilson M. Commensal communism and the oral cavity. J Dent Res 1998;77:1674-1683.
27. Sommer RF, Crowley M. Bacteriologic verification of roentgenographic findings in pulp involved teeth. J Am Dent Assoc 1940;27:723.
28. Morse FW, Yates MF. Root canal studies: Anaerobic cultures. J Dent Res 1942;21:5.
29. Morse FW, Yates MF. Follow-up studies of root filled teeth in relation to bacteriologic findings. J Am Dent Assoc 1941;28:956.
30. Teplitsky PE, Grieman R. History of formocresol pulpotomy. J Can Dent Assoc 1984;50:629-634.
31. Rosenthal MW. Historic review of the management of tooth hypersensitivity. Dent Clin North Am 1990;34:403-427.
32. Loevy HT, Kowitz AA. Histopathology according to G. V. Black. Quintessence Int 1991;22:33-39.
33. Rowe AH. An historical review of materials used for treatment up to the year 1900. J Br Endod Soc 1968;2:47-48.
34. Grossman LI. Endodontics: A peep into the past and the future. Oral Surg Oral Med Oral Pathol 1974;37:599-608.
35. Luebke RG, Grant T. The evolution of root canal therepy. LDAJ 1975;33:8-10.
36. Grossman LI. Endodontics, 1776-1976: A bicentennial history against the background of general dentistry. J Am Dent Assoc 1976;93:78-87.
37. Marmasse A. Root canal therapy from the time of Fauchard to the present time. Actual Odontostomatol (Paris) 1980;34:37-49.
38. Baldensperger R, Buquet J. History of endodontics from its origins to the beginning of this century. Bull Acad Natl Chir Dent 1984-1985;(30):49-65.
39. Gutmann JL. Sensitive dentine-arsenic and the treatment of the dental pulp. J. D. White, Dental Cosmos 6:388 Feb 1865. J Endod 1978;4:74.
40. Gutmann JL. The Herbst method of treating pulps. J Endod 1978;4:preceding 97.
41. Gutmann JL. A critical response to the Herbst method of treating pulps. J Endod 1978;4:133-134.
42. Cruse WP, Bellizzi R. A historic review of endodontics, 1689-1963, part 1. J Endod 1980;6:495-499.
43. Cruse WP, Bellizzi R. A historic review of endodontics, 1689-1963, part 2. J Endod 1980;6:532-535.
44. Bellizzi R, Cruse WP. A historic review of endodontics, 1689-1963, part 3. J Endod 1980;6:576-580.
45. Machtou P, Mandel E. The use of gutta percha in endodontics. Inf Dent 1986;68:1559, 1561, 1563 passim.
46. Rosenberg RJ, Schilder H. Endodontics: Controversial past, exciting present, incredible future. Alpha Omegan 2000;93:44-54.
47. Baume LJ. The biology of pulp and dentine. A historic, terminologic-taxonomic, histologic-biochemical, embryonic and clinical survey. Monogr Oral Sci 1980;8:1-220.
48. Baume LJ, Treccani A. Biology of the dental pulp and dentin: History of the histological discoveries (I). Riv Ital Stomatol 1983;52:799-803.
49. Baume LJ. The natural history of pulp and dentin. Ohio Dent J 1983;57:48-52.
50. Baume LJ. The centennial of the Dental School of Geneva. Pulp-dentin biology at the time of the establishment of the Dental School of Geneva (21 October 1881). Swiss Dent 1981;2:16-18, 20-22.
51. Sigron G. Centenary of the birth of the Swiss dental pulp researcher Walter Hess (1885-1980). Schweiz Monatsschr Zahnmed 1985;95:1130.
52. Finn SB (ed). Biology of the Dental Pulp Organ: A Symposium. Birmingham: University of Alabama Press, 1967.
53. Inoki R, Kudo T, Olgart L (eds). Dynamic Aspects of the Dental Pulp. New York: Chapman and Hall, 1990.
54. Proceedings of the Finnish Dental Society 1992; 88(Suppl 1).
55. Shimono M, Takahashi K (eds). Dentin/Pulp Complex. Tokyo: Quintessence, 1996.
56. Ishikawa T, Shimono M, Inoue T (eds). Dentin/Pulp Complex 2001. Proceedings of the International Conference on Dentin/Pulp Complex 2001. Tokyo: Quintessence, 2002.

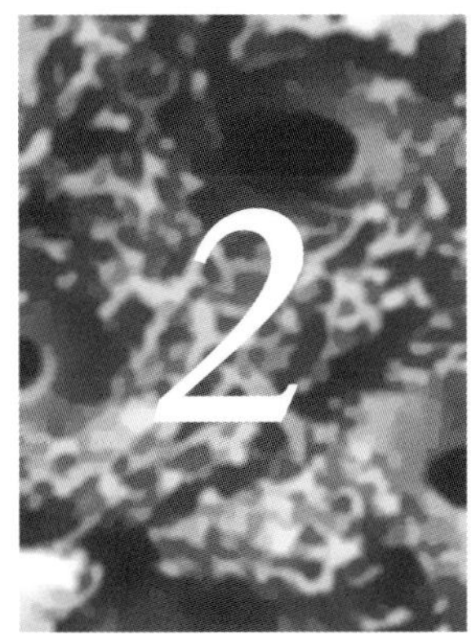

Development of the Pulpodentin Complex

Rena D'Souza, DDS, MS, PhD

Dentin is a unique, avascular mineralized connective tissue that forms the bulk of the tooth. It underlies enamel in the crown and cementum in the roots, providing structural support to these tissues and resilience to the tooth. In a mature tooth, dentin encloses a richly innervated and highly vascularized soft connective tissue, the dental pulp. Dentin and pulp are derived from the dental papilla, whose cells migrate to the first branchial arch from within the ectomesenchyme of the cranial neural crest. The tissues remain closely associated during development and throughout the life of an adult tooth and are hence most commonly referred to as the *pulpodentin complex*. It is this biologic intimacy that dictates the response of the pulpodentin complex to physiologic and pathologic stimuli.

Because the practice of dentistry often involves manipulation of both the dentin and the pulp, learning about the mechanisms that lead to their formation will provide the dentist with a better understanding of the response to and treatment of pulpal injuries. The purpose of this chapter is to provide a background for the succeeding chapters that discuss the biology of the mature pulpodentin complex during health and disease and in aging. This chapter reviews classic and current knowledge of the events in tooth development that lead to odontoblast differentiation. Attention is focused on the common themes that have emerged and on current knowledge about the influence of tooth-signaling molecules on the development of the pulpodentin complex. In addition, the chapter describes the general principles of dentin matrix formation, in particular the synthesis and secretion of extracellular matrix molecules. Examples of clinical applications of basic information are integrated throughout the chapter to emphasize the fundamental theory that developmental events are often reiterated in adult life.

Tooth Development (Odontogenesis)

For several decades, the developing tooth organ has served as a valuable paradigm for studying the fundamental processes involved in organogenesis. These processes are *(1)* the determination of position, when the precise site of tooth initiation is established, *(2)* the determination of form, or morphogenesis, when the size and shape of the tooth organ is set, and *(3)* cell differentiation, when organ-specific tissues are formed by defined cell populations, each with unique properties. The dental literature is enriched with excellent reviews on tooth development, and the reader is encouraged to study the topic in further detail.[1-6]

General features

Although the tooth is a unique organ, the principles that guide its development are shared in common with other organs, such as the lung, kidney, heart, mammary glands, and hair follicles.[7,8] The most important developmental events are those guiding epithelial-mesenchymal interactions, which involve a molecular crosstalk between the ectoderm and mesenchyme, two tissues that have a different origin. Although teeth are found only in vertebrates, their development involves genetic pathways that are also active in invertebrates. This conservation of a "molecular toolbox" for organogenesis throughout evolution proves that certain master regulatory molecules are critical to all tissue interactions during development.

New studies have also shown that tooth-signaling molecules are repeatedly used at various stages of development.[4,6] It is important that tooth morphogenesis and cell differentiation occur as a result of sequential interactions. Hence, it is not one biologic event involving a single molecule but rather a series of interactions involving several molecules that leads to the development of the pulpodentin complex.

Signaling is reciprocal; an exchange of information occurs in both directions from dental epithelium to mesenchyme and from dental mesenchyme to epithelium. For example, in experiments in which dental epithelium was separated from mesenchyme, cuspal patterning failed to occur. Similarly, in the absence of dental epithelium, odontoblasts are unable to differentiate from dental mesenchyme.[9-11]

It is only logical to apply these basic developmental principles to the current understanding of how the adult or mature pulpodentin complex responds in injury and repair. The latter clearly involves a series of molecules that operate in concert to dictate the outcome of pulpal disease and therapies. In the adult situation, whether certain cells and molecules can mimic the inductive influence of dental epithelium during development has yet to be definitively proven and remains a subject of interest in pulp biology research.

Stages of tooth development

Teeth develop in distinct stages that are easily recognizable at the microscopic level. Hence, stages of odontogenesis are described by the histologic appearance of the tooth organ. From early to late, these stages are described as the *lamina*, *bud*, *cap*, *early bell*, and *late bell* stages of tooth development.[12] Although the following description will use these common terms, modern literature uses functional terminology to describe odontogenesis as occurring in four phases: *initiation*, *morphogenesis*, *cell differentiation* (or *cytodifferentiation*), and *matrix apposition* (Fig 2-1). Figures 2-2a to 2-2e depict the morphologic stages of tooth development.

Lamina stage

The dental lamina is the first morphologic sign of tooth development and is visible at approximately 5 weeks of human development and at embryonic day 11 (E11) in mouse gestation. This thickening of the oral epithelium lining the frontonasal, maxillary, and mandibular arches occurs only at sites where tooth organs will develop. At the lamina stage, cells in the dental epithelium and underlying ectomesenchyme are dividing at different rates, the latter more rapidly. As will be explained later, the dental lamina has the full potential to induce tooth formation by dictating the fate of the underlying ectomesenchyme.[14]

Bud stage

As the dental lamina continues to grow and thicken to form a bud, cells of the ectomesenchyme proliferate and condense to form the dental

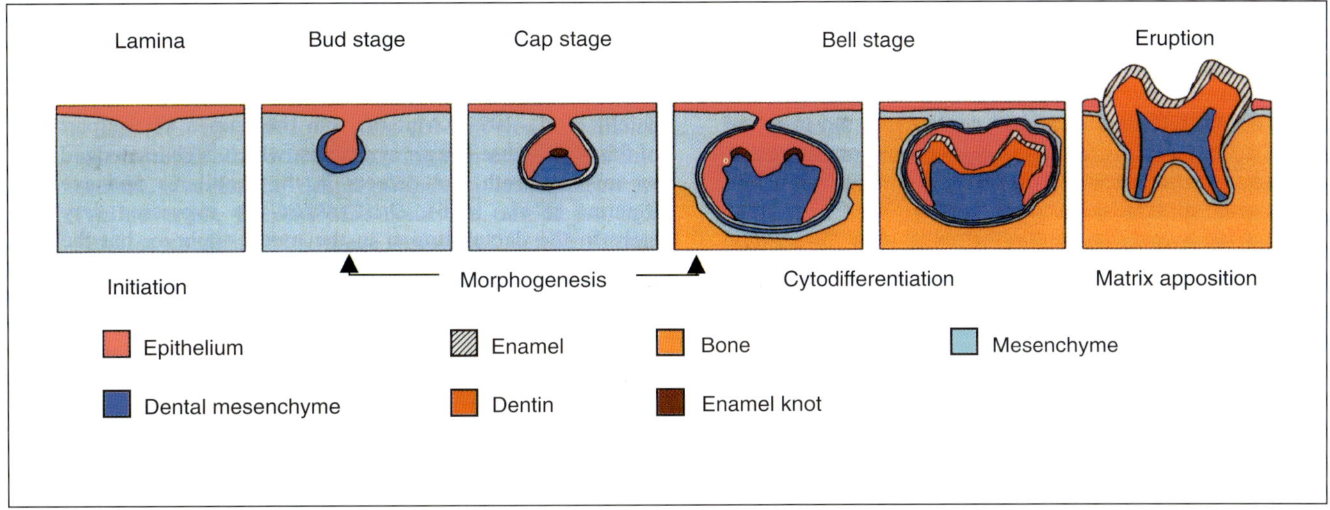

Fig 2-1 Stages of tooth development. Note the sequential transformation from the dental lamina to a distinctly shaped dental organ. The transient appearance of the enamel knot in the region of the forming cusp tips precedes the terminal differentiation of cells and the formation of specialized matrices. (Reprinted from Thesleff and Sharpe[13] with permission.)

papilla. At this stage, the inductive or tooth-forming potential is transferred from the dental epithelium to the dental papilla.

Cap stage

At this stage, the tooth bud assumes the shape of a cap that is surrounded by the dental papilla. The ectodermal compartment of the tooth organ is referred to as the *dental* or *enamel organ*. The enamel organ and dental papilla become encapsulated by another layer of mesenchymal cells, called the *dental follicle*, that separates the tooth organ papilla from the other connective tissues of the jaws.

The transition from the bud stage to the cap stage is an important step in tooth development, because it marks the onset of crown formation. Recent studies have pointed to the role of the enamel knot as an important organizing center that initiates cuspal patterning.[15,16] Formally described as a transient structure with no ascribed functions, the enamel knot is formed by the only cells within the central region of the dental organ that fail to grow. As will be described later, the enamel knot expresses a unique set of signaling molecules that influence both the shape of the crown and the development of the dental papilla. In incisors, the enamel knot initiates the first folding of dental epithelium. Secondary enamel knots determine the site of new cusps in molars.

Similar to signaling centers in other organizing tissues, such as the developing limb bud, the enamel knot undergoes programmed cellular death, or apoptosis, after cuspal patterning is completed at the onset of the early bell stage.

Early bell stage

The dental organ assumes the shape of a bell as cells continue to divide but at differential rates. A single layer of cuboidal cells, called the *external* or *outer dental epithelium*, lines the periphery of the dental organ; cells that border the dental papilla and are columnar in appearance form the *internal* or *inner dental epithelium*. The inner epithelium gives rise to the ameloblasts, cells responsible for enamel formation. Cells located in the center of the dental organ produce high levels of glycosaminoglycans that are able to sequester fluids as well as growth factors that lead to its expansion. This network of star-shaped cells is

Figs 2-2a to 2-2e Histologic survey of odontogenesis in a pig embryo. (Courtesy of the University of Houston, Health Science Center at Houston, Dental Branch.)

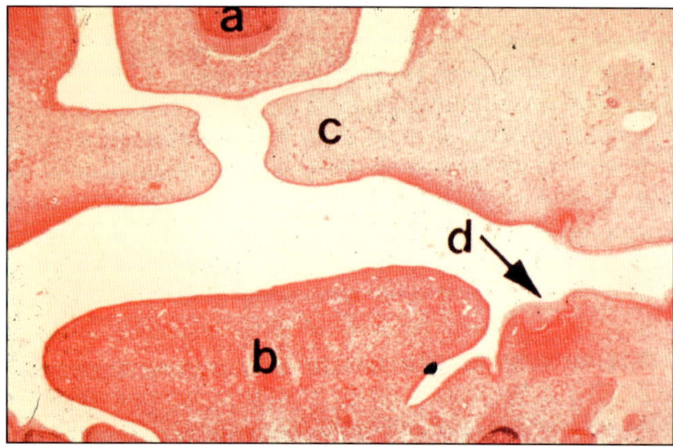

Fig 2-2a Lamina phase: a, nasal septum; b, tongue; c, palatal shelves; d, dental lamina (H&E stain).

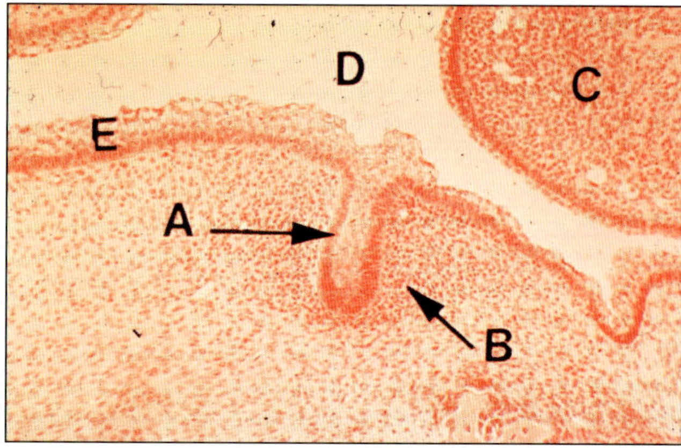

Fig 2-2b Bud stage: A, ectodermal outgrowth; B, dental mesenchyme; C, tongue; D, oral cavity space; E, oral ectoderm (H&E stain).

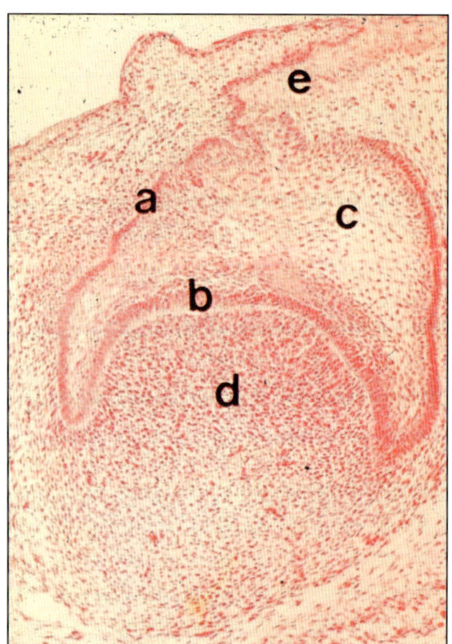

Fig 2-2c Cap stage or transition to early bell stage: a, outer dental epithelium; b, internal dental epithelium; c, stellate reticulum; d, dental papilla ectomesenchyme; e, dental lamina (H&E stain).

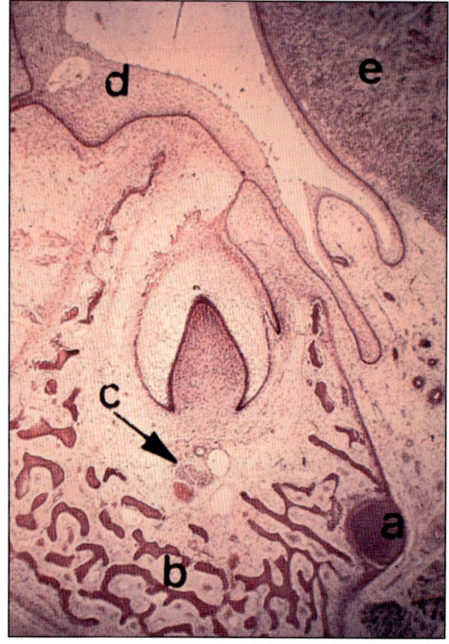

Fig 2-2d Late bell stage: a, nerve bundle; b, alveolar bone; c, vasculature; d, oral ectoderm; e, tongue. Note the extension of the dental lamina on the right aspect of the dental organ that will form the succedaneous incisor (H&E stain).

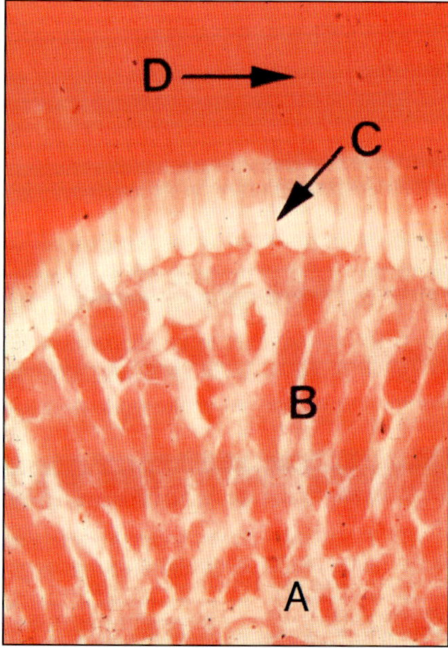

Fig 2-2e Onset of dentinogenesis: A, dental pulp; B, cluster of odontoblasts that appear crowded at the tip; C, odontoblast process; D, dentin.

named the *stellate reticulum*. Interposed between the stellate reticulum and the internal dental epithelium is a narrow layer of flattened cells, termed the *stratum intermedium*. These cells express high levels of alkaline phosphatase. The stratum intermedium is believed to influence the biomineralization of enamel. In the region of the apical end of the tooth organ, the internal and external dental epithelial layers meet at a junction called the *cervical loop*.[17-19]

At the early bell stage, each layer of the dental organ has assumed special functions. The reciprocal exchange of molecular information between the dental organ and dental papilla influences the important events that lead to cell differentiation at the late bell stage.

Late bell stage

The dental lamina that connects the tooth organ to the oral epithelium gradually disintegrates at the late bell stage. The cells of the internal dental epithelium continue to divide at different rates to determine the precise shape of the crown. Shortly after, cells of the internal dental epithelium at the sites of the future cuspal tips stop dividing and assume a columnar shape. The most peripheral cells of the dental papilla enlarge and become organized along the basement membrane at the tooth's epithelial-mesenchymal interface. These newly differentiated cells are called *odontoblasts*, cells that are responsible for the synthesis and secretion of dentin matrix. At this time, the dental papilla is termed the *dental pulp*.

After odontoblasts deposit the first layer of predentin matrix, cells of the internal dental epithelium receive their signal to differentiate further into ameloblasts, or enamel-producing cells. As enamel is deposited over dentin matrix, ameloblasts retreat to the external surface of the crown and are believed to undergo programmed cell death. In contrast, odontoblasts line the inner surface of dentin and remain metabolically active throughout the life of a tooth.

In summary, development of the tooth rudiment from the lamina to the late bell stages culminates in the formation of the tooth crown. As root formation proceeds, epithelial cells from the cervical loop proliferate apically and influence the differentiation of odontoblasts from the dental papilla as well as cementoblasts from follicle mesenchyme. This leads to the deposition of root dentin and cementum, respectively. The dental follicle that gives rise to components of the periodontium, namely the periodontal ligament fibroblasts, the alveolar bone of the tooth socket, and the cementum, also plays a role during tooth eruption, which marks the end phase of odontogenesis.

Experimental systems for studying tooth development

In the last decade, basic understanding of the molecules that control the events that lead to odontoblast differentiation and the formation of dental pulp has advanced significantly.[20] Most of the contemporary experimental approaches used in these studies have taken advantage of the mouse model because of its availability and ease of accessibility. The development of the dentition in mice closely parallels that in humans. Mice are the predominant system for genetic engineering approaches that have generated a volume of exciting data on tooth development.

Before a discussion of the families of signaling molecules is presented, it is important to understand modern experimental approaches and key techniques that are available for use in studies on tooth development. This section is intended to provide a simple description of these modern scientific tools for the dental student or endodontic resident interested in pursuing research in the area of pulp biology.

Tooth organ culture systems

Over the years, researchers have utilized various approaches to study and manipulate developing tooth organs.[21-23] In vitro systems include whole mandibular and maxillary explants as well as individually dissected molar organs that can be cultured in enriched serum by means of a Trowell-type system. The system involves placing the tooth

Figs 2-3a to 2-3c Tooth organ culture system. (Courtesy of Dr Richard Finkelman.)

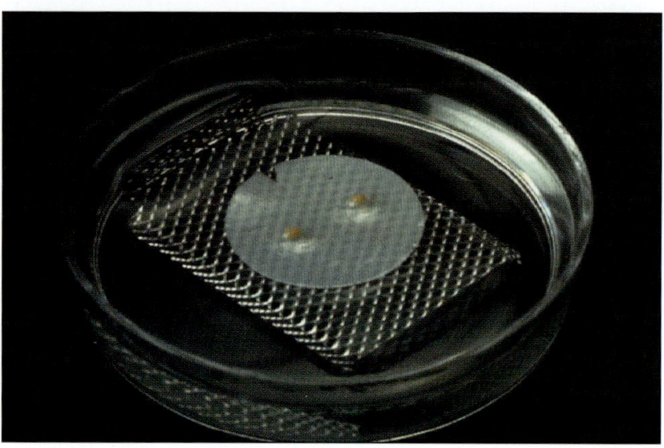

Fig 2-3a Trowell method showing two molar organs at the early cap stage placed on a filter on top of a metal grid within a culture dish.

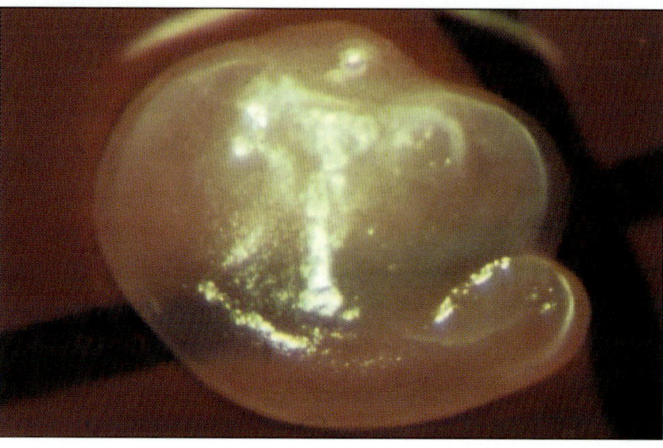

Fig 2-3b Molar organ after 12 days in culture. Note the formation of distinct cusps.

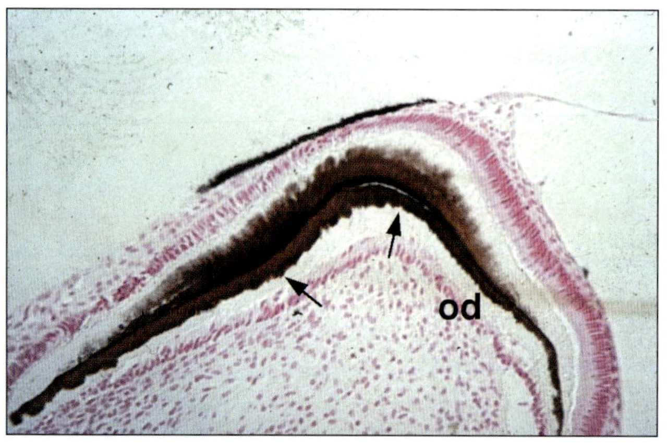

Fig 2-3c Histologic view of Fig 2-3b shows fully differentiated odontoblasts (od) and a layer of mineralized dentin *(arrows)* (von Kossa stain, original magnification ×10).

organ in the correct orientation on a filter that is supported by a metal grid at the gas-liquid interface within a culture well[24] (Figs 2-3a to 2-3c).

Another in vitro approach is the use of functional tooth organ recombination assays. Dental epithelium is separated from papilla mesenchyme by means of enzymes that degrade the basement membrane at the interface.[25,26] Isolated epithelium and mesenchyme can be cultured separately or recombined and then transplanted in vivo to study the effects on tooth development. Modifications of this approach include heterotypic recombinant cultures of epithelium and mesenchyme, in which each is derived from a different organ system, and heterochronic recombinations, in which tissues that are from the same organ system but at different stages of development are used (Fig 2-4).

Researchers interested in studying the effects of various molecules add these reagents in soluble form to the culture and then transplant the treated culture to the anterior chamber of the eye or the subcapsular region of the kidney in mice.[28] Overall, in vivo tooth organ explants that are cultured at in vivo ectopic sites advance further than do in vitro systems (Fig 2-5). In vivo cul-

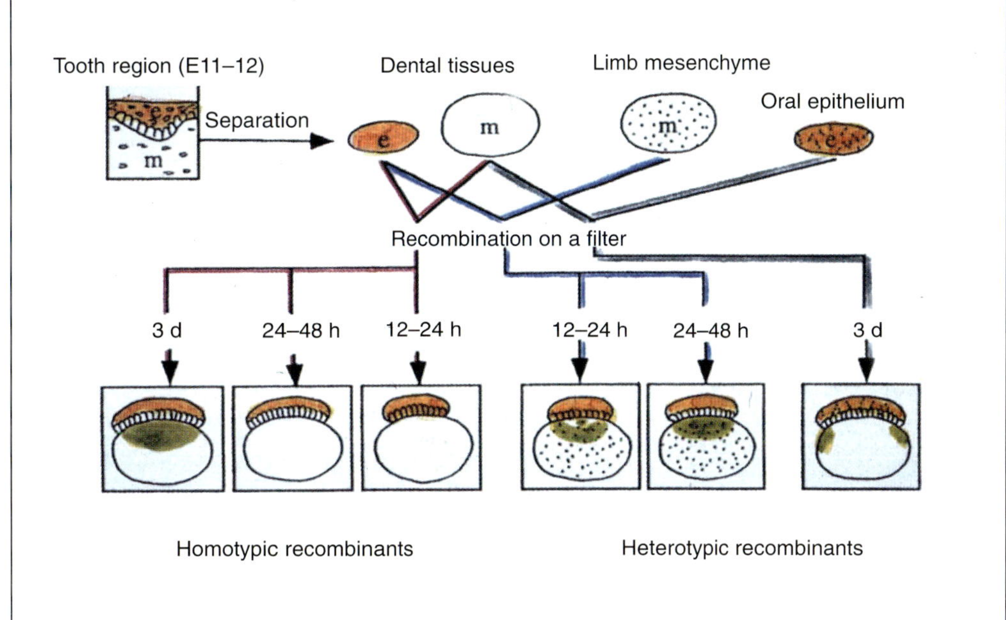

Fig 2-4 Strategy used for homotypic and heterotypic recombination assays: E11–12, days 11 to 12 of mouse embryonic development; e, epithelium; m, mesenchyme; h, hours in culture; d, days in culture. (Reprinted from Mitsiadis et al[27] with permission.)

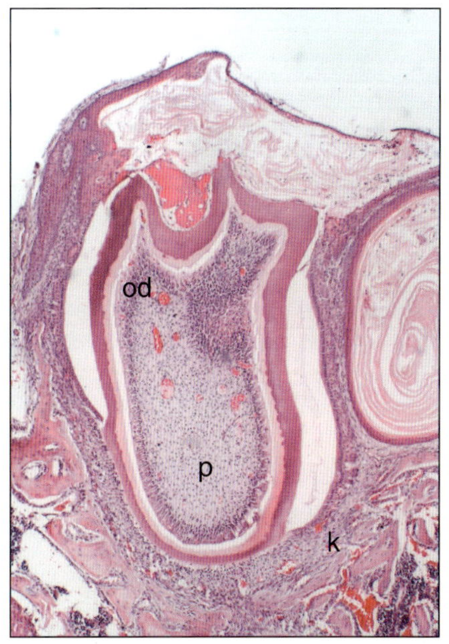

Fig 2-5 Microscopic view of a fully formed tooth that developed from the early cap stage after placement beneath the renal capsule: od, odontoblasts; p, dental pulp; k, kidney (H&E stain, original magnification ×4).

ture systems are also better suited for tooth organ dissections and recombinations that are performed at early stages of development.

An elegant experimental approach that has yielded important information on the nature of the signaling interactions between tooth epithelium and mesenchyme is the use of bead implantation assays.[29] Briefly, either heparin or agarose beads that are soaked in a known concentration of a growth factor are placed on separated dental mesenchyme. After approximately 24 hours in culture, the mesenchyme is analyzed for changes in gene or protein expression in the region surrounding the bead (Fig 2-6).

The availability of mouse strains with spontaneous mutations and genetically engineered "knockout" mice has further refined the use of the bead implantation assay.[31,32] When the reactions

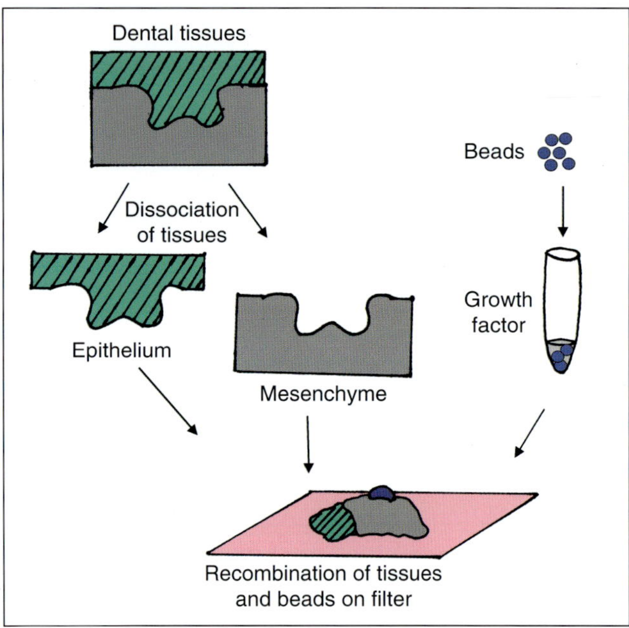

Fig 2-6 Principles of tooth tissue recombination and bead assays. (Modified from Thesleff and Sahlberg[30] with permission.)

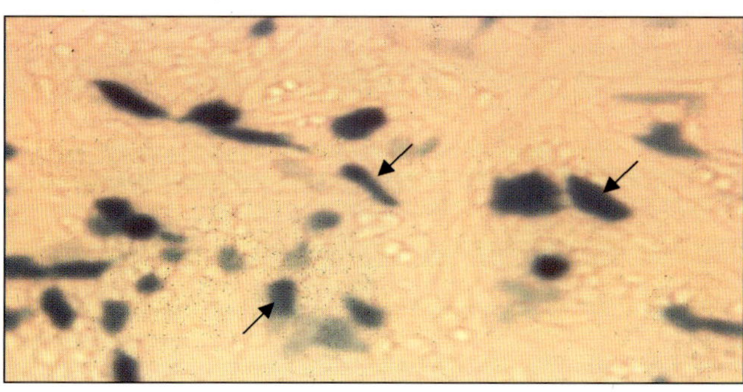

Fig 2-7 Odontoblast-like cells from the immortalized MDPC-23 cell line *(arrows)*. The blue staining detects the activity of the LacZ gene, which encodes for β-galactosidase activity. Blue cells have been successfully transfected with extra copies of the core-binding factor a1 (Cbfa1) gene, whose role is discussed later in the chapter (X-gal stain, original magnification ×40).

of mutant dental mesenchyme and wild-type (normal) mesenchyme are compared, it is possible to determine whether a certain molecule is needed for the expression of a second gene. This approach has led to new information about the relationships of tooth-signaling molecules within a genetic pathway.[6,33]

Odontoblast and dental pulp cell cultures

While tooth organ cultures have facilitated studies of early tooth development, the recent availability of odontoblast and pulp cell culture systems has made it possible to study late events that involve cell differentiation and matrix synthesis. An interesting approach is to utilize hemisectioned human teeth from which dental pulp has been carefully extirpated. The remaining layer of intact odontoblasts can then be cultured within the native pulp chamber, to which nutrient media and various growth factors or cytokines are added. Thick slices of human teeth with the odontoblastic layer left intact offer another useful approach to study the behavior of odontoblasts under conditions that simulate dental caries.[34,35]

The use of primary odontoblast cultures has been limited because intact cells are difficult to isolate in sufficient numbers and become phenotypically altered after several passages in culture. The recent development of cell immortalization procedures has made it possible to generate two established odontoblast-like cell lines. The MO6-G3 cell line was derived from an established murine odontoblast monolayer cell culture system that was infected with a temperature-sensitive Simian virus 40 (SV40).[36] MDPC-23 cells are a spontaneously immortalized cell line derived from mouse embryonic dental papilla that expresses dentin matrix proteins.[37] Clones of transformed cells can grow in selection media at 33°C for a period of 3 to 5 months and display the morphologic and biochemical characteristics of mature

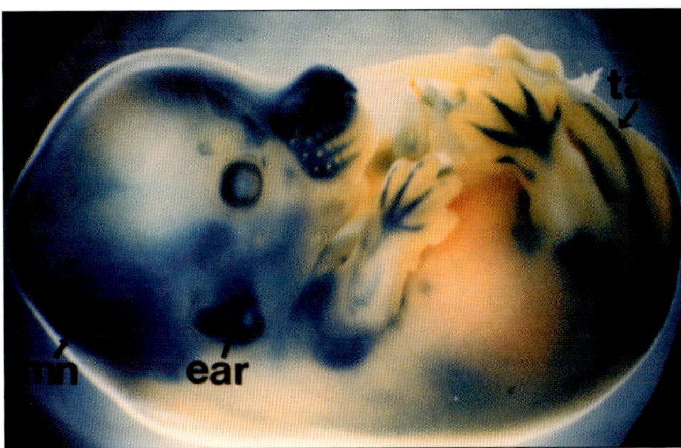

Fig 2-8a Whole-mount view of a developing transgenic mouse embryo in which expression of the LacZ reporter gene (blue staining) is driven by a type I collagen promoter. Expression of β-galactosidase is seen in all areas of the embryo that express type I collagen. mn, Meninges (β-gal stain). (Reprinted from Niederreither et al[42] with permission.)

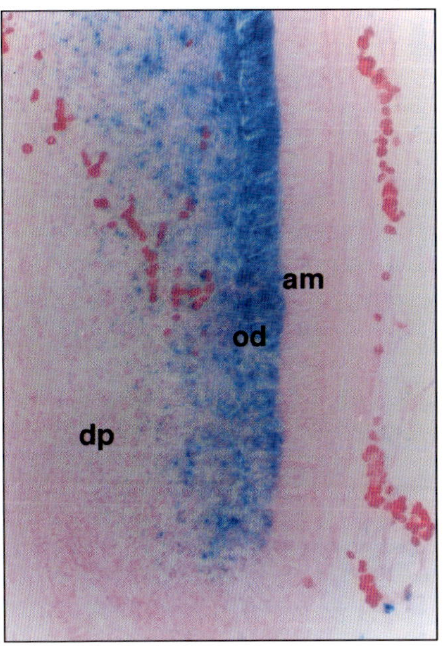

Fig 2-8b Section through the developing incisor at the neonatal stage showing activity of the transgene in differentiating odontoblasts (od) and some cells of the dental pulp (dp). Note the complete absence of staining for type I collagen in ameloblasts (am) (H&E stain, original magnification ×10).

odontoblasts (Fig 2-7). Dental pulp clones, the RPC-C2A and RDP 4-1 cell lines, which exhibit characteristics ranging from pulpal fibroblasts to preodontoblasts, are also available.[38,39]

The use of odontoblast and pulpal cell lines to test the biocompatibility of newly introduced dental materials has opened up an exciting dimension in pulp biology research. In addition, the MO6-G3 and MDPC-23 cell lines offer valuable systems for studying the regulation of genes that encode for dentin matrix proteins, thought to play critical roles in dentinogenesis.

Transgenic and knockout mice

The modern era of recombinant DNA technology and genetic engineering has made it possible to alter or mutate a gene of interest in vitro and then inject it into the pronucleus of a fertilized mouse egg.[40,41] Because knockout experiments have been used in many other dental pulp studies (see chapters 3, 5, 7, 11, and 17), the general method will be described in this chapter. The transgene, if successfully integrated into the host genome, can be transmitted through the germ line to the progeny. Transgenic and knockout mice thus offer a powerful means to study the role of molecules in their natural in vivo environment.

Transgenic mice generated through conventional technology can be designed to overexpress the gene of interest in cells or tissues where it is normally expressed (Figs 2-8a and 2-8b). When it is desirable to study the behavior of a gene at an ectopic site, the transgene of interest is placed behind the promoter of another gene that will drive expression in tissues where it is not normally expressed. In the case of a gene that is expressed in multiple tissues or organs, it is now possible to study activity at one particular site. This is achieved by driving the expression of the transgene with a tissue- or cell-specific promoter.

The following example illustrates the usefulness of a tissue-specific transgenic mouse model. As a means of assessing the precise role of transforming growth factor-β1 (TGF-β1) in odontoblast differentiation, transgenic mice that overexpress active TGF-β1 were generated.[43] Because TGF-β1 is also highly expressed in bone and other tissues, TGF-β1 overexpression was restricted to odontoblasts alone by using the promoter for dentin sialophosphoprotein (DSPP), a gene that is highly tooth specific. Overexpressors of TGF-β1 have defects in dentin that closely resemble dentinogenesis imperfecta, an inherited disorder of dentin. This model permitted an analysis of the direct role of TGF-β1 in dentin formation that was not confounded by its effect in bone and other tissues.[43] These results indicated an important role for TGF in dentin formation, a subject that will be discussed in further detail in chapter 3.

Knockout technology is used to generate lines of mice that lack a functional gene of interest throughout their lifespan. The targeted deletion of the gene is performed in embryonic stem cells that are derived from the inner cell mass of an early embryo. After these cells are cultured to select for the desired deletion, they are implanted into the cavity of a fertilized egg to generate a percentage of offspring that inherit the mutation.

Knockout mice offer a powerful means of assessing the biologic roles of a molecule in the context of a normal mouse. Certain knockout strains appear completely unaffected, indicating that the functions of the gene that are eliminated in vivo can be shared by other genes within the family, a phenomenon of biologic (functional) redundancy. Several knockout mice strains die during gestation or shortly after birth, indicating the importance of these genes in developmental processes. As a result, these mice have not proven to be informative about the role of the gene later in postnatal and adult life. Examples of this include the knockout mice that lack the genes for bone morphogenetic protein 2 (BMP-2) and 4 (BMP-4); these mice undergo embryonic lethality during early gestation. This problem is overcome by the use of conditional knockout technology, in which the inactivation of the gene occurs at a specific time and location.

Of relevance to pulp biology is the phenotype of the TGF-β1 mutant mouse. Teeth develop fully in TGF-β1 (–/–) mice and show no pathosis at birth or through the first 7 to 10 days of postnatal life compared to TGF-β1 (+/–) or TGF-β1 (+/+) littermates. By the end of the second week, TGF-β1 (–/–) mice develop a rapid wasting syndrome, characterized by multifocal inflammatory lesions with dense infiltration of lymphocytes and macrophages in major organs such as the heart and lungs, that eventually leads to death by the third week of life.[44] These observations supported a vast volume of research documenting a critical role for TGF-β1 as a potent immunomodulator.

To study the state of adult dentition in TGF-β1 (–/–) mice, their survival was prolonged with dexamethasone treatment.[44] The absence of a functional TGF-β1 gene resulted in significant destruction of pulp and periapical tissues as well as the hard tissues of the crown (Figs 2-9a and 2-9b). These data prove that no other TGF-β family members can substitute for the loss of TGF-β1. Clearly, the growth factor's dual role as a key modulator of pulpal inflammation and extracellular matrix (ECM) production is significant. Chapter 3 discusses in further detail the role of TGF-β1 in reparative dentinogenesis.

Laser capture microdissection

Among the new in vivo approaches available to analyze the behavior of cells under normal and diseased conditions, laser capture technology stands out as being most innovative. Laser capture microdissection was developed and applied in cancer biology to detect a mutant protein or gene in a single malignant cell[45] and to monitor in vivo differential gene expression levels in normal and malignant breast cell populations.[46]

Laser capture microdissection is being used in the Cancer Genome Anatomy Project to catalog the genes that are expressed during solid tumor progression and to construct complementary DNA (cDNA) libraries from normal and premalignant cell populations. Microarray panels[47] contain-

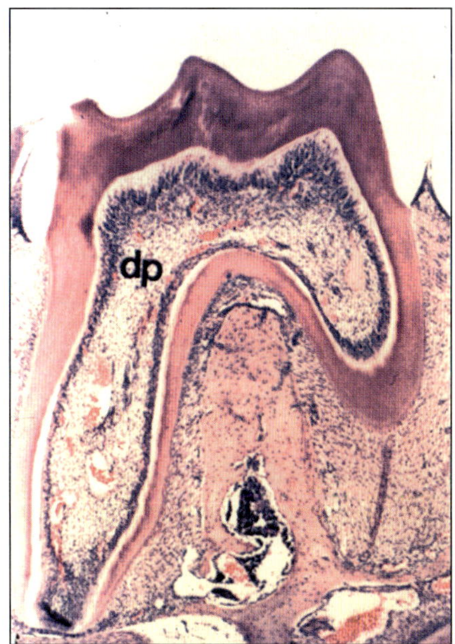

Fig 2-9a Normal mandibular first molar in a TGF-β1 (+/+) mouse at 50 days of postnatal life. dp, Dental pulp (H&E stain, original magnification ×10). (Reprinted from D'Souza et al[44] with permission.)

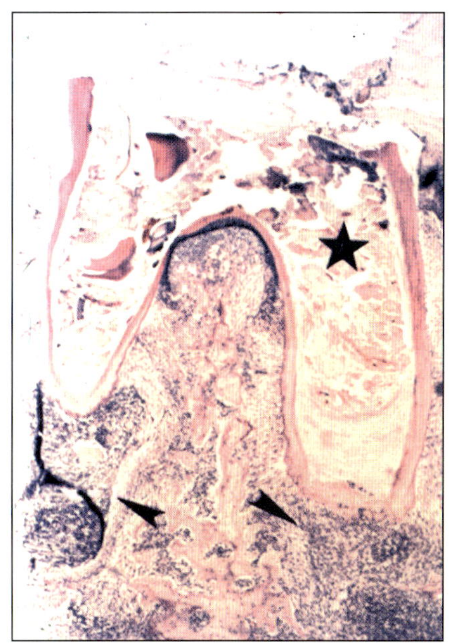

Fig 2-9b In a TGF-β1(–/–) animal whose survival was prolonged with dexamethasone, there is extensive damage to the hard and soft tissues of the molar: *arrowheads,* periapical inflammatory infiltrates; *star*, calcification within the pulp chambers and canals (H&E stain, original magnification ×10). (Reprinted from D'Souza et al[44] with permission.)

ing these index genes are being used to obtain gene expression patterns in human tissue biopsies. The fluctuation of expressed genes that correlate with a particular stage of disease is compared within or between individual patients. Such a fingerprint of gene expression patterns will provide important clues regarding etiology and contribute to diagnostic decisions and therapy.

Applications in this area will be particularly useful for dental pulp research, in which individual cell populations are difficult to access. The progress in understanding odontoblast differentiation has been slow because of serious limitations inherent to both in vivo and in vitro approaches. Pure populations of differentiating and mature odontoblasts are technically difficult to obtain from heterogenous dental papilla or pulp. Furthermore, immortalized odontoblast-like cell lines fail to fully reflect the molecular events that occur in the complex milieu of the tooth organ from which they are derived. Terminology used to describe odontoblast differentiation is sketchy, because it is unclear how morphologic change is reflected at the molecular cytogenetic level.

Initial studies of dentin ECM gene expression in differentiating odontoblasts have been promising (Figs 2-10a to 2-10d). Data from the future use of laser capture microdissection will provide a

Figs 2-10a to 2-10d Preliminary reverse transcriptase-polymerase chain reaction (RT-PCR) amplification of type I collagen from odontoblasts retrieved by laser capture microdissection.

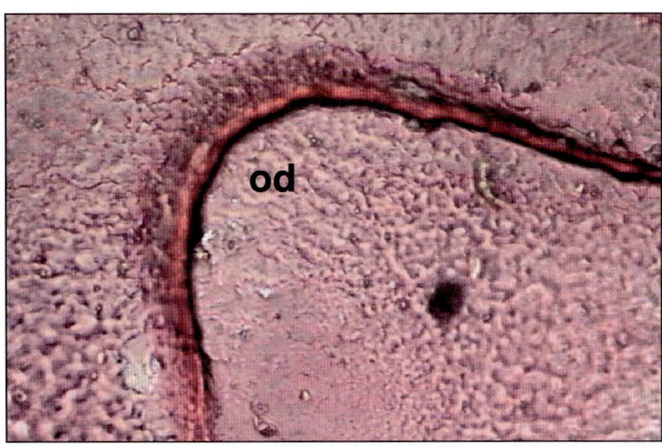

Fig 2-10a Thick, stained frozen section through the mesial cusp tip of a first molar from a newborn mouse prior to laser capture: od, odontoblasts (H&E stain, original magnification ×10).

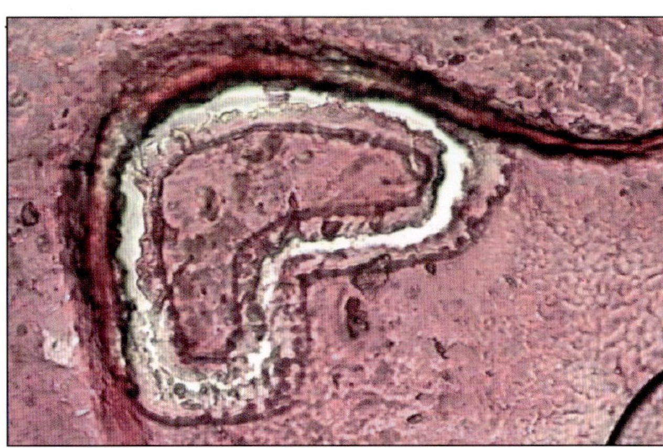

Fig 2-10b Outline of a zone of odontoblasts cut by the laser beam (H&E stain, original magnification ×10).

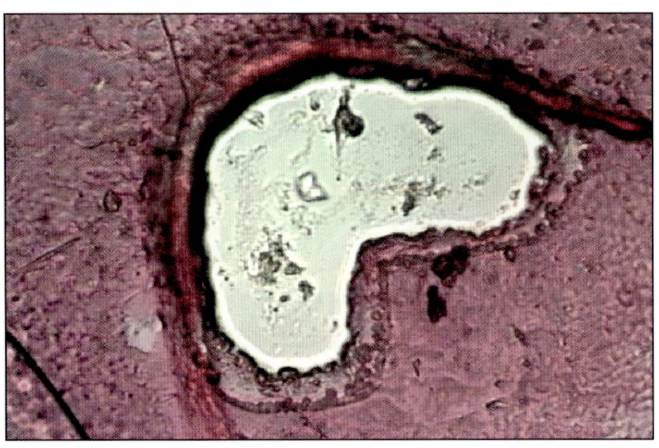

Fig 2-10c Hole created in tissue after catapulting of cells into the PCR tube (H&E stain, original magnification ×10).

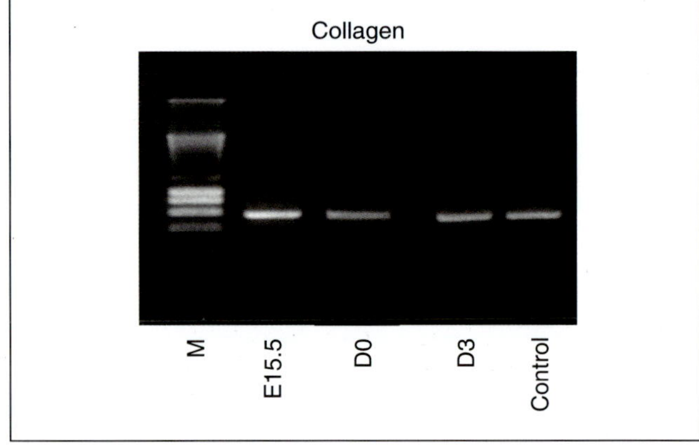

Fig 2-10d RT-PCR reaction showing type I collagen gene expression in odontoblasts at embryonic day 15.5 (E15.5), day 0 (D0), and day 3 (D3) of development: M, DNA markers; Control, MDPC-23 odontoblast-like cells.

correlation between the morphologic changes and the expression of known ECM genes during odontoblast differentiation. Information generated from this approach will also be valuable in developing a nomenclature that can be consistently used by researchers.

Moreover, known and unknown genes will be identified from the developmentally staged, odontoblast-specific cDNA libraries. Genes that are defined for each stage of primary dentin formation will provide important clues about temporal patterns of gene expression and the potential functions of encoded protein products in dentin mineralization. Such fundamental information will be useful in characterizing cells within the cell-rich zone of dental pulp, the identification of the replacement population of pulpal cells involved in reparative dentin formation, and

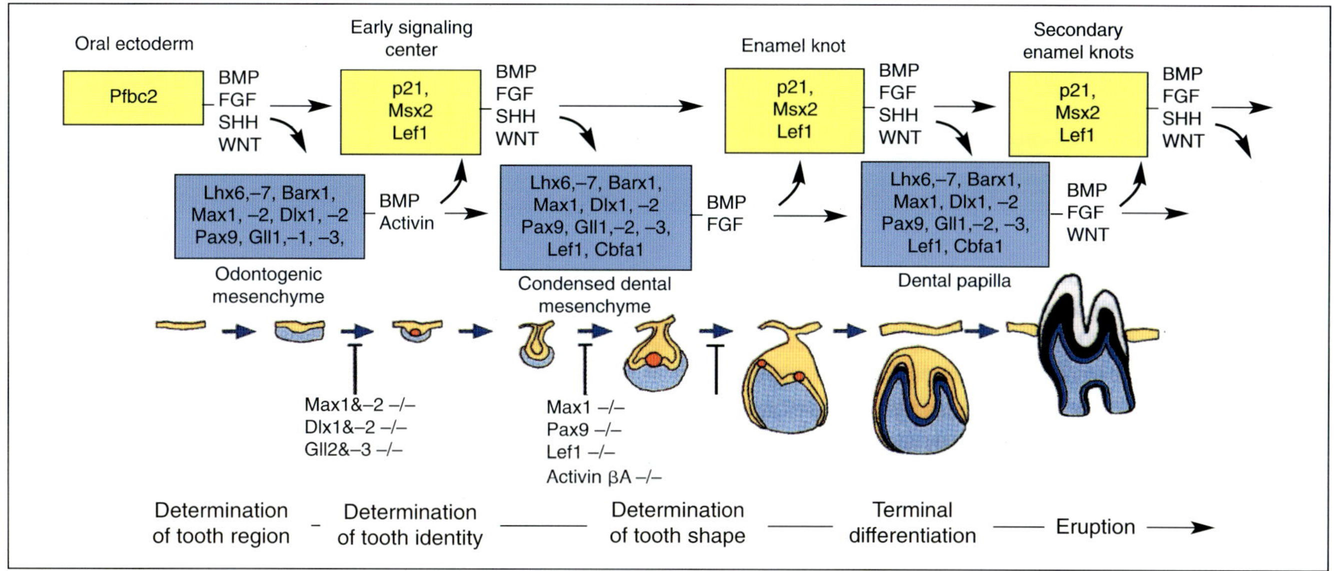

Fig 2-11 Molecules (transcription factors, growth factors, and other proteins) involved in epithelial-mesenchymal signaling interactions during tooth development. Little is known about molecules that influence the latest stages of terminal differentiation and tooth eruption. Note the time of arrest of tooth development in knockout mice that lack important transcription factors. (Reprinted from Jernvall and Thesleff[6] with permission.)

in the development of vital pulp therapies aimed at hastening the healing of the injured pulpodentin complex.

Signaling interactions that influence odontoblast differentiation and dental pulp formation

The combined use of conventional tooth organ culture and recombination techniques, as well as the application of modern molecular and genetic approaches, has significantly advanced the understanding of the genes responsible for tooth initiation and morphogenesis. An informative Internet site[48] presents a current catalog of all the molecules that are expressed in tooth organs.

The two principal groups of molecules that are involved in the reciprocal exchange of information between tooth epithelium and mesenchyme are transcription factors and growth factors (Fig 2-11). Transcription factors are proteins that bind to DNA near the start of transcription of a gene. They regulate gene expression by either facilitating or inhibiting the enzyme RNA polymerase in the initiation and maintenance of transcription. Transcription factors are rarely found in high amounts and are not secreted outside the cell. In general, they perform critical cell- or tissue-specific functions. Mutations involving transcription factors often result in defects of tooth formation.

Growth factors are secreted proteins that are capable of binding to specific receptors on the cell surface. Subsequent interaction with both membrane and cytoplasmic components leads to a complex series of intracellular events (signal transduction) that results in altered gene expression. These changes activate cell growth and differentiation. The majority of growth factors are synthesized at higher levels than transcription factors and perform versatile functions. In many instances, the functions of one growth factor overlap with those of a related family member, so that loss of function can be compensated for by biologic redundancy.

Molecular changes in dental mesenchyme are affected by the following families of molecules: the BMPs, fibroblast growth factors (FGFs), and WNT families; sonic hedgehog (Shh) as well as transcriptional molecules such as the Msx-1, Msx-2 homeobox genes; lymphoid enhancer-binding factor 1 (Lef-1); and Pax9, a member of the paired-box-containing transcription factor gene family. The actions and interactions of these molecules are complex and have been described eloquently in recent reviews.[6,13] The following discussion captures selected highlights.

The BMPs are among the best characterized signals in tooth development. In addition to directly influencing morphogenesis of the enamel organ (see the discussion on the enamel knot, later in the chapter), epithelial BMP-2 and BMP-4 are able to induce expression of Msx-1, Msx-2, and Lef-1 in dental mesenchyme, as shown in bead implantation assays.[29,31,49] The shift in BMP-4 expression from epithelium to mesenchyme occurs around embryonic day 12 and is coincident with the transfer of inductive potential from dental epithelium to mesenchyme.[29] In mesenchyme, BMP-4, in turn, requires Msx-1 to induce its own expression.[31] Figures 2-12a to 2-12d summarize the experiments performed on the role of the BMPs in dental mesenchyme.

The FGFs, in general, are potent stimulators of cell proliferation and division both in dental mesenchyme and epithelium. Expression of FGF-2, FGF-4, FGF-8, and FGF-9 is restricted to dental epithelium and can stimulate Msx-1 but not Msx-2 expression in underlying mesenchyme. FGF-8 is expressed early in odontogenesis (embryonic days 0.5 to 1.5), in presumptive dental epithelium, and can induce the expression of Pax9 in underlying mesenchyme. Interestingly, BMP-4 prevents this induction and may share an antagonistic relationship with the FGFs, similar to that observed in limb development.[50]

The expression of Shh, a member of the vertebrate family of hedgehog signaling proteins, is limited to presumptive dental epithelium. Recent studies by Hardcastle et al[51] have shown that Shh in beads cannot induce Pax9, Msx-1, or BMP-4 expression in dental mesenchyme but is able to stimulate other genes encoding the transmembrane protein patched (Ptc) and GO, a zinc finger transcription factor. Because neither FGF-8 nor BMP-4 can stimulate Ptc or GO, it can be assumed at the present time that the Shh signaling pathway is independent of the BMP and FGF pathways during tooth development.[51]

Several WNT genes are expressed during tooth development and may be required for the formation of the tooth bud.[13] These genes are believed to play a role in activating the intracellular pathway involving frizzled receptors, β-catenin, and nuclear transport of Lef-1. Other signaling molecules, including the Notch genes, epidermal growth factor, hepatocyte growth factor, and platelet-derived growth factor families, may also influence tooth development, although the exact nature of their involvement remains to be elucidated.

Mice genetically engineered with targeted mutations in transcription factor genes such as Msx-1, Lef-1, and Pax9 as well as activin-βA, a member of the TGF-β superfamily, have revealed important information. Knockouts of BMP-2, BMP-4, and Shh have proven less informative, largely because death occurs in utero prior to the onset of tooth development. In mutant strains deficient in Msx-1, Lef-1, Pax9, and activin-PA, tooth development fails to advance beyond the bud stage (Figs 2-13a to 2-13c). Thus, these molecules are important in directing the fate of the dental mesenchyme and its ability to influence the progress of epithelial morphogenesis to the cap stage.[52-55] Exciting discoveries in the field of human genetics have shown that mutations in MSX-1 and Pax9 are associated with premolar and molar agenesis, respectively (Frazier-Bowers and D'Souza, unpublished data, 2001; see Figs 2-13a to 2-13c).[56-58] These findings illustrate the importance of animal models in studies of human disease (Figs 2-14a to 2-14f).

More recently, mice lacking an important osteoblast-specific transcription factor, core-binding factor a1 (Cbfa1), were shown to completely

Figs 2-12a to 2-12d Bone morphogenetic protein (BMP) expression within the developing tooth organ. In situ hybridization pictures that have been digitized and processed. Red dots represent mRNA transcripts. (Reprinted from Thesleff and Sharpe[13] with permission.)

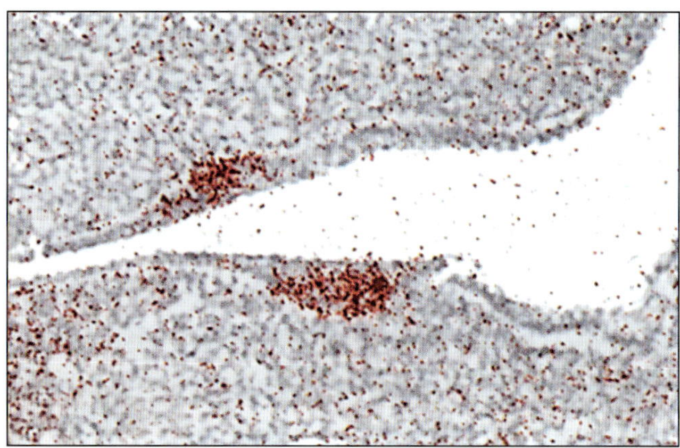

Fig 2-12a BMP-2 gene expression is highly restricted to the dental lamina.

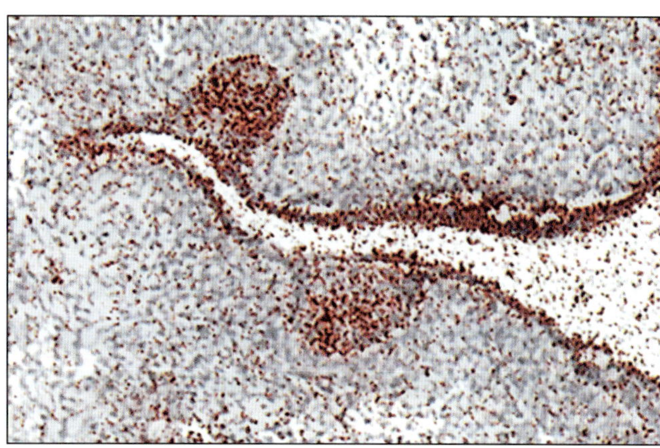

Fig 2-12b BMP-7 is coexpressed in the thickened dental epithelium.

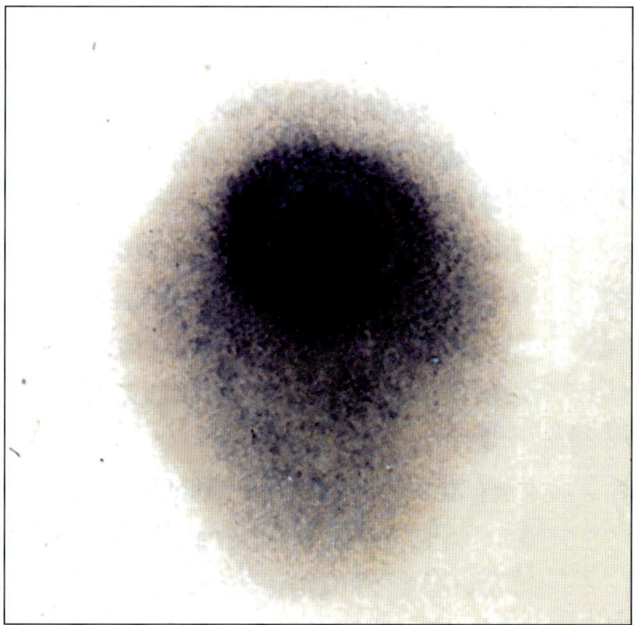

Fig 2-12c A bead that releases BMP-2 protein is capable of stimulating Msx-1 expression in dental mesenchyme.

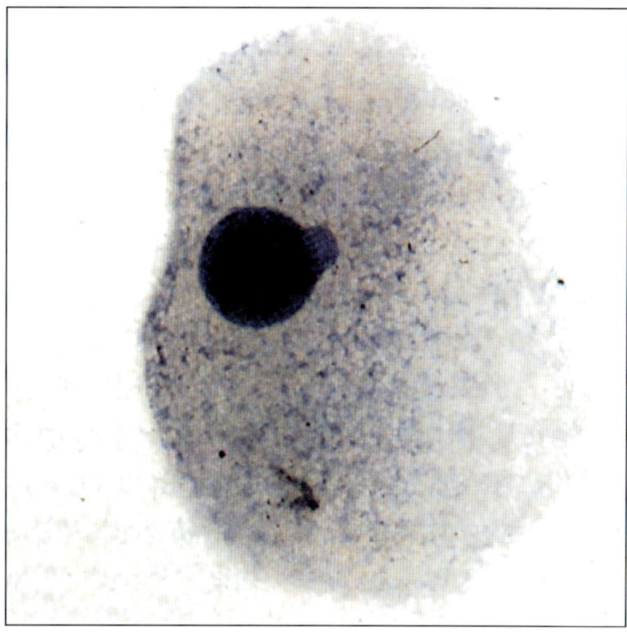

Fig 2-12d A control bead that has been soaked in bovine serum albumin is not capable of stimulating Msx-1 expression.

lack osteoblast differentiation and bone formation.[59] Mutations in Cbfa1 cause cleidocranial dysplasia, an inherited disorder in humans that is characterized by open fontanels in the skull, defective clavicles, multiple supernumerary teeth that fail to erupt, and various tooth matrix defects.[60,61] Molar organs that are Cbfa1 (-/-) arrest at the late cap or early bell stage of develop-

Figs 2-13a to 2-13c Role of Pax9 in the formation of the posterior human dentition.

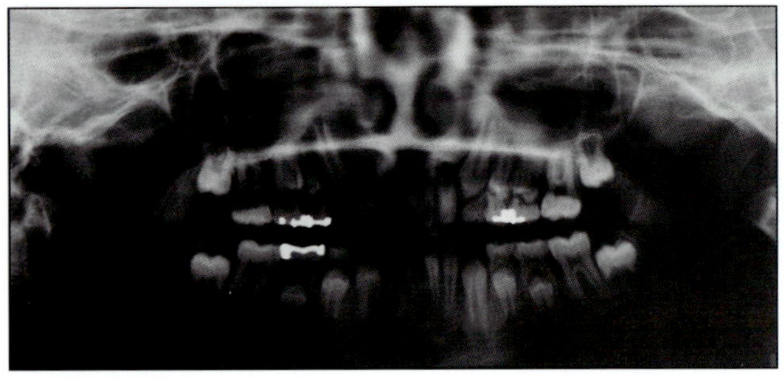

Fig 2-13a Panoramic radiograph of a normal dentition in an unaffected family member.

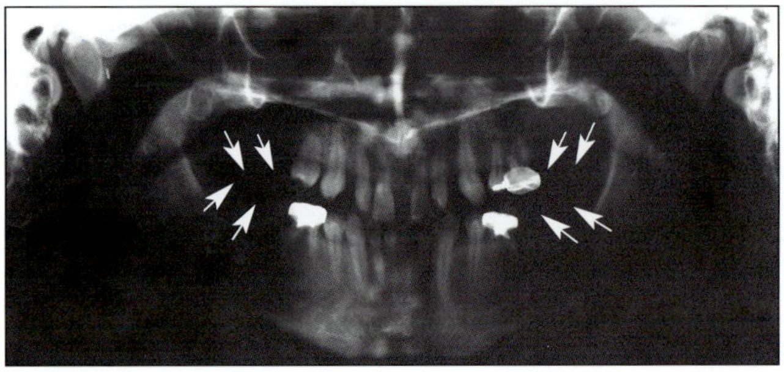

Fig 2-13b Panoramic radiograph of an affected individual who is missing molars *(arrows)*.

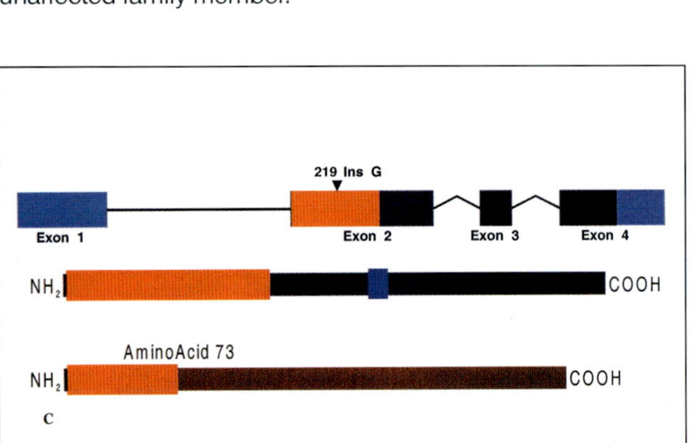

Fig 2-13c Insertion mutation of a single nucleotide, guanine, at residue 219. This defect caused a frameshift and a premature truncation site that resulted in a defective protein (compare bottom drawing to the normal protein in the center) that could not function like a normal Pax9 protein.

ment and appear hypoplastic and misshapen. Cbfa1-mutant incisors show defective odontoblasts and highly dysplastic dentin (see Figs 2-14a to 2-14f).[62]

One theory is that this transcription factor serves multiple functions in mineralizing tissue organs. In addition to playing an essential role in osteoblast differentiation, it is likely that Cbfa1 conditions the dental papilla mesenchyme to become responsive to epithelial signals. Once the molecular trigger from the enamel organ reaches the peripheral zone of dental papilla cells, Cbfa1 is down-regulated in dental papilla and odontoblast differentiation ensues. Thus, the presence of Cbfa1 in dental papilla can be viewed as a limiting factor of odontoblast differentiation; its presence in dental papilla at the bud and cap stages of odontogenesis has an osteogenic-like influence, while its removal from dental papilla triggers terminal events in odontoblast differentiation.

It can logically be concluded that certain cell populations within mature dental pulp retain an osteogenic phenotype and that after injury to the pulpodentin complex these are stimulated to form an osteodentin matrix rather than a true tubular dentin. Studies on this important mouse model of a human disease should provide important clues about the molecular mechanisms underlying how lineage diversity is established between osteoblasts and odontoblasts. Although it is clear that the two cell populations share a common pathway early in development, there is emerging evidence that their terminal differentiation into bone- and dentin matrix-producing cells involves different molecular pathways. As more information becomes available, researchers

Figs 2-14a to 2-14f Bone and tooth phenotype in mice genetically engineered to lack a functional Cbfa1 gene.

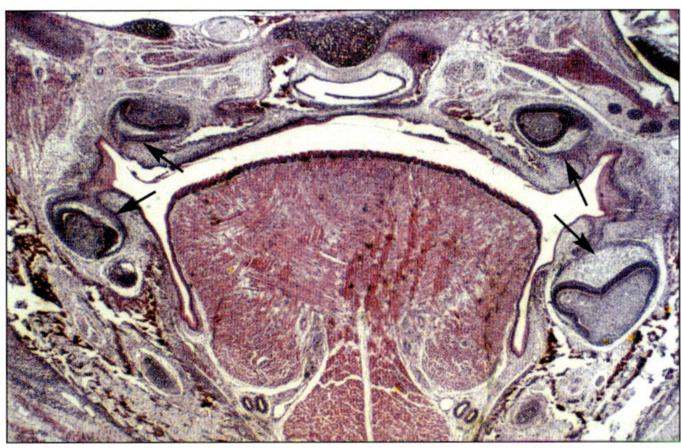

Fig 2-14a Coronal section through the molar region of a Cbfa1 (+/+) newborn mouse, revealing normal molar development *(arrows)* and formation of the alveolus (H&E stain, original magnification ×4).

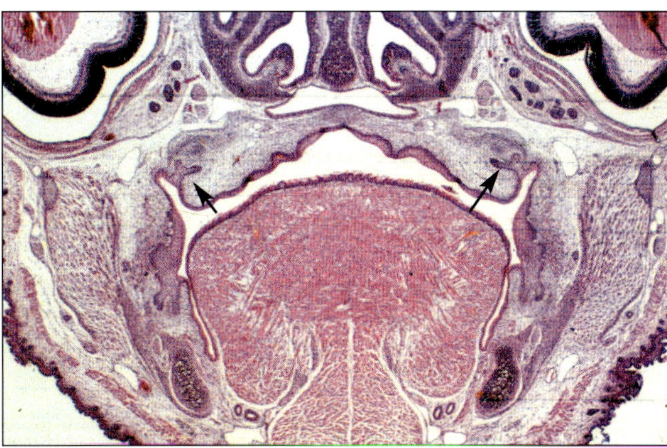

Fig 2-14b Extremely hypoplastic molar organs and a complete lack of bone in a Cbfa1 (–/–) mouse. *Arrows*, knockout tooth organs (H&E stain, original magnification ×4).

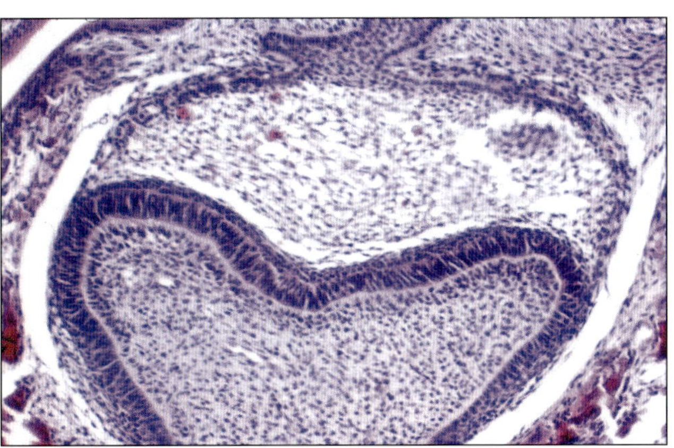

Fig 2-14c High-magnification view of a normal Cbfa1 (+/+) first molar (H&E stain, original magnification ×10).

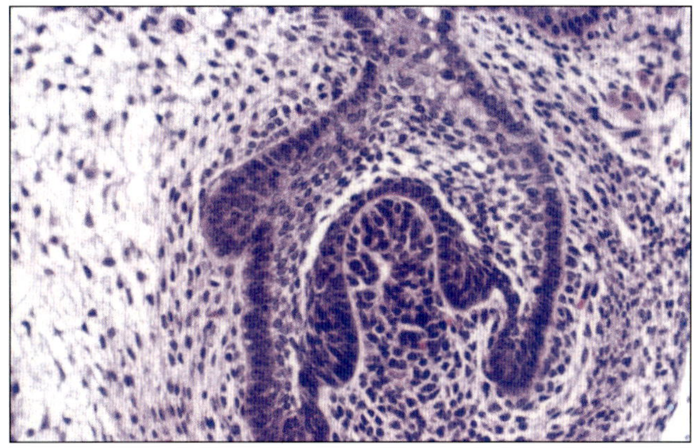

Fig 2-14d Higher-magnification view of a Cbfa1 mutant molar, which lacks normal cusp formation (H&E stain, original magnification ×10).

will be provided better clues on how to develop dentin-specific therapeutics capable of generating a true dentin matrix.

Enamel knots as signaling centers for cuspal morphogenesis

For more than a century, enamel knots were described as histologically distinct clusters of epithelial cells located first in the center of cap-stage tooth organs (primary) and then at the sites of future cusp tips (secondary). For years, it was speculated that these structures, appearing only transiently in odontogenesis, controlled the folding of the dental epithelium and hence cuspal morphogenesis. Recently, the morphologic, cellular, and molecular events leading to the formation and disappearance of the enamel knot have been described, thus linking its role to that of an organizing center for tooth morphogenesis.[16,63,64]

The primary enamel knot appears at the late bud stage, grows in size as the cap stage is reached, and is no longer visible at the early bell

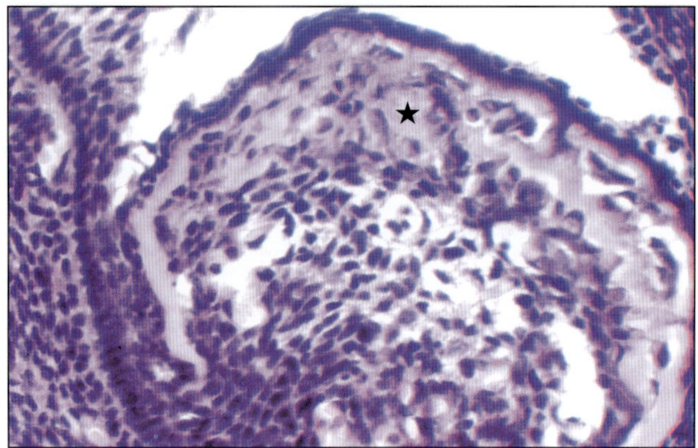

Fig 2-14e Newborn Cbfa1 (–/–) mouse with incisor organs that show defects in odontoblast differentiation and dentinal formation. The latter resembles an osteodentin matrix *(star)* (H&E stain, original magnification ×10).

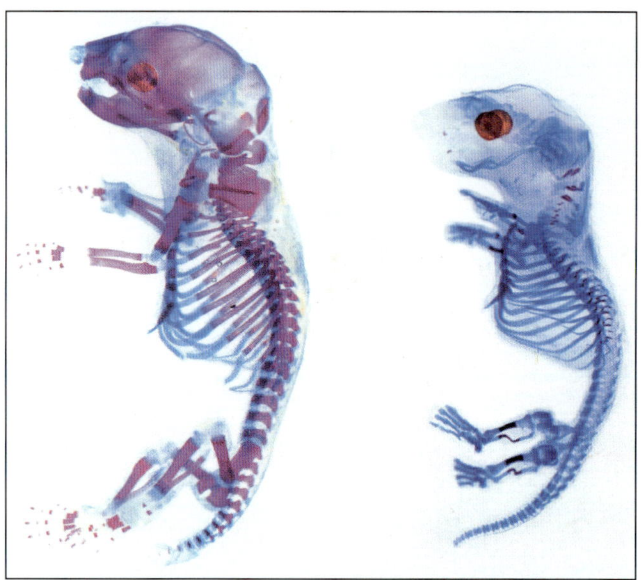

Fig 2-14f Whole-mount staining with alizarin red for bone and alcian blue for cartilage reveals the absence of bone in the mutant *(right)* compared to a normal littermate *(left)* (alizarin red stain for bone, alcian blue stain for cartilage, original magnification ×2). (Reprinted from the cover of Cell, vol 89, May 1997, with permission.)

stage (Figs 2-15a to 2-15d). Cells of the enamel knot are the only cells within the enamel organ that stop proliferating[15] and eventually undergo programmed cell death, or apoptosis.[65] Another intriguing finding has linked p21, a cyclin-dependent kinase inhibitor that is associated with terminal differentiation events, to apoptosis of the enamel knot.[64]

Although morphogens such as BMP-2, BMP-4, BMP-7,[63] FGF-9,[66] and Shh are expressed variantly throughout tooth morphogenesis, their co-localization within the primary enamel knot is strongly suggestive of its role as an organizing center for tooth morphogenesis. Notably, FGF-4 is exclusively expressed in the enamel knot,[15,67] either singly or in concert with FGF-9, to influence patterning or to regulate expression of downstream genes such as Msx-1 in underlying papilla mesenchyme. Because the instructive signaling influence lies with the dental mesenchyme prior to the development of the primary enamel knot, it is reasonable to assume that the dental mesenchyme is involved in the regulation of enamel knot formation. It is highly likely that signals from the enamel knot area influence gene expression in an autocrine and paracrine fashion, thus influencing the fate of the enamel organ and the dental papilla.

Role of the extracellular matrix in tooth morphogenesis and cytodifferentiation

Remodeling of the ECM is an important feature of epithelial morphogenesis, especially in branching organs such as salivary and mammary glands.[7,68] The ECM also regulates morphogenetic functions in a variety of craniofacial tissues.[69] Results of several functional in vitro studies have shown that the integrity of the ECM, in particular the basement membrane, influences the budding and folding of dental epithelium during morphogenesis.[11,70,71]

Molecules such as types I, III, and IV collagen, along with laminin and various proteoglycans, are differentially expressed in the basement membrane at the tooth epithelial-mesenchymal interface.[11,72,73] The presence of matrix metalloproteinases (MMPs) has been linked with the

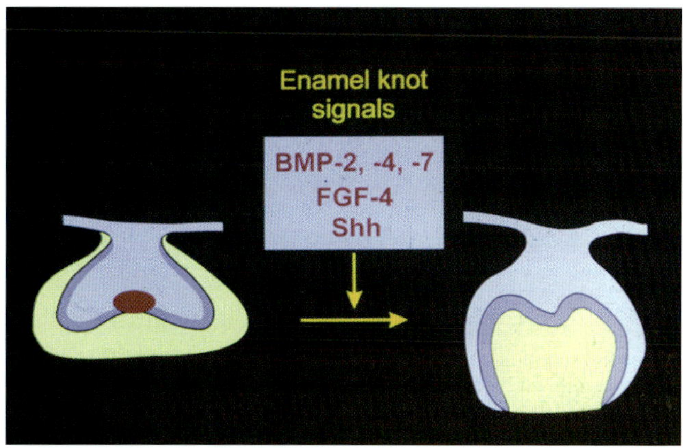

Fig 2-15a Role of the enamel knot as a signaling center for morphogenesis of the tooth cusp. (Courtesy of Dr I. Thesleff.)

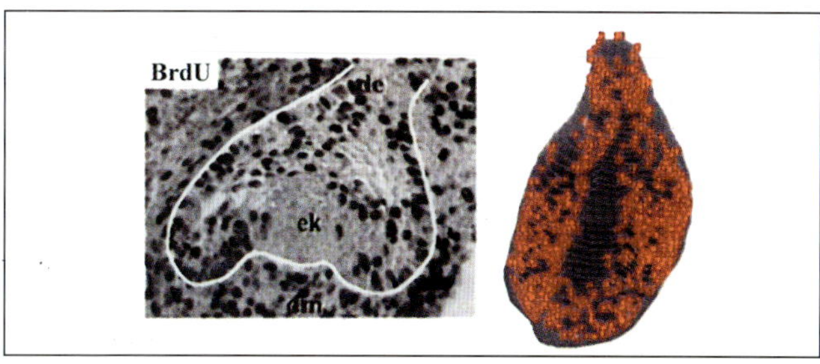

Fig 2-15b BrdU labeling identifies cells in the putative enamel knot that are negative for the stain and have left the cell cycle. (Reprinted from Thesleff and Sharpe[13] with permission.)

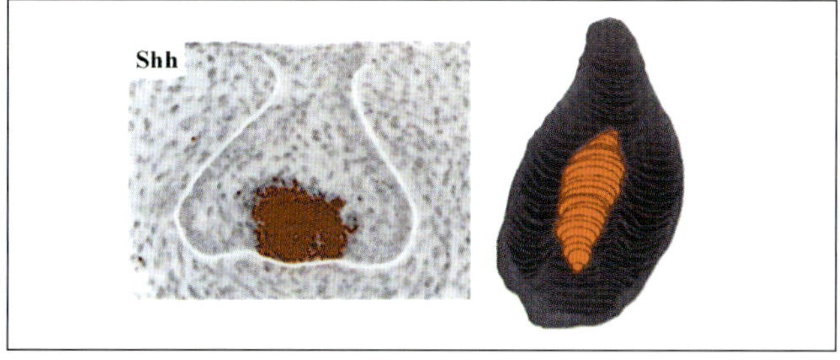

Fig 2-15c Same cell within the enamel knot expresses high levels of Shh (Reprinted from Thesleff and Sharpe[13] with permission.)

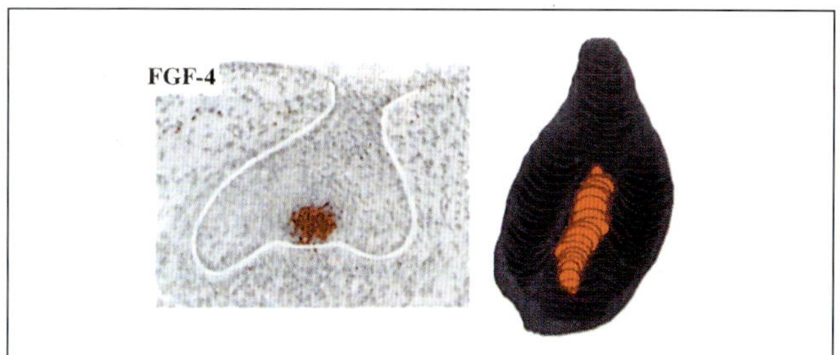

Fig 2-15d Same cell within the enamel knot expresses high levels of FGF-4. Three-dimensional reconstructions of serial sections (Figs 2-15b to 2-15d) illustrate the shape of the enamel knot. (Reprinted from Thesleff and Sharpe[13] with permission.)

morphogenesis of several epithelial-mesenchymal organs, including teeth.[74,75] Studies by Sahlberg et al[76] showed that gelatinase A, a MMP that cleaves type IV collagen increases in odontoblasts shortly after cuspal morphogenesis, contributes to the degradation of the basement membrane. The expression of protease inhibitors, tissue inhibitor of metalloproteinase 1, 2, and 3, also correlates with tooth morphogenesis (Sahlberg C et al, unpublished data, 2001). Earlier functional in vitro studies have shown that the integrity of the basement membrane influences the budding and folding of dental epithelium during morphogenesis and the spatial ordering of cells that undergo terminal differentiation.[11,70,77] The precise natures of the molecular interactions that influence morphogenesis at this dynamic interface are unknown.

Odontoblast differentiation

Odontoblast differentiation is initiated at the cusp tip in the most peripheral layer of dental papilla cells that align the epithelial-mesenchymal interface and follows three steps: induction, competence, and terminal differentiation. Inductive signals from the internal epithelial cells most likely involve members of the TGF-β family (BMP-2 and BMP-4; TGF-β1) that become partially sequestered in the basal lamina, to which peripher-

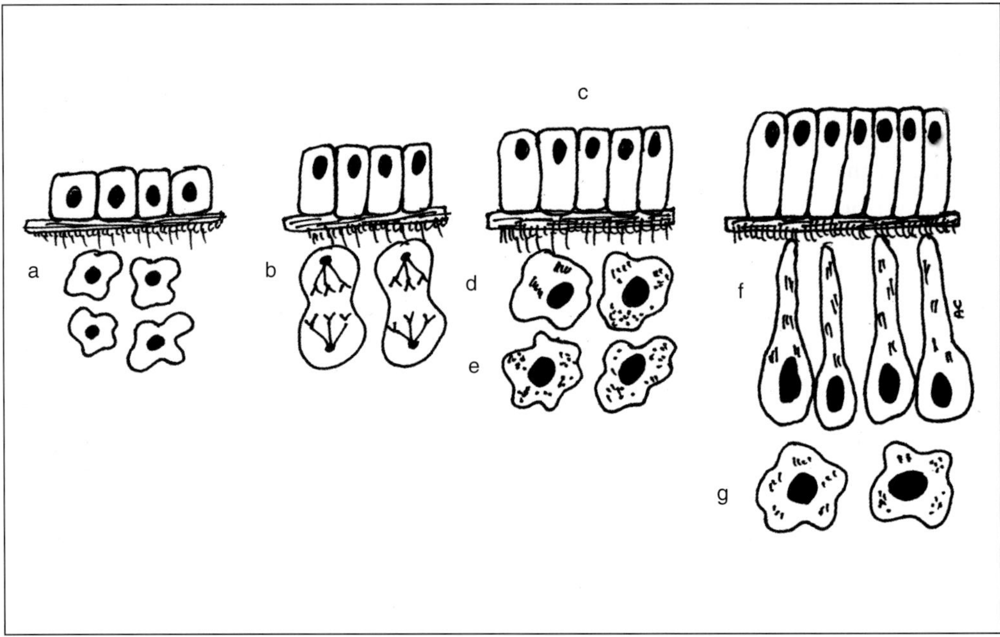

Fig 2-16 Terminal events in odontoblast differentiation: a, undifferentiated mesenchymal cells; b, committed dental mesenchymal cells that are in a state of mitosis or cell division; c, inner dental epithelium, which is important for driving the differentiation of cells nearest the basement membrane; d, basement membrane; e, daughter cells that are competent to become odontoblasts remain in the peripheral zone of the dental papilla; f, differentiated odontoblast with a polarized nucleus and cytoplasmic extensions; g, subodontoblastic cells.

al cells of the dental papilla become aligned. Competence is achieved after a predetermined number of cell divisions is complete and cells express specific growth factor receptors. In the final round of cell division, only the most peripheral layer of cells subjacent to the basal lamina respond to the signals from the internal dental epithelium to become fully differentiated into odontoblasts. The subodontoblastic layer of dental papilla cells thus represents dental papilla cells that are competent cells exposed to the same inductive signals as differentiated odontoblasts, but the competent cells lack the final signal (Fig 2-16).

Based on the information presented so far, it is clear that there has been considerable progress made in understanding the molecular events preceding the terminal differentiation of odontoblasts (see Fig 2-11). However, the final determinants of odontoblast differentiation remain to be characterized.

As is well documented in the literature, fully differentiated odontoblasts are postmitotic cells that are morphologically distinct from cells of the dental pulp. As differentiation proceeds in an apical direction, the round to cuboidal shape of these cells changes to a tall columnar appearance. On the subcellular level, cells acquire a synthetic and secretory apparatus by developing an extensive rough endoplasmic reticulum and golgi apparatus along with numerous lysosomes. To accommodate these organelles and to prepare for the secretion of dentin matrix components in an apical and unidirectional manner, the nucleus moves to the opposite pole of the cell in a position opposite to the inner dental epithelial cells. Nuclear repolarization is one of the hallmarks of odontoblast terminal differentiation.

Dentin matrix proteins and the biomineralization of dentin

The formation of dentin follows the same principles that guide the formation of other hard connective tissues in the body, namely, cementum and bone (see also chapter 3). The first requirement is the presence of highly specialized cells that are capable of synthesizing and secreting components of an organic matrix that is capable of accepting biologic apatite or mineral. Other prerequisites include a rich vascular supply and high levels of the enzyme alkaline phosphatase. At an alkaline pH, the latter is capable of cleaving phosphate ions from organic substrates and may play a role in ion transport through cell membranes.

As odontoblasts begin to secrete a predentin ECM, they retreat in a pulpal direction but remain connected to the matrix as it is being formed through cell extensions called *odontoblast processes*. The conversion of the organic predentin matrix, which is principally composed of type I collagen, into a mineralized layer of dentin is a highly complex process that begins at a distance away from the odontoblastic cell bodies.

The process of dentin mineralization is not well understood, and, for the past four decades, several researchers have attempted to answer the following questions[78,79]:

1. What is the exact composition of dentin matrix?
2. What biochemical features distinguish dentin from bone and cementum?
3. Are there dentin-specific markers and can they be used to characterize the nature of the replacement cell population responsible for forming reparative dentin?
4. How do the physical features and conformational structures of ECM molecules facilitate the calcification of dentin?
5. Do these macromolecules interact with each other during the mineralization of dentin, and do they form supramolecular complexes that promote the deposition of hydroxyapatite crystals?
6. What is the nature of the ECM molecules that modulate the initiation, rate, and extent of dentin deposition?
7. What is the nature of the genes that encode for dentin ECM molecules and are defects in these genes responsible for the inherited dentin disorders, namely, dentinogenesis imperfecta and dentin dysplasia?
8. What genes regulate the expression of key dentin ECM molecules?

Excellent reviews by Linde and Goldberg[80] and Butler and Ritchie[81] detail the composition of dentin matrix and the process of dentinogenesis. The following is a brief description of the principal components of the organic phase of dentin, which is composed of proteins, proteoglycans, lipids, various growth factors, and water.

Among the proteins, collagen is the most abundant and offers a fibrous matrix for the deposition of carbonate apatite crystals. The collagens that are found in dentin are primarily type I collagen (Figs 2-17a to 2-17d) with trace amounts of type V collagen and some type I collagen trimer. The importance of type I collagen as a key structural component of dentin matrix is illustrated by the inherited dentin disorder called dentinogenesis imperfecta (DGI), which is characterized by severe defects in dentin mineralization caused by a mutation in type I collagen. This form of dentinogenesis imperfecta is coupled with osteogenesis imperfecta-related bone diseases.

The other group of proteins is the noncollagenous proteins. Based on the classification of Butler and Ritchie,[81] dentin noncollagenous proteins are further grouped into five categories. The first and likely the most important group of dentin noncollagenous proteins are two proteins, originally classified as dentin-specific, dentin phosphoproteins (DPP), or phosphophoryns, and dentin sialoprotein (DSP) (see Figs 2-17a to 2-17d). After type I collagen, DPP is the most abundant of dentin matrix proteins and represents almost 50% of the dentin ECM. DPP is a polyionic macromolecule that is rich in phosphoserine and aspartic acid. Interestingly, DPP

Figs 2-17a to 2-17d Photomicrographs of in situ hybridization results showing dentin matrix gene expression in newly differentiated odontoblasts.

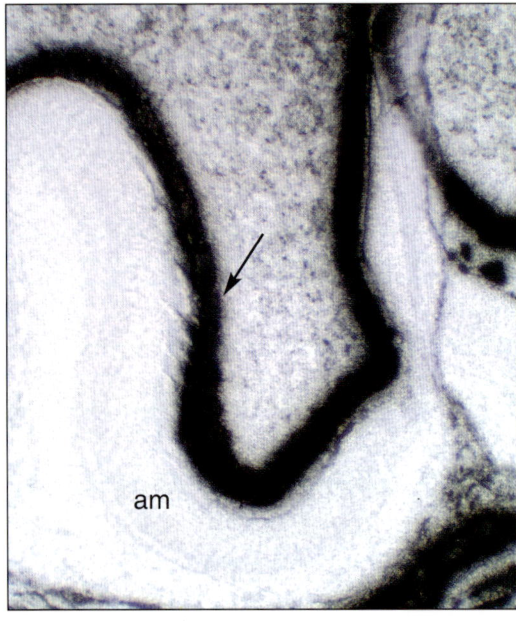

Fig 2-17a Brightfield view showing high levels of type I collagen messenger RNA transcripts in odontoblasts *(arrow)*. Opposing ameloblasts (am) are clearly negative, confirming the specificity of the α1 (I) collagen probe (H&E stain, original magnification ×10).

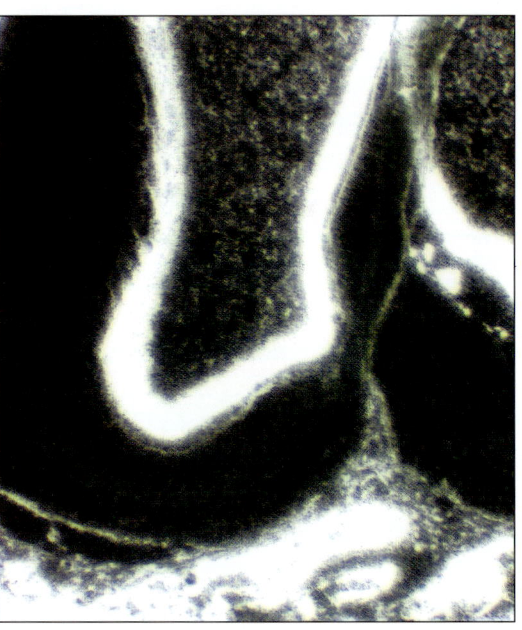

Fig 2-17b Darkfield view of type I collagen messenger RNA transcripts in odontoblasts (H&E stain, original magnification ×10).

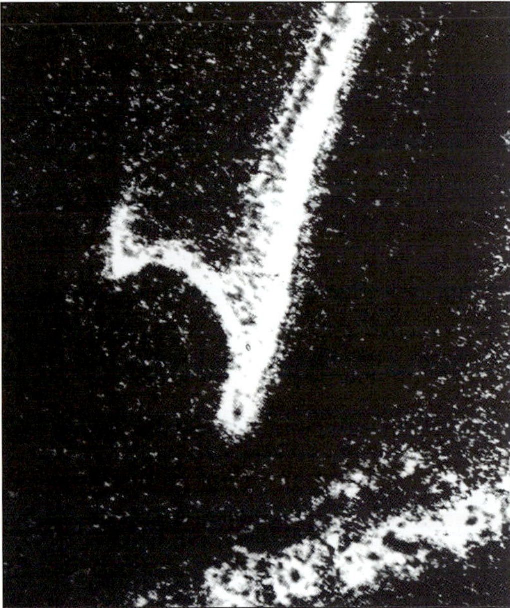

Fig 2-17c Dentin matrix protein1 is expressed at a lower level in odontoblasts and osteoblasts (H&E stain, original magnification ×10).

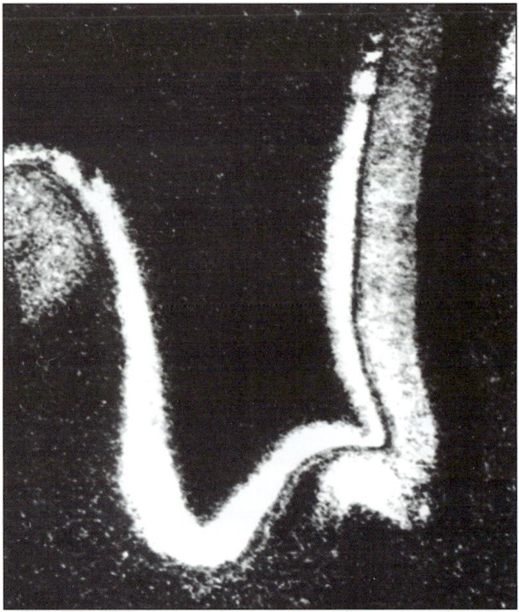

Fig 2-17d DSPP expression in odontoblasts and preameloblasts. Note that DSPP transcripts are not found in osteoblasts within the alveolar crypt (H&E stain, original magnification ×10).

Figs 2-18a to 2-18c Immunoreactive DSPP localized specifically in a rat molar tooth organ. Note the presence of DSPP in both physiologic and reparative dentin matrices.

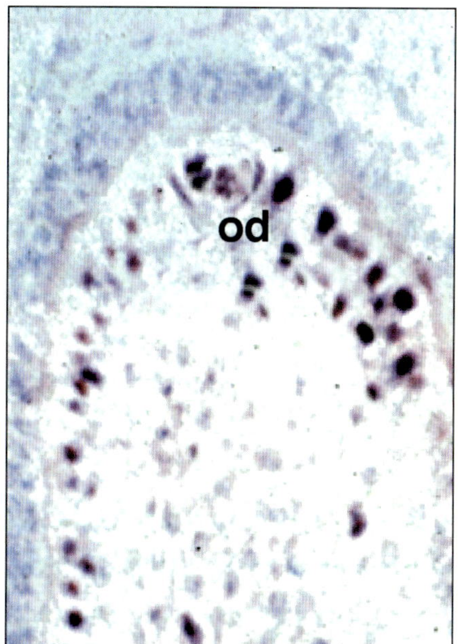

Fig 2-18a DSPP in differentiating odontoblasts (od).

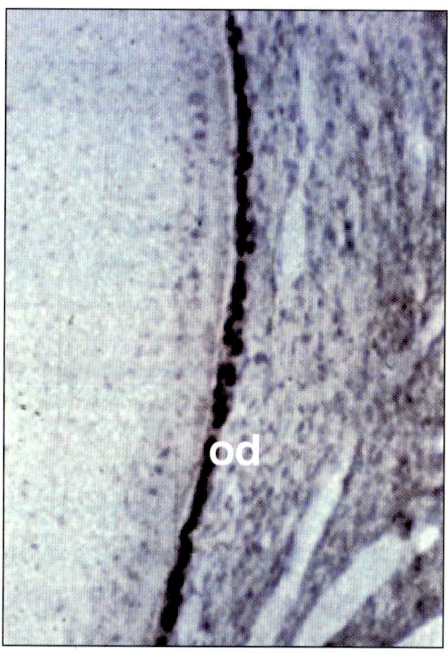

Fig 2-18b DSPP in mature or "resting" odontoblasts (od) lining circumpulpal dentin.

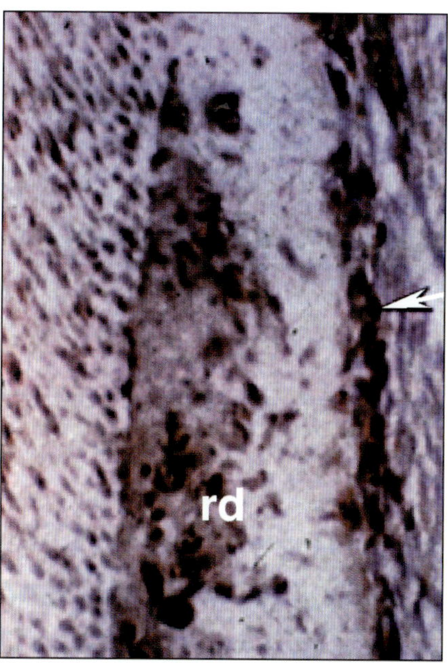

Fig 2-18c DSPP in a replacement population of odontoblasts aligning reparative dentin (rd). *Arrow*, replacement cells.

has a high affinity for type I collagen as well as calcium and is therefore considered a key protein for the initiation of dentin mineralization. Additionally, DPP may also affect the shape and size of apatite crystals.[82] DSP accounts for 5% to 8% of the dentin matrix and has a relatively high sialic acid and carbohydrate content. Because DSP closely resembled osteopontin and bone sialoprotein, researchers assumed that the protein played a role in cell attachment via an RGD sequence. However, further molecular analysis revealed the absence of such a sequence, leaving open questions about the potential role of DSP in dentinogenesis.

For several years it was believed that DSP and DPP were two independent proteins that were encoded by individual genes. Important studies by MacDougall et al[83] provided definitive evidence that the two proteins were specific cleavage products of a larger precursor protein that was translated from one large transcript. The single gene encoding for DSP and DPP was named *dentin sialophosphoprotein* (DSPP). In situ hybridization studies showed the co-localization of DSP and DPP transcripts in newly differentiated and fully functional odontoblasts in developing mouse molars, providing further proof that the two proteins were products of a single gene.[84] Immunolocalization studies using affinity-purified antibodies to DSP demonstrated the presence of the protein throughout the odontoblastic life cycle during primary, secondary (physiologic), and tertiary (reparative) dentinogenesis (Figs 2-18a to 2-18c).

The importance of DSPP in dentin formation was recently underscored with the discovery that mutations in this gene are responsible for the underlying dentinal defects in individuals with DGI.[85,86] Earlier studies had mapped the dentinogenesis imperfecta locus to human chromosome

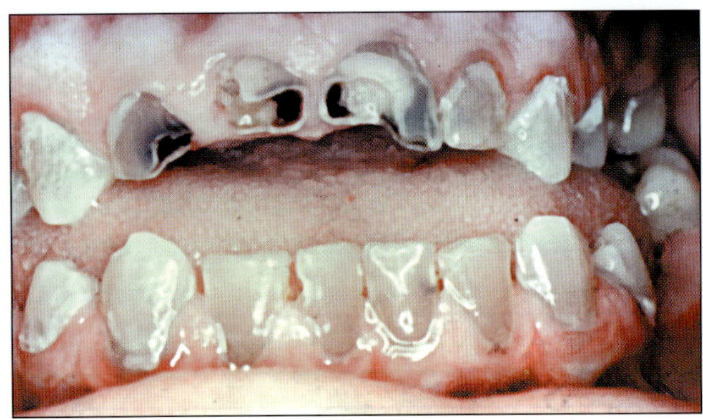

Fig 2-19a Patient afflicted with DGI. Note the discoloration and extensive loss of tooth structure. (Courtesy of Dr Nadarajah Vigneswaran.)

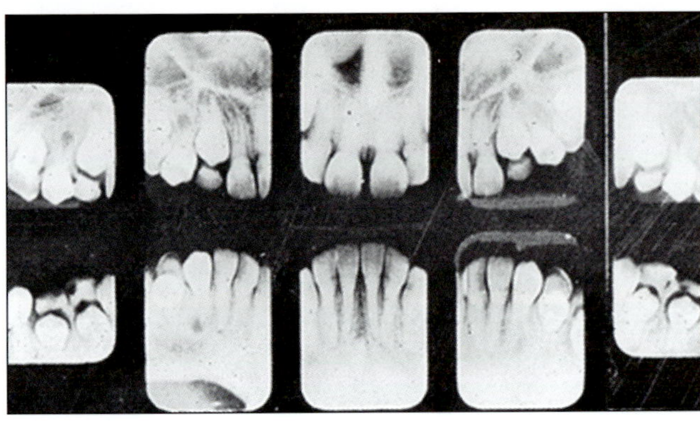

Fig 2-19b Radiograph of the affected teeth, revealing bulbous crowns, obliterated pulp chambers, and narrowed root canals. (Courtesy of Dr Nadarajah Vigneswaran.)

4 within the long arm region q13.21 (Figs 2-19a and 2-19b). Several important dentin ECM molecules, including DSPP, were also mapped to this critical region. Genetic studies of four independent families affected with varying forms of DGI led to the discovery of four different mutations in DSPP. Affected individuals in two of the four families showed a progressive hearing loss that was associated with DGI. Further analysis in mice revealed that DSPP is expressed in inner ear cells. This provides the first evidence that Dspp is not a dentin-specific gene.

A second category of noncollagenous proteins with calcium-binding properties is classified as mineralized tissue–specific, because these proteins are found in all the calcified connective tissues, namely, dentin, bone, and cementum. These include osteocalcin and bone sialoprotein. A serine-rich phosphoprotein, dentin matrix protein 1, whose expression was first described as being restricted to odontoblasts,[87] was later shown to be expressed by osteoblasts and cementoblasts[84] (see Figs 2-17a to 2-17d) and by brain cells.[88]

A third group of noncollagenous proteins that is synthesized by odontoblasts is found in soft connective tissues and organs. These include osteopontin and osteonectin. The fourth category of dentin noncollagenous proteins is not expressed in odontoblasts but is primarily synthesized in the liver and released into the circulation. An example of a serum-borne protein is α2HS glycoprotein. The fifth group of noncollagenous proteins is the various growth factors that appear to be sequestered within dentin matrix. They include the BMPs, insulin-like growth factors, and TGF-βs.

Future Directions in Research

Following the completion of the initial mapping of the human genome (Human Genome Project), it is anticipated that nearly every human disease gene will be identified and isolated. The current postgenomic era will stimulate new research on the nature of proteins and their defects. Gene discoveries will lead to genetic screening and prevention strategies, and it is highly likely that the genetic code for human dentition will be unraveled through the use of reverse genetics.

For pulp biology researchers, this era will undoubtedly provide challenging and exciting opportunities to explore several basic biologic issues that are not well understood. With the help of commercially available DNA microarrays (also referred to as *DNA chips* and *oligonucleotide arrays*) that allow screening of the entire human and mouse genomes, it will soon be possible to catalog the complete genetic and biochemical profile of odontoblasts (Fig 2-20). Through this method, odontoblast-specific and dental pulp-specific determinants during health and disease can be identified. Such knowledge can quickly be extrapolated to studies directed at understanding the nature of cells within the subodontoblastic layer as well as other pulpal cell populations. Furthermore, the underlying mechanisms of pulpitis and the molecular predictors of reversible versus irreversible pulpitis will be explored in depth.

Such new molecular data will be applied to tissue engineering and biomimetic approaches that are geared toward dentin regeneration after injury from caries and operative procedures. Basic science approaches directed toward understanding how key dentin matrix genes are regulated will lead to further studies on the molecules that control the terminal phases of odontoblast differentiation. Identification and isolation of growth factors and transcription factors will encourage the use of a multipronged approach for the treatment of injuries to the pulpodentin complex. This may require the use of genetically engineered mouse models before translational studies are performed on human teeth. Importantly, knowledge of these genes will generate a candidate list of genes whose role in inherited disorders of dentin, in particular the dentin dysplasias, can be analyzed in depth.

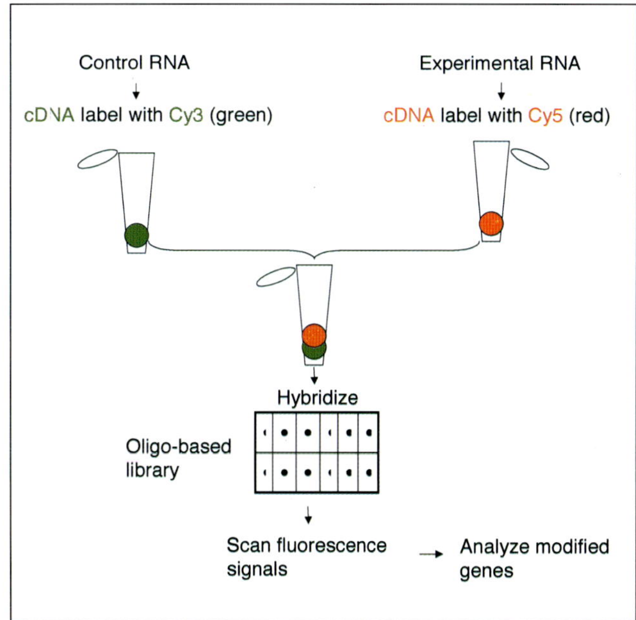

Fig 2-20 Experimental use of microarray technology. This technique is useful for studying differential levels of gene expression during development, disease, and repair. The identification of genes that are either up-regulated or down-regulated helps researchers understand the underlying mechanisms of gene expression.

References

1. Sharpe PT. Homeobox genes and orofacial development. Connect Tissue Res 1995;32:17-25.
2. Maas R, Bei M. The genetic control of early tooth development. Crit Rev Oral Biol Med 1997;8:4-39.
3. Peters H, Balling R. Teeth. Where and how to make them. Trends Genet 1999;15:59-65.
4. Thesleff I, Aberg T. Molecular regulation of tooth development. Bone 1999;25:123-125.
5. Tucker AS, Sharpe PT. Molecular genetics of tooth morphogenesis and patterning: The right shape in the right place. J Dent Res 1999;78:826-834.
6. Jernvall J, Thesleff I. Reiterative signaling and patterning during mammalian tooth morphogenesis. Mech Dev 2000;92:19-29.
7. Wessells NK. Tissue Interactions and Development. Menlo Park, NJ: Benjamin, 1977.
8. Thesleff I, Vaahtokari A, Kettunen P, Aberg T. Epithelial-mesenchymal signaling during tooth development. Connect Tissue Res 1995;32:9-15.
9. Kollar EJ, Baird GR. The influence of the dental papilla on the development of tooth shape in embryonic mouse tooth germs. J Embryol Exp Morphol 1969;21:131-148.
10. Kollar EJ, Baird GR. Tissue interactions in embryonic mouse tooth germs. 1. Reorganization of the dental epithelium during tooth-germ reconstruction. J Embryol Exp Morphol 1970;24:159-171.
11. Ruch JV. Determinisms of odontogenesis. Rev Biol Cellular 1987;14:1-99.
12. Ten Cate AR. Oral Histology: Development, Structure, and Function, ed 5. St Louis: Mosby, 1998.

13. Thesleff I, Sharpe P. Signalling networks regulating dental development. Mech Dev 1997;67:111–123.
14. Mina M, Kollar EJ. The induction of odontogenesis in non-dental mesenchyme combined with early murine mandibular arch epithelium. Arch Oral Biol 1987;32: 123–127.
15. Jernvall J, Kettunen P, Karavanova I, Martin LB, Thesleff I. Evidence for the role of the enamel knot as a control center in mammalian tooth cusp formation: Non-dividing cells express growth stimulating Fgf-4 gene. Int J Dev Biol 1994;38:463–469.
16. Jernvall J, Aberg T, Kettunen P, Keranen S, Thesleff I. The life history of an embryonic signaling center: BMP-4 induces p21 and is associated with apoptosis in the mouse tooth enamel knot. Development 1998;125: 161–169.
17. Pannese E. Observations on the ultrastructure of the enamel organ. 1. Stellate reticulum and stratum intermedium. Ultrastruct Res 1960;4:372.
18. Pannese E. Observations on the ultrastructure of the enamel organ. 2. Involution of the stellate reticulum. Ultrastruct Res 1961;5:328.
19. Pannese E. Observations on the ultrastructure of the enamel organ. 3. Internal and external enamel epithelia. Ultrastruct Res 1962;6:186.
20. Thesleff I, Vaahtokari A. The role of growth factors in determination and differentiation of the odontoblastic cell lineage. Proc Finn Dent Soc 1992;88(suppl 1): 357–368.
21. Szabó G. Studies on the cultivation of teeth in vitro. Anat 1954;88:31–44.
22. Hay MF. The development in vivo and in vitro of the lower incisor and molars of the mouse. Arch Oral Biol 1961;3:86–109.
23. Slavkin H, Bavetta LA. Organogenesis: Prolonged differentiation and growth of tooth primordia on the chick chorio-allantois. Experientia 1968;24:192–194.
24. Thesleff I. Differentiation of odontogenic tissues in organ culture. Scand J Dent Res 1976;84:353–356.
25. Vainio S, Thesleff I. Coordinated induction of cell proliferation and syndecan expression in dental mesenchyme by epithelium: Evidence for diffusible signals. Dev Dyn 1992;194:105–117.
26. Vainio S, Thesleff I. Sequential induction of syndecan, tenascin and cell proliferation associated with mesenchymal cell condensation during early tooth development. Differentiation 1992;50:97–105.
27. Mitsiadis TA, Lardelli M, Lendahl U, Thesleff I. Expression of Notch 1,2 and 3 is regulated by epithelial-mesenchymal interactions and retinoic acid in the developing mouse tooth and associated with determination of ameloblast cell fate. J Cell Biol 1995:130:407–418.
28. Kratochwil K. Tissue combination and organ culture studies in the development of the embryonic mammary gland. Dev Biol 1986;4:315–333.
29. Vainio S, Karavanova I, Jowett A, Thesleff I. Identification of BMP-4 as a signal mediating secondary induction between epithelial and mesenchymal tissues during early tooth development. Cell 1993;75:45–58.
30. Thesleff I, Sahlberg C. Organ culture in the analysis of tissue interactions. Methods Mol Biol 1999;97:23–31.
31. Chen Y, Bei M, Woo I, Satokata I, Maas R. Msx1 controls inductive signaling in mammalian tooth morphogenesis. Development 1996;122:3035–3044.
32. Bei M, Maas R. FGFs and BMP4 induce both Msx1-independent and Msx1-dependent signaling pathways in early tooth development. Development 1998;125: 4325–4333.
33. Bei M, Kratochwil K, Maas RL. BMP4 rescues a non-cell-autonomous function of Msx1 in tooth development. Development 2000;127:4711–4718.
34. Magloire H, Joffre A, Bleicher F. An in vitro model of human dental pulp repair. J Dent Res 1996;75:1971–1978.
35. Melin M, Joffre-Romeas A, Farges JC, Couble MIL, Magloire H, Bleicher F. Effects of TGF-β1 on dental pulp cells in cultured human tooth slices. J Dent Res 2000;79:1689–1696.
36. MacDougall M, Thiemann F, Ta H, Hsu P, Chen LS, Snead MIL. Temperature sensitive simian virus 40 large T antigen immortalization of murine odontoblast cell cultures: Establishment of clonal odontoblast cell line. Connect Tissue Res 1995;33:97–103.
37. Sun ZL, Fang DN, Wu XY, Ritchie HH, Begue-Kim C, Wataha JC, et al. Expression of dentin sialoprotein (DSP) and other molecular determinants by a new cell line from dental papillae, MDPC-23. Connect Tissue Res 1998;37: 251–261.
38. Kasugai S, Adachi M, Ogura H. Establishment and characterization of a clonal cell line (RPC-C2A) from dental pulp of the rat incisor. Arch Oral Biol 1988;33:887–891.
39. Kawase T, Orikasa M, Ogata S, Burns DM. Protein tyrosine phosphorylation induced by epidermal growth factor and insulin-like growth factor-1 in a rat clonal dental pulp-cell line. Arch Oral Biol 1995;40:921–929.
40. Young MF, Xu T. Creating transgenic mice to study skeletal function. In: Cowin S (ed). Bone Biomechanics Handbook. Orlando, FL: CRC Press, 1999.
41. Hogan BL, Horsburgh G, Cohen J, Hetherington CM, Fisher G, Lyon MF. Small eyes (Sey): A homozygous lethal mutation on chromosome 2 which affects the differentiation of both lens and nasal placodes in the mouse. J Embryol Exp Morphol 1986;97:95–110.
42. Niederreither K, D'Souza RN, de Crombrugghe B. Minimal DNA sequences that control the cell lineage-specific expression of the pro alpha 2(1) collagen promoter in transgenic mice. J Cell Biol 1992; 119:1361–1370.
43. Thyagarajan T, Sreenath T, Cho A, Wright JT, Kulkarni AB. Reduced expression of dentin sialophosphoprotein is associated with dysplastic dentin in mice overexpressing TGF-ß1 in teeth. J Biol Chem 2001;276:11016–11020.

44. D'Souza RN, Cavender A, Sood R, Tarnuzzer R, Dickinson DP, Roberts A, Letterio J. TGF-β1 is essential for the homeostasis of the dentin-pulp complex (Proceedings of the 5th International Conference of Tooth Morphogenesis and Differenctiation). Eur J. Oral Sci 1998;106(suppl 1): 185–191.
45. Schutze K, Lahr G. Identification of expressed genes by laser-mediated manipulation of single cells. Nat Biotechnol 1998;16:737–742.
46. Sgroi DC, Teng S, Robinson G, LeVangie R, Hudson JR Jr, Elkahloun AG. In vivo gene expression profile analysis of human breast cancer progression. Cancer Res 1999;59: 5656–5661.
47. DeRisi J, Penland L, Brown PO, Bittner ML, Meltzer PS, Ray M, et al. Use of a cDNA microarray to analyse gene expression patterns in human cancer. Nat Genet 1996; 14:457–460.
48. Thesleff I. Gene expression in tooth [online]. Available at: http://bite-it.helsinki.fi. Accessed January 22, 2002.
49. Kratochwil K, Dull M, Farinas I, Galceran J, Grosschedl R. Lef1 expression is activated by BMP-4 and regulates inductive tissue interactions in tooth and hair development. Genes Dev 1996;10:1382–1394.
50. Neubüser A, Peters H, Balling R, Martin GR. Antagonistic interactions between FGF and BMP signaling pathways: A mechanism for positioning the sites of tooth formation. Cell 1997;90:247–255.
51. Hardcastle Z, Mo R, Hui CC, Sharpe PT. The Shh signalling pathway in tooth development: Defects in Gli2 and Gli3 mutants. Development 1998;125:2803–2811.
52. Satokata I, Maas R. Msx1 deficient mice exhibit cleft palate and abnormalities of craniofacial and tooth development. Nat Genet 1994;6:348–356.
53. Van Genderen C, Okamura RM, Farinas I, Quo RG, Parslow TG, Bruhn L, et al. Development of several organs that require inductive epithelial-mesenchymal interactions is impaired in LEF-1-deficient mice. Genes Dev 1994;8:2691–2703.
54. Peters H, Neubüser A, Balling R. Pax genes and organogenesis: Pax9 meets tooth development. Eur J Oral Sci 1998;106(suppl 1):38–43.
55. Matzuk MM, Kumar TR, Bradley A. Different phenotypes for mice deficient in either activins or activin receptor type II. Nature 1995;374:356–360.
56. Vastardis H, Karimbux N, Guthua SW, Seidman JG, Seidman CE. A human MSX1 homeodomain missense mutation causes selective tooth agenesis. Nat Genet 1996;13: 417–421.
57. Goldenberg M, Das P, Messersmith M, Stockton DW, Patel PI, D'Souza RN. Clinical, radiographic, and genetic evaluation of a novel form of autosomal-dominant oligodontia. J Dent Res 2000;79:1469–1475.
58. Stockton DW, Das P, Goldenberg M, D'Souza RN, Patel PI. Mutation of PAX9 is associated with oligodontia. Nat Genet 2000;24:18–19.
59. Komori T, Yagi H, Nomura S, et al. Targeted disruption of Cbfa1 results in a complete lack of bone formation owing to maturational arrest of osteoblasts. Cell 1997;89: 755–764.
60. Otto F, Thornell AP, Crompton T, et al. Cbfa1, a candidate gene for cleidocranial dysplasia syndrome, is essential for osteoblast differentiation and bone development. Cell 1997;89:765–771.
61. Mundlos S, Otto F, Mundlos C, et al. Mutations involving the transcription factor CBFA1 cause cleidocranial dysplasia. Cell 1997;89:773–779.
62. D'Souza RN, Aberg T, Gaikwad J, Cavender A, Owen M, Karsenty G, et al. Cbfa1 is required for epithelial-mesenchymal interactions regulating tooth development in mice. Development 1999;126:2911–2920.
63. Vaahtokari A, Aberg T, Jernvall J, Keranen S, Thesleff I. The enamel knot as a signaling center in the developing mouse tooth. Mech Dev 1996;54:39–43.
64. Thesleff I, Jernvall J. The enamel knot: A putative signaling center regulating tooth development. Cold Spring Harb Symp Quant Biol 1997;62:257–267.
65. Vaahtokari A, Aberg T, Thesleff I. Apoptosis in the developing tooth: Association with an embryonic signaling center and suppression by EGF and FGF-4. Development 1996;122:121–129.
66. Kettunen P, Thesleff I. Expression and function of FGFs-4, -8, and -9 suggest functional redundancy and repetitive use as epithelial signals during tooth morphogenesis. Dev Dyn 1998;211:256–268.
67. Niswander L, Martin GR. Fgf-4 expression during gastrulation, myogenesis, limb and tooth development in the mouse. Development 1992;114:755–768.
68. Witty JP, Wright JH, Matrisian LM. Matrix metalloproteinases are expressed during ductal and alveolar mammary morphogenesis, and misregulation of stromelysin-1 in transgenic mice induces unscheduled alveolar development. Mol Biol Cell 1995;6:1287–1303.
69. Chin JR, Werb Z. Matrix metalloproteinases regulate morphogenesis, migration and remodeling of epithelium, tongue skeletal muscle and cartilage in the mandibular arch. Development 1997;124:1519–1530.
70. Hurmerinta K, Thesleff I, Saxen L. Inhibition of tooth germ differentiation in vitro by diazo-oxo-norleucine (DON). J Embryol Exp Morphol 1979;50:99–109.
71. Thesleff I, Pratt RM. Tunicamycin-induced alterations in basement membrane formation during odontoblast differentiation. Dev Biol 1980;80:175–185.
72. Lesot H, von der MK, Ruch JV. Immunofluorescent localization of the types of collagen synthesized in the embryonic mouse tooth germ. C R Acad Sci Hebd Seances Acad Sci D 1978;286:765–768.
73. Thesleff I, Stenman S, Vaheri A, Timpl R. Changes in the matrix proteins, fibronectin and collagen, during differentiation of mouse tooth germ. Dev Biol 1979;70: 116–126.

74. Reponen P, Sahlberg C, Huhtala P, Hurskainen T, Thesleff I, Tryggvason K. Molecular cloning of murine 72-kDa type IV collagenase and its expression during mouse development. J Biol Chem 1992;267:7856–7862.
75. Werb Z. ECM and cell surface proteolysis: Regulating cellular ecology. Cell 1997;91:439–442.
76. Sahlberg C, Reponen P, Tryggvason K, Thesleff I. Association between the expression of murine 72 kDa type IV collagenase by odontoblasts and basement membrane degradation during mouse tooth development. Arch Oral Biol 1992;37:1021–1030.
77. Thesleff I, Pratt RM. Tunicamycin inhibits mouse tooth morphogenesis and odontoblast differentiation in vitro. J Embryol Exp Morphol 1980;58:195–208.
78. Butler WT, Bhown M, Brunn JC, et al. Isolation, characterization and immunolocalization of a 53-kDal dentin sialoprotein (DSP). Matrix 1992;12:343–351.
79. Butler WT. Dentin matrix proteins and dentinogenesis. Connect Tissue Res 1995;33:59–65.
80. Linde A, Goldberg M. Dentinogenesis. Crit Rev Oral Biol Med 1993;4:679–728.
81. Butler WT, Ritchie H. The nature and functional significance of dentin extracellular matrix proteins. Int J Dev Biol 1995;39:169–179.
82. Fujisawa R, Kuboki Y. Preferential adsorption of dentin and bone acidic proteins on the (100) face of hydroxyapatite crystals. Biochim Biophys Acta 1991;1075(1):56–60.
83. MacDougall M, Simmons D, Luan X, Nydegger J, Feng J, Gu TT. Dentin phosphoprotein and dentin sialoprotein are cleavage products expressed from a single transcript coded by a gene on human chromosome 4. Dentin phosphoprotein DNA sequence determination. J Biol Chem 1997;272:835–842.
84. D'Souza RN, Cavender A, Sunavala G, Alvarez J, Ohshima T, Kulkarni AB, et al. Gene expression patterns of murine dentin matrix protein 1 (Dmp1) and dentin sialophosphoprotein (DSPP) suggest distinct developmental functions in vivo. J Bone Miner Res 1997;12:2040–2049.
85. Zhang X, Zhao J, Li C, et al. DSPP mutation in dentinogenesis imperfecta Shields type II. Nat Genet 2001;27:151–152.
86. Xiao S, Yu C, Chou X, et al. Dentinogenesis imperfecta 1 with or without progressive hearing loss is associated with distinct mutations in DSPP. Nat Genet 2001;27:201–204.
87. George A, Sabsay B, Simonian PA, Veis A. Characterization of a novel dentin matrix acidic phosphoprotein. Implications for induction of biomineralization. J Biol Chem 1993;268:12624–12630.
88. Hirst KL, Simmons D, Feng J, Aplin H, Dixon MJ, MacDougall M. Elucidation of the sequence and the genomic organization of the human dentin matrix acidic phosphoprotein 1 (DMP1) gene: Exclusion of the locus from a causative role in the pathogenesis of dentinogenesis imperfecta type II. Genomics 1997;42:38–45.

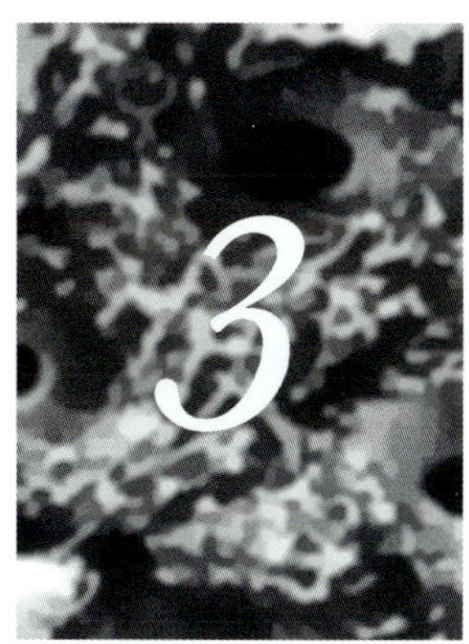

3 Dentin Formation and Repair

Anthony J. Smith, BSc, PhD

Classification of the orthodentin of mammals as primary, secondary, or tertiary[1] has provided a basis for understanding how dentin forms over the course of a lifetime (Fig 3-1). *Primary dentin* is the regular tubular dentin formed prior to eruption and completion of the apical region of the tooth, including the first formed mantle dentin. *Secondary dentin* is the regular circumpulpal orthodentin formed (in tubular continuity with the primary dentin) at a slower rate throughout the remaining life of the tooth. *Tertiary dentin* represents the more or less irregular dentin formed focally in response to noxious stimuli such as tooth wear, dental caries, cavity preparation, and restorative procedures. This category has been proposed to encompass a range of sometimes confusing terms, including *irregular secondary dentin*, *irritation dentin*, *reparative dentin*, *irregular dentin*, *reaction dentin*, *replacement dentin*, *defense dentin*, etc. Primary and secondary dentin, including mantle dentin, are the exclusive secretory products of the tightly packed layer of primary odontoblasts found on the formative surface of the tissue. Barring injury, these postmitotic cells generally survive for the life of the tooth and provide both vitality to the tissue and the ability to respond to a wide variety of environmental stimuli. An appreciation of odontoblast behavior throughout life is critical to our understanding of dentin formation.

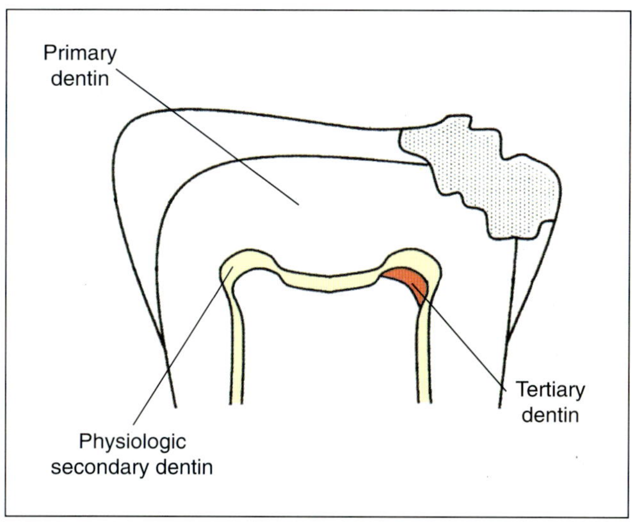

Fig 3-1 Schematic diagram of the locations of primary, physiologic secondary, and tertiary dentin in the human tooth.

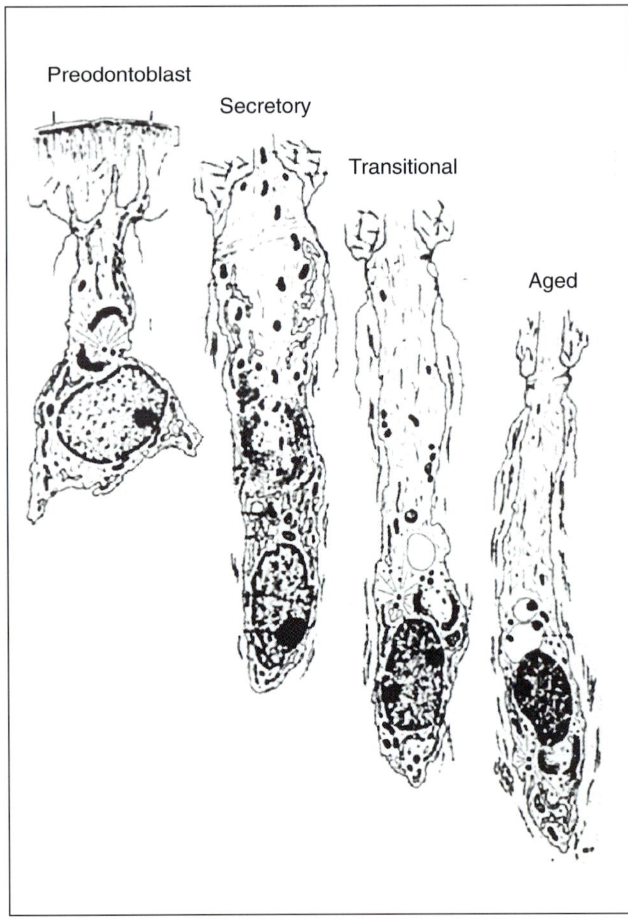

Fig 3-2 Diagram of the ultrastructural appearance of the human odontoblast throughout its life cycle. (Reprinted from Couve[4] with permission.)

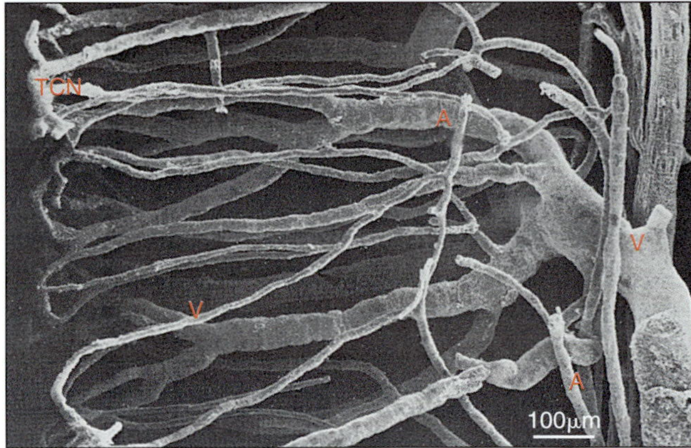

Fig 3-3 Resin cast of the subodontoblastic capillary plexus in a dog pulp: TCN, terminal capillary network beneath the dentin; A, terminal arteriole; V, venule. (Reprinted from Takahashi et al[14] with permission.)

Odontoblasts and Dentinogenesis

Odontoblasts and their relationship to the pulp

The traditional understanding of the morphology of the odontoblast is that of a tall, columnar secretory cell with a polarized, basal nucleus and a single cytoplasmic process. Although this concept holds true during active dentinogenesis, it is now clear that an odontoblast varies throughout its life cycle both in size and in content of cytoplasmic organelles, and that these changes are closely related to its functional activity (Fig 3-2).[2–5] The relationship between size and secretory activity of the cells is borne out by the differences in size between odontoblasts in the crown and those in the root of the tooth,[6] which may be related to the varying rate of dentinogenesis in these two areas of the tooth.

The phenotype of the odontoblast is defined both by its morphology and by its polarized secretion of a specific set of molecules[7] leading to deposition of a mineralizable matrix that has a regular tubular structure within which the odontoblast processes lie. These features may be important in considering the specificity of any repair responses seen after injury to the tooth.

However, the odontoblast cannot exist alone and requires the presence of other pulpal elements to survive and function. Attempts to culture odontoblasts in isolation have met with little success; organ cultures involving the entire dentin-pulp complex have been required for maintenance of their growth in vitro,[8,9] although immortalized pulp cell lines with odontoblast-like cell characteristics have been established.[10,11] The cell-rich layer of Höhl underlying the odontoblast layer shows some unique phenotypic characteristics in terms of cellular morphology[12] and may function to support odontoblast activity, being most conspicuous in the crown of the tooth during active dentinogenesis. During the last cell division of the pre-odontoblast prior to terminal differentiation, one of the daughter cells is positioned adjacent to the dental basement membrane and receives the inductive signal to differentiate to an odontoblast, while the other does not and may contribute to the cell-rich layer of Höhl. These cells may contribute to the progenitor cell population for odontoblast-like cell differentiation during tertiary dentinogenesis. Associated with this cell-rich layer is a rich capillary plexus that probably plays a key role in the transport of nutrients for secretion of the mineralized organic matrix during active dentinogenesis. Correlation of the blood supply of the developing tooth with the extent of mineralization[13] has demonstrated the intimate relationship between angiogenesis and dentinogenesis. The extensive vascular network in the coronal part of the pulp has been elegantly demonstrated in resin casts (Fig 3-3).[14] The importance of an adequate vascular supply to the odontoblasts for dentinogenesis is also highlighted during tertiary dentinogenesis when successful outcomes of the repair process generally require angiogenic activity at the injury site.

Secretory behavior of odontoblasts

The cytologic features of the active odontoblast have been well described[15] and reflect those of a secretory cell. Such features include a basal nucleus with parallel stacks of rough endoplasmic reticulum aligned parallel to the length of the cell, both on the apical side of the nucleus and at the apical end of the cell on either side of the prominent Golgi apparatus. The saccules are more distended on the mature aspect of the apparatus, and secretory granules, which are also found in apical areas of the cell and in the odontoblast process, are seen in the nearby cytoplasm. These sites are probably associated with exocytosis of the secretory granules. The terminal web, comprising transverse microfibrils, morphologically separates the cell body from the process, which has fewer cytologic features reflecting its secretory role.[16]

Use of radiolabeled proline and autoradiography has shown that the pathway of collagen synthesis and secretion is typical of most connective tissue cells. The radiolabel first appeared in the rough endoplasmic reticulum, then in the Golgi apparatus, and finally in the presecretory and secretory granules.[17,18] Label appeared in the predentin within 4 hours in the rat, presumably by exocytosis, but was not seen in the dentin until nearly a day after pulse-labeling. Similar pathways are responsible for secretion of the other matrix components of dentin, including phosphoproteins, glycoproteins, and proteoglycans, although these demonstrate much more rapid incorporation on the order of minutes rather than days.[19,20] This highlights possible differences in the control of secretion of the various components of dentin matrix, although much more needs to be learned about the control of odontoblast secretion.

The concept of two levels of secretion from the odontoblast has been proposed by Linde.[21] The major level of secretion is envisioned as being at the proximal end of the odontoblast cell body to form a matrix comprising collagen and proteoglycans, which reaches the advancing mineralization front after approximately 24 hours. The second, distal level of secretion is anticipated as being close to the mineralization front, where various tissue-specific noncollagenous matrix components, including phosphoproteins, are secreted (Fig 3-4). The latter components have been implicated in the mineralization process as nucleators for hydroxyapatite crystal formation,[22] and their secretion at this site could explain the mineralization of the collagenous predentin after a certain interval of time. Furthermore, this model might also explain the formation of peritubular dentin at this site, with its collagen-poor and noncollagenous rich matrix. Although very attractive, this model of dentin secretion should be recognized as merely hypothetical.

Complex matrix remodeling occurs during the transition of the matrix from predentin to

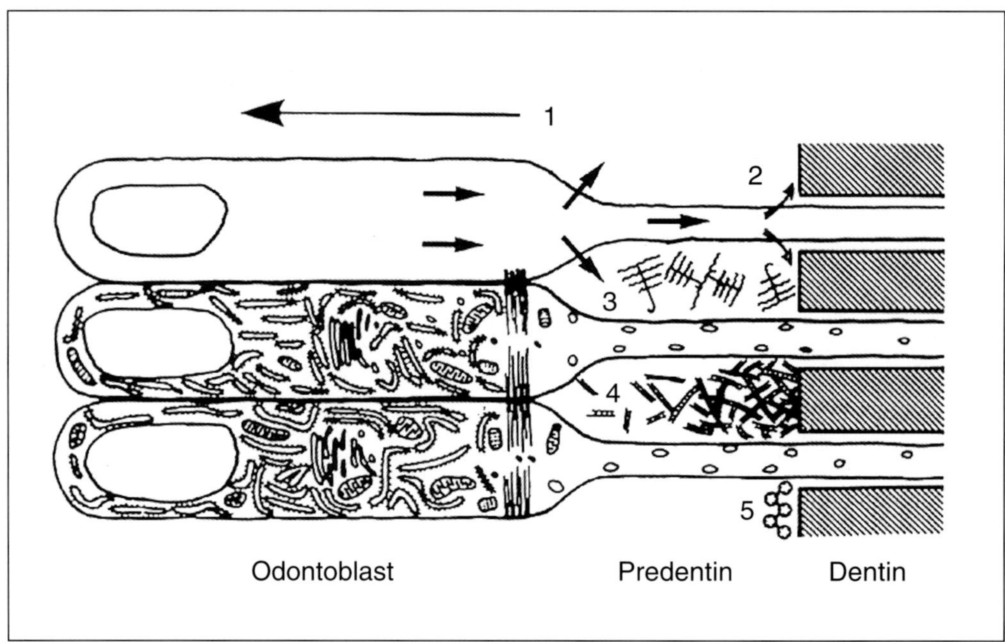

Fig 3-4 Schematic diagram of dentinogenically active odontoblasts with two proposed levels of secretion. Secretion of collagen (1) and proteoglycan (3) occurs at the proximal level and accumulates in the predentin (4), while secretion of noncollagenous components, including phosphoprotein, γ-carboxyglutamate–containing protein, and proteoglycan (5) occurs at the distal level (2) just prior to the mineralization front. (Reprinted from Linde[21] with permission.)

dentin, particularly in the proteoglycans. The matrix metalloproteinases (MMPs) are a complex family of matrix-degrading enzymes, and their expression by odontoblasts[23,24] and presence near the mineralization front is likely to be associated with the matrix remodeling taking place there. The involvement of this family of enzymes in dentinogenesis, which is just starting to be unraveled, should clarify our understanding of the maturation changes in the matrix during secretion and the mechanisms of mineralization.

Dentin has traditionally been regarded as a relatively inert tissue that does not undergo tissue remodeling to the same degree as is seen in bone. However, there is some ultrastructural evidence to indicate that limited endocytosis by the odontoblast does occur,[25] although the functional significance of this is still unclear. Nevertheless, what is clear is that the odontoblast maintains communication with deeper areas of the matrix through its process, which lies in the dentinal tubule. Numerous lateral branches from the processes permeating the dentin matrix can be observed (Fig 3-5), and these may connect with lateral branches of other odontoblasts. This level of communication between the cell and its matrix suggests that dentin may not be as inert as traditionally believed. The s-shaped primary curvature of the dentinal tubules in the crown of the tooth (Fig 3-6) is an effect of the crowding of odontoblasts as they move toward the center of the pulp. The result is a greater tubular density nearer to the pulp, but it also has consequences for the pulp region itself, which directly communicates with the outer surface of the dentin.

The mineralization of dentin requires the transfer of considerable quantities of mineral ions from the serum to the extracellular sites, where they are deposited as hydroxyapatite crystals. The subodontoblastic capillary plexus is well located for this transfer, although the transport of ions and the necessary regulation have to be addressed.

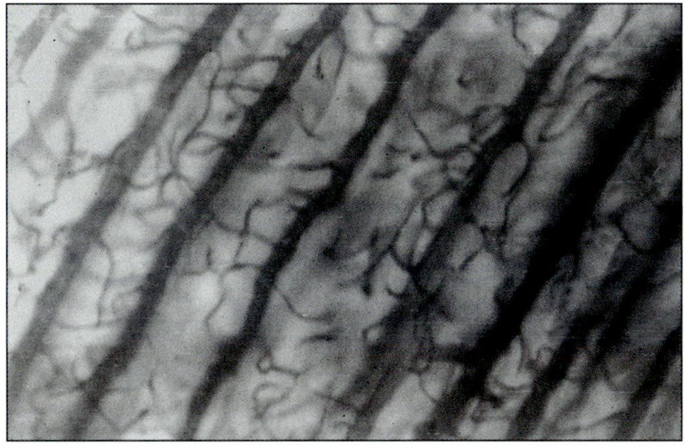

Fig 3-5 Odontoblast processes in human dentin with numerous lateral branches (original magnification ×2,000).

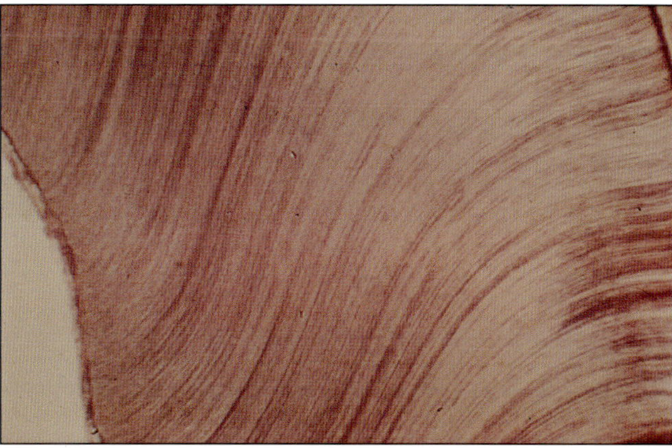

Fig 3-6 S-shaped primary curvature of the dentinal tubules in human crown dentin (H&E stain, original magnification ×80).

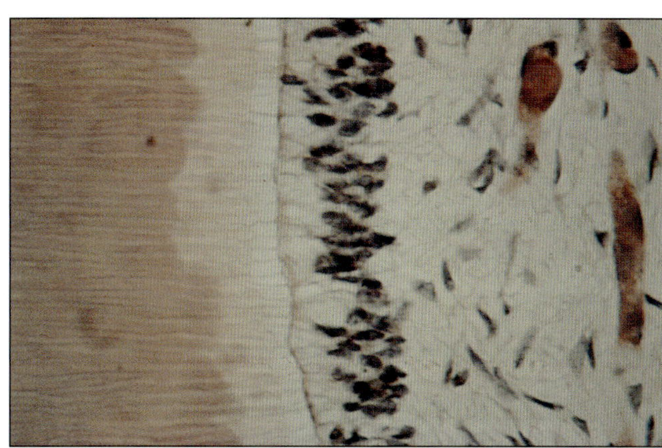

Fig 3-7 Globular appearance of the mineralization front in dentin arising from fusion of globules of hydroxyapatite or calcospherites (H&E stain, original magnification ×400).

While the odontoblast layer represents a relatively impermeable barrier, Nagai and Frank[26] found some evidence to suggest that calcium passes through the interodontoblastic space as well as through the odontoblast, accumulating in the Golgi apparatus and mitochondria but not in secretory vacuoles. High concentrations of calcium at the distal secretory pole of odontoblasts have been demonstrated by electron probe analysis,[27] supporting the concept of the latter route of calcium transport. A calcium transport system in which ions become associated with matrix components as they are synthesized and secreted could have energetic advantages for the cell as well as providing a means of regulation. However, a central role for the odontoblasts, in which calcium ions are transported through the cells themselves by different transmembranous ion-transporting mechanisms, has become apparent.[28] The possible nucleation of hydroxyapatite crystals on components of the organic matrix of dentin has long been suggested. The anionic nature of many of the matrix components has led to their implication in such a role,[22] but in vivo data implicating any single component are lacking. It is generally accepted that heterogeneous nucleation on organic matrix components is responsible for mineralization of circumpulpal dentin after mantle dentin formation and that the globular appearance of the mineralization front arises from the fusion of calcospherites (Fig 3-7). During mantle dentin formation at the initiation of dentinogenesis, mineralization is achieved through the mediation of matrix vesicles.[29] These are small mem-

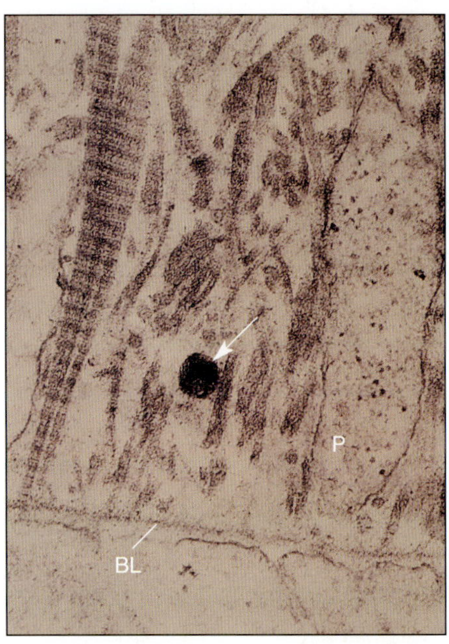

Fig 3-8 Matrix vesicle (*arrow*) adjacent to an odontoblast process (P) and beside the dental basement membrane (BL) in the early mantle dentin matrix. Large, coarse fibrils of collagen showing a typical striated appearance can be observed perpendicular to the basement membrane. (Reprinted from Eisenmann and Glick[29] with permission.)

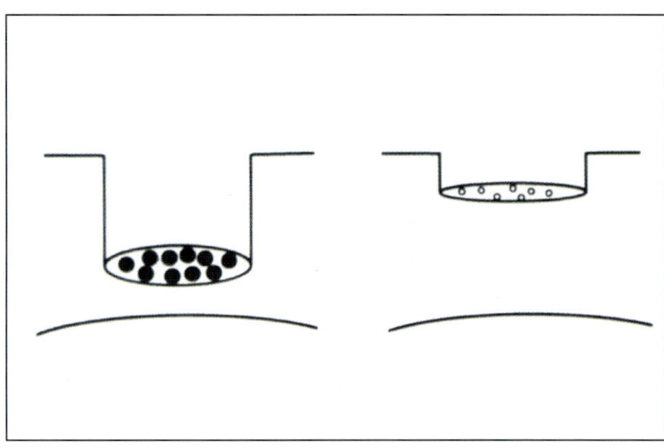

Fig 3-9 Schematic diagram of the differences in tubular density of the floor of a shallow *(right)* and deep *(left)* cavity prepared in dentin.

brane-bound vesicles rich in adenosine triphosphatase (ATPase) and phosphohydrolytic enzymes that arise by budding off from the odontoblast. The matrix vesicles are capable of concentrating mineral ions to overcome the solubility product to allow calcium phosphate crystal precipitation. These vesicles are present in the earliest mantle dentin matrix, adjacent to the large coarse fibrils of collagen lying perpendicular to the site of the dental basement membrane (Fig 3-8), but they are absent from the matrix subsequent to mantle dentin formation. The need for an alternative mechanism of mineralization during mantle dentin formation may relate to the fact that odontoblasts are still completing their terminal differentiation at this stage and may not be able to fully exhibit the odontoblast phenotype in terms of expression of dentin-specific matrix components. However, as soon as mantle dentin formation is completed and the odontoblasts are seen as a discrete, tightly packed layer of cells, mineralization proceeds in association with the extracellular matrix, and matrix vesicles can no longer be observed.

Primary Dentinogenesis

When mantle dentin formation is completed and the odontoblasts eliminate the extracellular compartment between them to form a tightly packed layer of cells, the matrix of dentin is produced exclusively by the odontoblasts. Elaboration of this matrix involves secretion of collagen fibrils that are smaller in dimension than are those in mantle dentin and associated noncollagenous organic matrix or ground substance. The odontoblasts lie on the formative surface of this matrix and move pulpally as the matrix is secreted, leaving a single cytoplasmic process embedded within a dentinal tubule in the matrix. These tubules, which increase in density nearer to the pulp, con-

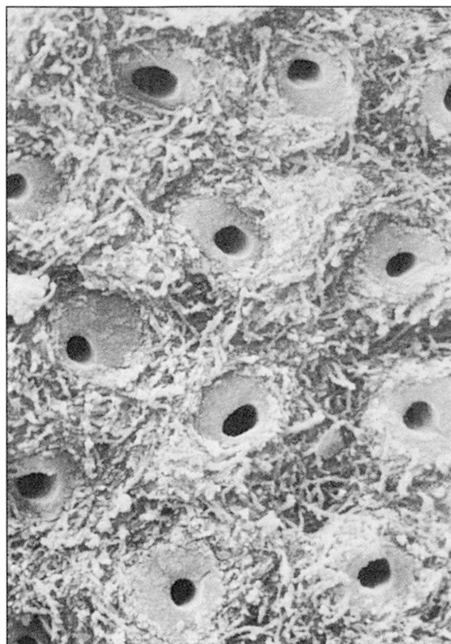

Fig 3-10 Scanning electron micrographic appearance of dentin showing the dentinal tubules cut in cross-section, each with a surrounding collar of peritubular dentin matrix, which has a homogeneous nonfibrillar appearance. The fibrillar, collagenous matrix of the intertubular dentin contrasts in appearance and composition with the peritubular dentin. (Reprinted from Scott et al[77] with permission.)

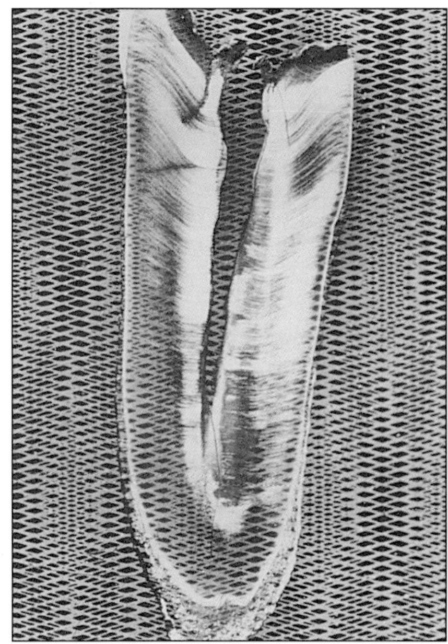

Fig 3-11 Apical sclerotic dentin in a ground section of an old tooth, the translucent appearance of which allows visualization of the mesh pattern underlying it. (Reprinted from Ten Cate[78] with permission.)

fer the property of permeability on the dentin. The gradient of tubular density as the dentin is traversed (Fig 3-9) has clinical implications related to the depth of cavity preparation and tissue permeability.[30] This intertubular dentin matrix comprises the bulk of the circumpulpal dentin. As this matrix forms, a matrix with a rather different composition, known as the peritubular dentin matrix, is secreted around the tubule perimeter. Peritubular dentin is more highly mineralized than the intertubular dentin matrix, contains few collagen fibrils, and is rich in noncollagenous matrix components (Fig 3-10). Its continued deposition throughout primary dentinogenesis leads to regional differences in its thickness through the dentin matrix. The dentinal tubules are tapered structures because of peritubular dentin formation, and they vary in diameter from approximately 2.5 μm near the pulp to 0.9 μm near the amelodentinal junction. Complete occlusion of dentinal tubules can be observed. The translucent appearance of areas of matrix containing such tubules has been described as sclerotic dentin, which appears to be age-related and shows a preferential distribution in the apical third of the root, the crown midway between the pulpal and outer surface of the tooth, and on the pulpal surface of the dentin (Fig 3-11). The derivation of this sclerotic dentin may be varied. Its presence in root dentin of adolescent premolars in the absence of any external influence is suggestive of a physiologic response involving continued secretion of peritubular dentin. However, it might also arise from deposition of mineral within the tubule in the absence of peritubular dentin formation, from diffuse calcification within a viable process or from calcification of both the process and the tubular contents.[7] Whatever the derivation, the presence of sclerosis will reduce the permeability of dentin and has obvious clinical significance in terms of dentinal sensitivity and the potential transport of irritants along the tubules.

The secretion of dentin occurs rhythmically, showing alternate phases of activity and quiescence, and this leads to formation of incremental growth lines in dentin perpendicular to the dentinal tubules. Both a daily and a 5-day rhythmic pattern of incremental lines, the latter showing a 20-μm periodicity, can be observed in dentin, though there has been confusion over the nomenclature associated with these lines. Control of this rhythmic dentin deposition has been suggested to be associated with the circadian rhythmic activity of peripheral adrenergic neurons that produce variations in blood flow to the odontoblasts.[31] However, this explanation does not correspond with the different periodicity observed for these lines in the crown and root of the tooth. The rate of dentin deposition is slower in the root than in the crown, and yet circadian rhythms are likely to influence cell secretion similarly in both areas.

This raises a critical question: what are the mechanisms controlling odontoblast secretion? Odontoblast secretion proceeds rapidly throughout primary dentin formation (with differences in rate between the crown and root of the tooth) with a clear blueprint for both the crown and the root. Once these parts of the tooth have been completed, the rate of secretion abruptly decreases. Such control will also be fundamental to our understanding of the factors controlling tertiary dentin secretion during repair after injury to the pulpodentin complex. The control mechanisms for physiologic dentin secretion remain elusive, but various growth factors, hormones, and transcription factors have been implicated in the regulation of odontoblast secretory activity (reviewed by Smith and Lesot[32]). Identification of various growth factors, particularly the transforming growth factor-β (TGF-β) family, and of signal transduction pathways provides some clues as to how odontoblast secretion may be regulated. Both paracrine and autocrine control of expression of these growth factors may have a strong regulatory effect on odontoblast secretion. Although such signaling molecules may be capable of regulating odontoblast secretion, it is unclear what determines their control to up- and down-regulate specific phases of dentinogenesis. Modulation of their activity by extracellular matrix (ECM) molecules[33] perhaps indicates a "chicken and egg" situation whereby growth factors can influence ECM secretion and ECM molecules in turn modulate growth factor activity. Transcriptional control of growth factor expression may also provide a key mode of regulation. Some form of pre-programming of odontoblasts to regulate their secretory activity cannot be excluded. Programming is a feature of cell death or apoptosis, and it appears to occur to some extent in odontoblasts,[34] though to a lesser degree than in most tissues. However, the ability to up-regulate odontoblast secretion during tertiary dentinogenesis suggests that for the majority of the primary odontoblast population, local cellular signaling mechanisms can override any pre-programming of cellular secretory activity. Clearly, the physiologic regulation of odontoblast secretion will provide many challenges to researchers and will represent a key topic of study for the future.

Physiologic Secondary Dentinogenesis

Physiologic secondary dentinogenesis represents the slower-paced deposition of dentin matrix that continues after completion of the crown and root of the tooth and spans a lifetime (see Fig 3-1). While secondary dentin is deposited all around the periphery of the tooth, its distribution is asymmetric, with greater amounts on the floor and roof of the pulp chamber. This leads to pulp recession, the extent of which will depend on the age of the individual. Thus, secondary dentinogenesis may potentially increase the difficulty of endodontic procedures. Historically, there has been considerable confusion over what constitutes physiologic secondary dentin and use of the term *secondary dentin* to describe tertiary dentin formed in response to an external influence. Differences between the composition of glycosaminoglycans and that of other glycoconjugates for secondary dentin have been reported on the basis of histochemical stains,[35] although it is unclear whether these differences can be ascribed to true physiologic secondary dentin.

The tubules of the secondary dentin matrix are largely continuous with those of the primary dentin, suggesting that the same odontoblasts are responsible for primary and secondary dentin secretion. However, down-regulation of the secretory activity of these cells means that secondary dentin is deposited relatively slowly. The wide-ranging rates (from less than 1 to 16 μm per day) of secondary dentin deposition that have been reported perhaps reflect in part the unclear identification of secondary and tertiary dentins. However, early studies from Hoffman and Schour[36] in the rat molar provide insight into both the dynamics and the gradients of secondary dentin secretion. In the pulp horns, a daily rate of 16 μm observed at 35 to 45 days had declined to 1.25 μm per day at 500 days. On the roof and floor of the pulp cavity, the rate was 2.5 μm per day at 125 to 135 days and declined to 0.69 μm at 500 days. Thus, the rate of formation varies in different areas of the tooth and appears to slow with age to a rate of only about 8% to 25% of that observed at a younger age. However, if the greater rate of secretion in the pulp horns reflects a response to attrition, at least in part, then some of this secretion represents strictly tertiary dentinogenesis. This highlights the need to use terminology describing the different phases of dentinogenesis only as a means of understanding the processes taking place and not as an inflexible classification system.

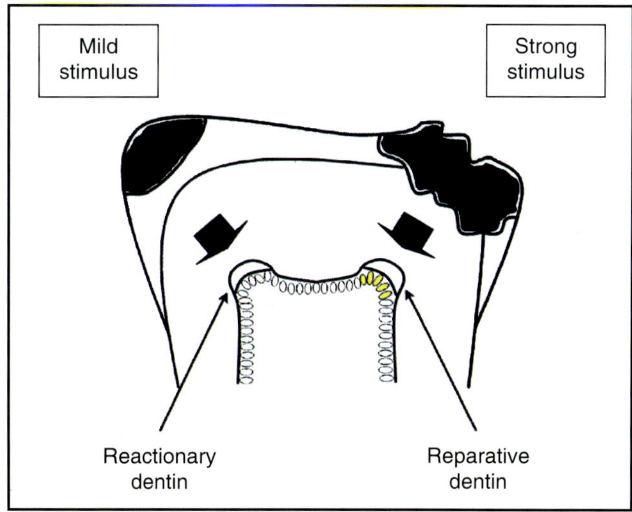

Fig 3-12 Schematic diagram of reactionary (secreted by surviving postmitotic primary odontoblasts) and reparative (secreted by a new generation of odontoblast-like cells after death of the primary odontoblasts) variants of tertiary dentinogenesis. (Reprinted from Smith et al[38] with permission.)

Tertiary Dentinogenesis

To overcome the plethora of confusing terms used to describe the focal secretion of dentin in response to external influences—including such as dental caries, tooth wear, trauma, and other tissue injury—Kuttler[1] proposed the concept of tertiary dentin formation. Tertiary dentin encompasses a broad spectrum of responses, ranging from secretion of a regular, tubular matrix that differs little from primary and secondary dentins, to secretion of a very dysplastic matrix that may even be atubular. The cellular and molecular processes responsible for this spectrum of responses also may show a number of differences. Tertiary dentin has been subclassified as either *reactionary* or *reparative*[37,38] as a means of distinguishing the different sequences of biologic events taking place in situations of milder and stronger external stimuli responsible for initiation of the response (Fig 3-12).

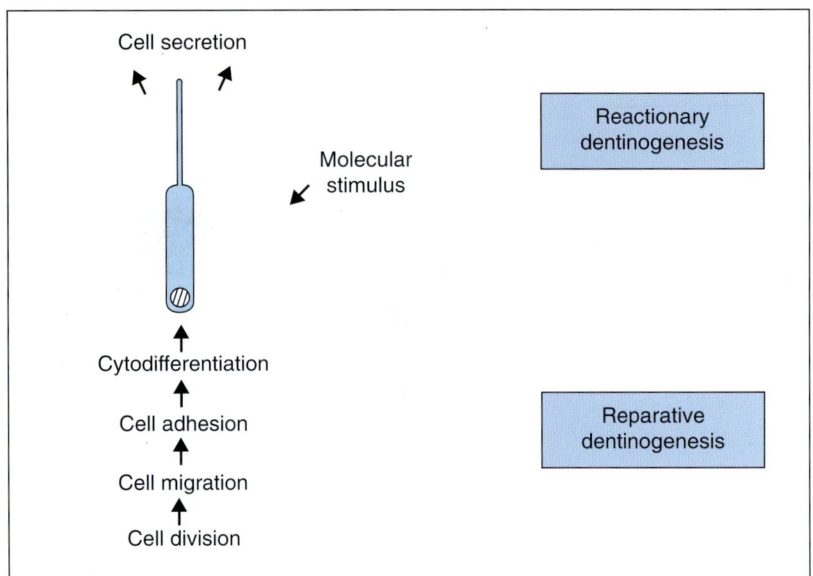

Fig 3-13 Schematic diagram of biologic processes taking place during reactionary and reparative dentinogenesis. (Reprinted from Smith et al[38] with permission.)

Reactionary dentin is defined as a tertiary dentin matrix secreted by surviving postmitotic odontoblast cells in response to an appropriate stimulus. Typically, such a response will be made to milder stimuli and represents up-regulation of the secretory activity of the existing odontoblast responsible for primary dentin secretion. In contrast, *reparative dentin* is defined as a tertiary dentin matrix secreted by a new generation of odontoblast-like cells in response to an appropriate stimulus after the death of the original postmitotic odontoblasts responsible for primary and physiologic secondary dentin secretion. Such a response will normally be made to stronger stimuli and represents a much more complex sequence of biologic processes. Reparative dentin actually encompasses a broad range of responses, some of which appear to be relatively specific while others are classified as tertiary dentinogenesis only because they occur in the pulpodentin complex.

It is appropriate to consider these two variants of tertiary dentinogenesis individually in view of the diversity of the biologic processes taking place (Fig 3-13), although it must be recognized that reparative dentinogenesis will often be a sequel to reactionary dentinogenesis and that both variants may be observed within the same lesion.

Reactionary dentinogenesis

Reactionary dentin is, by definition, secreted by surviving primary odontoblasts. Therefore, to determine cell survival, its identification requires chronologic information on the postinjury events within the pulpodentin complex. While such information is often lacking in histologic studies of pulpal responses following dental injury, the presence of tubular continuity between physiologic secondary and tertiary dentin matrices has been suggested as characteristic of this response.[39]

The biologic processes responsible for reactionary dentinogenesis represent focal up-regulation of the secretory activity of the surviving odontoblasts. As such, this response might be considered an extension of the physiologic behavior of these odontoblasts, and the rationale for identification of a tertiary dentinogenic response would be the nature of the initiating stimulus, ie, injury to the tissues. This distinction is probably important in that control of up-regulation of secretion is determined by the stimulus and may show differences to physiologic regulation of cell secretory behavior. The intensity of the response will reflect both the degree and the duration of the stimulus, although the extent of the response is limited to those cells in direct tubular communication with the initiating stimulus. Thus, beneath a cavity preparation, the reactionary dentinogenic response is generally limited to those areas where the dentinal tubules communicate with the cavity. In unetched preparations, variable plugging of the tubules may lead to differential stimulation of individual odontoblasts beneath the preparation and an irregular interface between the reactionary dentin and odontoblasts, possibly with finger-like projections of matrix (Fig 3-14).

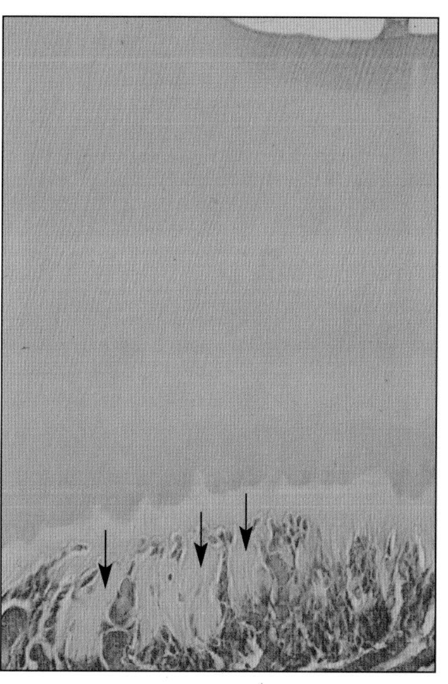

Fig 3-14 Reactionary dentinogenic response beneath an unetched and unexposed cavity *(top)* prepared in a ferret canine tooth in which a lyophilized preparation of isolated dentin matrix proteins have been implanted. Reactionary dentin secretion is restricted to that area in which the dentinal tubules are in direct communication with the cavity. Note the finger-like projections of reactionary dentin matrix *(arrows)* due to differential stimulation of individual odontoblasts beneath the preparation.

The molecular basis of odontoblast up-regulation during reactionary dentinogenesis has only recently received much attention. Traditionally, it has been suggested that "irritation" from plaque bacterial products during caries or leaching of components from restorative materials beneath preparations may be responsible for the stimulus. However, these hypotheses have never really identified the molecular signaling processes responsible for cellular up-regulation. An in vivo study, in which isolated dentin matrix components were implanted in the base of unexposed cavities that had been carefully prepared in ferret teeth to ensure primary odontoblast survival, has shown that bioactive molecules in these isolated matrix preparations are capable of stimulating reactionary dentinogenesis.[40] These findings indicate that the signaling molecules for reactionary dentinogenesis may be derived and released by diffusion of the injurious agent through the dentin matrix. Partial purification of the isolated matrix preparations to enrich their growth factor content, particularly of the TGF-β family, has implicated these molecules in the cellular signaling responsible for reactionary dentinogenesis.[38] Direct application of the TGF-β1 and TGF-β3 isoforms to the odontoblast layer on agarose beads in cultured tooth slices has demonstrated their ability to up-regulate odontoblast secretion.[41] Similar findings were made after application of a solution of TGF-β1 to cultured tooth slices using small Perspex tubes glued to the dentin matrix that allowed diffusion of the growth factor through the dentinal tubules.[42] TGF-β1, TGF-β2, and TGF-β3 isoforms are expressed by odontoblasts,[43] and TGF-β1 becomes sequestrated within the dentin matrix.[44] Thus, considerable endogenous tissue pools of this growth factor are found within the dentin matrix, and these are available for release if the matrix is solubilized or degraded.

During caries, plaque bacterial acids diffusing through and demineralizing the dentin matrix might be expected to solubilize some of this tissue pool of growth factor. In cavity preparation, the use of etchants or cavity conditioning agents may also release these molecules. A number of commonly used etchants have been found to solubilize TGF-β1 and various noncollagenous matrix components from dentin, the most effective of these being ethylenediaminetetraacetic acid (EDTA) (Smith and Smith, unpublished data, 1998). Restorative materials may also stimulate reactionary dentinogenesis through similar mechanisms. Calcium hydroxide can solubilize TGF-β1 and noncollagenous matrix components from dentin (Smith et al, unpublished data, 1995), a finding that provides new insight into the action of this widely used material. Thus, a variety of factors associated both with the injury process to the tissue and its subsequent restoration may fortuitously contribute to defense reactions of repair.

A role for the TGF-βs in tertiary dentinogenesis is supported by studies with TGF-β1 (-/-) mice, in which there appears to be decreased "secondary" (tertiary) dentin formation.[45] Although release of TGF-β1 from the dentin matrix may provide an explanation for the cellular signaling of reactionary dentinogenesis, it must be recognized that other growth factors are also sequestrated within the dentin matrix. Insulin-like growth factors (IGFs) -I and -II,[46] bone morphogenetic proteins (BMPs),[47] and a number of angiogenetic growth factors[48] have been reported in dentin matrix. This diverse group of growth factors provides a powerful cocktail of bioactive molecules that may be released and participate in cellular signaling during injury and repair to the pulpodentin complex. The presence of angiogenic growth factors in dentin may explain the stimulation of angiogenesis at sites of tertiary dentin formation, but the range of cellular effects arising from release of some of the other growth factors remains to be elucidated. The concept of dentin as an inert tissue must therefore be questioned, and a variety of cellular effects arising from solubilization of its matrix remain to be identified.

Factors Influencing Reactionary Dentinogenesis

A tertiary dentinogenic response beneath a caries lesion is easily recognized.[49] A reactionary response is often associated with small, slowly progressing lesions,[50] whereas in more active lesions death of the primary odontoblasts is more likely to occur, and reparative dentinogenesis will be seen if the prevailing tissue conditions allow. However, even in more slowly progressing lesions, the response may be a mixture of reactionary and reparative dentinogenesis.[50] Thus, the activity of a caries lesion will have a strong influence on the nature of the tertiary dentinogenic response.

Various factors associated with cavity preparation and restoration can influence the tertiary dentinogenic response: the method of cavity preparation, the dimensions of the cavity, the residual dentin thickness (RDT) of the cavity, etching of the cavity, and the nature of the dental materials used and the method of their application for the restoration. Many studies have described the pulpal changes in response to these various factors, and the consensus is that cavity restoration events can influence the underlying pulpal cell populations to a degree that is proportionally greater than the differences in cytotoxicity of cavity restoration materials themselves.[51-55] This highlights the need for careful control of cavity preparation conditions in studies of pulpal responses. Use of animal models[52] for assessment of pulpal responses to restorative factors can allow more reproducible control of these factors, while in vitro organ culture approaches offer opportunities to examine some of these factors in the absence of inflammation and bacteria.[55,56] Nevertheless, it is still important to assess human dental responses to these factors to overcome possible species variations and to attempt to quantify their relative importance. The complex interplay between the various factors makes it difficult to unravel their involvement during different phases of the injury and repair responses.

Histomorphometry of reactionary dentinogenesis beneath standardized cavity preparations in a relatively young population of human teeth with subsequent statistical analysis showed a strong correlation between reactionary dentin secretion and RDT, patient age, and cavity floor surface area and restoration width.[53] RDT was apparently the most significant factor determining the secretion of reactionary dentin, which is increased in area by 1.187 mm^2 for every 1-mm decrease in the RDT beneath the cavity. Increases in reactionary dentin area were also correlated with increases in the dimensions of other cavity preparation variables. A weaker correlation was observed between choice of restoration material and reactionary dentinogenesis; however, zinc oxide- eugenol appeared to have no effect on reactionary dentinogenesis compared with calcium hydroxide/amalgam types of restorations.

Similar observations on the quantitative relationship between RDT and reactionary dentinogenesis were made in a larger study of 217 human teeth.[54] Reactionary dentin secretion was seen beneath cavities with an RDT above 0.5 mm or below 0.25 mm; however, maximum reactionary dentinogenesis (approximately fourfold greater) was observed beneath cavities with an RDT between 0.5 and 0.25 mm. Reduced reactionary dentin secretion beneath cavities with an RDT below 0.25 mm appeared to be associated with reduced odontoblast survival, presumably as a result of irreversible cell damage during cavity cutting. Choice of restoration material influenced reactionary dentin secretion, as well as odontoblast survival, to a significant but lesser degree than did RDT. In terms of their influence on reactionary dentinogenesis, calcium hydroxide had the greatest influence, followed by resin composite, resin-modified glass ionomer, and zinc oxide-eugenol. This ranking reflected a combination of the effects of the materials on odontoblast cell survival and stimulation of reactionary dentinogenesis. A schematic diagram of the relationship between RDT and reactionary dentinogenesis may offer guidance in treatment planning (Fig 3-15).

We can now start to understand how the various restorative factors influence reactionary dentinogenesis on a mechanistic basis. RDT after cavity cutting has the potential to influence odontoblast cell survival: in deep (RDT less than 0.25 mm) cavities, little more than 50% odontoblast survival may be seen,[54] whereas in shallower cavities, odontoblast survival is about 85% or greater, and despite the likely cutting of the odontoblast process, the cells respond by secretion of reactionary dentin. Although little is known about how the cell responds to cutting of its process, it is generally assumed that such breaks in the membrane integrity are soon restored. Receptors to TGF-βs have been demonstrated on odontoblasts,[57] and ultrastructural immunolabeling studies have suggested their presence on the odontoblast process as well, especially nearer to the pulp (Murray et al, unpublished data, 2001). Receptors to other growth factors may also be present, and therefore localization studies are required. With shallower cavities, the amount of reactionary dentin that is secreted can be corre-

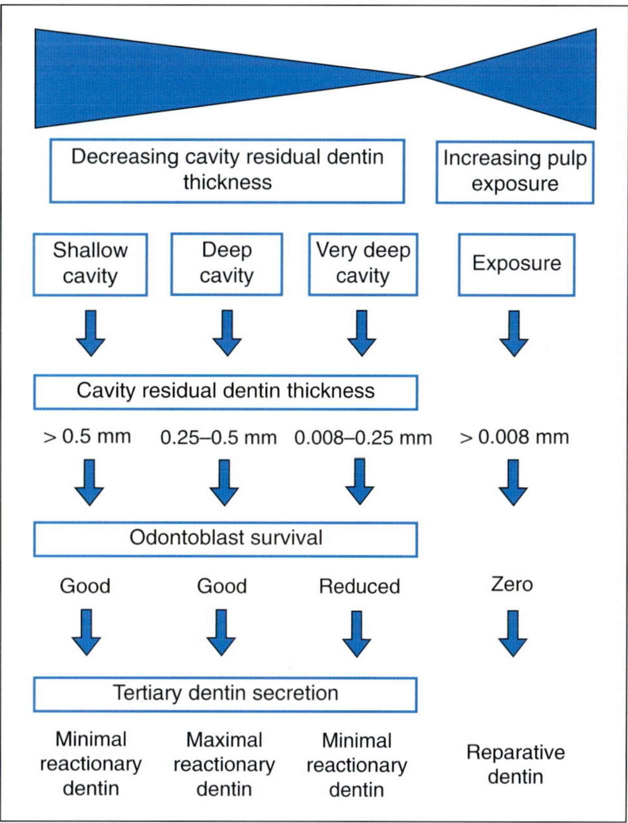

Fig 3-15 Schematic diagram of the relationship between cavity residual dentin thickness, odontoblast survival, and tertiary dentinogenesis.

lated with the RDT, which suggests that distance of diffusion of cell-signaling molecules is a determining factor.

Cavity etching can positively influence the secretion of reactionary dentin. Treatment with EDTA[55] for 0 seconds, 60 seconds, and 120 seconds led to a ranking of 60 seconds > 120 seconds > 0 seconds for reactionary dentin secretion. Reduced reactionary dentinogenesis after 0 or 120 seconds of treatment was associated with decreased odontoblast survival. The stimulatory effect of EDTA treatment on reactionary dentinogenesis might be ascribed to the ability of this chemical to release growth factors from the dentin matrix during its solubilizing action, which could then diffuse down the dentinal tubules and bind to receptors on the odontoblasts for signaling of a reactionary dentinogenic response. Other etchants such as phosphoric acid have less of a stimulatory effect on reactionary dentinogenesis, perhaps reflecting their less effective action in solubilizing matrix-bound growth factors. Such a sequence for cellular signaling of reactionary dentinogenesis would be expected to be dependent on the distance of diffusion of the growth factor molecules, and this would be in accord with the observations on the importance of RDT to the amount of reactionary dentin secreted. Restorative materials that are capable of stimulating reactionary dentinogenesis, such as calcium hydroxide, may have similar actions on the dentin matrix–releasing growth factors, which then diffuse to the odontoblasts and prompt their up-regulation. Clearly, complex events take place during cavity preparation and restoration involving the interplay of many factors, but odontoblast cell survival and release of endogenous matrix-bound pools of growth factors and other bioactive molecules in the tooth may be critical to the signaling of reactionary dentinogenesis.

Reparative dentinogenesis

In nonexposed pulps, reparative dentinogenesis may be a sequel to reactionary dentinogenesis (Fig 3-16), or it may occur independently in the absence of reactionary dentin if the injury is of sufficient intensity (eg, an active caries lesion). The reparative response of tertiary dentinogenesis will always take place at sites of pulp exposure because of the loss of odontoblasts and the need for dentin bridge formation. Reparative dentinogenesis involves a much more complex sequence of biologic events than reactionary dentinogenesis in that progenitor cells from the pulp must be recruited and induced to differentiate into odontoblast-like cells before their secretion may be up-regulated to form the reparative dentin matrix (Fig 3-17).

The matrices secreted during reparative dentinogenesis show a broad spectrum of appearances ranging from a regular, tubular matrix to a very dysplastic, atubular matrix (Fig 3-18) sometimes with cellular inclusions present. This heterogeneity in matrix morphology is often paralleled in the morphology and secretory behavior of the odontoblast-like cells responsible for its secretion, leading to considerable variations in matrix structure and composition (Fig 3-19).

Though all of these responses may generally be categorized as reparative dentinogenesis, they nonetheless show considerable heterogeneity. This heterogeneity may reflect the specificity of the dentinogenic processes taking place. These processes may resemble physiologic dentinogenesis or, instead, represent nonspecific matrix secretion. Nonspecific secretion can occur from cells with few phenotypic characteristics of odontoblast-like cells, and is believed to represent part of a more generalized wound-healing response. The differences in tubularity observed in a reparative dentin matrix (Fig 3-20) will have consequences for the permeability of the matrix to provide pulpal protection from the possible effects of bacteria and restorative materials. Maintenance of the tubular physiologic structure of dentin may be a sensible goal in tissue regeneration generally, but it must be considered in relation to the tissue environment created by a restoration. Where there is a need to provide pulpal protection from the effects of bacterial microleakage and components of restorative materials,

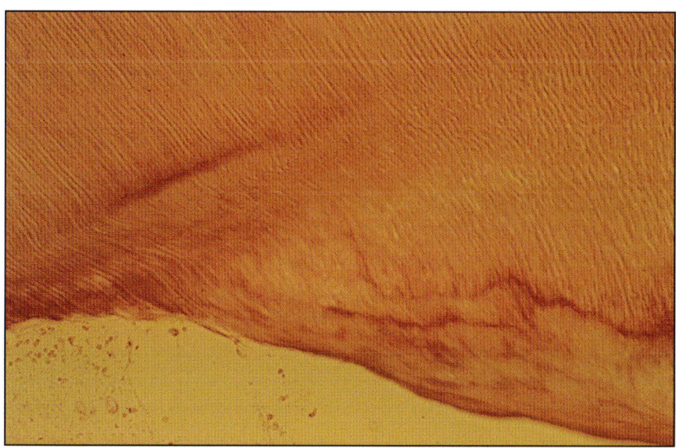

Fig 3-16 Tertiary dentinogenic response beneath a caries lesion in a human tooth showing an initial reactionary dentinogenic response adjacent to the physiologic dentin with a subsequent reparative dentinogenic response, the matrix of which shows heterogeneity in its tubularity (periodic acid–Schiff stain, original magnification ×250).

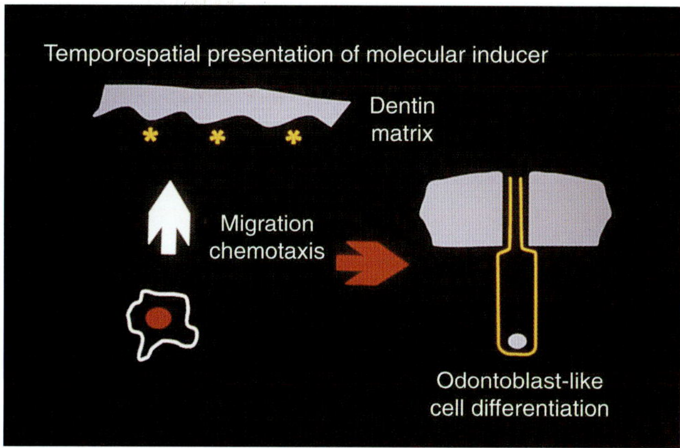

Fig 3-17 Schematic diagram of biologic events during reparative dentinogenesis showing progenitor cell recruitment through chemotaxis and migration and temporospatial presentation of the molecular signal for induction of odontoblast-like cell differentiation on the surface of existing dentin matrix prior to secretion of reparative dentin matrix. (Reprinted from Smith et al[79] with permission.)

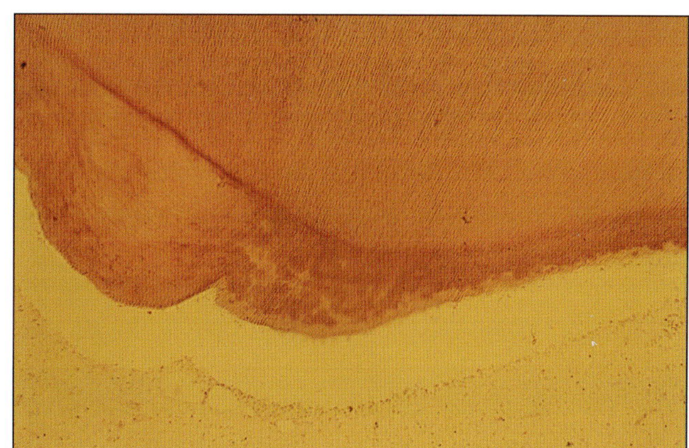

Fig 3-18 Reparative dentin secreted beneath and demarcated from physiologic dentin by a darker-staining calciotraumatic line underlying a caries lesion in a human tooth. Note the considerable heterogeneity in the reparative dentin ranging from a tubular *(right)* to an atubular *(left)* matrix (periodic acid–Schiff stain, original magnification ×100).

the presence of a tubular, reparative matrix will increase permeability and may therefore be disadvantageous.

Reparative dentinogenesis will often be preceded by secretion of a fibrodentin matrix,[12] which is atubular and is associated with rather cuboidal cells with poorly developed organelles on its formative surface. Deposition of tubular matrix by polarized cells is then seen later on the surface of this fibrodentin. Whether fibrodentin deposition represents a specific dentinogenic response or a nonspecific connective tissue wound-healing response is uncertain. Data on the molecular phenotype of these cells are not available, but the morphology of the cells responsible for its synthesis and secretion point to a relatively nonspecific response. Nevertheless, it may play an important role in the signaling of true reparative dentinogenesis by providing a substrate upon which signaling molecules for odontoblast-like cell differentiation may become immobilized. In this way, it could mimic the role of the dental basement membrane for odontoblast differentiation during tooth development, where it has been suggested that growth factors derived from the inner dental epithelium become temporospatially

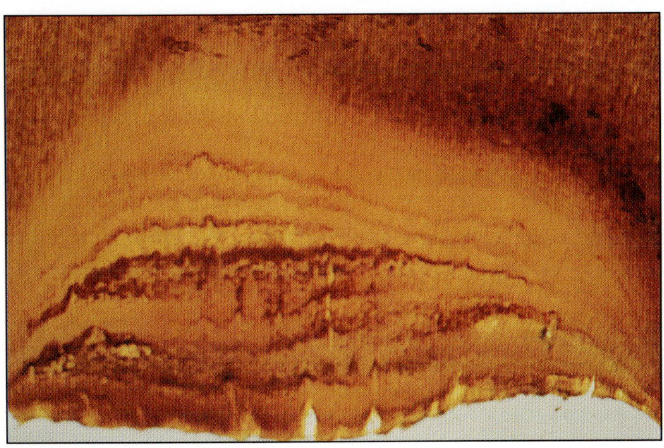

Fig 3-19 Reparative dentin matrix secreted beneath a caries lesion in a section of a human tooth stained with silver colloid to demonstrate phosphoproteins. Note considerable heterogeneity in the staining intensity of these matrix components reflecting variations in odontoblast-like cell behavior during secretion (original magnificatoin ×250).

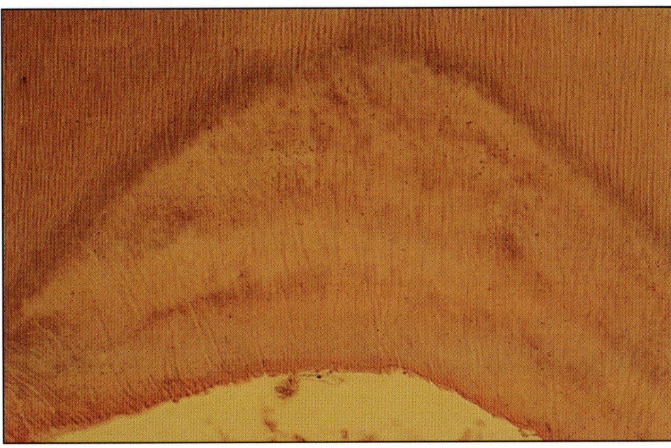

Fig 3-20 Reparative dentin matrix secreted beneath a caries lesion in a human tooth, showing a less tubular structure than the adjacent physiologic dentin, which will reduce the permeability of this tissue (H&E stain, original magnificatoin ×250).

immobilized on the basement membrane for presentation to the pre-odontoblasts to signal their terminal differentiation.[58]

Recapitulation of embryonic events leading to tooth development during tertiary dentinogenesis has been proposed, and indeed, many common features of the two processes can be observed.[32] The need for progenitor cell recruitment, induction of differentiation, and up-regulation of secretory activity are common to both processes (Fig 3-21), although the absence of physiologic regulation of the biologic events during repair may lead to more diversity in the cellular secretions seen. Progenitor cell recruitment, signaling of odontoblast-like cell differentiation, and subsequent up-regulation of matrix secretion by these cells are the three critical steps for reparative dentinogenesis. While up-regulation of matrix secretion is common to reactionary dentinogenesis, the first two steps distinguish the process of reparative dentinogenesis.

Progenitor cell recruitment

The derivation of the progenitor cells recruited for odontoblast-like cell differentiation during reparative dentinogenesis is still unclear. However, the neural crest origin of the ectomesenchymal cells of the dental papilla giving rise to the odontoblasts is likely to be important to their phenotype. Isolated pulpal cells from adult human teeth show many similarities in their molecular phenotype to bone marrow stem cells but appear to show different behavior both in vitro and after transplantation into immunocompromised mice in vivo.[59] Thus, the pulpal derivation of these cells appears to confer specificity on their developmental potential. However, this study was not able to identify the nature or localization of the cell population from which these pulpal cells were isolated.

The undifferentiated mesenchymal cells in the cell-rich zone of Höhl adjacent to the odontoblast layer have been suggested as progenitors,[60] and they are attractive candidates since they will have experienced a developmental history similar to that of the primary odontoblasts. During tooth development, pre-odontoblasts align themselves perpendicular to the dental basement membrane during the final mitotic division. One daughter cell is exposed to the epithelial-derived epigenetic signal for induction of odontoblast differentiation and the other is not[58] and is generally assumed to join the cells in the cell-rich zone of Höhl instead. However, cells from elsewhere in the pulp have also been implicated as progenitors for the odontoblast-like cell. These include perivascular cells, undifferentiated mesenchymal cells, fibroblasts, etc.[61] What the relative contribution from any of these cell populations is to progenitor recruitment for odontoblast-like cell differentiation is unclear, but the possibility suggests opportunities for heterogeneity in the nature of the response. Aging may influence the survival of some of these possible progenitor cell populations, and their different phenotypic characteristics may contribute to the specificity of the process if they are involved in reparative dentinogenesis. Thus, depending on the age of the patient and the survival of cells following injury to the dentin-pulp complex, considerable heterogeneity may be seen in the cellular response. Stem cells are pluri-potent, and their presence in tissues can offer opportunities for regeneration in response to growth and differentiation signals. There are many genes that control the behavior and expression potential of stem cells, including the highly conserved Notch signaling pathway, which can enable equivalent precursor cells to adopt different cell potentials.[62] Such genetic control may be important in determining progenitor cell recruitment during reparative dentinogenesis. Reappearance of Notch in subodontoblast cells during reparative responses to injury and in association with vascular structures in apical areas of the root of the tooth[63] may indicate the role of cells in these areas to contribute to reparative dentinogenesis. If this is the case, then both undifferentiated mesenchymal cells and pericytes may be progenitors of odontoblast-like cells.

Migration of progenitor cells in the pulp to the site of injury for reparative dentinogenesis requires an appropriate chemotactic attractant. Isolated human dentin matrix components have been found to be chemotactic in vitro to pulpal cells showing characteristics of pericytes (Murray et al, unpublished data, 2001), and dissolution of dentin matrix at sites of injury could provide such a stimulus. Although the specific components in the matrix that are responsible for these effects remain to be identified, TGF-β1 is known to be chemotactic for fibroblasts, macrophages, neutrophils, and monocytes during dermal wound healing.[64] Attraction of inflammatory cells to the site of injury may further enhance the chemotaxis of other cells, including pulpal progenitor cells, since many will also produce TGF-βs and other growth factors. TGF-β1 has also been reported to be mitogenic for cells in the subodontoblast layer,[42] and thus may provide both a migratory stimulus for progenitor cells and stimulate their proliferation to expand the available population of progenitor cells.

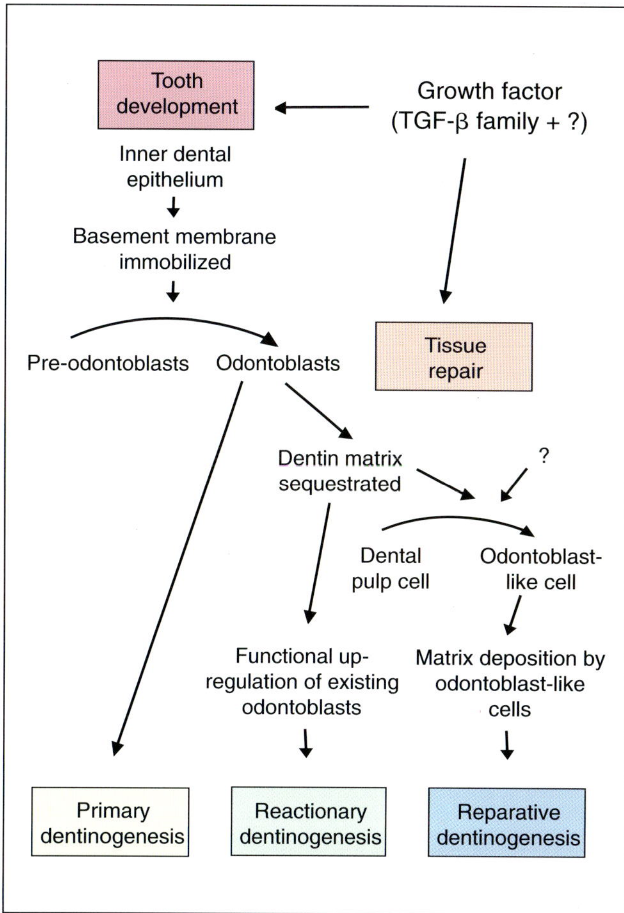

Fig 3-21 Schematic comparison of events during tooth development and dental tissue repair highlighting the many similarities among the processes taking place. (Reprinted from Smith and Lesot[32] with permission.)

Signaling of odontoblast-like cell differentiation

Following recruitment of progenitor cells to the site of injury, signaling of odontoblast-like cell differentiation has to be achieved before reparative dentin secretion can commence. While an epithelial-derived, temporospatially regulated epigenetic signal is responsible for induction of odontoblast differentiation during tooth development,[58] the absence of epithelium in the mature tooth requires an alternative derivation for this signal.

Dentin matrix can be autoinductive, and the various reports of its ability to induce odontoblast-like cell differentiation[65] concur with the histopathologic reports of matrix growth from dentin chips pushed into the pulp during cavity preparation. Implantation of isolated dentin matrix components, including fractions derived from both the soluble and the insoluble matrix compartments, in exposed cavities prepared in ferret teeth gave rise to a reparative dentinogenic response, with secretion of a regular tubular matrix by polarized, columnar odontoblast-like cells in the absence of a fibrodentin precursor matrix.[66] Culture of dissociated embryonic dental papillae with the same dentin matrix preparations induced a physiologic gradient of odontoblast differentiation, which could be inhibited by inclusion of antibodies to TGF-β1.[67] Similar effects were observed when the dentin matrix components were substituted by recombinant TGF-β1 immobilized with heparin, and the odontoblast-like cells showed most of the molecular phenotypic characteristics of physiologic odontoblasts.[67,68] Thus, the epigenetic signaling of odontoblast differentiation by growth factors may be recapitulated during repair in adult tissues. Experimental application of recombinant TGF-β1 to adult pulp tissue in dogs has confirmed the ability of this growth factor to signal odontoblast-like cell differentiation.[69] TGF-β3 may also exert similar effects since application of agarose beads soaked in this growth factor at sites of needle-punch injury in cultured tooth slices led to alignment of columnar odontoblast-like cells on the bead surface in a number of cultures.[41] Other members of the TGF-β family of growth factors, including the BMPs, have also been implicated in signaling of odontoblast-like cell differentiation during reparative dentinogenesis.[70-72] These findings provide new opportunities to exploit endogenous pools of growth factors sequestrated in dentin matrix and to develop novel biomaterials containing growth factors for use in pulp-capping.

The presence of growth factors, particularly the TGF-βs, in both the soluble and insoluble tissue compartments of dentin matrix[44,48] provides opportunities for cellular interaction with these molecules in several ways. Release of growth factors from the soluble tissue compartment may arise from tissue demineralization by bacterial acids during caries. Further release of these molecules during cavity preparation and restoration may also arise from the action of cavity-etching agents and diffusion of components leached from restorative materials. Diffusion of these soluble growth factors to the pulp may provide a chemotactic attraction for progenitor cells to the injury site and a mitogenic stimulus to expand this cell population. It is unclear whether the signaling of odontoblast-like cell differentiation may involve the soluble or insoluble tissue pools of these growth factors. However, if developmental events are recapitulated, it seems likely that immobilized matrix-bound growth factors may provide the signal for differentiation. This tissue pool of growth factors appears to be masked by mineral and other matrix components and requires exposure before they can participate in signaling processes. Ultrastructural immunolabeling of untreated cut dentin surfaces for TGF-β showed absence of reactivity.[73] However, treatment of the cut surface with cavity etchants unmasked the TGF-β in the matrix to varying degrees, with the different etchants demonstrating variable ability to expose these molecules (Fig 3-22). It is therefore apparent that conventional restorative procedures can act on the dental tissues in ways not previously appreciated and may contribute significantly to cellular events involved in repair after injury.

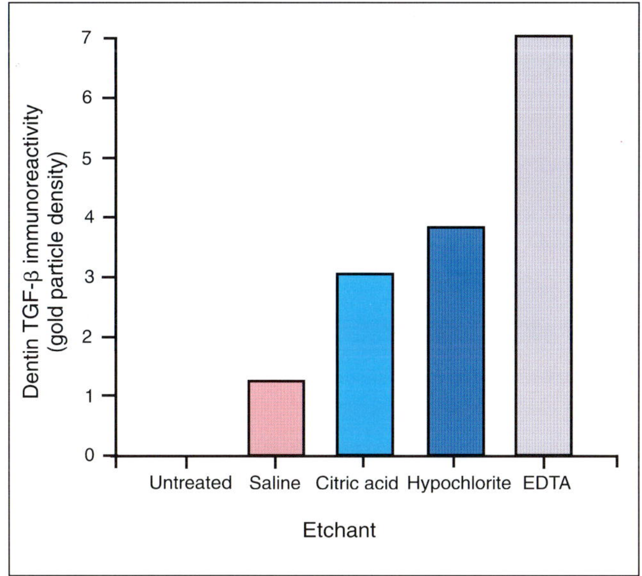

Fig 3-22 Comparison of immunoreactivity of cut human dentin matrix for TGF-β1 after treatment with various etchants. EDTA, ethylenediaminetetraacetic acid. (Data from Zhao et al.[73])

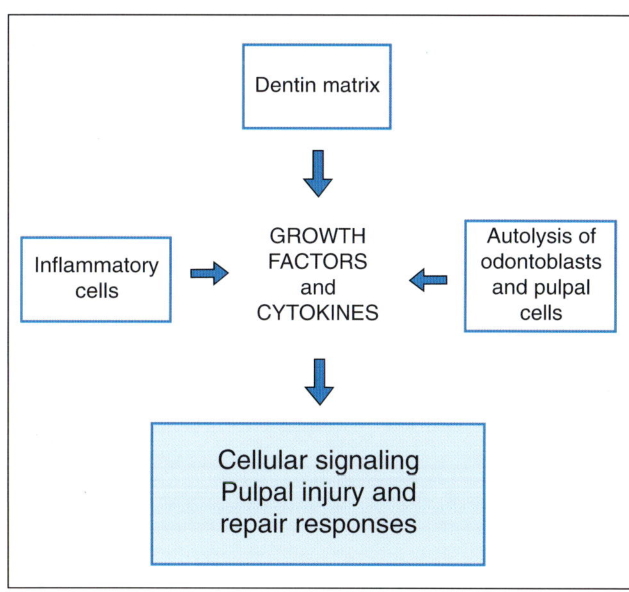

Fig 3-23 Schematic diagram of possible derivations of signaling molecules contributing to pulpal injury and repair responses.

It is also important to recognize that a variety of cell-signaling molecules may be present in the extracellular milieu at sites of injury in the pulp. Even though the greatest focus recently has been on TGF-βs derived from the dentin matrix, it must be remembered that a cocktail of growth factors is present within this matrix. The effects of some of the individual molecules on pulpal cells remain to be determined, and little attention has been paid to any synergistic effects that combinations of these molecules may have. Thus, it is possible that a variety of biologic effects arising from dentin matrix dissolution may yet be identified. Clearly, pulpal injury, cavity preparation, and restoration procedures may all influence these biologic effects through differential solubilization of various matrix-bound bioactive molecules. Injury events within the pulp may also directly give rise to bioactive molecules from cells, which may influence subsequent cellular events. Death of odontoblasts and other pulpal cells may release intracellular contents at the site of injury. Inflammatory cells attracted to the site of injury will also give rise to cytokines and growth factors, which will modulate cellular events both directly and indirectly. Thus, a complex interplay between signaling molecules in the pulp can be anticipated after injury (Fig 3-23), which may result in a range of responses.

Dentin bridge formation

At sites of pulp exposure, dentin continuity may be restored through dentin bridge formation across the exposure. There have been reports of bridging after pulp-capping with a variety of agents, the most common being calcium hydroxide (although resin composites are gaining in usage; see also chapters 13 and 14). Dentin bridge formation is not distinct from reparative dentinogenesis but rather represents a particular situation under which reparative dentin is formed. However, the extent of the injury and the reparative processes required may influence the quality or structure of the new matrix secreted within the bridge. Divergence from the normal, regular

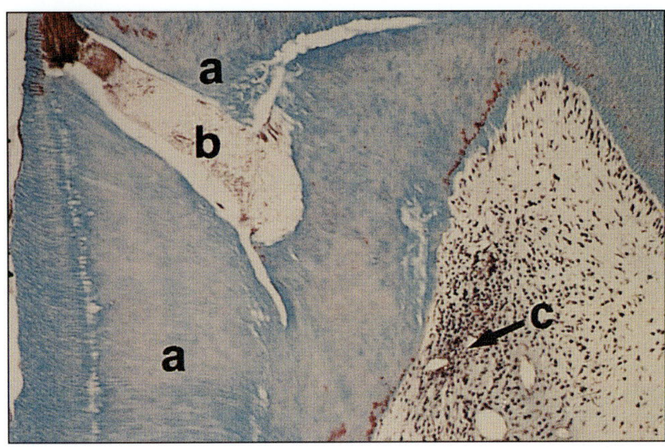

Fig 3-24 Tunnel defect containing debris (b) within a reparative dentin bridge (a) of a Dycal (Dentsply, York, PA) direct-capped exposure at 2 years. Chronic inflammatory cells, some with ingested Dycal particles (c), are present below the bridge in the pulp (Masson stain, original magnification ×41.4). (Reprinted from Cox et al[76] with permission.)

tubular structure of dentin may be common. This must lead us to question the specificity of the dentinogenic response in some situations.

New dentin bridge formation is often regarded as an indication of successful pulp-capping treatment, although this is probably true only where the bridge provides an effective bacteriometic seal. Mjör[74] cautioned that the presence of a dentin bridge may not be a suitable criterion for assessment of successful pulp healing, especially during capping of young healthy pulps. Many bridges are permeated by pulpal tissue and operative debris. The concept of dentin bridges has been questioned because of the presence of imperfections in many bridges.[75] These imperfections, called *tunnel defects* (Fig 3-24), involve multiple perforations that allow communication between the pulp and capping material interface. An incidence of 89% for multiple tunnel defects in dentin bridges after calcium hydroxide pulp capping has been reported,[76] and 41% of these bridges were associated with recurring pulpal inflammation or necrosis and with the presence of inflammatory cells and stained bacterial profiles. The patency of these tunnel defects prevents a hermetic seal that would protect the pulp against recurring infection from bacterial microleakage. This highlights the need to use materials capable of providing long-term bacteriometic sealing over capped pulps and opportunities for developing new capping materials that stimulate more specific dentinogenic responses during pulpal healing.

References

1. Kuttler Y. Classification of dentin into primary, secondary and tertiary. Oral Surg 1959;12:996.
2. Takuwa S, Nagai N. Ultrastructure of rat odontoblasts in various stages of their development and maturation. Arch Oral Biol 1971;16:993.
3. Fox AG, Heeley JD. Histological study of pulps of human primary teeth. Arch Oral Biol 1980;25:103–110.
4. Couve E. Ultrastructural changes during the life cycle of human odontoblasts. Arch Oral Biol 1986;31:643–651.
5. Romagnoli P, Mancini G, Galeotti F, Franchi E, Piereoni P. The crown odontoblasts of rat molars from primary dentinogenesis to complete eruption. J Dent Res 1990; 69:1857–1862.
6. Frank RM, Nalbandian J. Structure and ultrastructure of dentine. In: Berkovitz BKB, Boyde A, Frank RM, Höhling HJ, Moxham BJ, Nalbandian J, Tonge CH (eds). Teeth. Berlin: Springer-Verlag, 1989:173.
7. Butler WT. Dentin matrix proteins. Eur J Oral Sci 1998; 106(Suppl 1):204–210.
8. Magloire H, Joffre A, Bleicher F. An in vitro model of human dental pulp repair. J Dent Res 1996;75:1971–1978.
9. Sloan AJ, Shelton RM, Hann AC, Moxham BJ, Smith AJ. An in vitro approach for the study of dentinogenesis by organ culture of the dentine-pulp complex from rat incisor teeth. Arch Oral Biol 1998;43:421–430.
10. MacDougall M, Thiemann F, Ta H, Hsu P, Chen LS, Snead ML. Temperature sensitive simian virus 40 large T antigen immortalization of murine odontoblast cell cultures: Establishment of clonal odontoblast cell line. Connect Tissue Res 1995;33:97–103.
11. Thonemann B, Schmalz G. Bovine dental papilla-derived cells immortalized with HPV 18 E6/E7. Eur J Oral Sci 2000;108:432–441.
12. Baume LJ. The biology of pulp and dentine. A historic, terminologic-taxonomic, histologic-biochemical, embryonic, and clinical survey. Monog Oral Sci 1980;8:1–220.
13. Tobin CE. Correlation of vascularity with mineralization in human fetal teeth. Anat Rec 1972;174:371–379.
14. Takahashi K, Kishi Y, Kim S. A scanning electron microscope study of the blood vessels of dog pulp using corrosion resin casts. J Endod 1982;8:131–135.

15. Leblond CP, Weinstock M. Comparative study of dentin and bone formation. In: Bourne GH (ed). The Biochemistry and Physiology of Bone. Vol 4: Calcification and physiology, ed 2. New York: Academic Press, 1976:Ch 12.
16. Fromme HG, Höhling HJ, Riedel H. Elektronen-mikroskopische studien über die Dentin-bildung II. [Electron microscopic studies of dentin formation 2. Autoradiographic studies on the function of odontoblasts.] Dtsch Zahnärztl Z 1972;27:6-13.
17. Weinstock A, Leblond CP. Synthesis, migration and release of precursor collagen by odontoblasts as visualized by radioautography after [3H] proline administration. J Cell Biol 1974;60:92.
18. Frank RM. Electron microscopy autoradiography of calcified tissues. Int Rev Cytol 1979;56:183-253.
19. Weinstock A, Weinstock M, Leblond CP. Autoradiographic detection of 3H-fucose incorporation into glycoprotein by odontoblasts and its deposition at the site of the calcification front in dentin. Calcif Tissue Res 1972;8: 181-190.
20. Weinstock A, Leblond CP. Radioautographic visualization of the deposition of a phosphoprotein at the mineralization front in the dentine of the rat incisor. J Cell Biol 1973;56:838.
21. Linde A. Noncollagenous proteins and proteoglycans in dentinogenesis. In: Linde A (ed). Dentin and Dentinogenesis, vol II. Boca Raton: CRC Press, 1984:55.
22. Linde A. Dentin matrix proteins: Composition and possible functions in calcification. Anat Rec 1989;224: 154-166.
23. Llano E, Pendas AM, Knäper V, et al. Identification and structural and functional characterization of human enamelysin (MMP-20). Biochemistry 1997;36:15101-15108.
24. Caron C, Xue J, Bartlett JD. Expression and localization of membrane type 1 matrix metalloproteinase in tooth tissues. Matrix Biol 1998;17:501-511.
25. Linde A, Goldberg M. Dentinogenesis. Crit Rev Oral Biol Med 1993;4:679-728.
26. Nagai N, Frank RM. Electron microscopic autoradiography of Ca45 during dentinogenesis. Cell Tissue Res 1974;155:513-523.
27. Boyde A, Reith EJ. Quantitative electron probe analysis of secretory ameloblasts and odontoblasts in the rat incisor. Histochemistry 1977;50:347.
28. Linde A, Lundgren T. From serum to the mineral phase. The role of the odontoblast in calcium transport and mineral formation. Int J Dev Biol 1995;39:213-222.
29. Eisenmann DR, Glick PL. Ultrastructure of initial crystal formation in dentin. J Ultrastruct Res 1972;41:18-28.
30. Trowbridge HO. Dentistry today. Dentistry 1982;22(4): 22-29.
31. Larson PA, Linde A. Adrenergic vessel innervation in the rat incisor pulp. Scand J Dent Res 1971;79:7.
32. Smith AJ, Lesot H. Induction and regulation of crown dentinogenesis–embryonic events as a template for dental tissue repair. Crit Rev Oral Biol Med 2001;12:425-437.
33. Smith AJ, Matthews JB, Hall RC. Transforming growth factor-β1 (TGF-β1) in dentine matrix: Ligand activation and receptor expression. Eur J Oral Sci 1998;106(Suppl 1): 179-184.
34. Franquin JC, Remusat M, Abou Hashieh I, Dejou J. Immunocytochemical detection of apoptosis in human odontoblasts. Eur J Oral Sci 1998;106 (Suppl1):384-387.
35. Symons NBB. The microanatomy and histochemistry of dentinogenesis. In: Miles AEW (ed). Structural and Chemical Organization of Teeth, vol I. New York: Academic Press, 1967:285.
36. Hoffman MM, Schour I. Quantitative studies in the development of the rat molar, I. The growth pattern of the primary and secondary dentin (from birth to 500 days of age). Anat Rec 1940;78:233.
37. Lesot H, Bègue-Kirn C, Kubler MD, Meyer JM, Smith AJ, Cassidy N, Ruch JV. Experimental induction of odontoblast differentiation and stimulation during reparative processes. Cells Mater 1993;3:201.
38. Smith AJ, Cassidy N, Perry H, Begue-Kirn C, Ruch JV, Lesot H. Reactionary dentinogenesis. Int J Dev Biol 1995; 39:273.
39. Mjör IA. Dentin and pulp. In: Mjör IA (ed). Reaction Patterns in Human Teeth. Boca Raton: CRC Press, 1983:63.
40. Smith AJ, Tobias RS, Cassidy N, Plant CG, Browne RN, Begue-Kirn C, et al. Odontoblast stimulation in ferrets by dentine matrix components. Arch Oral Biol 1994;39:13.
41. Sloan AJ, Smith AJ. Stimulation of the dentine-pulp complex of rat incisor teeth by transforming growth factor-β isoforms 1-3 in vitro. Arch Oral Biol 1999;44:149-156.
42. Melin M, Joffre-Romeas A, Farges JC, Couble ML, Magloire H, Bleicher F. Effects of TGF-β1 on dental pulp cells in cultured human tooth slices. J Dent Res 2000;79: 1689-1696.
43. Sloan AJ, Perry H, Matthews JB, Smith AJ. Transforming growth factor-B isoform expression in mature human molar teeth. Histochem J 2000;32:247-252.
44. Cassidy N, Fahey M, Prime SS, Smith AJ. Comparative analysis of transforming growth factor-Beta (TGF-β) isoforms 1-3 in human and rabbit dentine matrices. Arch Oral Biol 1997;42:219-223.
45. D'Souza RN, Cavender A, Dickinson D, Roberts A, Letterio J. TGF-β1 is essential for the homeostasis of the dentin-pulp complex. Eur J Oral Sci 1998;106(Suppl1):185-191.
46. Finkelman RD, Mohan S, Jennings JC, Taylor AK, Jepsen S, Baylink DJ. Quantitation of growth factors IGF-I, SGF/IGF-II and TGF-β in human dentin. J Bone Miner Res 1990;5: 717-723.
47. Bessho K, Tanaka N, Matsumoto J, Tagawa T, Murata M. Human dentin-matrix-derived bone morphogenetic protein. J Dent Res 1991;70:171-175.
48. Roberts-Clark D, Smith AJ. Angiogenic growth factors in human dentine matrix. Arch Oral Biol 2000;45:1013-1016.
49. Magloire H, Bouvier M, Joffre A. Odontoblast response under carious lesions. Proc Finn Dent Soc 1992;88(suppl 1):257-274.

50. Bjørndal L, Darvann T. A light microscopic study of odontoblastic and non-odontoblastic cells involved in tertiary dentinogenesis in well-defined cavitated carious lesions. Caries Res 1999;33:50–60.
51. Lee SJ, Walton RE, Osborne JW. Pulpal responses to bases and cavity depths. Am J Dent 1992;5:64–68.
52. Cox CF, White KC, Ramus DL, Farmer JB, Snuggs HM. Reparative dentin: Factors affecting its deposition. Quintessence Int 1992;23:257–270.
53. Murray PE, About I, Lumley PJ, Smith G, Franquin JC, Smith AJ. Post-operative pulpal responses and dental repair. J Am Dent Assoc 2000;131:321–329.
54. Murray PE, About I, Lumley PJ, Franquin J-C, Remusat M, Smith AJ. Human cavity remaining dentin thickness and pulpal activity. Am J Dent (in press).
55. Murray PE, Lumley PJ, Smith AJ. Comparison of operative procedure variables on in vitro pulpal viability. Am J Dent (in press).
56. Murray PE, Lumley PJ, Ross HF, Smith AJ. Tooth slice organ culture for cytotoxicity assessment of dental materials. Biomaterials 2000;21:1711–1721.
57. Sloan AJ, Matthews JB, Smith AJ. TGF-β receptor expression in human odontoblasts and pulpal cells. Histochem J 1999;31:565
58. Ruch JV, Lesot H, Bègue-Kirn C. Odontoblast differentiation. Int J Dev Biol 1995;39:51–68.
59. Gronthos S, Mankani M, Brahim J, Gehron Robey P, Shi S. Postnatal human dental pulp stem cells (DPSCs) in vitro and in vivo. Proc Natl Acad Sci USA 2000;97:13625–13630.
60. Cotton WR. Pulp response to cavity preparation as studied by the method of thymidine ^{3}H autoradiography. In: Finn SB (ed). Biology of the Dental Pulp Organ. Tuscaloosa, AL: Univ Alabama Press, 1968:69.
61. Fitzgerald M, Chiego JD, Heys DR. Autoradiographic analysis of odontoblast replacement following pulp exposure in primate teeth. Arch Oral Biol 1990;35:707–715.
62. Artavanis-Tsakonas S, Matsuno K, Fortini ME. Notch signaling. Science 1995;268:225–232.
63 Mitsiadis T, Fried K, Goridis C. Reactivation of Delta-Notch signaling after injury: Complementary expression patterns of ligand and receptor in dental pulp. Exp Cell Res 1999;246:312–318.
64. Pierce GF, Tarpley J, Yanagihara D, Mustoe TA, Fox GM, Thomason A. Platelet-derived growth factor (BB homodimer), transforming growth factor-beta 1, and basic fibroblast growth factor in dermal wound healing. Neovessel and matrix formation and cessation of repair. Am J Pathol 1992;140:1375–1388.
65. Tziafas D, Kolokuris I. Inductive influences of demineralized dentin and bone matrix on pulp cells: An approach of secondary dentinogenesis. J Dent Res 1990;69:75–81.
66. Smith AJ, Tobias RS, Plant CG, Browne RM, Lesot H, Ruch JV. In vivo morphogenetic activity of dentine matrix proteins. J Biol Buccale 1990;18:123–129.
67. Bègue-Kirn C, Smith AJ, Ruch JV, Wozney JM, Purchio A, Hartmann D, Lesot H. Effects of dentin proteins, transforming growth factor beta 1 (TGF-beta 1) and bone morphogenetic protein 2 (BMP2) on the differentiation of odontoblast in vitro. Int J Dev Biol 1992;36:491–503.
68. Bègue-Kirn C, Smith AJ, Loriot M, Kupferle C, Ruch JV, Lesot H. Comparative analysis of TGF betas, BMPs, IGF1, msxs, fibronectin, osteonectin and bone sialoprotein gene expression during normal and in vitro-induced odontoblast differentiation. Int J Dev Biol 1994;38:405–420.
69. Tzaifas D, Alvanou A, Papadimitriou S, Gasic J, Komnenou A. Effects of recombinant basic fibroblast growth factor, insulin-like growth factor-II and transforming growth factor-β1 on dog dental pulp cells in vivo. Arch Oral Biol 1998;43:431–444.
70. Rutherford RB, Wahle J, Tucker M, Rueger D, Charette M. Induction of reparative dentine formation in monkeys by recombinant human osteogenic protein-1. Arch Oral Biol 1993;38:571–576.
71. Rutherford RB, Spangberg L, Tucker M, Rueger D, Charette M. The time-course of the induction of reparative dentine formation in monkeys by recombinant human osteogenic protein-1. Arch Oral Biol 1994;39:833–838.
72. Nakashima M. Induction of dentin formation on canine amputated pulp by recombinant human bone morphogenetic proteins (BMP)-2 and -4. J Dent Res 1994;73:1515–1522.
73. Zhao S, Sloan AJ, Murray PE, Lumley PJ, Smith AJ. Ultrastructural localisation of TGF-β exposure in dentine by chemical treatment. Histochem J 2000;32:489–494.
74. Mjör IA. Pulp reaction to calcium hydroxide-containing materials. Oral Surg Oral Med Oral Pathol 1972;33:961–965.
75. Walton RE, Langeland K. Migration of materials in the dental pulp of monkeys. J Endod 1978;4:167–177.
76. Cox CF, Sübay RK, Ostro E, Suzuki S, Suzuki SH. Tunnel defects in dentin bridges: Their formation following direct pulp capping. Oper Dent 1996;21:4–11.
77. Scott DB, Simmelink JW, Nygaard V. Structural aspects of dental caries. J Dent Res 1974;53:175.
78. Ten Cate R. Oral Histology: Development, Structure, and Function, ed 5. St Louis: Mosby Text-book, 1998:158.
79. Smith AJ, Sloan AJ, Matthews JB, Murray PE, Lumley P. Reparative processes in dentin and pulp. In: Addy M, Embery G, Edgar WM, Orchardson R (eds). Tooth Wear and Sensitivity. London: Martin Dunitz, 2000:53–56.

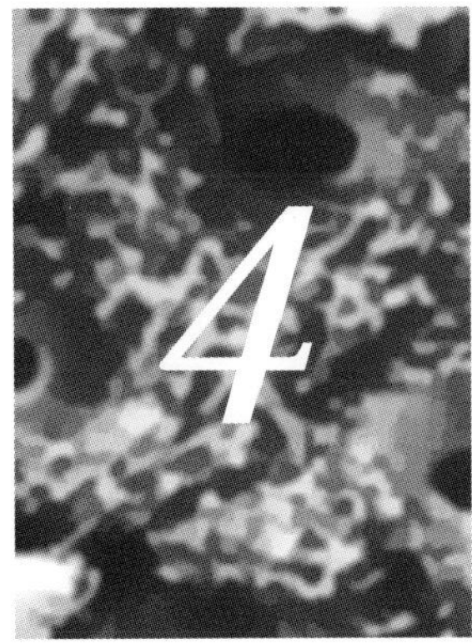

Pulpodentin Complex

David Pashley, DMD, PhD

The previous chapters have dealt with the developmental aspects of dentin and the pulp, the various types of dentinogenesis, and mineralization. This chapter describes the structure of dentin, its chemical and physical properties, and some of its mechanical properties. This topic is clinically significant in that the permeability properties of dentin regulate the rate of diffusion of irritants that initiate pulpal inflammation. Because of this interaction, the pulp and dentin are often discussed together as a functional unit, the pulpodentin complex.

Structure of the Pulpodentin Complex

There is a great deal of evidence that dentin and the pulp are functionally coupled and hence integrated as a tissue. For example, when normal intact teeth are stimulated thermally, dentinal fluid expands or contracts faster than does the volume of the tubules that contain the fluid, which causes hydrodynamic activation of intradental nerves. If the external tissues that seal dentin (eg, enamel and cementum) are lost for any reason, the normal compartmentalization of the two tissues is lost and they become functionally continuous. Under these pathologic conditions, the dentin surface to the pulp becomes a fluid-filled continuum. It is through this fluid medium that bacterial substances may diffuse across dentin to produce pulpal reactions.[1-8] The pulp responds to these chemical stimuli in the short term by mounting an acute inflammatory response, which produces an outward movement of both fluid[9-12] and macromolecules.[13-15] In the long term, pulpal tissues produce tertiary dentin as a biologic response in an attempt to reduce the permeability of the pulpodentin complex and to restore it to its original sequestration[16] (see also chapter 3). In vivo, radioactive tracer experiments demonstrate the continuity of the dentinal fluid–pulpal fluid circulation in exposed dentin and the importance of pulpal blood flow in clearing pulpal interstitial fluids of exogenous material.[17,18] Thus, the pulpodentin complex functions as an integrated unit.[19]

Odontoblasts are highly differentiated cells that form the tubular dentin matrix (chapter 3). Their cell bodies reside in the pulp chamber (Fig 4-1), but their processes pass various distances

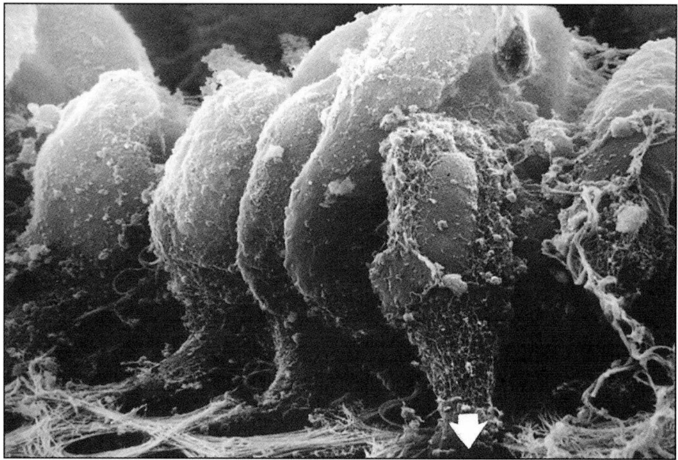

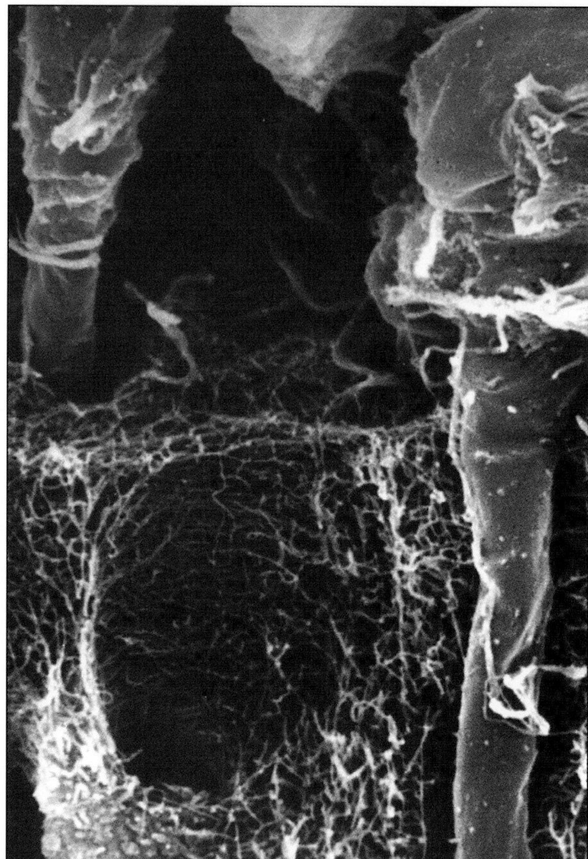

Fig 4-1 *(above)* Human odontoblast layer at the junction of the pulp and predentin. Each cell sends an odontoblast process *(arrow)* through the predentin toward the periphery. (Reprinted from Jean et al[20] with permission.)

Fig 4-2 *(right)* After removal of odontoblasts and their processes, the predentin can be seen to be woven from collagen fibrils approximately 100 nm in diameter. These fibrils polymerize perpendicular to the cell process, forcing the network to form circumferentially around the process. (Reprinted from Jean et al[20] with permission.)

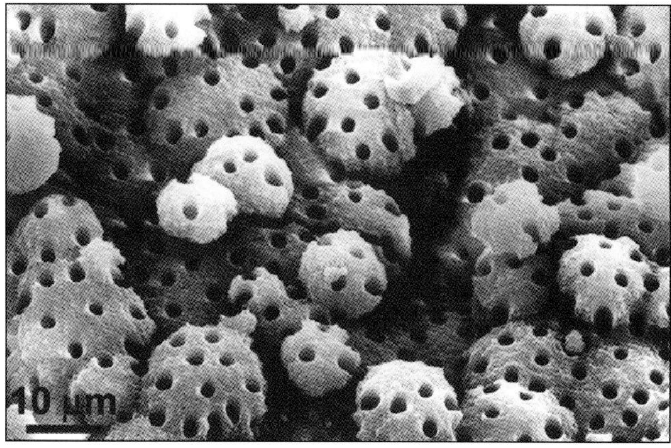

Fig 4-3 When the predentin is removed by NaOCl treatment, the underlying mineralizing dentin matrix can be seen, organized into hemispherical units called calcospherites. Note that each calcospherite contains many dentinal tubules. (Courtesy of Dr Franklin Tay, University of Hong Kong.)

through the unmineralized, freshly secreted predentin into the mineralized matrix.[20] Detailed information about the structure and function of odontoblasts may be found in recent reviews.[21,22] If the odontoblast layer is removed, the odontoblast processes are sometimes removed from the unmineralized tubules of predentin as well (Fig 4-2).[23] This dentin matrix is not yet mineralized and contains tubular openings 3 µm in diameter where no peritubular dentin matrix has yet been formed. When the predentin is removed by treatment with 5% NaOCl, one can see the underlying mineralized tubules that are almost 3 µm in diameter (Fig 4-3). At this relatively low magnification (×500), the spherical surface of calcospherites[24] can be seen (Fig 4-3).

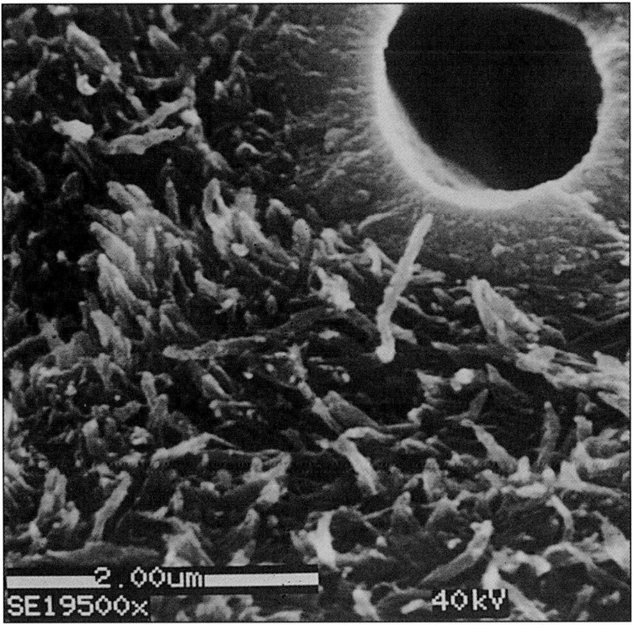

Fig 4-4 Fractured dentin showing a single dentinal tubule lined by hypermineralized, collagen-poor peritubular dentin, more accurately called *intratubular dentin*. Note that the dentin surrounding the tubules (ie, intertubular dentin) has a different texture due to the presence of collagen fibrils, whose presence is masked by apatitic crystallites (original magnification ×19,500). (Reprinted from Pashley[19] with permission.)

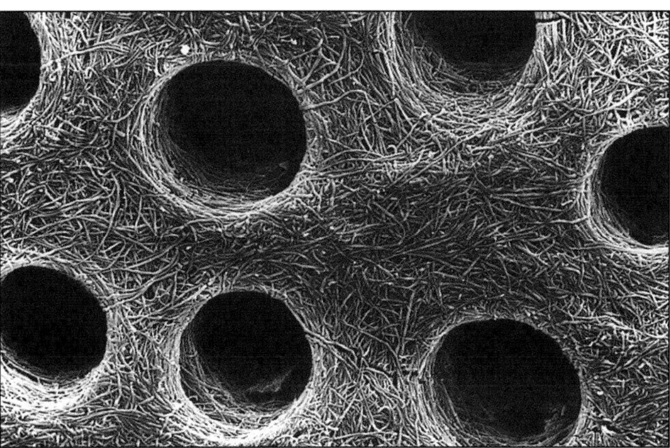

Fig 4-5 Acid etching dentin removes the peritubular dentin matrix and strips the crystallites off the collagen fibrils, permitting the true fibrillar nature of the dentin matrix to be seen (original magnification ×10,000). (Courtesy of Dr Jorge Perdigâo, University of Minnesota.)

Dentin

Dentin morphology

Dentin is a porous biologic composite made up of apatite crystal filler particles in a collagen matrix (Fig 4-4). This mineralized matrix was formed developmentally by odontoblasts, which began secreting collagen at the dentinoenamel junction (DEJ) and then grew centripetally while trailing odontoblast processes. Acid etching or ethylenediaminetetraacetic acid (EDTA) chelation removes the peritubular dentin matrix, thereby enlarging the tubule orifice, and removes the mineral crystallites from around the collagen fibrils, exposing the fibrillar nature of the dentin matrix (Fig 4-5).

There are three types of dentin: primary, secondary, and tertiary. *Primary dentin* is the original tubular dentin largely formed prior to eruption of a tooth. The outer layer of primary dentin, called *mantle dentin*, is slightly less mineralized (about 4%) than is regular circumferential dentin. Mantle dentin is about 150 µm wide and comprises the first dentin laid down by newly differentiated odontoblasts.[25] These cells may not be completely differentiated, or they may have had relatively short odontoblast processes providing slightly less than ideal mineralization. *Secondary dentin* is the same circumpulpal dentin as primary dentin, but secondary dentin is formed after completion of root formation. The major difference between primary and secondary dentin is that the latter is secreted more slowly than primary dentin. Because the same odontoblasts form both types of dentin, the tubules remain continuous. Over decades, a large amount of secondary dentin is formed on the roof and floor of the pulp chamber, causing the chamber to become more shallow. Similarly, secondary dentin formation

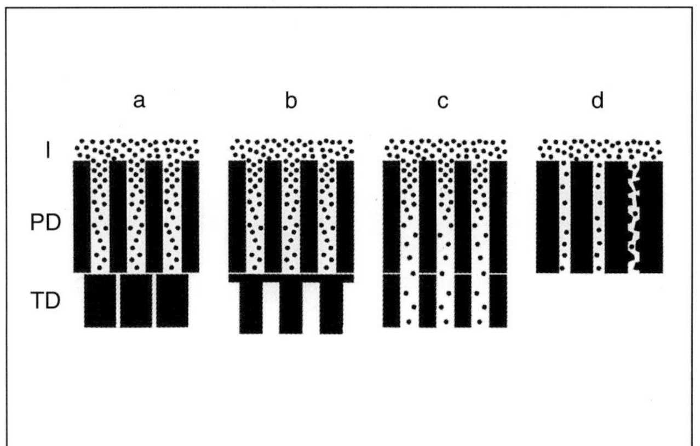

Fig 4-6 Schematic showing the tubular nature of various types of dentin. *(a)* Primary dentin (PD) is shown above less tubular tertiary dentin (TD). The small dots indicate the concentration of a potentially noxious substance diffusing across dentin. The original odontoblasts were destroyed, but the newly differentiated odontoblasts in the reparative dentin did not line up with the original primary dentin, greatly lowering its permeability. *(b)* Sometimes the newly formed odontoblasts lack a process and form a layer of atubular dentin that can reduce the permeability to near zero. *(c)* Injured odontoblasts sometimes do not die but simply make more dentin at a fast rate, thereby increasing dentin thickness and reducing its permeability. *(d)* Intraluminal crystalline deposits (I) in tubules may lower dentin permeability. (Modified from Tziafas et al[16] with permission.)

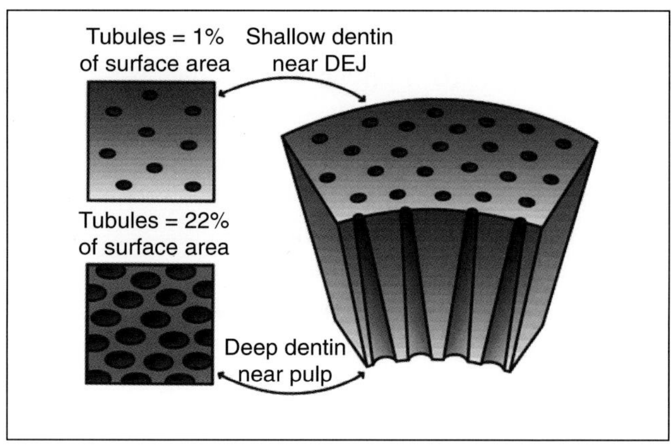

Fig 4-7 Each dentinal tubule is an inverted cone with the largest diameter at the pulp chamber or root canal and the smallest diameter at the cementodentinal junction (CDJ) or DEJ due to the progressive formation of more peritubular dentin. (Courtesy of Parkell, Biomaterials Division, Farmingdale, NY.)

causes the dimensions of the root canal to become increasingly smaller with age. The presence of cellular processes on odontoblasts makes primary and secondary dentin tubular in nature. The third type of dentin, *tertiary dentin* (also known as irritation dentin, irregular secondary dentin, reactionary dentin, or reparative dentin[16,26]) (Fig 4-6) is found only in dentin that has been subjected to trauma or irritation (eg, exposed hypersensitive cervical dentin, carious dentin, traumatic cavity preparation).

Because the circumference of the most peripheral part of the crown or root of a tooth is much larger than the circumference of the final pulp chamber or root canal space, the odontoblasts are forced closer together as they continue to lay down dentin, developing a pseudostratified columnar layer in parts of the coronal pulp, especially over pulp horns.[27,28] They are cuboidal in the root canal[24] and become flat near the apex.[22] The convergence of dentinal tubules toward the pulp creates a unique structural organization to dentin that has profound functional consequences, as will be discussed below. This convergence in the density of tubules has been estimated to be 5:1[29-31] in coronal dentin. It is less in root dentin but still more than 2:1.

Each individual dentinal tubule is an inverted cone with the smallest dimensions at the DEJ and the largest dimensions at the pulp (Fig 4-7). Originally, each tubule had a diameter of nearly 3 μm. However, within each tubule is a collagen-poor, hypermineralized cuff of intertubular dentin (see Fig 4-4), called *peritubular dentin* in many texts. It is actually periluminal dentin or, more accurately, intratubular dentin.[32] Its formation narrows the lumen of the tubule from its original 3 μm to as little as 0.6 to 0.8 μm in superficial dentin. This large amount of peritubular dentin in superficial dentin near the DEJ is due in part to the fact that it is "older" than middle or deep dentin. Thus, the width of intratubular (peritubular) dentin decreases as tubules are followed inward toward the pulp, with the exception that there is no peritubular dentin in intraglobular dentin.[33] Very close to the pulp, where there is no intratubular or peritubular dentin, the tubule (luminal) diameter is almost 3 μm.[34] Thus, most of the narrowing of the tubule lumen as one observes dentin more peripherally is due to deposition of peritubular dentin.[21,35,36] Although there have been reports of giant tubules 5 to 40 μm in diameter in human permanent and primary teeth,[37] they number fewer than 30 giant tubules per tooth. They extend from the pulp chamber to the incisal DEJ, but there is some question as to their patency. Similar developmental defects in incisal regions have been reported.[38,39]

The composition of collagen-poor and mineral-rich peritubular dentin is different from that of intertubular dentin (see Fig 4-4). The mineral is in the form of small calcium-deficient, carbonate-rich hydroxyapatite crystals, which have a higher crystallinity and are almost 5 times harder than intertubular dentin.[40] Little is known about the biologic control of peritubular dentin apposition. Although it is a very slow process, it can be accelerated by occlusal abrasion[41] and other forms of pulpal irritation and may be more rapid in primary[42] than in permanent teeth.

Although the complete composition of dentinal fluid is unknown, it presumably contains an ion product of calcium and phosphate near or above the solubility product constants for a number of forms of calcium phosphate.[43–45] This fluid tends to form mineral deposits in dentinal tubules, which may take many forms[38,39] (see Fig 4-6), for the outward movement of dentinal fluid presents a larger amount of mineral ions to the walls of the tubules than could occur by diffusion in sealed tubules. This principle has been used experimentally to slow the depth of demineralization of dentin in vivo under simulated caries-forming conditions.[46]

The permeability properties of dentinal tubules indicate that they have functionally much smaller dimensions than their actual microscopic dimensions.[47,48] Although the microscopic diameter of dentinal tubules at the DEJ has been reported to be 0.5 to 0.9 μm, they function as though they are 0.1 μm in diameter. Dentin can remove 99.8% of a bacterial suspension of streptococci that are approximately 0.5 μm in diameter when pressure is applied to the solution,[49] which tends to prevent infection of the pulp even when patients masticate on infected carious dentin. This phenomenon is why there are no bacteria in the tubules at the extreme front of the carious attack.[38] Although bacteria can invade dentinal tubules,[50] they do not invade as fast or as far in vital dentin,[51,52] presumably because dentinal fluid moving outward contains immunoglobulins.[53] Fluid shifts across dentin may occur, but the fluid is virtually sterile because of the presence of intratubular deposits of mineral and collagen fibrils that form multiple constrictions within the tubule to dimensions less than those of most microorganisms. In one study, 65% of the dentinal tubules in occlusal coronal dentin contained large collagen fibrils.[54] These would tend to trap any suspended bacteria as fluid flows through the tubules. The long-term effects of having bacteria trapped in tubules depend upon their source of nutrition and the effects of immunoglobulins from the pulp.

Extent of the odontoblast process

Controversy continues regarding the extent of the odontoblast process. Developmentally, odontoblast processes extend from the odontoblast cell body, through mineralized dentin matrix, to the dentin-enamel junction at the bell stage of tooth development. However, as dentin thickens, the cellular processes must elongate. Because there are no supporting cells or blood vessels in the tubules, the ability of the odontoblast cell body to support a long cytoplasmic process is questionable. In human teeth, the thickness of dentin is about 3 to 3.5 mm. Although nerve axons can be more than 1 m in length, they are not 3 mm from supporting cells or capillaries. In the absence of any evidence for cytoplasmic

Table 4-1 Dentinal tubule density and diameter at various distances from the pulp and the calculated areas of fluid-filled tubules, peritubular dentin, and intertubular dentin

Distance from pulp	Number* of tubules $\times 10^6/cm^2$	Radius* of tubules $\times 10^4/cm^{-4}$	Areas† Fluid-filled tubules (A_t)	Peritubular dentin (A_p)	Intertubular dentin (A_i)
0	4.5	1.25	22.10	66.25‡	11.65
0.1–0.5	4.3	0.95	12.19	36.58	51.23
0.6–1.0	3.8	0.80	7.64	22.92	69.44
1.1–1.5	3.5	0.60	3.96	11.89	84.15
1.6–2.0	3.0	0.55	2.85	8.55	88.60
2.1–2.5	2.3	0.45	1.46	4.39	94.15
2.6–3.0	2.0	0.40	1.01	3.01	95.98
3.1–3.5	1.9	0.40	0.96	2.86	96.18

*Data calculated from Garberoglio and Brännström.[34]

†$A_t = \pi r^2 N(100)$, where N = number of tubules per square cm. A_t, although an area, is also the percent of surface area occupied by water. $A_p = \pi N(R^2 - r^2)(100)$, where R = 2r and r = tubule radius. $A_i = 100 - (A_p - A_t)$.

‡There is no peritubular dentin at the pulpal surface, but it begins close to the pulpal surface.

streaming analogous to axon transport, it seems unlikely that any odontoblast could maintain such a long process.

The length of processes of most odontoblasts, regardless of dentin thickness, is between 0.1 and 1.0 mm.[55-61] The extent varies somewhat with species and position within the tooth.[55-57] The extent of the odontoblast process is important for a number of reasons. If odontoblasts participate directly in the mechanism of dentin sensitivity to surface stimuli, then these stimuli must interact with a cytoplasmic process. When cavities are prepared in deep dentin for restorative procedures, the odontoblast processes are amputated, thereby irritating the cell body residing in the pulp. Most studies[23,55-59,62] have shown that the process does not extend more than one third the length of the tubule under normal conditions. Based on this analysis, the odontoblast is probably not directly involved in dentin sensitivity.[63] Branching of dentinal tubules into multiple smaller lateral branches is extensive at the DEJ, minimal in middle dentin, and almost absent near the pulp.[64] In addition, branching of tubules is highest in the apical region and lowest in the coronal region.[26]

Changes in dentin structure with depth

The area occupied by the lumina of dentinal tubules can be calculated as the product of the cross-sectional area of a single tubule, πr^2, and N, the number of tubules per cm^2. The term *r* is the radius of the tubule. Because both the radius of dentinal tubules and their number per unit area increase[31,65,66] as one examines dentin from the DEJ to the pulp, the area occupied by tubule lumina also increases. Garberoglio and Brännström measured the tubule radius by carefully correcting for shrinkage artifact.[34] Table 4-1 uses their data and provides calculations for the area occupied by tubule lumina at the DEJ and near the pulp.[67,68] Because this area is occupied by dentinal fluid, which is 95% water, these areas are also approximately equal to their tubular water content. That is, the water content of dentin near the DEJ is about 1% (volume percent), while that of dentin near the pulp is about 22%, a 20-fold variation. Textbooks list the water content of dentin at approximately 10% by weight or 20% by volume,[69] but that is an average value (Table 4-2).

The difficulty in bonding to deep dentin is caused, in part, by its high water content, which competes with resin monomers for the surfaces

Table 4-2 Chemical composition of dentin

	Mineral wt% (vol%)	Organic wt% (vol%)	Water wt% (vol%)
LeGeros[69]	70 (47)	20 (30)	10 (21)
Kinney et al[82]	65 (45)	35 (48)	— (7)
Frank et al[83]	70 (47)	20 (32)	10 (21)

of collagen fibrils.[70,71] Fortunately, the water content can be controlled in nonvital dentin, which facilitates bonding to endodontically treated dentin. This phenomenon may become more important in endodontics as the use of adhesive resins for secondary seals increases in popularity. It is well known that loss or leakage of the access-opening temporary restorative material can lead to bacterial contamination of root canal fillings.[72-77] To avoid such contamination, several investigations have recommended the use of secondary seals on the floor of the pulp chamber that extend over the orifice of the filled canal.[78-81] This technique not only protects the root canal filling from leakage but also seals off any accessory canals that might exist on the pulpal floor. The use of transparent, unfilled resins is preferred because they permit observation of the underlying gutta-percha and are soft enough to remove easily should retreatment be necessary.

Chemical composition of dentin

The composition of bulk dentin (see Table 4-2) has been reported to be 70% mineral, 20% organic, and 10% water.[21] Due to the high density of dentin (ranging between 2.05 and 2.30 g/cm^{-3}), the weight percentage is much higher than volume percentage.[84]

The mineral phase of dentin is a calcium-deficient carbonate-rich apatite with platelike crystals of intertubular dentin 50 to 60 nm long,[85] 36.4 ± 1.5 nm wide, and 10.3 ± 0.3 nm thick.[86] This small size, relative to large apatite crystals in enamel, is thought to be responsible for the high critical pH of dentin (pH 6.7). This crystal size is clinically significant because root dentin demineralizes at less than 10% of the hydrogen ion concentration required for enamel demineralization (pH 6.7 vs 5.5), making dentin more susceptible to caries than enamel once root surfaces become exposed.[87] Trace elements are also found in dentin.[69,88,89] About 90% of the organic portion of the dentin matrix is made up of type I collagen; noncollagenous protein growth factors and proteoglycans make up the remainder.[90-92] The water content of dentin varies with location, but bulk dentin has been reported to be between 8% and 16% water,[89] most of which is unbound water that can be removed by heating to 120°C. A small fraction of the water (probably less than 1%) is associated with apatite crystals and with collagen.

Physical characteristics of dentin

Dentin is a heterogeneous composite material that contains micrometer-diameter tubules surrounded by highly mineralized (about 95 vol% mineral phase) peritubular dentin embedded within a partially mineralized (about 30 vol% mineral phase) collagen matrix (intertubular dentin).[93,94] The bulk of tooth structure is made up of dentin, which is the vital part of the tooth (Table 4-3).

Dentin is much softer than enamel (Knoop hardness of 68 vs 343 kg/mm^{-2}). The softness of dentin makes it wear much faster than enamel[95] and permits efficient endodontic instrumentation with hand or rotary files.[96] Dentin is also more elastic than enamel (modulus of elasticity of about 11 to 20 vs 86 GPa). This greater elasticity makes dentin tougher than enamel, and it also supports dentin's stress-breaking or shock-absorbing function for the overlying enamel.

Recent modifications to the atomic force microscope (AFM) permit measurement of both nanohardness and the modulus of elasticity of intertubular and peritubular dentin.[40] Peritubular dentin has a greater nanohardness than intertubular dentin (250 KHN vs 52 KHN). In addition, deep dentin tends to be more elastic than superficial dentin (modulus of elasticity of about 17 vs 21 GPa). The shear strength of dentin also varies by

Table 4-3 Mechanical properties of dentin

Mechanical properties	Dentin* Bulk	Peritubular	Intertubular
Compressive strength (MPa)	217–300[95]	–	–
Young's modulus (GPa)	11–19.9[99,101]	29.8–30[94]	16–21.1[94]
Shear strength (MPa)	45–132[97,98]	–	–
Tensile strength (MPa)	31–106[99,101]	–	–
Microhardness (kg/mm^{-2})	40–70[96]	–	–
Nanohardness (GPa)	–	2.2–2.5[94]	0.12–0.52[94]

*Because dentin is not homogeneous, values are given in ranges.

region, with superficial dentin having greater shear strength than deep dentin (132 vs 45 MPa).[97] Although measured using a different technique, the shear strength of middle dentin is reported to be about 72.4 to 86.9 MPa.[98]

The ultimate tensile strength of human dentin has been reported to range from 36 to 100 MPa, with the larger value derived from recent studies using smaller specimens.[99-101] The bulk modulus of elasticity (ε) of human dentin has been reported to range from 11 to 19 GPa, with a value of 14 GPa derived from recent studies using smaller specimens.[99-101]

Due to wide variation in the microscopic structure of dentin, one would expect the mechanical properties of dentin to vary across regions. Indeed, the values given for the bulk mechanical properties of dentin are generally listed as a range because they are not uniform. For instance, microhardness values in the crown fall from 350 kg/mm^{-2} in enamel to 50 kg/mm^{-2} in dentin just beneath the DEJ, rise to 70 kg/mm^{-2} within 1 mm from the DEJ, and then decline slowly to the pulp (40 to 50 kg/mm^{-2} near the pulp).[102] Similar distributions are found for the modulus of elasticity.[103] Thus, mantle dentin and the zone of interglobular dentin about 200 μm from the DEJ are less mineralized,[25] less stiff regions compared with the stiffer inner core of dentin. Root dentin has an even lower microhardness as it is measured from the cementoenamel junction (CEJ) (about 30 kg/mm^{-2}), rises to 52 kg/mm^{-2} about halfway across, and then falls to 40 to 45 kg/mm^{-2} near the pulp.[102] This variation in mechanical properties of dentin plays a critical role in the distribution of mechanical forces through a tooth.

Mechanics of root dentin

What have been needed in dental mechanics are techniques that can show the distribution of stresses and strains in dental hard tissues under load. Modeling techniques such as the use of model teeth constructed of photoelastic materials[104,105] or the use of finite element stress analysis[106] have been questioned because they assume uniform mechanical properties. Alternative techniques measure the distribution of stress or strain applied to whole teeth.[107] For example, grids used to support tiny tissue sections for transmission electron microscopy have been used to transfer microscopic patterns to tooth surfaces. This permits multiple measurements of regional microstrains by measuring distortions in the grid.[108] A more sophisticated approach involves the application of Moiré gratings (200 lines/mm^{-1}) to longitudinal sections of teeth, permitting measurement of two-dimensional strain fields.[109] Under these conditions, most of the strain was found in the low-modulus, 200-μm-thick region just below the DEJ and at the CEJ, suggesting that these low-modulus zones act as stress buffers or cushions. An even more sensitive method, called Moiré interferometry, uses laser light and a grating with 2,000 lines/

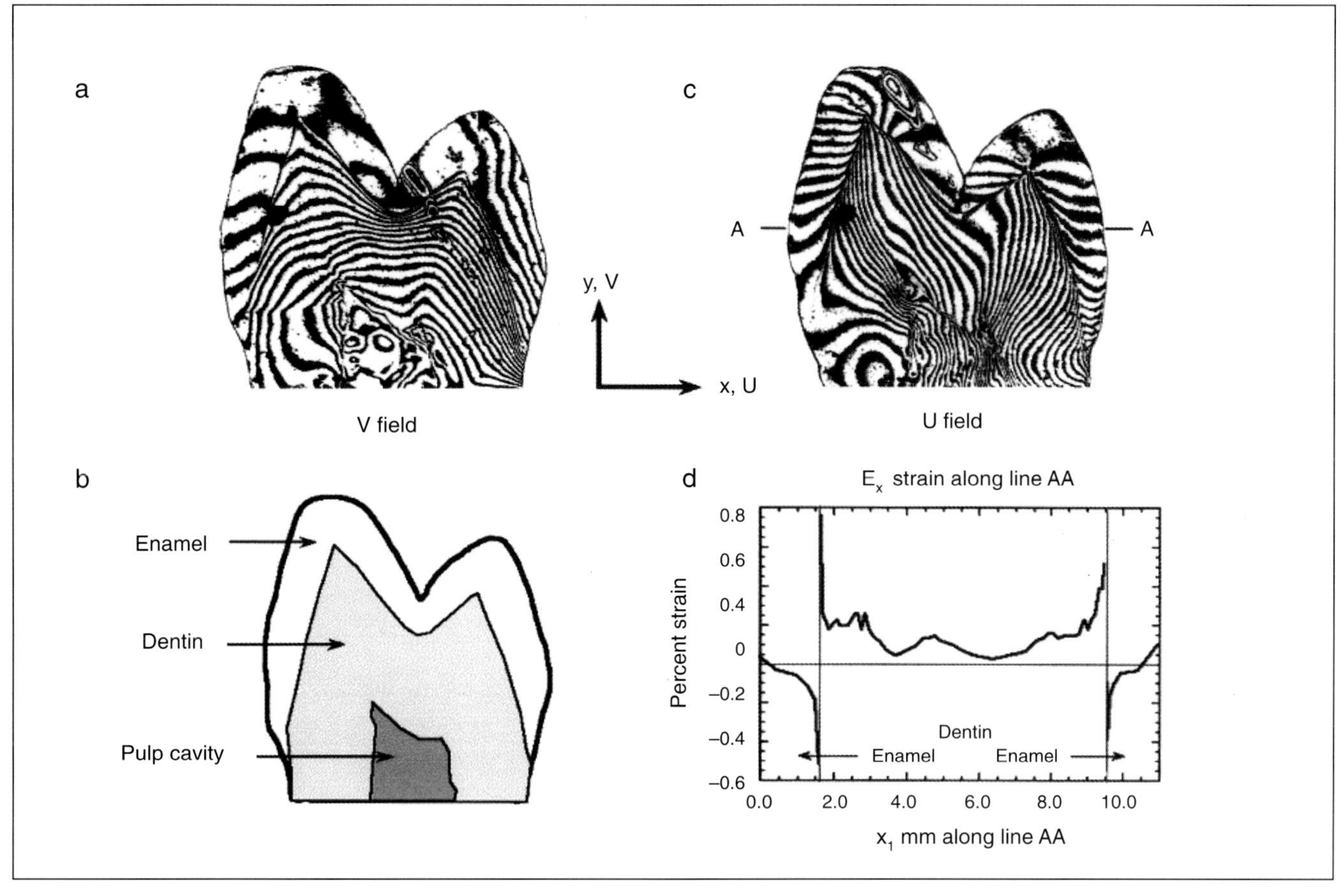

Fig 4-8 Plane-field strain patterns in a longitudinally sectioned tooth. A diffraction grating with 2,000 lines/mm was transferred to the polished surface while the tooth was dry, and the tooth was allowed to rehydrate. When viewed in a Moiré interferometer, there was little strain (ie, few fringes) in the specimen when it was dry (not shown). The higher water content of dentin and its much lower modulus of elasticity than enamel permitted more strain (ie, more interference fringes) to develop in dentin than in enamel. Similar strains can be induced by compressive forces. *(a)* Plane strain in the longitudinal or y-axis. *(b)* Schematic diagram showing longitudinally sectioned tooth. *(c)* Same specimen showing strain in the x-axis. *(d)* Graph of percent strain versus distance along line AA. Negative strain is compression. Clinically, dentin is usually moist but is then often air dried, which produces the same qualitative graph, though inverted. (Courtesy of Dr Judy Wood, Clemson University.)

mm^{-2} (Fig 4-8). Few interference fringes were apparent when the grid was placed on the relatively dry longitudinally sectioned tooth, but after allowing the specimen to rehydrate, the dentin gained more moisture than the enamel and hence expanded, creating negative (eg, compressive) strains, the magnitude of which is shown in the closeness of the fringes (see Fig 4-8). Changes in full-field microstrains can be quantitated by taking sequential photographs of the changing fringe patterns, followed by quantitative image analysis.[110,111]

Because of the regional differences in mineral distribution, hardness, and elastic modulus within root dentin,[112] such two-dimensional studies need to be done in the x, y, and z planes. For example, multiple rosette strain gauges were placed on the buccal plate of bone over a maxillary central incisor at the cervical, middle, and apical thirds of the root in a patient undergoing surgery.[113] The tooth was then loaded, and strains induced in the overlying bone were measured. Maximum strain was found in the bone over the cervical region, intermediate strain in the bone over the middle third, and no strain in the bone over the apical third. In another patient who had lost buccal bone to periodontal disease, the same procedures were

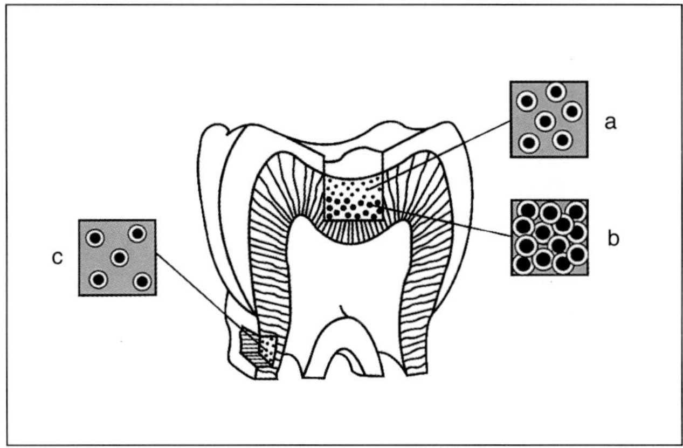

Fig 4-9 Schematic representation of cavities prepared on the occlusal surface of coronal dentin *(a,b)* and at the cervical region of the root surface *(c)*. Note that there are fewer tubules in superficial dentin *(a)* than in deep dentin *(b)* and that the tubules are not only closer together in deep dentin but larger in diameter. This combination is responsible for the exponential increase in dentin permeability with depth. (Reprinted from Pashley[19] with permission.)

repeated with rosette strain gauges fixed to the cervical, middle, and apical thirds of root dentin. The strains in root dentin were much lower than in bone, and the distribution of shear strain on the bone surface was nearly constant. In these studies, most of the axial bite forces were distributed along the cervical and middle thirds of the root and of the supporting bone, thereby relieving the apical region of stress and strain. This distribution of forces may protect blood vessels entering the root apex from occlusal forces that might transiently cut off venous outflow.[113]

The ideal approach to evaluating the mechanical properties of teeth under function is to use three-dimensional quantitative microscopic X-ray tomography.[114,115] Such studies will permit quantitative 3-D microstrains in teeth under functional loads before and after endodontic therapy, cementation of posts, etc.

Permeability of coronal dentin

The tubular structure of dentin provides channels for the passage of solutes and solvents across dentin. The number of dentinal tubules per square millimeter varies from 15,000 at the DEJ to 65,000 at the pulp.[26,28,30,34,66] Because both the density and diameter of the tubules increase with dentin depth from the DEJ, the permeability of dentin is lowest at the DEJ and highest at the pulp (Fig 4-9; see also Table 4-1). However, at any depth, the permeability of dentin in vitro is far below what would be predicted by the tubule density and diameters due to the presence of intratubular material such as collagen fibrils, mineralized constrictions of the tubules, etc.[116] The permeability of dentin is highest for small molecules (Fig 4-10) such as water, lower for larger molecules such as albumin and immunoglobulins, and still lower for molecules with MW over 10^6 such as endotoxins. The details of methods used to measure dentin permeability may be found elsewhere.[48]

Dentin permeability is divided into two broad categories: *(1)* transdentinal movement of substances through dentinal tubules, such as fluid shifts in response to hydrodynamic stimuli, and *(2)* intradentinal movement of exogenous substances into intertubular dentin, as occurs with infiltration of hydrophilic adhesive resins into demineralized dentin surfaces during resin bonding (Fig 4-11) or demineralization of intertubular dentin by acids.[82,118]

Dentin may be regarded both as a barrier and as a permeable structure, depending on its thickness, age, and other variables.[119] Dentin's tubular structure makes it very porous. The minimum porosity of normal peripheral coronal dentin is about 15,000 tubules per square millimeter. Once uncovered by trauma or tooth preparation, these tubules become diffusion channels from the surface to the pulp. The rate of diffusional flux of exogenous material across the dentin to the pulp is highly dependent upon dentin thickness and the hydraulic conductance of dentin.[48,120] Thin dentin permits much more diffusional flux than

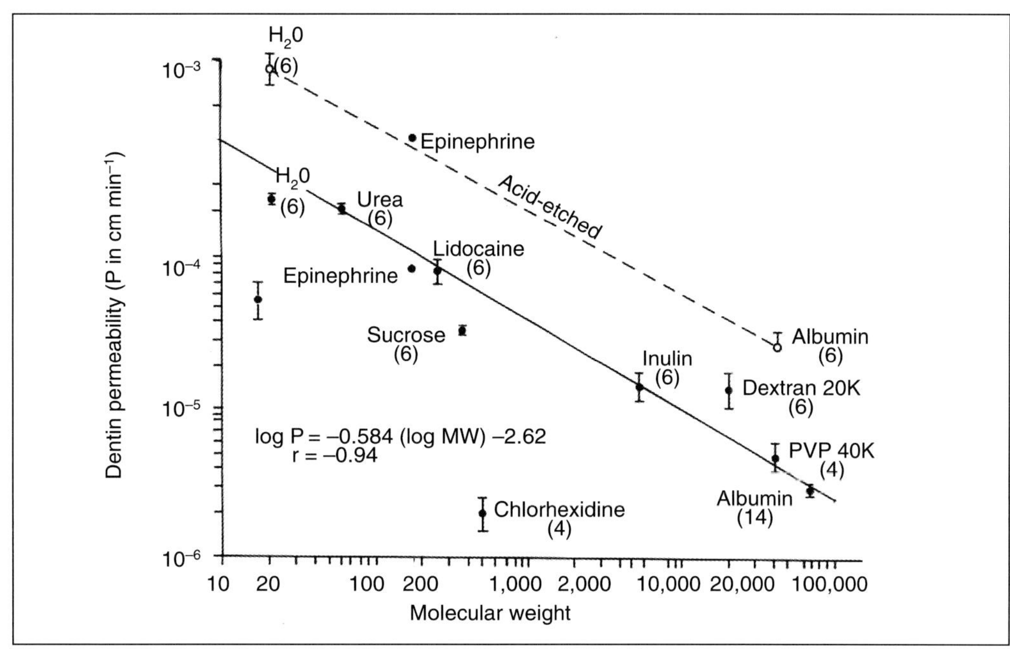

Fig 4-10 Permeability of dentin for various substances. Permeability decreases as a function of molecular weight (MW), or more accurately, with the cube root of MW. The solid line indicates the results obtained with smear-layer–covered dentin; the dashed line indicates the higher permeability of acid-etched dentin. (Reprinted from Pashley and Livingston[117] with permission.)

does thick dentin. However, in exposed vital dentin with open tubules, the inward diffusional flux of materials competes with the rinsing action of outward convective fluid transport.[12,121] This competition may serve a protective function in mitigating the inward flux of potentially irritating bacterial products into exposed, sensitive dentin.

The permeability of dentin is not uniform but varies widely, especially on occlusal surfaces, where perhaps only 30% of the tubules (Fig 4-12) are in free communication with the pulp.[123] Scanning electron microscopic examination of acid-etched occlusal dentin reveals that all the tubules are exposed, but functional studies of the distribution of fluid movement across the occlusal dentin reveal that the tubules that communicate with the pulp are located over pulp horns and that the central region is relatively impermeable. Apparently, intratubular materials such as collagen fibrils[54] and mineralized deposits restrict fluid movement even though the peripheral and central ends of the tubules are patent. Even microscopically, within any 100 × 100 μm field, only a few tubules are patent from the periphery to the pulp.[124]

Axial dentin is much more permeable than occlusal dentin.[125,126] The gingival floor, proximal boxes, or gingival extension of finish lines in crown preparations often ends in regions of high dentin permeability.[127] As many as 4 million exposed dentinal tubules are found in a surface area of approximately 1 cm^2 in full-crown preparations on posterior teeth.[68] Although the tubules are occluded by smear layers and/or cement following placement of castings, both cement and smear layers have finite solubilities and may permit some tubules to become exposed over time, most likely occurring at the most peripheral extensions of restorations, where diffusion distances to the pulp are shortest.

The permeability of sclerotic dentin is very low,[128] regardless of whether the sclerosis was due to physiologic or pathologic processes, because the tubules become filled with mineral deposits. Indeed, this reaction is fortuitous in that

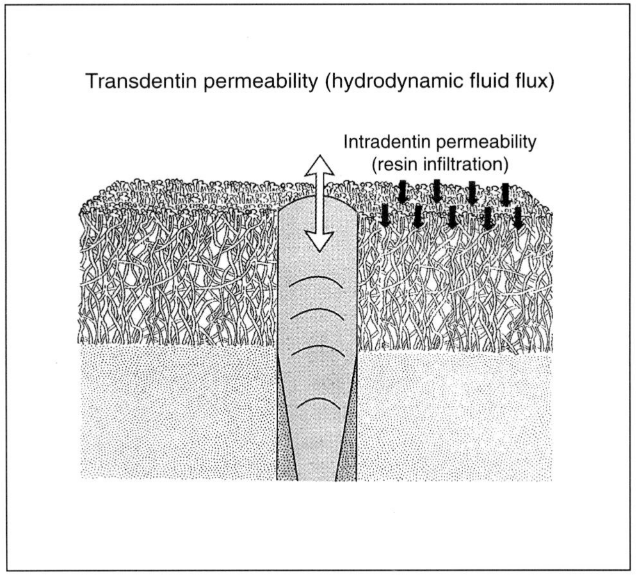

Fig 4-11 Schematic diagram contrasting transdentinal permeablity due to movement of materials within tubules and intradentin permeability in which materials diffuse into porosities created between tubules by demineralization. (Reprinted from Pashley[19] with permission.)

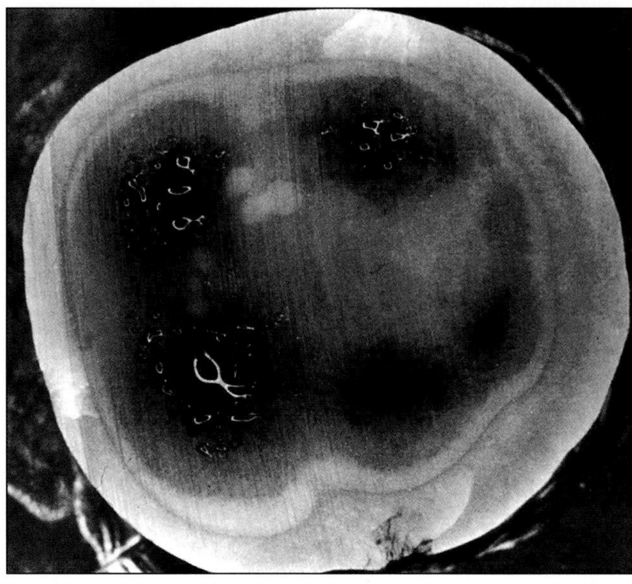

Fig 4-12 Photograph showing fluid moving across dentin from the underlying pulp chamber in vitro under a simulated pulpal pressure of 20 cm H_2O. Note that the dentin is most permeable over the pulp horns, where the tubules have their largest diameters and densities. (Reprinted from Pashley et al[123] with permission.)

it slows the caries process and tends to protect the pulp. Most pulpal reactions to cavity preparations or restorative materials used on carious dentin are due to changes that occur across adjacent normal dentin rather than the almost impermeable caries-affected dentin.

Permeability of root dentin

As in coronal dentin, the permeability of root dentin depends upon dentin thickness, the number of tubules/mm^2, and the diameter and patency of the tubules.[48,68,120] There are more tubules/mm^2 in deep dentin near the canal than in peripheral dentin because the outer circumference of the root is larger than the circumference of the root canal (Fig 4-13). The number of tubules (and odontoblasts) remains constant from the outer root dentin to the root canal, but the tubules become crowded together at the canal.[129] Although a number of authors have reported tubule densities in various regions of teeth, few have been specific about the exact location. For example, the greater concavity of buccal or lingual walls, compared with mesial or distal walls, increases tubule density. In premolars, dentinal tubule densities of the pulpal wall at the level of the CEJ are higher on the lingual side than the mesial or distal side (72,000 vs 44,000 tubules/mm^2).[28] There is less concavity in third molars (ie, the crown is more square in outline), and the corresponding dentinal tubule densities are more similar (66,000 vs 61,000 tubules/mm^2). Given these values for tubule density (72,000 tubules/mm^2) and known values for the radius of each tubule (2.5 μm), one can calculate the percentage of dentin surface area occupied by tubule lumina.[31,66,68,130] By this calculation, 35% of the area of the buccal wall of the coronal pulp chamber of premolars is occupied by tubules. Although the permeability of dentin should be proportional to the area occupied by dentinal tubules, quantitative comparisons of the theoretical or calculated permeability versus the actual measured permeability revealed the latter to be less than 3% of the

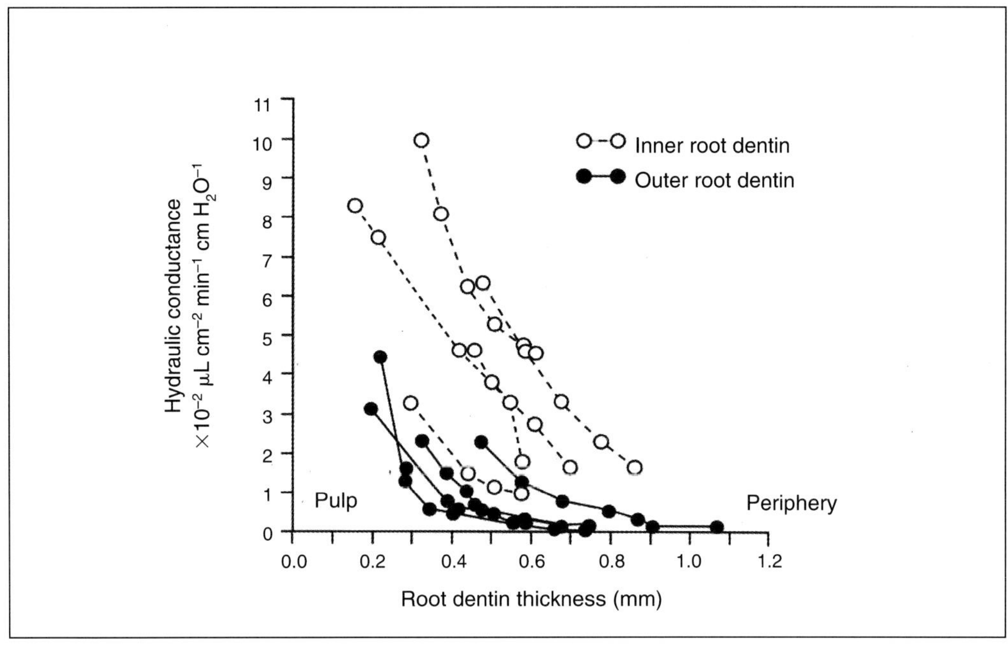

Fig 4-13 Permeability of inner and outer root dentin as a function of dentin thickness. Flat root surfaces were split longitudinally into outer and inner halves, each about 1.1 mm thick. The permeability of the outer half *(solid circles)* was low even after removal of cementum (from 1.1 to 0.9 mm) and then only slowly increased as the dentin was made thinner by grinding the periphery. The rate of increase of root dentin permeability was much higher in inner dentin *(open circles)*. (Modified from Fogel et al[129] with permission.)

theoretical value.[110] This finding is explained by the fact that dentinal tubules are not smooth bore tubes but contain a good deal of intratubular material such as mineralized nodules and collagen fibrils.[54,131]

Dentinal permeability has numerous clinical implications. For example, NaOCl is a commonly used irrigant in endodontic procedures. Soaking dentin disks in 5% NaOCl for 1 hr produces a 105% increase in the hydraulic conductance of human cervical dentin.[132] In contrast, soaking dentin disks with even 35% H_2O_2 for 1 hr produces a 16% decrease in permeability.

During endodontic instrumentation of root canals, the softest inner dentin is removed.[96] The increase in the diameter of the root canal leads to a decrease in the number of tubules/mm^2 (the exact opposite of what occurs in operative dentistry when drilling from the enamel toward the pulp). In addition, the root dentin is made slightly thinner.[133] These two phenomena tend to influence root dentin permeability oppositely, with the reduction in thickness being more dominant. However, the shaping of the canal also creates long smear plugs[134] and thick smear layers[62,129] on the instrumented surface that decrease the permeability of dentin.

Smear layers and smear plugs

Smear plugs are composed of grinding debris whose particle sizes are smaller than tubule orifices (Figs 4-14 to 4-16). Although most smear plugs in coronal or radicular dentinal tubules are only 1 to 3 µm long, smear plugs in instrumented root canals are up to 40 times longer (40 µm), because the tubule diameters are so much larger at the pulp chamber.[128] The presence of grinding debris in the tubule orifices and on the dentin surface also lowers the permeability of dentin.[67,135,136] Treatment of smear layers with NaOCl

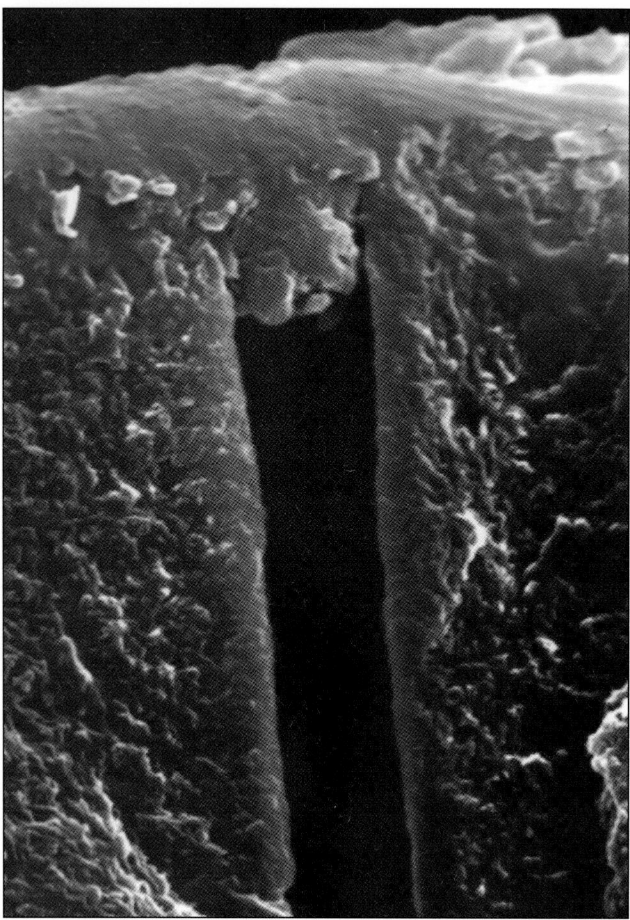

Fig 4-14 SEM of the fractured edge of smear-layer–covered dentin showing that the smear layer is about 0.5 μm thick and continuous with the smear plug, shown here to be about 1 μm deep. The smear layer and plugs function as a unit to lower permeability. (Reprinted from Pashley[19] with permission.)

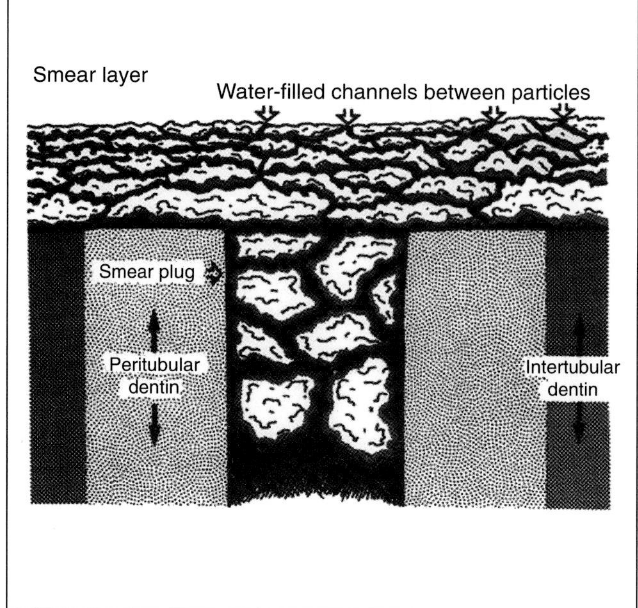

Fig 4-15 Schematic diagram illustrating that smear layers and smear plugs are made up of submicron pieces of grinding or cutting debris burnished together and to the underlying dentin. Although it looks solid in Fig 4-14, isotope tracer studies have shown the debris to be permeable to water-soluble materials (see Fig 4-10) via water-filled channels around constituent particles. (Reprinted from Pashley et al[144] with permission.)

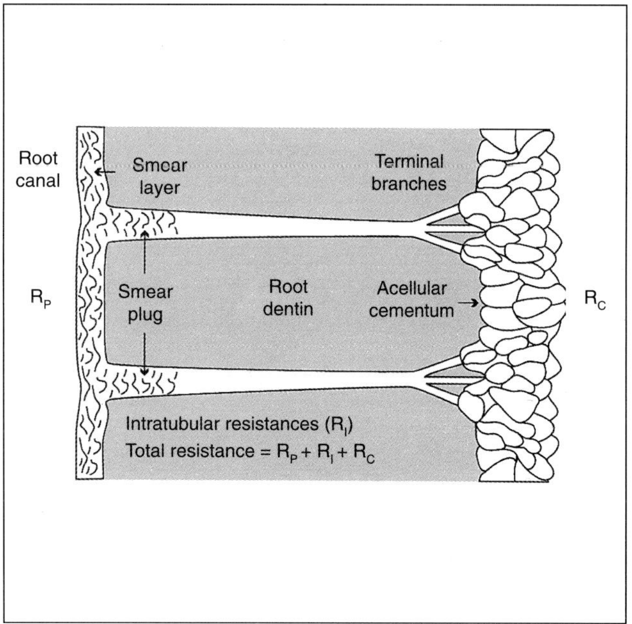

Fig 4-16 Schematic diagram illustrating that instrumented radicular dentin is occluded on the inside by a smear layer and smear plugs and on the outside by cementum. The tubules in root dentin taper to submicron terminal branches that reduce radicular permeability. The total resistance to fluid flow across root dentin is the sum of the pulpal resistance due to the presence of a smear layer and smear plugs (R_P); intratubular resistance due to the presence of intratubular collagen fibrils, mineralized nodules, etc (R_I); and the peripheral cemental resistance (R_C).

does not remove the smear layer[137] because most of the organic component is masked by mineral. Only after removal of the mineral with EDTA or acids can NaOCl remove the organic portion.[138] This restriction is the rationale for the sequential use of NaOCl and EDTA as endodontic irrigants for removal of the smear layer.

Any instrument placed in contact with the root canal or pulp chamber will create a smear layer. For example, instrumentation with K-files decreases the permeability of root dentin by 49%.[139] The presence of the smear layer and smear plugs prevents the entry of sealer[140] or thermoplasticized gutta-percha[141] into dentinal tubules. However, the critical seal is in the apical third, a region where it is difficult to remove the smear layer. It is important to understand that the mere presence of dental materials (eg, sealer or gutta-percha "tags") in tubules does not ensure a perfect seal. For example, in resin bonding studies, the presence of long resin tags in dentinal tubules was not correlated with lack of microleakage because most of the tags were loose.[142]

Moreover, even the absence of a smear layer on the dentinal surface may not necessarily correlate with increased dentinal permeability.[143] To evaluate this possibility, the canals of single-rooted teeth were endodontically instrumented, filled with radioactive water, and the diffusional flux of the water was measured before and after removal of the smear layer. Removal of the smear layer with 0.5 mol/L EDTA and 5% NaOCl resulted in a 34% decrease in permeability. When the measurements were repeated after soaking the specimens in water for 2 months, the permeability of roots to tritiated water had increased 81% above the previously measured values. Apparently, during the treatment of root canals with EDTA, the concentration of ionized calcium and phosphate in tubular fluid increases to high levels, allowing the formation of precipitates in the tubules that actually lower the permeability of dentin, even though SEM studies of these surfaces indicate that the smear layer has been removed. Over the next 2 months, these precipitates slowly dissolved, leading to an increase in permeability.

Table 4-4 Comparison of coronal vs radicular hydraulic conductance of dentin*

Thickness (mm)	Lp ($\mu L\ cm^{-2}\ minute^{-1}\ cm\ H_2O^{-1}$)	
	Coronal	Radicular
0.9	0.1210	0.0005
0.7	0.1850	0.0204
0.6	0.390	0.0304
0.2	—	0.0701
0.1	1.500	0.0801

*Reprinted from Pashley[122] with permission.

Thus, SEM studies demonstrating smear layer removal may not indicate an increase in dentin permeability because they fail to show subsurface changes that can have a profound effect on dentin permeability.

The permeability of root dentin and coronal dentin is not uniform.[143] When measured for hydraulic conductance, root dentin has a permeability that is only about 3% to 8% as great as that of coronal dentin (Table 4-4). It is likely that the relative impermeability of root dentin protects the periodontal tissues from the wide variety of potentially cytotoxic compounds that historically have been placed in root canals to sterilize them.[129,145,146] Similarly, the low permeability of root dentin prevents sulcular endotoxins[147] from diffusing into the pulp. Part of the barrier properties of the root are due to the low permeability of cementum,[148] although this characteristic may increase in periodontally involved teeth.

Cementum serves as a "surface resistor" in series with root dentin to reduce permeability (see Fig 4-16). For example, the outer half of root dentin slabs, covered peripherally by cementum, has a very low permeability as compared with the inner half slabs (see Fig 4-13).[129] Even after removal of all of the cementum, the permeability remains low until more than 200 µm of outer dentin is removed because there is no sharp demarcation between cementum and root dentin,[149] and multiple branches in the tubules of root dentin[26] often modify the hydraulic conduc-

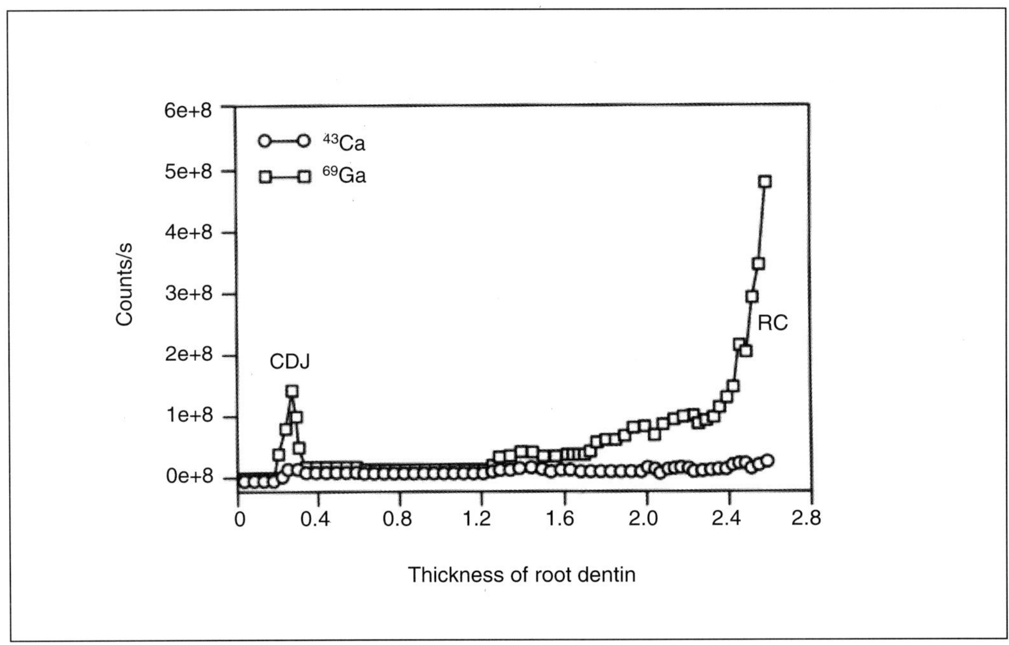

Fig 4-17 Root canal filled with 1 mol/L citrate-chelated gallium nitrate for 1 week in vitro in an attempt to permeate gallium from the root canal space to the cemental surface, where it could inhibit osteoclast-induced external resorption. The root was split-mounted on a stage and subjected to continuous laser ablation (266 nm). The plume of dentin "dust" was swept into an inductively coupled plasma mass spectrometer to quantitate the amount of gallium and calcium across the thickness of root dentin. The y-axis represents counts/sec of ^{69}gallium or ^{43}calcium, both naturally occurring, nonradioactive isotopes. Note that the concentration of ^{43}Ca was constant across the thickness of the root (2.4 mm) but that the concentration of gallium was very high near the canal (RC), fell as the tubules became smaller, and increased again at the CDJ due to low barrier properties of cementum.

tance of dentin.[150] After removal of the most external root dentin, the permeability of the outer half of the root dentin slabs increases rapidly (see Fig 4-13). Other studies have confirmed the importance of cementum in reducing the permeability of root dentin. In one study,[133] two groups of single-rooted teeth underwent endodontic instrumentation. One group had all of the cementum and some external root dentin removed (about 0.5 mm) along with the smear layer on the instrumented external surface, and the second group had intact cementum layers sealing the external surfaces. The group without cementum showed significant increases in permeability during extirpation of the pulp, cleaning and shaping with NaOCl, and removal of the smear layer with EDTA. In another study, gallium nitrate, a substance known to inhibit osteoclasts,[151] was placed in the canal of extracted teeth as a therapeutic dressing for 1 week. It was then removed, the root was sectioned longitudinally, and the amount of gallium taken up by root dentin was quantitated by laser ablation combined with inductively coupled plasma mass spectrometry.[152] The gallium concentration was highest adjacent to the canal but fell off as the more peripheral dentin was sampled. At the extreme periphery near the cementum, the gallium concentration rose (Fig 4-17). This finding was interpreted to confirm previous observations that cementum has a lower permeability than root dentin.[148,153,154] Thus, cementum and the low permeability of peripheral root dentin protect the periodontium from chemicals that are used during root canal therapy.

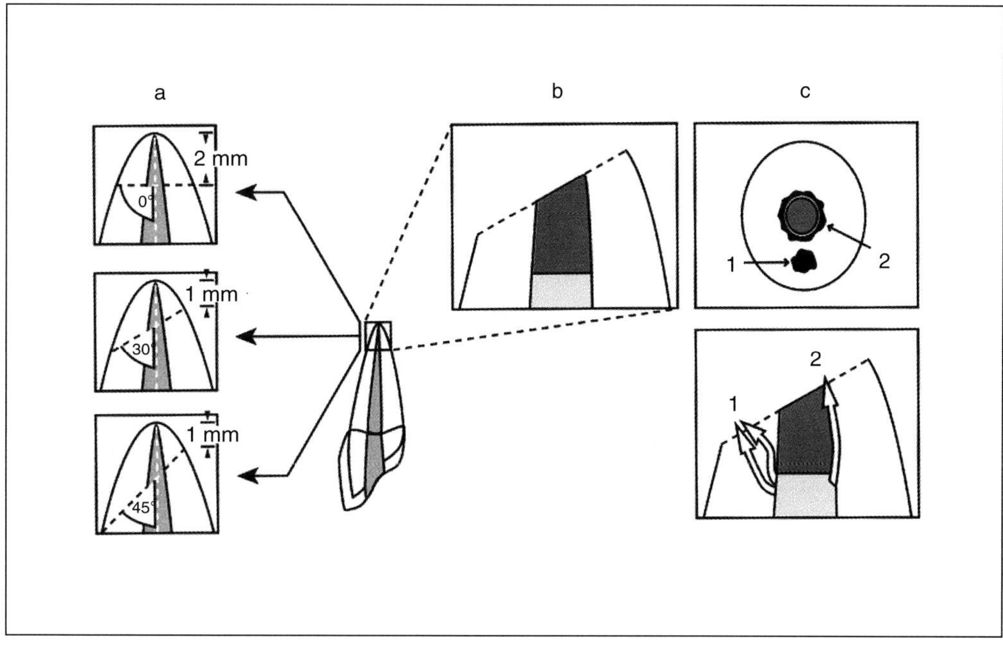

Fig 4-18 Schematic diagram showing the influence of apical bevel angle on the depth of the reverse filling required to prevent leakage of substances through exposed dentinal tubules. *(a)* Possible angles of resection. *(b)* Reverse filling. *(c)* Routes of leakage via gaps around the filling (2) or via tubules that were not sealed by filling (1). (Modified from Gilheany et al[163] with permission.)

Upon closer examination, the permeability of root dentin itself is not uniform but displays regional differences along its axial length. Cervical and middle root dentin have higher permeabilities than apical dentin,[133,145,154,155] consistent with their higher tubule density as compared with apical dentin.[156] The permeability of the floor of the pulp chamber in the region of the furcation has been reported to be high because of the presence of accessory canals.[157-160] However, subsequent studies examining the floor of the pulp chamber in 100 unerupted third molars found only one tooth with a patent accessory canal.[161] The higher incidence of accessory canals reported in earlier studies may have been due to soaking specimens in 5% NaOCl, which may have removed organic material in accessory canals, thereby exaggerating their incidence. Although it is possible that the use of third molars may have underestimated the incidence of accessory canals, other studies using SEM to examine the pulpal floors of human molars revealed only two accessory canals out of 87 human molars.[24] Thus, the current findings clearly demonstrate that coronal and middle root dentin have greater permeability than apical dentin, with permeability of the pulpal floor being largely influenced by the presence of patent accessory canals.

Endodontists need to be especially aware of the tubule density of apical dentin because this region may be beveled during apical surgery. During such surgery, the resection of the root at an oblique angle may be favored to facilitate visibility and the placement of a reverse filling. However, this angled resection may expose dentinal tubules beneath the retrofilling material, thereby introducing the possibility of tubule leakage (Fig 4-18). The greater the angle of the root resection, the greater the potential for microleakage.[162,163] Thus, minimally angled resections have been advocated along with placement of the reverse filling below the edge of the bevel to prevent

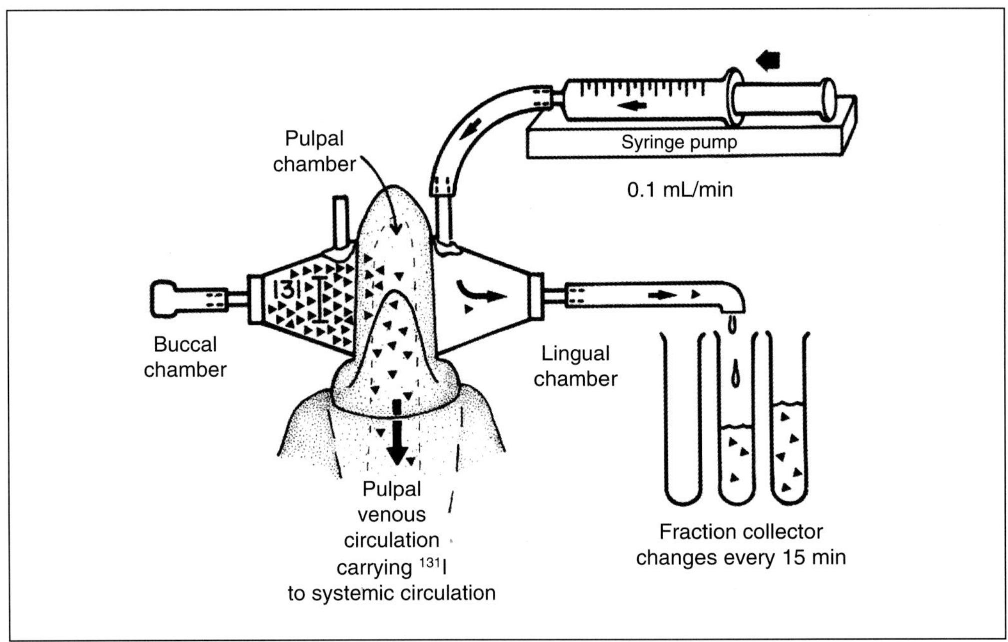

Fig 4-19 Schematic diagram illustrating how dual chambers were placed on both buccal and lingual surfaces of dog molars to measure both systemic absorption of substances applied to dentin and changes in pulpal interstitial fluid concentration of substances. Triangles indicate radioactive iodide. (Reprinted from Pashley[17] with permission.)

leakage through dentinal tubules exposed by the bevel (see Fig 4-18). The steeper the bevel, the deeper the reverse filling must be to prevent this leakage. In addition to apical root resection with near-zero-degree bevels, others have proposed sealing the resected surface with resin, eliminating the need for a reverse filling.[164–166] Several quantitative and qualitative studies have evaluated dentinal tubules in apical dentin.[156,167–171] As described above, the tubule density is much lower in apical dentin than in coronal dentin, and the density of apical dentinal tubules can be further reduced with age, becoming nearly translucent over time due to increased deposition of mineral crystals.

Balance between permeation of noxious substances across dentin and clearance

There is a balance (Fig 4-19) between the rate at which materials permeate exposed dentin to reach the pulp and the rate at which they are cleared from interstitial fluid by the pulpal microcirculation and lymphatic vessels.[17,19,119,120] This is shown in Fig 4-19, where conical chambers were placed on the buccal and lingual surfaces of a dog molar in vivo. Radioactive iodide (triangles in Fig 4-19) was placed in the buccal chamber. The lingual chamber was perfused with samples collected by a fraction collector. Blood samples, drawn every 10 minutes, revealed that the pulpal circulation cleared almost all of the iodide that permeated the buccal dentin. Little iodide showed up in the rinsing fluid of the lingual chamber (open triangles in Fig 4-20) until epinephrine was added to the buccal chamber, causing cessation of pulpal blood flow and accumulation of iodide in the pulp, as indicated by the large increase in iodide diffusing across the lingual dentin. Procedures that reduce pulpal blood flow (eg, activation of pulpal sympathetic nerves, administration of vasoconstrictor agents with local anesthetics) (see Fig 4-20) upset this balance, permitting higher interstitial fluid concentrations of extrinsic material to exist than

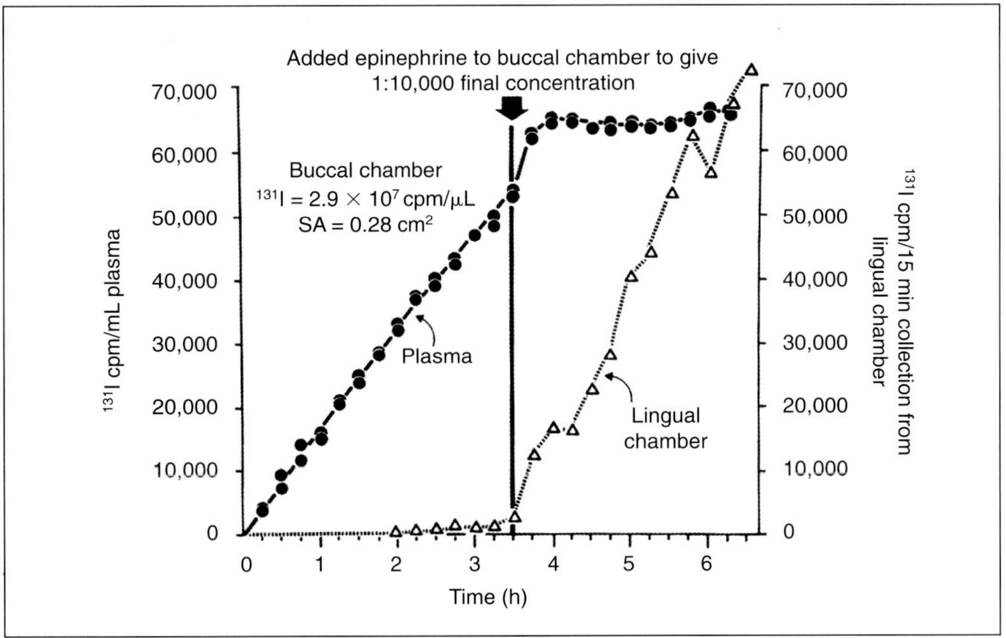

Fig 4-20 Effects of topical epinephrine on pulpal interstitial fluid iodide concentration. Over the first 3.5 hours, the plasma iodide concentration rose linearly as iodide permeated the buccal dentin into the pulp where the microcirculation cleared it so efficiently that little iodide ever showed up in rinsings from the lingual chamber. However, as soon as epinephrine was added to the buccal chamber, the pulpal clearance stopped, and the insterstitial fluid concentration rose and began diffusing across the lingual dentin into the lingual chamber. (Reprinted from Pashley[17] with permission.)

would occur at normal levels of capillary flow.[119] The control of pulpal blood flow is covered in detail in chapter 6.

Interventions that stimulate pulpal blood flow can lead to reduced interstitial levels of materials due to reduced permeability of dentinal tubules and increased clearance by the pulpal microvasculature. For example, electrical stimulation of the inferior alveolar nerve in cats causes an increase in pulpal blood flow and an increase in outward dentinal fluid movement.[11,172-174] This increase shifts the inflow-outflow balance in the opposite direction, leading to a reduction in pulpal levels of materials. This response is believed to be due to axon reflex activity. That is, antidromic stimulation of the inferior alveolar nerve causes simultaneous depolarization of all of the nerve terminals providing sensory innervation of the teeth. This release of neuropeptides from the terminals causes both increased pulpal blood flow and extravasation of plasma proteins from the microcirculation.[13,173]

Alterations in pulpal blood flow may alter diffusion of substances through dentinal tubules by varying the rate of dentinal fluid outflow. Matthews and Vongsavan[172] speculated that hydrodynamic stimulation of exposed dentin (for instance, mechanically) evoked the release of neuropeptides from nerve terminals, thereby increasing local blood flow, tissue pressure, and stimulation of outward flow of fluid in dentinal tubules.[174] This outward fluid flow might rinse the tubules free of inward-diffusing noxious substances by "solvent drag." Indeed, Vongsavan et al[9-12] demonstrated that Evans blue dye would not diffuse into exposed dentin in vivo but would do so in vitro. They speculated that the outward fluid flow in vivo blocked inward diffusion. This notion was tested in vitro by quantitation of the decrease in the inward flux of radioactive iodide when a

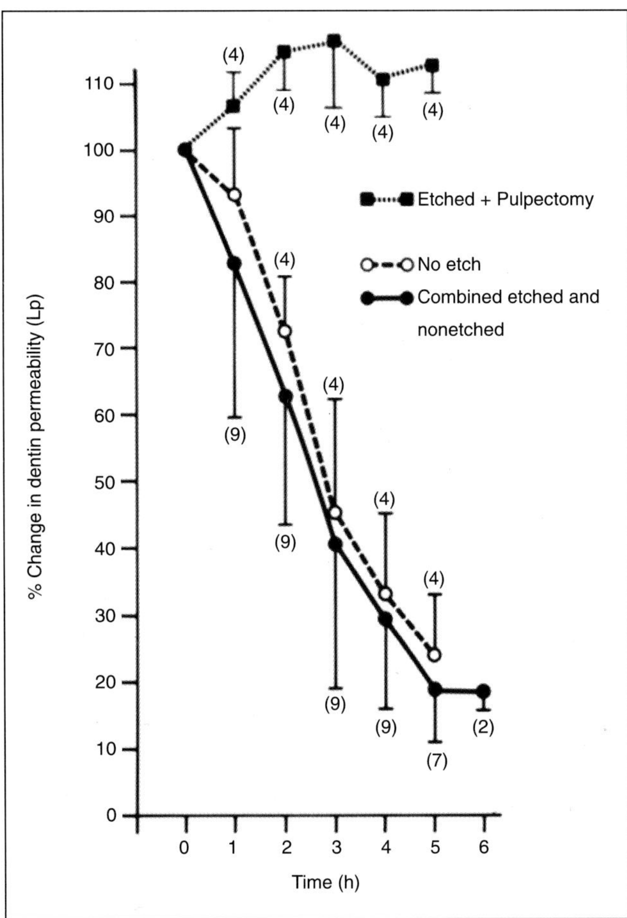

Fig 4-21 Changes in dentin permeability of dog dentin in vivo as a function of time. Dashed line indicates the data obtained from unetched cavities; solid line indicates the combined acid-etched and unetched data in intact teeth; dotted line indicates the data obtained in pulpectomized teeth. Numbers in parentheses are the number of teeth studied. (Reprinted from Pashley[120] with permission.)

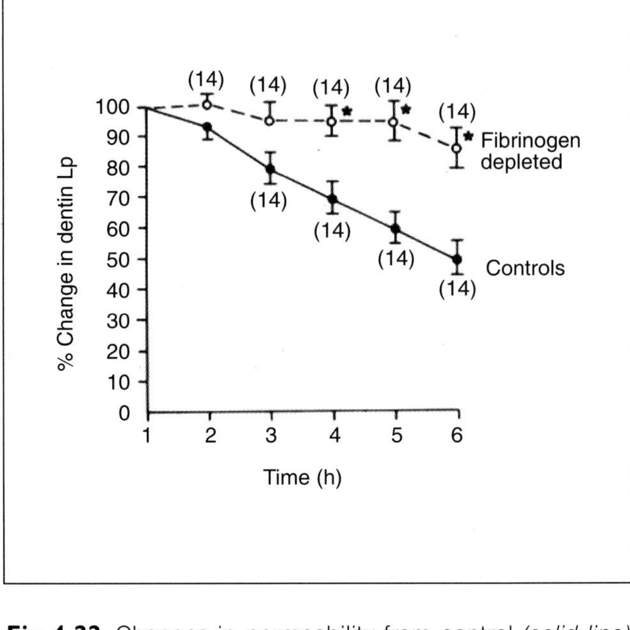

Fig 4-22 Changes in permeability from control *(solid line)* and fibrinogen-depleted dogs *(dashed line)* as a function of time following cavity preparation. Asterisks indicate experimental time periods where significant differences ($P < .05$) were noted. (Reprinted from Pashley[120] with permission.)

simulated outwardly directed 15-cm H_2O pulpal pressure was applied to dentin disks. This outward fluid movement produced a 50% to 60% reduction in the inward diffusion of radioactive iodide across acid-etched dentin in vitro.[121] Thus, stimulation of dentin with open tubules (ie, hypersensitive dentin) should produce higher rates of outward fluid flow and less inward diffusion of bacterial toxins than nonstimulated dentin. This protective effect is diminished in the presence of a smear layer.[121] Under these conditions, the inward flux of noxious substances may increase and permit higher interstitial fluid concentrations[17,120] to be achieved than would occur if there was more outward fluid movement. However, such partial occlusion may be of therapeutic advantage to the increase in pulpal concentrations of topically applied agents.[175]

In exposed dentin, the outward fluid flow through tubules is a first line of defense against the inward diffusion of noxious substances. Dentinal fluid also contains plasma proteins (eg, albumin, globulins) that bind or agglutinate some materials and may play a protective role.[53] A second defensive reaction occurs in freshly exposed dentin that causes the permeability of dentin to fall after cavity preparation (Fig 4-21) in vital dog teeth but not in nonvital teeth.[120] Further, in experiments in which there was a continuous inward-directed bulk fluid movement, the rate of decrease in dentin permeability was due to the slow outward movement of some unidentified substance. These experiments were repeated on dogs treated with an enzyme that depleted fibrinogen from their blood. Under these conditions, cavity preparation produced a much smaller reduction in dentin permeability (Fig 4-22). Apparently the outward movement of fluid is associated with an outward flux of plasma proteins,[14] including fibrinogen.[175] Although attempts to recover fibrinogen in dentinal fluid have been unsuccessful (Pashley, unpublished observation), labeled fibrinogen has been detected in the dentin of rat molars.[176] This finding may be because the dentin thickness in rat molars following cavity preparation is only about 100 µm. Bergenholtz et al[4,177,178] found fibrinogen only in very deep cavities prepared in monkey or human teeth. Pashley et al[175] reported that dentin removed 61% of fibrinogen as it passed through a 1.0-mm disk. Presumably, even larger amounts of fibrinogen in vivo would be removed because the tubules contain odontoblast processes at their terminations, which further reduces the sizes of the channels through which this high-molecular-weight molecule must move. This molecule may be responsible for reducing dentin permeability, especially at the pulpal terminations of the tubules, where it may polymerize into fibrin. Thus, there are multiple physiologic mechanisms regulating the inward diffusions of substances through dentinal tubules.

Effects of restorative procedures and caries on dentin permeability and pulp

Traumatic cavity preparations and hydrodynamic activation of exposed cervical dentin are often associated with more rapid dentinogenesis,[179] which may be due to intratubular fluid shifts that activate intrapulpal nerves. These nerves have been shown to release neuropeptides such as substance P and calcitonin gene-related peptide (CGRP) in the pulp, where they have many effects. For example, CGRP increases the in vitro expression of bone morphogenetic protein (BMP) -2 transcripts in human pulpal cells.[180] When this expression leads to more dentin formation, it also tends to lower dentin permeability by making the tubules longer.

As dentin matrix is synthesized, secreted, and mineralized, several growth factors are trapped in its structure[181-186] (see chapter 3). For example, growth factors such as bone morphogenetic protein-2 (BMP-2), fibroblast growth factor (FGF), epidermal growth factor, insulin-like growth factor-1, transforming growth factor-β, vascular endothelial growth factor (VEGF), and others may be incorporated into mineralized dentin matrix. These growth factors may be released during carious invasion of dentin or pulpal inflammation.[182,183,187] The release of these preformed growth factors may permit their diffusion into the pulp, where they can bind to their receptors on odontoblasts[188-190] and activate appropriate genes to initiate repair processes.[188-190]

It may be possible to apply growth factors onto intact dentin that, following inward diffusion, will stimulate dentinogenesis. To test this hypothesis, Smith et al[191] created Class V cavities in ferret canines using an atraumatic technique. They then applied an EDTA extract containing a complex mixture of growth factors solubilized from dentin to the cavity preparation.[192,193] In young adult ferrets, the reparative dentin resembled normal primary tubular dentin; in older animals it resembled osteodentin in that it was atubular and displayed cellular inclusions. This finding was the first unequivocal report of the activation of dentinogenesis by molecules applied to intact dentin. The response was less in cavities with thicker dentin between the cavity floor and the pulp chamber than with thinner dentin. Interestingly, dentin matrix formation was sometimes so rapid that cells became trapped within the matrix. The rate of dentinogensis seemed to become slower as more dentin was formed. As more dentin is formed, the amount of growth factors diffusing from the floor of the cavity to the pulp is expected to decrease, which in turn slows matrix secretion. The details of which factors are important, their dose-response relationships, possible synergism, and location of receptors and second messengers need to be explored.[188] In one study, various concentrations of soluble osteogenic protein-1 (OP-1) were applied to the floors of Class V cavities prepared in monkey teeth.[194] Control cavities received no treatment while experimental cavities received either calcium hydroxide paste or OP-1 at concentrations of 0.01, 0.1, 1, or 10 μg/μL. The lower two concentrations of OP-1 were found to be ineffective at stimulating reparative dentin formation when the tissue was examined 2 months later. In both experimental groups (calcium hydroxide and OP-1), more reparative dentin was formed in cavities where the remaining dentin thickness was 0.2 mm. These results suggest either the receptors for osteogenic proteins are located on the cell body of the odontoblasts, rather than on the odontoblast process, or that the process is extremely short.[188] The lack of response in pulps beneath thicker dentin may have been due to dissipation of the concentration of the growth factor to levels that were below its therapeutic concentration or to nonspecific binding of the protein to the walls of the tubules.[195]

From a clinical perspective, it would be advantageous to induce odontoblast-like cells to produce atubular dentin following the topical application of growth factors to dentin, which would seal the pulp from hydrodynamic and bacteriologic insult. It would also interfere with further diffusion of growth factors to the pulp and would therefore be self-limiting. However, this technique may not be possible if the odontoblasts are normal, for the odontoblast phenotype results in the production of tubular dentin. Apparently, only less differentiated odontoblastoid cells without processes can form atubular dentin. Whether fully differentiated odontoblasts can be transiently induced to dedifferentiate into more primitive phenotypes to produce atubular dentin remains to be seen.

Dynamics of the Pulpodentin Complex

Dentin is a living tissue that can and does react to changes in its environment.[19,135] It is the only innervated hard tissue of the tooth.[15,196] Normally, dentin is covered coronally by enamel and on its root surfaces by cementum. Dentin exposed to the oral environment is subjected to large chemical, mechanical, and thermal stimuli. The exposed, fluid-filled tubules permit minute fluid shifts across dentin whenever dentin is exposed to tactile, thermal, osmotic, or evaporative stimuli, which in turn activate mechanoreceptors in the pulp. These fluid shifts can directly stimulate odontoblasts, pulpal nerves, and subodontoblastic blood vessels by applying large shear forces on their surfaces as the fluid streams through narrow spaces. In rats, exposure of dentin irritates the pulp and causes the release of neuropeptides such as CGRP or substance P from the pulpal nerves to create a local neurogenic inflammatory condition.[15,197,198] These stimuli also produce changes in pulpal blood vessels, leading to increased flow of plasma fluid and plasma proteins from vessels into pulpal tissue spaces and out into dentinal tubules.[9-11,13,15,167] This extravasation of plasma can also cause increases in local pulpal tissue pressure,[174,199] which tends to increase firing of sensitized neurons.[15,198] The outward fluid flow may have a protective, flushing action that may reduce the inward diffusion of noxious bacterial products in both exposed cervical dentin (Fig 4-23) and perhaps even in leaking restorations.[10,12,119,121] Additional information on this topic is found in chapters 6, 7, and 8.

Reactions to cavity preparations: Fluid shifts

Although most dentists regard cavity preparation as a minor, routine restorative procedure, it is a crisis from the perspective of the pulp. The use of cutting burs in handpieces produces vibrations, inward fluid shifts (caused by frictional heat generation on the end of a poorly irrigated cutting bur), outward fluid shifts due to evaporative water loss (if only air cooling is used), and slight inward fluid shifts due to osmotic movement of cooling water into dentin.[201] When air blasts are directed on smear layer–covered dentin, the evaporative water loss induces an outward fluid flow equivalent to that produced by applying a negative pressure of 247 cm H_2O to dentin.[202] Thus, simple restorative procedures may have profound effects on the pulp. These fluid shifts occur in both directions at various stages of cavity preparation. Outward fluid shifts accompany the application of hypertonic conditioners, primers, varnishes, or bonding agents,[144] and then, during light curing of adhesive resins, additional inward fluid shifts occur due to heat generated during polymerization of adhesive resins and resin composites.[203]

All of these fluid shifts create a barrage of hydrodynamic stimuli across dentin into the pulp, causing pain in the unanesthetized patient. Further, these stimuli will evoke peripheral release of neuropeptides, causing local pulpal neurogenic inflammation under the irritated tubules,[187,204] alterations in pulpal blood flow,[205] and increases in tissue pressure.[174] Although the fluid shifts would still occur in patients following administration of local anesthesia, fewer nerves would fire, resulting in less release of neuropeptides and generally less neurogenic inflammation.[15,197,204]

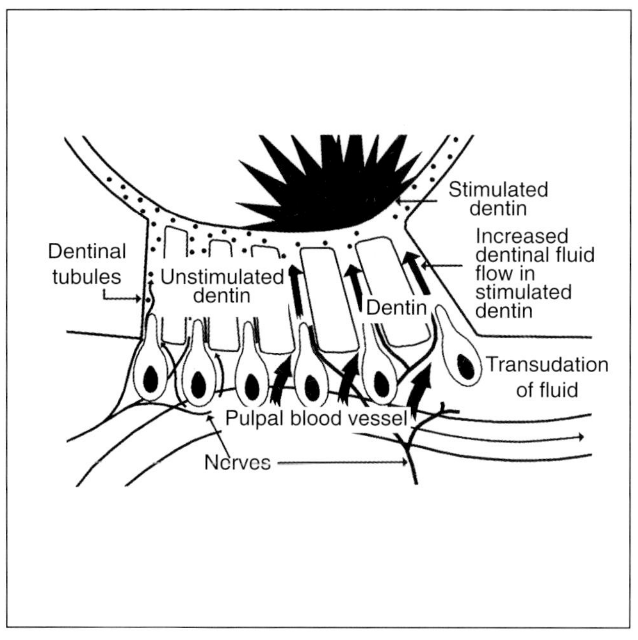

Fig 4-23 Schematic diagram showing the inward diffusion of noxious material *(small solid circles)* opposed by the outward movement of dentinal fluid in response to axon-reflex-induced release of neuropeptides causing vasodilation, transudation, and increased capillary permeability. (Reprinted from Pashley[200] with permission.)

Disruption of odontoblast layer

Restorative dental procedures can also damage odontoblasts. Deep cavity preparation in rat molars causes aspiration of odontoblasts[15] and nerves[206]; more shallow cavity preparation causes disruption of junctional complexes between odontoblasts,[207] which decreases their barrier properties,[208-210] allowing large molecules (eg, horseradish peroxidase) from the blood stream to penetrate dentin.[210,211] The loss of gap junctions may interfere with the ability of the odontoblasts to secrete a collagen matrix in a synchronous, coordinated manner due to the loss of cell signaling between adjacent cells. The proteins that make up gap junctions are called *connexins*.[212,213] How long it takes odontoblasts to re-establish the continuity of gap junctions and to revert to tissue rather than cellular function is unknown. Presumably, bacterial substances in plaque and saliva could easily move from the oral cavity into the pulp after such operative procedures.[3,4,6-8] Mechanisms responsible for the disruption of rat odontoblasts during cavity preparation have not been studied but probably arise from the rapid, outward movement of dentinal fluid in response to evaporative water loss from dentin during cavity preparation. As subodontoblastic capillaries pass into the odontoblast layer, disruption of the layer will also cause direct damage to capillaries that sustain the odontoblasts, leading to microhemorrhages. They may leak plasma proteins[176] such as fibrinogen into tissue spaces that are in communication with dentinal fluid. As described above (see Figs 4-21 and 4-22), this leakage of fibrinogen may mediate the reduction in dentinal permeability observed after cavity preparations because depletion of circulating fibrinogen greatly attenuates reduction in dentin permeability.[119,120]

Several investigators have measured the flux of plasma proteins across dentin following cavity preparation.[14,177,178,214,215] They reported that several plasma proteins, including albumin, could be detected in relatively high concentrations immediately after cavity preparations in monkeys and humans,[215] but concentrations fell over the next few hours to days. These plasma proteins contain immunoglobulins that may inactivate some bacterial products. Bacterial or salivary products possibly activate complement, which would also contribute to pulpal inflammation. Many of these reactions to cavity preparation are immediate and short term. Displacement of odontoblasts into tubules disrupts their internal cytoskeleton and causes cell death.[207,216] These cells undergo autolysis over the next few days and are replaced by mesenchymal reserve cells that begin to differentiate into new odontoblasts. The cell signals responsible for this process are now beginning to be understood (see chapter 3).

Displacement of odontoblasts and their replacement by new cells[217] is associated with very little pulpal inflammation if the environment is sterile and if the dentin is well sealed. It is possible for cavities in teeth to be prepared with no pulpal inflammation or formation of reparative dentin[186,191] using copious air-water spray; light, intermittent cutting forces; and sharp burs. However, when the dentin is not sealed (ie, cervical abrasion) or when the restored cavity exhibits microleakage, the pulpodentin complex will undergo long-term reactions that are the result of continual leakage and permeation of bacterial substances around gaps in restorations and through unsealed dentinal tubules into the pulp.[4,119] This condition converts acute pulpal reactions associated with cavity preparation or dentin exposure into chronic pulpal reactions.

Bacteria and their products have been shown to produce severe pulpal reactions.[1,4-8] The argument over whether bacterial or chemical irritants cause more pulpal inflammation has been going on for decades. Early germ-free animal studies demonstrated minimal pulpal reactions to materials.[218,219] These findings have been confirmed more recently by studies in rat and monkey teeth, where restorative materials were placed directly on pulpal soft tissues followed by surface sealing.[220-223] The pulpal reactions seen in most dental materials usage studies seem to be the result of bacterial colonization of gaps between restorative materials and tooth structures. These colonies continually shed bacterial products that cause continual pulpal irritation. The extensive experimental work supporting this conclusion has been recently reviewed.[4,222,224-226]

An intricate network of contact between pulpal microvessels and nerve fibers provided by the cellular processes of dendritic cells (specialized antigen-presenting cells) was demonstrated by Jontell et al[227,228] (see chapter 5). They also showed that low concentrations (10^{-9} mol/L) of substance P stimulated T-cell mitogenesis in vitro when pulp cells were used as accessory cells; CGRP produced inhibition under the same conditions. These findings indicate that immunocompetent cells, peripheral nerve terminals, and the pulpal vasculature may interact and provide significant defensive functions at multiple levels in pulpal defense. These defenses may be compromised by some restorative materials if they are applied to pulp exposures.[229-231]

Conclusion

The pulpodentin complex is an important concept in understanding the pathobiology of dentin and pulp. Developmentally, pulpal cells produce dentin, nerves, and blood vessels. Although dentin and pulp have different structures and compositions, once formed they react to stimuli as a functional unit. Exposure of dentin through attrition, trauma, or caries produces profound pulpal reactions that tend to reduce dentin permeability and stimulate formation of additional dentin. These reactions are brought about by changes in fibroblasts, nerves, blood vessels, odontoblasts, leukocytes, and the immune system. Recent discoveries of the effects of nerves on pulpal blood vessels and vice versa have produced a new appreciation for the interaction of these two systems in response to stimuli applied to dentin.

Too often, for technical or experimental reasons, the individual components of the pulpodentin complex are studied independently. However, it is becoming clear that the individual components are very interactive and that each modifies the activity of the other. Thus, where we used to speak of neurovascular interactions, we now must consider neurovascular-immuno-odontoblast interactions.[227]

Acknowledgments

The author is grateful to Michelle Burnside for outstanding secretarial support. This work was supported in part by grant DE 06427 from the National Institute of Dental and Craniofacial Research.

References

1. Bergenholtz G. Effects of bacterial products on inflammatory reactions in the dental pulp. Scand J Dent Res 1977; 85:122-129.
2. Bergenholtz G. Inflammatory responses of the dental pulp to bacterial irritation. J Endod 1981;7:100-104.
3. Bergenholtz G. Pathogenic mechanisms in pulpal disease. J Endod 1990;16:98-101.
4. Bergenholtz G. Evidence for bacterial causation of adverse pulpal responses in resin-based dental restorations. Crit Rev Oral Biol Med 2000;11:467-480.
5. Bergenholtz G, Warfvinge J. Migration of leukocytes in dental pulp in response to plaque bacteria. Scand J Dent Res 1982;90:354-362.
6. Warfvinge J, Bergenholtz G. Healing capacity of human and monkey dental pulps following experimentally induced pulpitis. Endod Dent Traumatol 1986;2:256-262.
7. Hanks CT, Syed SA, Craig SA. Modeling bacterial damage to pulpal cells, in vitro. J Endodon 1991;17:21-25.
8. Pissiotis E, Spängberg L. Dentin permeability to bacterial proteins in vitro. J Endod 1994;20:118-122.
9. Vongsavan N, Matthews B. The permeability of cat dentine in vitro and in vivo. Arch Oral Biol 1991;36:641-646.
10. Vongsavan N, Matthews B. Fluid flow through cat dentine in vivo. Arch Oral Biol 1992;37:175-185.
11. Vongsavan N, Matthews B. Changes in pulpal blood flow and fluid flow through dentine produced by autonomic and sensory nerve stimulation in the cat. Proc Finn Dent Soc 1992;88(suppl 1):491-497.
12. Vongsavan N, Matthews RW, Matthews B. The permeability of human dentine in vitro and in vivo. Arch Oral Biol 2000;45:931-935.
13. Raab WH-M. Zar entstehung des plasmaextravasates in der zahnpulpa. Dtsch Zahnärztl Z 1989;44:686-688.
14. Maita E, Simpson MD, Tao L, Pashley DH. Fluid and protein flux across the pulpodentin complex of the dog, in vivo. Arch Oral Biol 1991;36:103-110.
15. Byers MR, Närhi MOV. Dental injury models: Experimental tools for understanding neuroinflammatory interactions and polymodal nociceptor functins. Crit Rev Oral Biol Med 1999;10:4-39.
16. Tziafas D, Smith AJ, Lesot H. Designing new treatment strategies in vital pulp therapy. J Dent 2000;28:77-92.
17. Pashley DH. The influence of dentin permeability and pulpal blood flow on pulpal solute concentration. J Endod 1979;5:355-361.
18. Potts TV, Cunningham T, Finkelstein MJ, Silverberg-Strumfeld L. The movement of radioactive molecules across dentine in vivo in the dog. Arch Oral Biol 1985;30: 353-357.
19. Pashley DH. Dynamics of the pulpodentin complex. Crit Rev Oral Biol Med 1996;7:104-133.
20. Jean A, Kerebel B, Kerebel L-M. Scanning electron microscope study of the predentin-pulpal border zone in human dentin. Oral Surg 1986;61:392-398.
21. Frank RM, Nalbandian J. Structure and ultrastructure of dentin. In: Berkovitz BKB, Boyde A, Frank RM, et al (eds). Teeth. New York: Springer-Verlag, 1989: 212.
22. Ten Cate R. Oral Histology: Development, Structure and Function, ed 5. St. Louis: Mosby, 1998: 166.
23. Brännström M, Garberoglio R. The dentinal tubules and the odontoblast process. Acta Odontol Scand 1972;30: 291-311.
24. Marion D, Jean A, Hamel H, Kerebel L-M, Kerebel B. Scanning electron microscopic study of odontoblasts and circumpulpal dentin in a human tooth. Oral Biol 1991;72: 473-478.
25. Herr P, Holz J, Baume LJ. Mantle dentine in man: A quantitative microradiographic study. J Biol Buccale 1986;14: 139-146.
26. Mjör IA, Nordahl I. The density and branching of dentinal tubules in human teeth. Arch Oral Biol 1996;41:401-412.
27. Couve E. Ultrastructural changes during the life cycle of human odontoblasts. Arch Oral Biol 1986;31:643-651.
28. Schellenberg U, Kreg G, Bosshardt D, Nair PNR. Numerical density of dentinal tubules at the pulpal wall of human permanent premolars and third molars. J Endod 1992;18:104-109.

29. Hoppe WF, Stüben J. Über die Messung des Volumens der Dentinkanälchen und über des Kanalvolumens zum Gesamtdentinvolumen. Stoma 1965;65:38–45.
30. Walton RE, Outhwaite WC, Pashley DH. Magnification, an interesting optical property of dentin. J Dent Res 1976; 55:639–642.
31. Fosse G, Saele PK, Eide R. Numerical density and distributional pattern of dentin tubules. Acta Odontol Scand 1992;50:201–210.
32. Linde A, Goldberg M. Dentinogenesis. Crit Rev Oral Biol Med 1993;45(5):679–728.
33. Blake GC. The peritubular translucent zones in human dentine. Br Dent J 1958;104:57–59.
34. Garberoglio R, Brännström M. Scanning electron microscopic investigation of human dentinal tubules. Arch Oral Biol 1976;21:355–362.
35. Mjör IA. Reaction Patterns in Human Teeth. Boca Raton, FL: CRC Press, 1983: 86.
36. Mjör IA. Dentin-predentin complex and its permeability: pathology and treatment overview. J Dent Res 1985;64 (special issue):621–627.
37. Hals E. Observations on giant tubules in human coronal dentin by light microscopy and microradiography. Scand J Dent Res 1983;91:1–7.
38. Tronstad L. Optical and microradiographic appearance of intact and worn human coronal dentine. Arch Oral Biol 1972;17:847–858.
39. Miller J. Large tubules in dentine. J Dent Child 1981;48: 269–271.
40. Kinney JH, Balooch M, Marshall SJ, Marshall GW, Weihs TM. Hardness and Young's modulus of peritubular and intertubular dentine. Arch Oral Biol 1996;41:9–13.
41. Mendis BRRN, Darling AI. A scanning electron microscopic and micrographic study of closure of human coronal dentinal tubules related to occlusal attrition and caries. Arch Oral Biol 1979;24:725–733.
42. Hirayama A, Yamada M, Miake K. Analytical electron microscope studies on the dentinal tubules of human deciduous teeth [abstract 65]. J Dent Res 1985;64:743.
43. Rasmussen P. The concentration of calcium, inorganic phosphate and protein in the interstitial fluid of rats. Calcif Tiss Res 1970;6:197–203.
44. Larsson PA, Howell DS, Pita JC, Blanco LN. Aspiration and characterization of predentin fluid in developing rat teeth by means of a micropuncture and micro-analytical technique. J Dent Res 1988;67:870–875.
45. Lundgren T, Nannmark U, Linde A. Calcium ion activity and pH in the odontoblast-predentin region: Ion-selective microelectrode measurements. Calcif Tiss Int 1992;50: 134–136.
46. Shellis RP. Effects of a supersaturated pulpal fluid on the formation of caries-like lesions on the roots of human teeth. Caries Res 1994;28:14–20.
47. Michelich V, Pashley DH, Whitford GM. Dentin permeability: A comparison of functional versus anatomical tubular radii. J Dent Res 1978;57:1019–1024.
48. Pashley DH. Dentin permeability: Theory and practice. In: Spängberg L (ed). Experimental Endodontics. Boca Raton, FL: CRC Press, 1990:19–49.
49. Michelich VJ, Schuster GS, Pashley DH. Bacterial penetration of human dentin, in vitro. J Dent Res 1980;59: 1398–1403.
50. Lundy T, Stanley HR. Correlation of pulp histopathology and clinical symptoms in human teeth subjected to experimental irritation. Oral Surg 1969;27:187–201.
51. Olgart L, Brännström M, Johnson G. Invasion of bacteria into dentinal tubules. Acta Odontol Scand 1974;32:61–70.
52. Nagoaka S, Miyazaki Y, Liu H, Iwamoto Y, Kitano M, Kawagoe M. Bacterial invasion into dentinal tubules of human vital and nonvital teeth. J Endod 1995;21:70–73.
53. Hahn C-L, Overton B. The effects of immunoglobulins on the convective permeability of human dentine in vitro. Arch Oral Biol 1997;42:835–843.
54. Dai X-F, Ten Cate AR, Limeback H. The extent and distribution of intratubular collagen fibrils in human dentin. Arch Oral Biol 1991;36:775–778.
55. Holland GR. The extent of the odontoblast process in the cat. J Anat 1976;120:133–149.
56. Holland GR. The odontoblast process: Form and function. J Dent Res 1985;64(special issue):499–514.
57. Holland GR. Morphological features of dentine and pulp related to dentine sensitivity. Arch Oral Biol 1994;39 (suppl):35–115.
58. Thomas HF. The extent of the odontoblast process in human dentine. Arch Oral Biol 1979;28:465–469.
59. Thomas HF. The dentin-predentin complex and its permeability: Anatomical overview. J Dent Res 1985;64(special issue):607–612.
60. Byers MR, Sugaya A. Odontoblast processes in dentin revealed by fluorescent Di-I. J Histochem Cytochem 1995;43:159–168.
61. Weber DF, Zaki AL. Scanning and transmission electron microscopy of tubular structures presumed to be human odontoblast processes. J Dent Res 1986;65:982–986.
62. LaFleche RG, Frank RM, Steuer P. The extent of the human odontoblast process as determined by transmission electron microscopy: The hypothesis of a retractable suspensor system. J Biol Bucc 1985;13:293–305.
63. Brännström M. Etiology of dentin hypersensitivity. Proc Finn Dent Soc 1992;88(suppl 1):7–14.
64. Weber DE. An improved technique for producing casts of the internal structure of hard tissues including some observations on human dentine. Arch Oral Biol 1983; 28:885–891.
65. Olsson S, Olio G. The structure of dentin surfaces exposed for bond strength measurements. Scand J Dent Res 1993;101:180–184.

66. Dourda AO, Moule AJ, Young WG. A morphometric analysis of the cross-sectional area of dentine occupied by dentinal tubules in human third molar teeth. Int Endod J 1994;27:184–189.
67. Pashley DH. Smear layer: Physiologic considerations. Oper Dent 1984; 9(suppl 3):13–29.
68. Pashley DH. Clinical correlations of dentin structure and function. J Prosthet Dent 1991;66:777–781.
69. LeGeros RZ. Calcium Phosphate in Oral Biology and Medicine, vol 15, Monographs in Oral Science. New York: Karger, 1991.
70. Pashley DH, Carvalho RM. Dentine permeability and adhesive bonding. J Dent 1997;25:355–372.
71. Eick JD, Gwinnett AJ, Pashley DH, Robinson SJ. Current concepts on adhesion to dentin. Crit Rev Oral Biol Med 1997;8:306–335.
72. Swanson K, Madison S. An evaluation of coronal microleakage in endodontically treated teeth. Part I: Time periods. J Endod 1987;13:56–59.
73. Madison S, Swanson K, Chiles SA. An evaluation of coronal microleakage in endodontically treated teeth. Part II: sealer types. J Endod 1987;13:109–112.
74. Wilcox LR, Diaz-Arnold A. Coronal microleakage of permanent lingual access restorations in endodontically treated anterior teeth. J Endod 1989;15:584–587.
75. Torabinejad M, Ung B, Kettering JD. In vitro bacterial penetration of coronally unsealed endodontically treated teeth. J Endod 1990;16:566–569.
76. Magura ME, Kafrawy AH, Brown LE, Newton CW. Human saliva coronal microleakage in obturated root canals: An in vitro study. J Endod 1991;17:324–331.
77. Khayat A, Lee S-J, Torabinajad M. Human saliva penetration of coronally unsealed obturated root canals. J Endod 1993;19:458–461.
78. Wolanek GA, Loushine RJ, Weller RN, Kimbrough WF, Volkmann KR. In vitro bacterial penetration of endodontically treated teeth coronally sealed with a dentin bonding agent. J Endod 2001;27:354–357.
79. Belli S, Zhang Y, Periera PNR, Pashley DH. Adhesive sealing of pulp chambers. J Endod 2001;27:521–526.
80. Galvan RR, West LA, Liewehr FR, Pashley DH. An evaluation of coronal microleakage of five materials in the pulp chamber of endodontically treated teeth. J Endod (in press).
81. Wells JD, Loushine RJ, Weller RN, Kimbrough WF, Pashley DH. Coronal sealing ability of two dental cements. J Endod (in press).
82. Kinney JH, Marshall GW, Marshall SJ. Three-dimensional mapping of mineral densities in carious dentin: Theory and method. Scan Micros 1994;8:197–205.
83. Frank RM, Nalbandian J. Structure and ultrastructure of dentine. In: Berkovitz BKB, Boyde A, Frank RM, et al (eds). Teeth. New York: Springer-Verlag, 1989:175.
84. Manly RS, Hodge HC. Density and refractive index studies of dental hard tissues. I. Methods for separation and determination of purity. J Dent Res 1939;18:133–141.
85. Johansen E. Microstructure of enamel and dentin. J Dent Res 1964;43:1007–1020.
86. Frank RM, Voegel JC. Dissolution mechanisms of the apatite crystals during dental caries and bone resorption. In: Berlin RD, Herrmann H, Lepow IH, Tanzer JM (eds). Molecular Basis of Biological Degradative Processes and Structure and Ultrastructure of the Dental Pulp. New York: Academic Press, 1978:277–311.
87. Hoppenbrouwers, PMM, Driessens FCM, Borggreven JMPM. The vulnerability of unexposed human dental roots to demineralization. J Dent Res 1986;65:955–958.
88. Retief DH, Cleaton-Jones PE, Turkstra J, DeWet WJ. The quantitative analysis of the elements in normal human enamel and dentine by neutron activation analysis and high resolution gamma spectroscopy. Arch Oral Biol 1971;16:1257–1267.
89. Weatherall JA, Robinson C. The inorganic composition of teeth. In: Zipkin I (ed). Biological Mineralization, vol 3. New York: Wiley, 1973:43–74.
90. Butler WT. Dentin matrix proteins. Eur J Oral Sci 1998; 106(suppl 1):204–210.
91. Veis A. Mineral-matrix interactions in bond and dentin. J Bone Miner Res 1993;8(suppl 2):S493–S497.
92. Goldberg M, Takagi M. Dentin proteoglycans: Composition, ultrastructure and functions. Histochem J 1993; 25:781–806.
93. Marshall GW. Dentin microstructure and characterization. Quintessence Int 1993;24:606–617.
94. Marshall GW, Marshall SJ, Kinney JH, Balooch M. The dentin substrate: Structure and properties related to bonding. J Dent 1997;25:441–458.
95. Craig RG. Restorative Dental Materials, ed 10. St. Louis: Mosby, 1996:89.
96. Pashley DH, Okabe A, Parham P. The relationship between dentin microhardness and tubule density. Endod Dent Traumatol 1985;1:176–179.
97. Smith DC, Cooper WEG. The determination of shear strength: A method using a micropunch apparatus. Br Dent J 1971;130:333–337.
98. Watanabe LG, Nguyen T, Garner M, Kilbourne AM, Marshall SJ, Marshall GW. Dentin shear strength relative to tubule orientation: Effects of tubule orientation and intratooth location. Dent Mater 1996;12:109–115.
99. Bowen RL, Rodriguez MS. Tensile strength and modulus of elasticity of tooth structure and several restorative materials. J Am Dent Assoc 1962;64:378–387.
100. Lehman ML. Tensile strength of human dentin. J Dent Res 1967;46:197–201.
101. Sano H, Ciucchi B, Matthews WG, Pashley DH. Tensile properties of mineralized and demineralized human and bovine dentin. J Dent Res 1994;73:1205–1211.

102. Wang R, Weiner S. Human root dentin: Structural anisotropy and Vickers microhardness isotrophy. Connect Tissue Res 1998;39:269–279.
103. Meredith N, Sherriff M, Setchell DJ, Swanson SAV. Measurements of the microhardness and Young's modulus of human enamel and dentin using an indentation technique. Arch Oral Biol 1996;41:539–545.
104. Mahler DB, Peyton FA. Photoelasticity as a research techique for analyzing stresses in dental structures. J Dent Res 1955;34:831–838.
105. Lehman ML, Meyer RL. Relationship of dental caries and stress concentrations in teeth as revealed by photoelastic tests. J Dent Res 1966;45:1706–1714.
106. Versluis A, Tantbirojn D, Douglas WH. Why do shear bond tests pull out dentin? J Dent Res 1997;76:1298–1307.
107. Panitvisai P, Messer HH. Cuspal deflection in molars in relation to endodontic and restorative procedures. J Endod 1995;21:57–61.
108. Palamara JEA, Wilson PR, Thomas CDL, Messer HH. A new imaging technique for measuring the surface strains applied to dentine. J Dent 2000;28:141–146.
109. Wang RZ, Weiner S. Strain-structure relations in human teeth using Moiré fringes. J Biomech 1998;31:135–141.
110. Wood JD, Wang R, Weiner S, Pashley DH. Mapping of tooth deformation caused by moisture change using Moiré interferometry. Dent Mater (in press).
111. Wood JD, Pashley DH. Nonlinear mechanical properties of dentin [abstract 1749]. J Dent Res 2000;79 (special issue):363.
112. Kishen A, Ramamurty U, Asundi A. Experimental studies on the nature of property gradients in the human dentine. J Biomed Mater Res 2000;57:650–659.
113. Asundi A, Kishen A. A strain gauge and photoelastic analysis of in vivo strain and in vitro stress distributions in human dental supporting structures. Arch Oral Biol 2000;45:543–550.
114. Dowker SE, Davis GR, Elliott JC. X-ray microtomography: Nondestructive three-dimensional imaging for in vitro endodontic studies. Oral Surg 1997;83:510–516.
115. Engelke K, Karolczak M, Lutz A, Seibert U, Schaller S, Kalander W. Micro-CT technology and application for assessing bone structure. Radiologie 1999;39:203–212.
116. Koutsi V, Noonan RG, Horner JA, Simpson MD, Matthews WG, Pashley DH. The effect of dentin depth on the permeability and ultrastructure of primary molars. Pediatr Dent 1994;16:29–35.
117. Pashley DH, Livingston MJ. Effect of molecular size on permeability coefficients in human dentine. Arch Oral Biol 1978;23:391–395.
118. Kinney JH, Balooch M, Haupt DL, Marshall SJ, Marshall GW. Mineral distribution and dimensional changes in human dentin during demineralization. J Dent Res 1995;74:1179–1184.
119. Pashley DH, Pashley EL. Dentin permeability and restorative dentistry. Am J Dent 1991;4:5–9.
120. Pashley DH. Dentin-predentin complex: Physiological overview. J Dent Res 1985;64 (special issue):613–620.
121. Pashley DH, Matthews WG. The effects of outward forced convective flow on inward diffusion in human dentine, in vitro. Arch Oral Biol 1993;38:577–582.
122. Pashley DH. Considerations of dentin permeability in cytotoxicity testing. Int Endod J 1988;21:143–154.
123. Pashley DH, Andringa HJ, Derkson GD, Derkson ME, Kalathoor S. Regional variability in dentine permeability. Arch Oral Biol 1987;32:519–523.
124. Macpherson JV, Beeston MA, Unwin PR, Hughes NP, Littlewood D. Scanning electrochemical microscopy as a probe of local fluid flow through porous solids: Application to the measurement of convective rates through a single dentinal tubule. J Chem Soc Faraday Trans 1995; 91:1407–1410.
125. Richardson DW, Tao L, Pashley DH. Dentin permeability: effects of crown preparation. Int J Prosthodont 1991;4:219–225.
126. Maroli S, Khea SC, Krell KV. Regional variation in permeability of young dentin. Oper Dent 1992;17:93–100.
127. Garberoglio P. The ratio of the densities of dentinal tubules on the cervical and axial walls in cavities. Quintessence Int 1994;25:49–52.
128. Tagami J, Hosoda H, Burrow MF, Nakajima M. Effect of aging and caries on dentin permeability. Proc Finn Dent Soc 1992;88(suppl 1):149–154.
129. Fogel HM, Marshall FJ, Pashley DH. Effects of distance from the pulp and thickness on the permeability of human radicular dentin. J Dent Res 1988;67:1381–1385.
130. Paul SJ, Scharer P. Factors in dentin bonding. Part I: A review of the morphology and physiology of human dentin. J Esthetic Dent 1993;5(1):5–9.
131. Szabó J, Szabó I, Trombitas K. Interodontoblastic fibers in human dentine observed by scanning electron microscopy. Arch Oral Biol 1985;30:161–165.
132. Barbosa SV, Savavi KE, Spängberg LSW. Influence of sodium hypochlorite on the permeability and structure of cervical human dentine. Int Endod J 1994;27:309–312.
133. Tao L, Anderson TW, Pashley DH. Effect of endodontic procedures on root dentin permeability. J Endod 1991; 17:583–588.
134. Mader CL, Baumgartner JC, Peters DD. Scanning electron microscopic investigation of the smeared layer on root canal walls. J Endod 1984;10:477–483.
135. Pashley DH. Dentin: A dynamic substrate: A review. Scan Microsc 1989;3:161–176.
136. Pashley DH, Livingston MJ, Greenhill JD. Regional resistances to fluid flow in human dentine, in vitro. Arch Oral Biol 1978;23:807–810.

137. Goldman LB, Goldman M, Kvonman JH, Lin PS. The efficacy of several irrigating solution for endodontics: A scanning electron microscope study. Oral Surg 1981; 52:197-204.

138. Goldman M, Goldman LB, Cavaleri R, Bogis J, Lin PS. The efficacy of several endodontic irrigating solutions: A scanning electron microscopic study. Part 2. J Endod 1982;8:487-482.

139. Fogel HM, Pashley DH. Dentin permeability: Effects of endodontic procedures on root slabs. J Endod 1990;16: 442-445.

140. White RR, Goldman M, Lin PS. The influence of the smeared layer upon dentinal tubule penetration by endodontic filling materials. Part II. J Endod 1987;13: 369-374.

141. Evans JT, Simon JHS. Evaluation of the apical seal produced by injected thermoplasticized gutta-percha in the absence of smear layer and root canal sealer. J Endod 1986;12:101-107.

142. Iwaku M, Nakamichi I, Horie K, Suiza S, Fusayama T. Tags penetrating dentin of a new adhesive resin. Bull Tokyo Med Dent Univ 1981;28:45-51.

143. Galvan DA, Ciarlone AE, Pashley DH, Kulild JC, Primack PD, Simpson MD. Effect of smear layer removal on the diffusion permeability of human roots. J Endod 1994; 20:83-86.

144. Pashley DH, Horner JA, Brewer PD. Interactions of conditioners on the dentin surfaces. Oper Dent 1992;17 (suppl 5):137-150.

145. Marshall FJ, Massler M, Dute HL. Effects of endodontic treatments on permeability of root dentine. Oral Surg 1960;13:203-223.

146. Martin H, LaSala A, Michanowicz A. Permeability of the apical third of the root to drugs used in endodontic therapy: An in vitro study. J Oral Ther 1968;4:451-455.

147. Nissan R, Segal H, Stevens RH, Pashley DH, Trowbridge HO. The ability of bacterial endotoxin to diffuse through human dentin. J Endod 1995;21:62-64.

148. Petelin M, Skaleri U, Ceve P, Schara M. The permeability of human cementum in vitro measured by electron paramagnetic resonance. Arch Oral Biol 1999;44: 259-267.

149. Furseth R. The structure of peripheral root dentin in young human premolars. Scand J Dent Res 1974;82: 557-561.

150. Merchant VA, Livingston MJ, Pashley DH. Dentin permeation: Comparison of diffusion with filtration. J Dent Res 1977;56:1161-1164.

151. Liewehr FR. A Comparison of the Effects of Etidronate, Clodronate and Gallium Nitrate on Dentin Resorption by Osteoclast-like Cells, in Vivo [thesis]. Augusta: Medical College of Georgia, 1993.

152. Ghazi AM, Shuttleworth S, Angulo SJ, Pashley DH. Gallium diffusion in human root dentin: Quantitative measurements by pulsed Nd:YAG laser ablation combined with an inductively coupled plasma mass spectrometer. J Clin Laser Med Surg 2000;18:173-183.

153. Abbott PV, Hume WR, Heithersay GS. Barriers to diffusion of Ledermix paste in radicular dentin. Endod Dent Traumatol 1989;5:98-104.

154. Wiebkin OW, Cardaci SC, Heithersay GS, Pierce AM. Therapeutic delivery of calcitonin to inhibit external inflammatory root resorption. I. Diffusion kinetics of calcitonin through the dental root. Endod Dent Traumatol 1996a; 12:265-271.

155. Guignes P, Faure J, Maurette A. Relationship between endodontic preparations and human dentin permeability measured in situ. J Endod 1996;22:60-67.

156. Carrigan PJ, Morse DR, Furst L, Sinai IH. A scanning electron microscopic evaluation of human dentinal tubules according to age and location. J Endod 1984; 10:359-363.

157. Lowman JV, Burke RS, Pellen GV. Patient accessory canals: Incidence on molar furcation region. Oral Surg 1973;36:580-584.

158. Vertucci FJ, Williams RG. Furcation canals in the human mandibular first molar. Oral Surg 1974;38:308-314.

159. Burch JG, Hulen SA. Study of the presence of accessory foramina and the topograph of molar furcations. Oral Surg 1974;38:451-455.

160. Koenigs JF, Brillant JD, Foreman DW. Preliminary scanning electron microscopic investigations of accessory foramina in the furcation areas of human molar teeth. Oral Surg 1974;38:773-783.

161. Rapp R, Matthews G, Simpson M, Pashley DH. In vitro permeability of furcation dentin in permanent teeth. J Endod 1992;18:444-447.

162. Vertucci FJ, Beatty RG. Apical leakage associated with retrofilling techniques: A dye study. J Endod 1986;12: 331-336.

163. Gilheany PA, Figdor D, Tyas MJ. Apical dentin permeability and microleakage associated with root end resection and retrograde filling. J Endod 1994;20:22-26.

164. Rud J, Munksgaard EC, Andreasen JO, Rud V. Retrograde root filling with composite and a dentin-bonding agent. 2. Endod Dent Traumatol 1991;7:126-131.

165. Andreasen JO, Munksgaard EC, Fredebo L, Rud L. Periodontal tissue regeneration including cementogenesis adjacent to dentin-bonded retrograde composite fillings in humans. J Endod 1993;19:151-153.

166. Rud J, Rud V, Munksgaard EC. Long-term evaluation of retrograde root filling with dentin-bonded resin composite. J Endod 1996;22:90-93.

167. Nalbandian J, Gonzales F, Sognnaes RF. Sclerotic age changes in root dentin of human teeth as observed by optical, electron, and x-ray microscopy. J Dent Res 1960;39:598-607.

168. Weber DF. Human dentine sclerosis: A microradiographic survey. Arch Oral Biol 1974;19:163–169.
169. Vasiliadis L, Darling AI, Levers BGH. The histology of sclerotic human root dentine. Arch Oral Biol 1983;28: 693–700.
170. Tidmarsh BG, Arrowsmith G. Dentinal tubules at the root ends of apicected teeth: A scanning electron microscopy study. Int Endod J 1989;22:184–189.
171. Quevedo J, Spängberg L, Safavi K, Hand A. The numerical density of dentinal tubules at the apical pulpal wall [abstract PR 38]. J Endod 1997;23:276.
172. Matthews B, Vongsavan N. Interactions between neural and hydrodynamic mechanisms in dentine and pulp. Arch Oral Biol 1994;39(suppl):87S–97S.
173. Olgart L, Kerezoudis NP. Nerve pulp interactions. Arch Oral Biol 1994;39(suppl):47S–54S.
174. Heyeraas KJ, Berggreen E. Interstitial fluid pressure in normal and inflamed pulp. Crit Rev Oral Biol Med 1991;10:328–336.
175. Pashley DH, Galloway SE, Stewart FP. Effects of fibrinogen in vivo on dentine permeability in the dog. Arch Oral Biol 1984;29:725–728.
176. Chiego DJ. An ultrastructural and autoradiographic analysis of primary and replacement odontoblasts following cavity preparation and wound healing in the rat molar. Proc Finn Dent Soc 1992;88(suppl):243–256.
177. Bergenholtz G, Jontell M, Tuttle A, Knutsson G. Inhibition of serum albumin flux across exposed dentine following conditioning with GLUMA primer, glutaraldehyde or potassium oxalate. J Dent 1993;21:330–337
178. Bergenholtz G, Knutsson G, Okiji T, Jontell M. Albumin flux across dentin of young human premolars following temporary exposure to the oral environment. In: Shimono M, Takahashi K (eds). Dentin/Pulp Complex. Tokyo: Quintessence, 1996:51–57.
179. Cox CF, White KC, Ramus DL, Farmer JB, Snuggs HM. Reparative dentin: Factors affecting its deposition. Quintessence Int 1992;23:257–270.
180. Calland JW, Harris SE, Carnes DL. Human pulp cells respond to calcitonin gene-related peptide in vitro. J Endod 1997;23:485–489.
181. Finkelman RD, Mohan S, Jennings JC, Taylor AK, Jepsen S, Baylink DJ. Quantitation of growth factors IGF-I, SGF/IGF-II and TGF-β in human dentin. J Bone Miner Res 1990;5:717–723.
182. Magloire H, Bouvier M, Joffre A. Odontoblast response under carious lesions. Proc Finn Dent Soc 1992;88 (suppl 1):257–274.
183. Magloire H, Joffre A, Bleicher F. An in vitro model of human dental pulp repair. J Dent Res 1996;75: 1971–1978.
184. Cassidy N, Fahey M, Prime SS, Smith AJ. Comparative analysis of transforming growth factor-b isoforms 1–3 in human and rabbit dentin matrices. Arch Oral Biol 1997;42:219–223.
185. Roberts-Clark DJ, Smith AJ. Angiogenic growth factors in human dentine matrix. Arch Oral Biol 2000;45: 1013–1016.
186. Smith AJ, Sloan AJ, Matthews JB, Murray PE, Lumley P. Reparative processes in dentine and pulp. In: Addy M, Embery G, Edgar WM, Orchardson R (eds). Tooth Wear and Sensitivity. London: Martin-Dunitz, 2000:53–66.
187. Melin M, Joffre-Romeas A, Farges I-C, Couble M-L, Magloire H, Bleicher F. Effects of TGF-β1 on dental pulp cells in cultured human tooth slices. J Dent Res 2000; 79:1689–1696.
188. Sloan AJ, Matthews JB, Smith AJ. TGF-β receptor expression in human odontoblasts and pulpal cells. Histochem J 1999;31:565–569.
189. Sloan AJ, Smith AJ. Stimulation of the dentin-pulp complex of rat incisor teeth by transforming growth factor-β isoforms 1–3 in vitro. Arch Oral Biol 1999;44:149–156.
190. Sloan AJ, Perry H, Matthews JB, Smith AJ. Transforming growth factor-β isoform expression in mature healthy and carious molar teeth. Histochem J 2000;32:247–252.
191. Smith AJ, Tobias RS, Cassidy N, et al. Odontoblast stimulation in ferrets by dentine matrix components. Arch Oral Biol 1994;39:13–22.
192. Smith AJ, Tobias RS, Plant CG, Browne RM, Lesot H, Ruch JV. In vivo morphogenic activity of dentine matrix proteins. J Biol Bucc 1990;18:123–129.
193. Smith AJ, Cassidy N, Perry H, Begue-Kirn C, Ruch J-V, Lesot H. Reactionary dentinogenesis. Int J Dev Biol 1995;39:273–280.
194. Rutherford B, Spängberg L, Tucker M, Charette MC. Transdentinal stimulation of reparative dentin formation by osteogenic protein-1 in monkeys. Arch Oral Biol 1995;40:681–683.
195. Weibkin OW, Cardaci SC, Heithersay GS, Pierce AM. Therapeutic delivery of calcitonin to inhibit external inflammatory root resorption. II. Influence of calcitonin binding to root mineral. Endod Dent Traumatol 1996b;12: 272–276.
196. Byers MR. Dental sensory receptors. Int Rev Neurobiol 1984;25:39–44.
197. Olgart L. Neurogenic components of pulp inflammation. In: Shimono M, Takahashi K (eds). Dentin/Pulp Complex. Tokyo: Quintessence, 1996:169–175.
198. Närhi M, Yamamoto H, Ngassapa D. Function of intradental nociceptors in normal and inflammed teeth. In: Shimono M, Takahashi K (eds). Dentin/Pulp Complex. Tokyo: Quintessence, 1996:136–140.
199. Berggreen H, Heyeraas KJ. The role of sensory neuropeptides and nitric oxide on pulpal blood flow and tissue pressure in the ferret. J Dent Res 1999;78: 1535–1543.
200. Pashley DH. Dentine permeability and its role in the pathobiology of dentine sensitivity. Arch Oral Biol 1994;39(suppl):73S–80S.

201. Horiachi H, Matthews B. In vitro observations on fluid flow through human dentine caused by pain-producing stimuli. Arch Oral Biol 1973;18:275–294.
202. Pashley DH, Matthews WG, Zhang Y, Johnson M. Fluid shifts across human dentine in vitro in response to hydrodynamic stimuli. Arch Oral Biol 1996;11: 1065–1072.
203. Hussey DL, Biagioni PA, Lamey PJ. Thermographic measurements of temperature change during resin composite polymerization in vivo. J Dent 1995;25:267–271.
204. Olgart L. Involvement of sensory nerves in hemodynamic reactions. Proc Finn Dent Soc 1992;88(suppl 1): 403–410.
205. Olgart L. Neural control of pulpal blood flow. Crit Rev Oral Biol Med 1996;7:159–171.
206. Byers MR, Närhi MV, Mecifi KB. Acute and chronic reactions of dental sensory nerves to hydrodynamic stimulation or injury. Anat Rec 1988;221:872–883.
207. Ohsima H. Ultrastructural changes in odontoblasts and pulp capillaries following cavity preparation in rat molars. Arch Histol Cytol 1990;53:423–428.
208. Bishop MA. An investigation of pulp capillaries and tight junctions between odontoblasts in cats. Anat Embryol 1987;177:131–138.
209. Bishop MA. Extracellular fluid movement in the pulp: the pulp/dentin permeability barrier. Proc Finn Dent Soc 1992;88(suppl 1):331–336.
210. Turner D, Marfurt C, Sattelburg C. Demonstration of physiological barrier between pulpal odontoblasts and its perturbation following routine restorative procedures: A horseradish peroxidase tracing study in the rat. J Dent Res 1989;68(8):1262–1268.
211. Turner DF. Immediate physiological response of odontoblasts. Proc Finn Dent Soc 1992;88(suppl 1): 55–63.
212. Pinero GJ, Parker S, Rundus V, Hertzberg EL, Minkoff R. Immunolocalization of connexin 43 in the tooth germ of the neonatal rat. Histochem J 1994;26:765–770.
213. George CH, Kendall JM, Evans WH. Intracellular trafficking pathways in the assembly of connexins into gap junctions. J Biol Chem 1999;274;8678–8685.
214. Pashley DH, Nelson R, Williams EC, Kepler EE. Use of dentine-fluid protein concentrations to measure pulp capillary reflection coefficients in dogs. Arch Oral Biol 1981;26:703–706.
215. Knutsson G, Jontell M, Bergenholtz G. Determination of plasma proteins in dentinal fluid from cavities prepared in healthy young human teeth. Arch Oral Biol 1994;39: 185–190.
216. Eda S, Saito T. Electron microscopy of cells displaced into the dentinal tubules due to dry cavity preparation. J Oral Path 1978;7:326–335.
217. Fitzgerald M. Cellular mechanisms of dentinal bridge repair using 3H-thymidine. J Dent Res 1979;58: 2198–2206.
218. Kakehashi S, Stanley HR, Fitzgerald RJ. The effects of surgical exposure of dental pulps in germ-free and conventional laboratory rats. Oral Surg 1965;20:340–349.
219. Kobayashi C, Yoshida H. Wound healing of the exposed pulp in germ-free and conventional rats. Jpn J Conserv Dent 1981;24:747–753.
220. Cox CF, Bergenholtz G, Heys DR, Syed M, Fitzgerald M, Heys RJ. Pulp capping of dental pulp mechanically exposed to oral microflora: A 1-2 year observation of wound healing in the monkey. J Oral Pathol 1985;14: 156–158.
221. Cox CF, Keall CL, Keall HJ, Ostro E, Bergenholtz G. Biocompatibility of surface sealed dental materials against exposed pulps. J Prosthet Dent 1987a;57:1–8.
222. Cox CF. Biocompatibility of dental materials in the absence of bacterial infection. Oper Dent 1987b;12: 146–152.
223. Inoue T, Shimono M (1992). Repair dentinogenesis following transplantation into normal and germ-free animals. Proc Finn Dent Soc 1992;88(suppl):183–194.
224. Browne RM, Tobias RS. Microbial microleakage and pulpal inflammation: A review. Endod Dent Traumatol 1986; 2:177–183.
225. Cox CF, Suzuki S. Re-evaluating pulp protection: Calcium hydroxide liners versus cohesive hybridization. J Am Dent Assoc 1994;125:823–831.
226. Camps J, Dejou J, Remusat M, About I. Factors influencing pulpal response to cavity restorations. Dent Mater 2000;16:432–440.
227. Jontell M, Okiji T, Dahlgren U, Bergenholtz G. Interaction between perivascular dentitic cells, neuropeptides, and endothelial cells in the dental pulp. In: Shimono M, Takahashi K (eds). Dentin/Pulp Complex. Tokyo: Quintessence, 1996:182–187.
228. Jontell M, Okiji T, Dahlgren U, Bergenholtz G. Immune defense mechanisms of the dental pulp. Crit Rev Oral Biol Med 1998;9:179–200.
229. Jontell M, Hanks CT, Bratel J, Bergenholtz G. Effects of unpolymerized resin components on the function of accessory cells derived from the rat incisor pulp. J Dent Res 1995;74:1162–1167.
230. Rakich DR, Wataha JC, Lefebvre CA, Weller RN. Effects of dentin bonding agents on macrophage mitochondrial activity. J Endod 1998;24:528–533.
231. Rakich DR, Wataha JC, Lefebvre CA, Weller RN. Effects of dentin bonding agents on the secretion of inflammatory mediators from macrophages. J Endod 1999;25: 114–117.

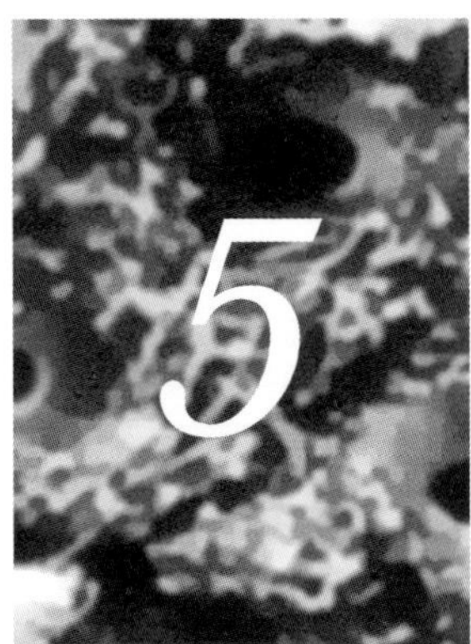

Pulp As a Connective Tissue

Takashi Okiji, DDS, PhD

Dental pulp is a connective tissue uniquely situated within the rigid encasement of mineralized dentin. Although dental pulp shares many properties with other connective tissues of the body, the peculiar location of dental pulp imposes several special characteristics on it. It is apparent that the composition and structure of the pulp are quite different from those of the dentin. However, the two tissues exist in intimate embryologic and functional relation, which is why the dentin and pulp are usually considered together as an undissociable functional complex, termed the *pulpodentin complex*.

General Properties of Connective Tissue

Connective tissue is the supporting tissue widely distributed throughout the body. The major constituent of connective tissue is its extracellular matrix, which is mainly composed of fibriller proteins and ground substance. Connective tissue cells are scattered within the extracellular matrix. Fibriller proteins form an extensively meshed network of long, slender polymers that are arranged in an amorphous hydrated gel of ground substance. There are two types of fibriller proteins: collagen and elastin. Collagen is the more abundant type and is the main component of collagen fibers, which confer strength of the tissue. Elastin is the main component of elastic fibers, which provide elasticity to the tissue. In the pulp, elastic fibers are distributed only in the walls of larger blood vessels. Ground substance is responsible primarily for the viscoelasticity and filtration function of connective tissue. It is mainly composed of macromolecules called *proteoglycans*, which consist of a protein core and a varying number of large, unbranched polysaccharide side chains called *glycosaminoglycans*. Extracellular matrix also contains adhesive glycoproteins such as fibronectin, which primarily function to mediate cell-matrix interactions.

Fibroblasts are the principal cells in connective tissue. They form a network within extracellular matrix and produce a wide range of extracellular matrix components already described. They are also responsible for degrading the extracellular elements and thus are essential in the remodeling of connective tissue. Other cellular elements

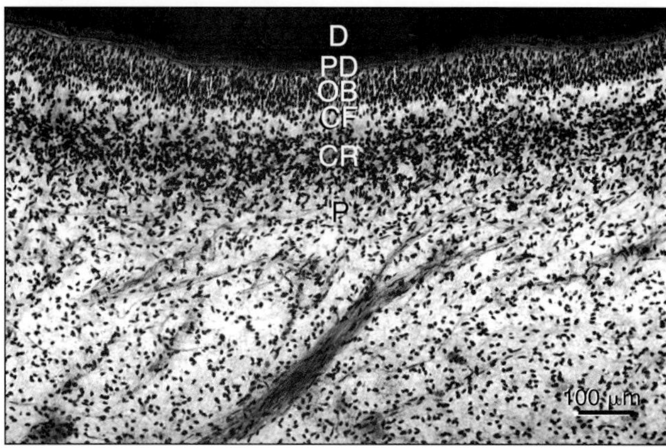

Fig 5-1 Light micrograph of mature coronal pulp (human third molar). D, dentin; PD, predentin; OB, odontoblast layer; CF, cell-free zone; CR, cell-rich zone; P, pulp proper.

include blood-derived defense cells, such as macrophages, whose primary function is to cope with infection.

There are several types of connective tissue that differ in their relative composition of the basic elements already described. Connective tissue proper is divided broadly into two classes: *(1)* loose connective tissue, which is rich in ground substance and contains relatively fewer fibers, and *(2)* dense connective tissue, which is characterized by a clear predominance of collagen fibers and fewer cells. Dental pulp is classified as a loose connective tissue.

The major function of connective tissue is to provide a matrix that binds cells and organs and ultimately gives support to the body. Connective tissue is also responsible for various activities that initiate and orchestrate reactions to pathogenic invasion, and thus it serves as an essential site of host defense. Connective tissue also has a remarkable capacity to repair damaged tissue in the form of scarring.

Structural Organization of the Pulp

In the central core of the pulp, the basic components already described are arranged in a manner similar to that found in other loose connective tissues. However, a characteristic cellular arrangement can be seen in the peripheral portion of the pulp (Fig 5-1).

A layer of odontoblasts, the specialized cells that elaborate dentin, circumscribes the outermost part of the pulp. They form a single layer lining the most peripheral portion of the pulp, with cell bodies in the pulp and long cytoplasmic processes, the odontoblast processes, extending into the dentinal tubules (Fig 5-2). The shape of the cell body of odontoblasts is not uniform, rather these cells are tall and columnar in the coronal pulp, short and columnar in the midportion of the tooth, and cuboidal to flat in the root portion. A network of capillaries, termed the *terminal capillary network*, exists within the odontoblast layer.[1] There also exist nerve fibers (terminal axons that exit from the plexus of Raschkow) that pass between the odontoblasts as free nerve endings[2] (Fig 5-3). Moreover, this layer is populated by a substantial number of Class II major histocompatibility complex (MHC) molecule-expressing dendritic cells that may be responsible for detecting transdentinal antigenic stimuli.[3,4] Collagen fibrils,[5-8] proteoglycans,[9,10] and fibronectin[11,12] are identified between odontoblasts. They seem to be part of the interodontoblastic fibrous structure, the Korff fibers, which may be demonstrated by means of silver impregnation.

Subjacent to the odontoblast layer, an area relatively free of cells is seen. This area is known as the cell-free zone or zone of Weil. Major constituents of this zone include the rich network of mostly unmyelinated nerve fibers (see Fig 5-3), blood capillaries, and processes of fibroblasts. This zone is often inconspicuous when the odontoblasts are actively forming dentin.

More deeply situated pulpward is the cell-rich zone, which has a relatively high density of cells. The constituents of this zone are basically the

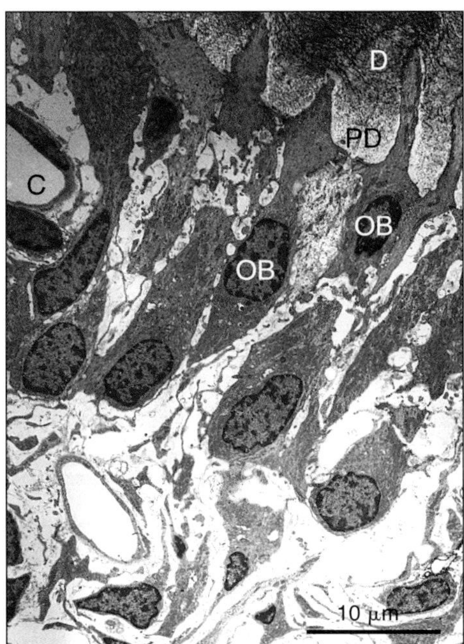

Fig 5-2 Electron micrograph of the odontoblast layer of a rat molar. D, dentin; PD, predentin; OB, odontoblast; C, capillary.

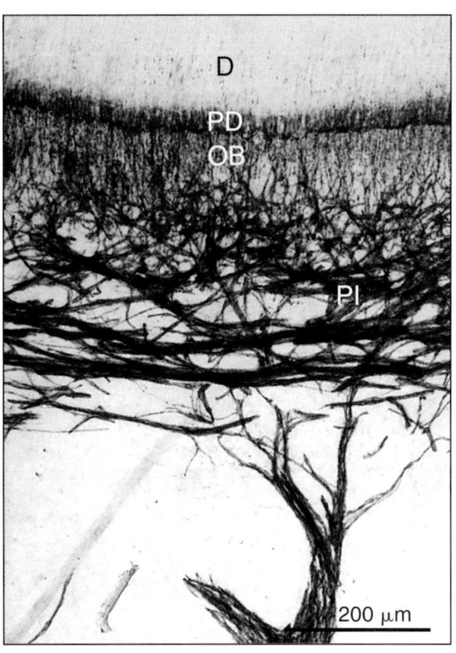

Fig 5-3 Distribution of neural elements (nerve fibers and Schwann cells) in a human third molar. Immunoperoxidase staining using a monoclonal antibody directed against nerve growth factor receptor. D, dentin; PD, predentin; OB, odontoblast layer; PI, plexus of Raschkow.

same as those in the pulp proper, ie, fibroblasts, undifferentiated mesenchymal cells, defense cells (macrophages and lymphocytes), blood capillaries, and nerves. This zone is discernible due to its higher density of fibroblasts than the pulp proper and is much more prominent in the coronal pulp than in the root pulp. It has been suggested that this zone is a source of cells that differentiate into secondary (replacement) odontoblasts upon injury to primary odontoblasts (see chapter 3).

From the cell-rich zone inward is the central connective tissue mass known as pulp proper or pulp core. This zone contains fibroblasts, the most abundant cell type; larger blood vessels; and nerves. Undifferentiated mesenchymal cells and defense cells such as macrophages are frequently located in the perivascular area. Collagen-fiber bundles are much more numerous in the root pulp than in the coronal pulp. The clinical implication of this higher density of collagen-fiber bundles in the apical region is the use of a barbed broach during pulpectomies. The most efficient removal of pulp tissue is achieved when the broach is passively placed apically to engage these large collagen bundles.

Pulp As the Soft Tissue Component of the Pulpodentin Complex

As already stated, the pulp is usually considered together with the dentin as the pulpodentin complex due to anatomic, developmental, and functional relationships. Structurally, pulpal elements such as odontoblast processes and neuronal terminals extend into the dentin. Functional coupling between pulp and dentin is exemplified in several aspects: *(1)* pulp is capable of elaborating dentin both physiologically and in response to external stimuli; *(2)* pulp carries nerves that give dentin its sensitivity; *(3)* pulpal connective tissue is able to respond to dentinal injuries, even when it is not directly stimulated; and *(4)* encapsulation in dentin creates a low-compliance environment that influences the defense potential of the pulp.

Low-compliance environment

The most restrictive anatomic feature characteristic of the connective tissue of pulp is that it is encased in rigid mineralized tissue. This provides the pulp a low-compliance environment in which nutrition for the tissue is almost entirely supplied via vessels traversing the narrow apical foramen. Recognition of this physiologic restriction was the historical basis for the so-called self-strangulation theory that stigmatized the pulp as a connective tissue with a low capacity for defense or repair. According to the theory, increased tissue pressure, resulting from even modest increases in vasodilation and plasma exudation during inflammation, caused blood vessel compression and resultant ischemia and pulp necrosis. Some studies indeed showed a dramatic and sustained decrease of pulpal blood flow following application of inflammatory mediators.[13] However, more recent studies indicate that the pulp has physiologic feedback mechanisms that act to oppose increases in tissue pressure (ie, increased lymph flow and absorption of interstitial fluid into capillaries in noninflamed areas).[14] This may be why inflammation of the pulp is usually long-standing within a confined area but heals following appropriate treatment measures. See chapter 6 for a detailed description of this point.

Dentin permeability

As described extensively in chapter 4, dentin is not a barrier that completely prevents the invasion of external noxious substances, eg, bacteria and their by-products, in the underlying pulp. This is due to its tubular structure, through which irritants may diffuse and affect the pulp in a number of clinical situations. A clear example is the effect of Class V cavity preparations in monkey teeth. Neutrophil infiltration was evident in the area of the pulp below the cut dentin when bacterial products were sealed within the cavities, whereas little or no inflammation was seen when the bacterial products were not applied.[15,16] Responses of the connective tissue of the pulp to several types of injuries, including caries and operative procedures, are thus highly dependent on the degree of dentinal damage and resultant status of dentin permeability.[17–20]

Dentin permeability is influenced by pathophysiologic conditions of the neural and vascular systems of the underlying pulp. Microcirculatory changes of the pulp under the low-compliance environment can determine the status of pulpal blood flow, plasma exudation, and intradental tissue pressure, and thus may influence the amount and direction of dentinal fluid movement.[13,21,22] As described below, excitation of intradental nerves causes release of vasoactive neuropeptides that potentially influence pulpal circulation.[20,22–24]

Sensory innervation

The extremely rich sensory innervation (see Fig 5-3) likely influences the defense reactions in the connective tissue of the pulp (see also chapter 7). A large portion of the sensory fibers contains neuropeptides, such as substance P and calcitonin gene-related peptide (CGRP),[2,25] which are stored in the nerve terminals and may be released upon depolarization. These neuropeptides are known to modulate vasodilation and increase in vascular permeability (neurogenic inflammation). Several researchers have actually demonstrated that stimulation of pulpal sensory nerves induces blood-flow increases and vascular leakage of proteins, which are most likely mediated by the release of neuropeptides.[21,26,27] Immunomodulatory effects of these neuropeptides have also been suggested.[28]

Substance P and CGRP exert trophic effects on the growth of pulp fibroblasts in vitro.[29,30] Moreover, inferior alveolar nerve sectioning and capsaicin treatment, both of which caused a decrease in the number of nerves containing substance P

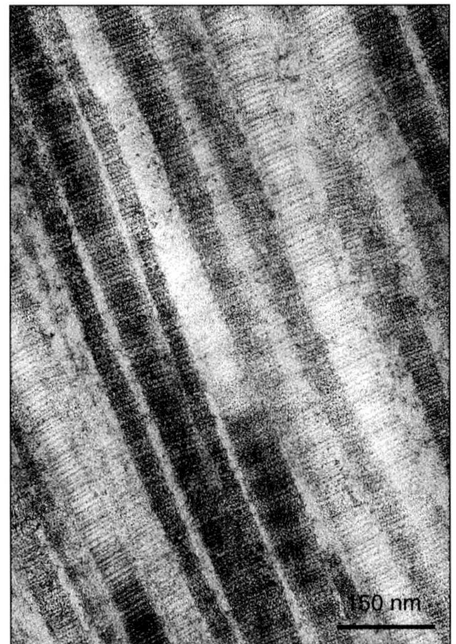

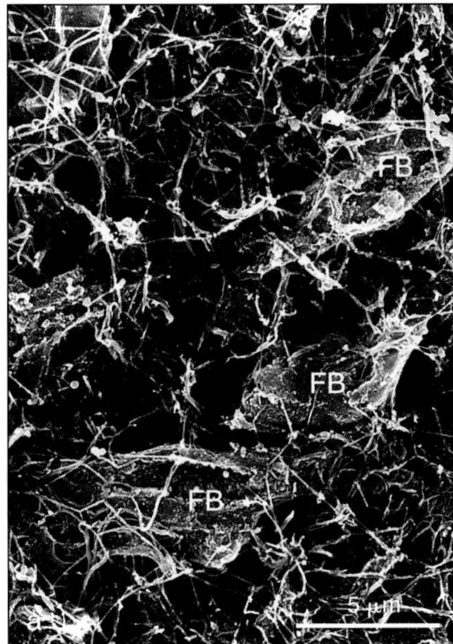

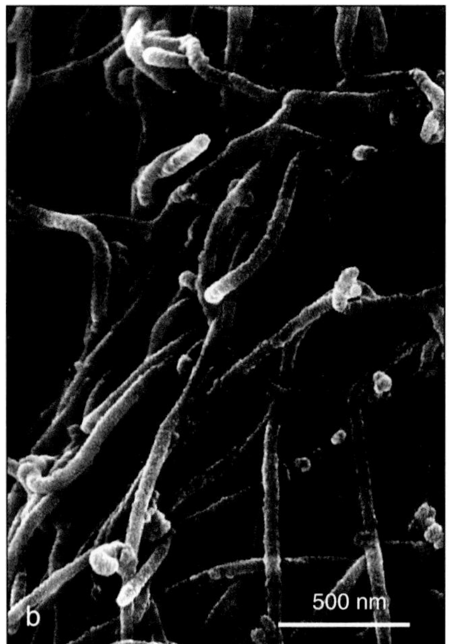

Fig 5-4 Transmission electron micrograph (TEM) of collagen fibrils in the central portion of the coronal pulp of a rat molar. Characteristic striations are visible.

Fig 5-5 Scanning electron micrograph (SEM) of the central portion of the coronal pulp of a rat molar. *(a)* Low-power view showing network of collagen fibrils. Fibroblasts (FB) are embedded. *(b)* High-power view showing striations of the fibrils.

and CGRP, resulted in reduced secondary dentin deposition in rat molars.[31] These findings suggest that sensory nerves play a role in the modulation of extracellular matrix production and secondary dentinogenesis. Thus, pulpal sensory neurons have afferent (ie, pain-detecting) and efferent (ie, neurogenic inflammation, immunomodulatory, and healing) functions.

Extracellular Matrix of the Pulp

Collagen overview

Collagen is an extracellular structural protein that represents the major constituent of all connective tissues. Its structure is characterized by the presence of the triple-helical domain, which is formed by an assembly of three polypeptide chains (α chains) bound by hydrogen bonds and hydrophobic interactions. Chemically, collagen contains two characteristic amino acids: hydroxyproline and hydroxylysine. Glycine, proline, and hydroxyproline are the three main amino acid components, but there are at least 15 collagen types that differ in chemical composition, morphology, distribution, and function.[32] Cells responsible for the synthesis of collagen include fibroblasts, chondroblasts, osteoblasts, cementoblasts, and odontoblasts.

Collagen type I is the most common form and occurs in a variety of tissues, including skin, tendon, bone, dentin, and dental pulp. Type I collagen is the major component of macromolecular structures, designated as collagen fibers. The collagen fibers are made up of fibrils in which the basic collagen molecules are aggregated in a highly organized structure. The fibrils display characteristic striations at intervals of 67 nm, determined by the stepwise overlapping arrangement of the molecules, and are a hallmark for identification of collagen fibrils under the electron microscope (Figs 5-4 and 5-5). The common molecular species contains two genetically distinct α chains that differ in their amino acid composition and sequence in a ratio of 2 to 1. This molecular arrangement is designated as $[\alpha 1(I)]_2\alpha 2(I)$. Small amounts of homotrimers ($[\alpha 1(I)]_3$) occur in some circumstances.

The biosynthesis of collagen involves a highly organized sequence of unique posttranslational modifications of the original polypeptides. These modifications proceed through the following steps: *(1)* formation of polypeptide chains by the polyribosomes of rough endoplastic reticulum; *(2)* hydroxylation of proline and lysine residues; *(3)* glycosylation of hydroxylysine residues; *(4)* assembly of polypeptide chains to form procollagen with a triple-helix configuration; *(5)* transportation to the Golgi complex, where procollagen molecules are packaged in secretory vesicles; *(6)* secretion of procollagen molecules into the extracellular space, where the terminal telopeptide is cleaved to form collagen molecules; *(7)* aggregation to form collagen fibrils; and *(8)* reinforcement and insolubilization of the fibrillar structure by cross-linking.

Collagen fibers are inelastic but have great tensile strength, giving the tissue its consistency and strength. Dense connective tissue such as tendon contains many collagen fibers assembled to form collagen bundles. However, loose connective tissue, such as dental pulp, contains fewer collagen fibers.

Differences in the combinations and linkages of the polypeptide chains making up collagen molecules are responsible for the different types of collagen. Based on their supramolecular structures, the collagens are divided into two main classes: fibriller collagens (types I to III, V, and XI) and nonfibriller collagens. Collagen type II ($[\alpha 1(II)]_3$) mainly occurs in cartilage and forms only thin fibrils, which do not aggregate into fibers. This type does not occur in the pulp. Type III ($[\alpha 1(III)]_3$) usually codistributes with type I collagen in a variety of unmineralized tissues and is a main component of reticular fibers, which form a loose mesh of extremely fine fibers particularly rich during embryogenesis, inflammatory processes, and wound healing. Type IV (occurs as $[\alpha 1(IV)]_2\alpha 2(VI)$, $[\alpha 1(IV)]_3$, or $[\alpha 2(IV)]_3$) and type VII ($[\alpha 1(VII)]_3$) are present in the basement membranes. Type V occurs as $[\alpha 1(V)]_2\alpha 2(V)$, $[\alpha 1(V)]_3$, or $\alpha 1(V)\alpha 2(V)\alpha 3(V)$ and is widely distributed in a variety of unmineralized tissues. Type VI is a heterotrimer of three distinct chains, $\alpha 1(VI)$, $\alpha 2(VI)$, and $\alpha 3(VI)$, and is widely distributed in the body as interfibrillar filaments.

Collagen in pulp

Collagen is a major organic component in the pulp, although the pulp appears to contain relatively lower concentrations of collagen compared with other collagenous connective tissues. The amount of collagen in dried human pulp is 25.7% in premolars and 31.9% in third molars.[33] These percentages are much higher than those reported for pulp in other species, such as 10.3% of the total protein in rabbit incisor pulp.[34] The content is higher in the radicular part of the pulp than in the coronal part.

Of the collagen molecules occurring in the pulp, types I and III represent the bulk of the tissue collagen.[35-37] Type I is the predominant type and may contribute to the establishment of the architecture of the pulp. It is found mainly in thick, striated fibrils distributed in varying numbers and density throughout the connective tissue of the pulp. The relative proportion of type III collagen in the pulp is also high.[35-40] It has been reported that type III collagen constitutes 42.6% of total collagen in human pulp[33] and over 40% in bovine pulp.[36] This high level may provide the pulp a certain measure of elasticity.[41] Type III collagen usually forms thinner fibrils than type I. In the pulp proper, type III collagen appears as fine-branched filaments, whose distribution is similar to that of reticular fibers.[37] In both cell-free and cell-rich zones, type III collagen is richly distributed.[42]

The composition of collagen types in dentin and predentin differs considerably from that of pulp. Dentin and predentin collagens are almost exclusively composed of type I,[38,43] although some investigators detected the presence of type III[42,44] and type V[45,46] collagens in predentin. Pulp fibroblasts can produce both type I and type III collagens, whereas the majority of collagen molecules produced by odontoblasts are type I.[47] This finding supports the idea that dentin collagen originates from odontoblasts and is not a combined product of odontoblasts and pulp fibroblasts.

Collagen fibers between odontoblasts were originally described as coarse argyrophilic fibers, the so-called Korff fibers, arising from the pulp, passing spirally between the odontoblasts, and entering the predentin. These fibers are particularly evident during early dentinogenesis, suggesting that they are implicated in odontoblast differentiation and formation of the mantle dentin. Ten Cate et al, however, reported that there was no electron microscopic evidence of collagen bundles of the size of Korff fibers between odontoblasts.[48,49] Yet later electron microscopic studies detected interodontoblastic collagen fibers, some of which were continuous from the predentin to the pulp, possibly corresponding to the Korff fibers.[5–8,50] These fibers are mainly composed of collagen types I[51] and III.[44,51,52]

Collagen type V[39,40,46] and type VI[40,46,53] have been observed in the pulp forming a dense meshwork of thin microfibrils throughout the stroma of the connective tissue of the pulp. Corkscrew fibers of collagen type VI have been found between fully differentiated odontoblasts toward the predentin, suggesting that these fibers are a component of Korff fibers.[40] In addition, collagen type IV is identified as a component of basement membranes of pulpal blood vessels.[40,54]

Turnover of collagen fibers in normal pulp is fairly high as compared with that of other dental tissues.[55] This activity is mostly associated with fibroblasts, which are able to both synthesize and degrade collagen (see Fibroblasts of the Pulp below). Upon bacterial infection and inflammation, collagen degradation may be accelerated, an observation supported by the findings that pulps collected from teeth diagnosed with suppurative pulpitis showed elevated collagenolytic activity[56] and that no structure showing immunoreactivity to collagen type III was detected in the area of inflammatory infiltrates in pulpitic human teeth.[57] Collagenase produced by bacteria and/or neutrophils may be primarily responsible for such accelerated collagen degradation. However, in vitro studies have suggested that fibroblasts also up-regulate production of collagenolytic enzymes in response to infection and inflammation.[58–60]

Collagen synthesis in the pulp is accelerated during the reparative process, exemplified in the process of dentin bridge formation following application of calcium hydroxide to exposed vital pulps (see also chapter 13). Calcium hydroxide initially induces the formation of a superficial necrotic zone due to its high pH. Following infiltration of inflammatory cells, fibroblast-like cells (including progenitors of secondary odontoblasts) proliferate and migrate to the injury site. This action is followed by the formation of new collagen that is arranged in contact with the superficial necrotic zone and contains cellular inclusions.[61] Thus the application of calcium hydroxide results in an accelerated collagen formation. During the early phase of reparative dentinogenesis, collagen fibrils show an interodontoblastic arrangement comparable to that of Korff fibers. However, these fibers become thinner and fewer following establishment of a firm layer of secondary odontoblasts.[62,63] It has thus been postulated that these fibers give support to the precursors of secondary odontoblasts before the formation of the regular odontoblastic layer.

Elastin

Elastin molecules are joined to form a random coil structure that expands and contracts like a rubber band. This characteristic confers a pronounced elasticity to these fibers. Elastic fibers are first formed in bundles of thin microfibrils called *oxytalan fibers*. Elastin is then deposited between oxytalan fibers to form elastic fibers. In the pulp, elastic fibers are always associated with larger blood vessels. Fine oxytalan fibril-like, nonstriated filaments interspersed between collagen fibrils have been observed[64]; however, a later immunoelectron microscopic study reported that these filaments represent type III collagen.[37]

Glycosaminoglycogens and proteoglycans

Glycosaminoglycans are long, unbranched polymers of repeating disaccharide units (70 to 200 residues). The disaccharides usually consist of a hexosamine (glucosamine or galactosamine), which may contain ester sulfate groups, and a uronic acid (D-glucuronic acid or L-iduronic acid) with a carboxyl group. There are four main types of glycosaminoglycans that differ in the composition of the disaccharides and in tissue distribution: chondroitin sulfate/dermatan sulfate, heparin sulfate/heparin, keratin sulfate, and hyaluronic acid. Hyaluronic acid is not sulfated and exists as free chains. The other glycosaminoglycans are present as constituents of proteoglycans, which consist of a central protein core to which side chains of glycosaminoglycans are covalently linked. The structure of proteoglycans is greatly heterogeneous in terms of the size of the core protein and the size and number of glycosaminoglycan chains. In general, the three-dimensional structure of proteoglycans can be portrayed as an interdental brush, with the wire stem representing the protein core and the bristles representing the glycosaminoglycans.

Because of the abundance of carboxyl groups, sulfated hexosamines, and hydroxyl groups in glycosaminoglycan chains, proteoglycans are intensely hydrophilic and act as polyanions. The long glycosaminoglycan chains form relatively rigid coils constituting a network in which a large amount of water is held. Thus, proteoglycans are present as a characteristic gel that occupies a large space relative to their weight and provides protection against compression of connective tissue. Given their spatial organization and high negative charge, proteoglycans prevent diffusion of larger molecules but attract cationic material. Importantly, most extracellular matrix proteins and many growth factors such as transforming growth factor-β have binding sites for glycosaminoglycans. Thus, proteoglycans regulate tissue organization by linking together several extracellular matrix components (which serve as cellular binding sites) and may act as a reservoir for bioactive molecules. Some proteoglycans, such as syndecan, are located on the cell membrane. These feature an extracellular domain that is able to bind to extracellular glycoproteins (collagen, fibronectin, tenascin, etc) and a cytoplasmic domain that links with the cytoskeleton. Thus they are cell-surface receptors that connect extracellular matrix molecules to the cell's cytoskeleton and control the cell's functions.[32]

The pulp contains several types of glycosaminoglycans that normally occur in other connective tissues.[38,65] In human pulp, chondroitin sulfate, dermatan sulfate, and hyaluronic acid are consistently found.[66–69] A variety of proteoglycans are also identified in the connective tissue of the pulp by means of immunohistochemistry.[9,10] Predentin possesses various types of glycosaminoglycans and proteoglycans, whereas dentin mainly contains chondroitin sulfate.[9,38,70,71]

Glycosaminoglycans and proteoglycans are thought to play an important role during dentinogenesis. They show an affinity for collagen and thus influence its fibrinogenesis, which takes place before the period of mineralization. Chondroitin sulfate, the major glycosaminoglycan present in teeth with active dentinogenesis, has a strong capacity to bind calcium[72] and may be involved in maintaining calcium phosphate during mineralization.[73] An in vitro study has demonstrated that glycosaminoglycan may also be involved in the maintenance of the polarized state of cultured odontoblasts.[74] In a recent study employing human teeth, decorin, a small chondroitin–dermatan sulfate proteoglycan consisting of a core protein and a single glycosaminoglycan chain, was immunolocalized in odontoblast cell bodies and its processes located within predentin and along the calcification front and dentinal tubules (Fig 5-6).[10] This finding suggests that decorin is synthesized by odontoblasts and transported through the odontoblast processes, where an accumulation along the calcification front may be involved in mineral nucleation.

During infection and inflammation, the high viscosity of proteoglycans may present a mechan-

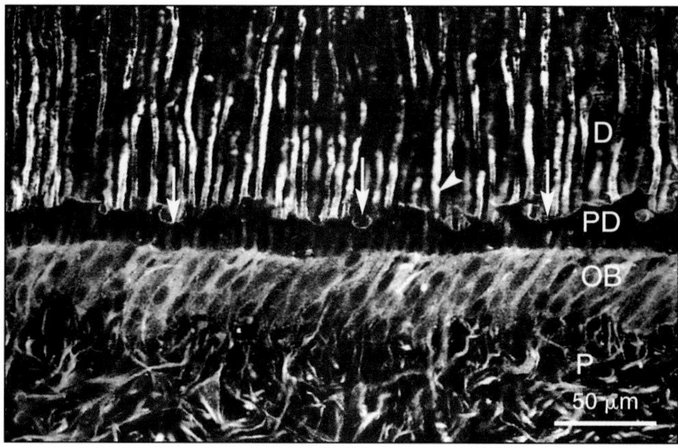

Fig 5-6 Distribution of the small proteoglycan decorin in the pulpodentin complex of a human tooth. Immunofluorescence staining using an antiserum against decorin. Intense immunoreactivity extends along the calcification front *(arrows)* and dentinal tubules. Odontoblast cell bodies (OB) and their processes *(arrowhead)* in predentin (PD) also express specific antibody reaction. D, dentin; P, pulp. (Reprinted from Yoshiba et al[10] with permission.)

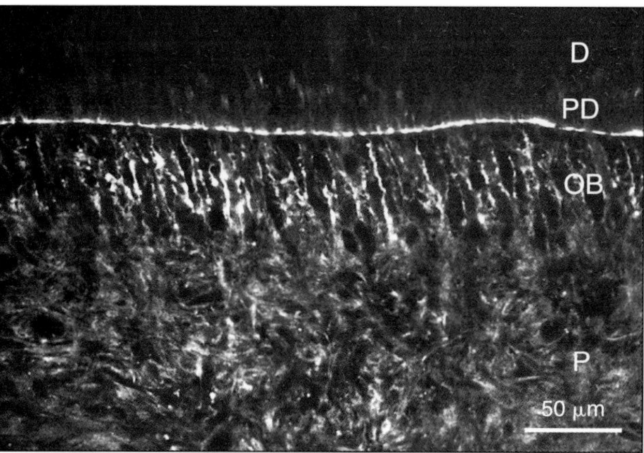

Fig 5-7 Distribution of fibronectin in the pulpodentin complex of a human tooth. Immunofluorescence staining using an antifibronectin antibody. Between odontoblasts (OB), fibrous structures, some of which extend into predentin, show specific antibody reaction. A fluorescent line is visible at the border between odontoblast cell bodies and predentin (PD). D, dentin; P, pulp. (Reprinted from Yoshiba et al[11] with permission.)

ical barrier to bacteria. However, several bacterial species, such as some strains of streptococci, produce hyaluronidase as a spreading factor. This enzyme reduces the viscosity of the barrier by hydrolyzing glycosaminoglycans and thus contributes to bacterial penetration of connective tissues. By virtue of this ability, hyaluronidase is presumed to be a factor promoting the destruction of periodontal tissues.[75] The enzyme activity has been detected in bacterial isolates from infected root canals,[76] although its relevance to pulpal pathosis is not completely understood.

Fibronectin

Fibronectin is a multifunctional stromal glycoprotein that exists as *(1)* a circulating plasma protein, *(2)* a protein that attaches on the surface of cells, and *(3)* insoluble fibrils forming part of the extracellular matrix. This molecule, with a molecular weight of 440,000, features sites binding collagen, glycosaminoglycans, and several cell adhesion molecules such as integrens. By virtue of this ability, fibronectin acts as a mediator for cell-cell and cell-matrix adhesion and thus has a major effect on the proliferation, differentiation, and organization of cells.

Fibronectin is ubiquitously distributed in the extracellular matrix of the pulp. In the pulp proper, it forms a reticular network of fibrils, with an increased concentration around the blood vessels.[42,77-79] Fibronectin is also immunolocalized in the odontoblast layer, where it forms corkscrew fibers passing from the pulp into predentin parallel to the long axis of odontoblasts[11,12,78] (Fig 5-7), which suggests that fibronectin is a constituent of Korff fibers. Fibronectin at this position is believed to mediate the interaction between fully differentiated odontoblasts and extracellular fibers and may contribute to the maintenance of the specific morphology of these cells.[11,12] Immunoreactivity of fibronectin is also seen at the border between odontoblast cell bodies and predentin, suggesting that fibronectin may contribute to the maintenance of a tight seal at this site.[11,12]

Fibronectin is implicated in the terminal differentiation and polarization of primary odontoblasts.[80,81] Preodontoblasts in the dental papilla are initially surrounded by fibronectin associated with the dental basement membrane. During terminal differentiation of odontoblasts, however, fibronectin is restricted to distribution around the apical pole of polarizing odontoblasts. Consequently, a 165-kDa nonintegrin protein, presumably representing a membrane fibronectin receptor, accumulates at the apical pole.[82] It has been postulated that an interaction between extracellular fibronectin and this protein modulates the shape and polarity of the odontoblasts through reorganization of the cytoskeleton.

As in other connective tissues, fibronectin may be involved in cell migration and anchorage in the wound-healing process of the connective tissue of the pulp. Moreover, it is implicated in reparative dentinogenesis as well. In exposed human pulps capped with calcium hydroxide, fibronectin is immunolocalized in the zone of initial dystrophic calcification located just beneath the superficial necrotic layer. Progression of odontoblast differentiation has been seen beneath this zone.[83] In another study in which cavity preparation was made in rat molars, fibronectin was shown to accumulate first in the exudative lesion below the cavity and then distributed in newly formed predentin.[84] These findings suggest that fibronectin regulates the migration and differentiation of secondary odontoblasts.

Fibronectin is recognized by most adherent cells via integrins, a group of heterodimeric cell-surface glycoprotein receptors. The integrins are composed of two noncovalently linked polypeptide chains, α and β. Eight α subunits and 15 β subunits have been identified. The various combinations of α and β subunits constitute about 30 different integrin molecules that differ in their ligand-binding specificity and expression on different types of cells. Each subunit contains a large extracellular domain, a transmembrane segment, and usually a short cytoplasmic domain. The extracellular domain, where the α and β subunits are bound, interacts with their ligands. The cytoplasmic domain forms links with the cytoskeleton through a series of linked proteins. Thus, integrins are transmembrane receptors that link the intracellular actin network with extracellular matrix.[85] Besides fibronectin, there are various other integrin ligands, including extracellular proteins (collagen, laminin, tenascin), adhesion molecules belonging to the immunoglobulin superfamily, fibrinogen, coagulation factors, complement factor C3b, and some bacterial and viral proteins. Fibroblasts from human pulp have been reported to express $\alpha 1$, $\alpha 3$, $\alpha 5$, $\alpha 6$, αv, and $\beta 1$ integrin subunits, although subunits responsible for fibronectin binding have not yet been determined.[86,87]

Basement membrane

At the epithelial-mesenchymal interface, there exists a sheet-like arrangement of extracellular matrix proteins known as the basement membrane. Under conventional electron microscopy, the sheet resolves into two layers: an electron-dense "lamina densa" and an electron-lucent "lamina lucida." The basement membrane is a combined product of connective tissue and epithelium and is mainly composed of type IV collagen, the adhesive glycoprotein laminin, fibronectin, and heparian sulfate. The dental basement membrane, found at the interface between the inner enamel epithelium and the dental papilla, also expresses these molecules.[88] Type IV collagen molecules aggregate to form a flexible meshwork, with binding sites for the rest of the basement membrane components, and thus they form the skeleton for several adhesive proteins. Laminin binds not only to the basement membrane components but also to epithelial cells, thereby anchoring these cells to the sheet of type IV collagen. Besides providing anchorage, the basement membrane acts as a molecular sieve that controls the passage of molecules between epithelial cells and connective tissue. Moreover, the basement membrane controls cell organization and differentiation by the mutual interaction of extracellular matrix molecules and cell-surface receptors. This type of action is well exemplified in the process of odontoblast differentiation during tooth development (see chapter 2). In mature pulp, basement membranes are distributed at the cell-connective tissue interfaces of endothelial cells and Schwann cells, as demonstrated by immunohistochemistry to laminin and type IV collagen.[40,54]

Cells of the Pulp

Odontoblasts

Odontoblast structure and function

Odontoblasts, the most highly differentiated cells of the pulp, are postmitotic neural crest-derived cells. They produce the components of the organic matrix of predentin and dentin, including collagens (mainly type I) and proteoglycans. Odontoblasts also synthesize various noncollagenous proteins, including bone sialoprotein, dentin sialoprotein, phosphophoryn, osteocalcin, osteonectin, and osteopontin. Dentin sialoprotein and phosphophoryn are considered to be dentin-specific.[89] These molecules are secreted at the apical end of the cell body as well as along the cytoplasmic processes within the tubules of the predentin. Moreover, odontoblasts may intracellularly transport calcium ions to the mineralization front.[90] In addition, they may also have the capacity to degrade organic matrix.[91] Odontoblasts are most active during the early period of primary dentin formation. The cell body of actively synthesizing odontoblasts is columnar, 5 to 7 µm in diameter and approximately 40 µm in length. Following the completion of primary dentin formation, the odontoblasts become less active and appear rather flat.

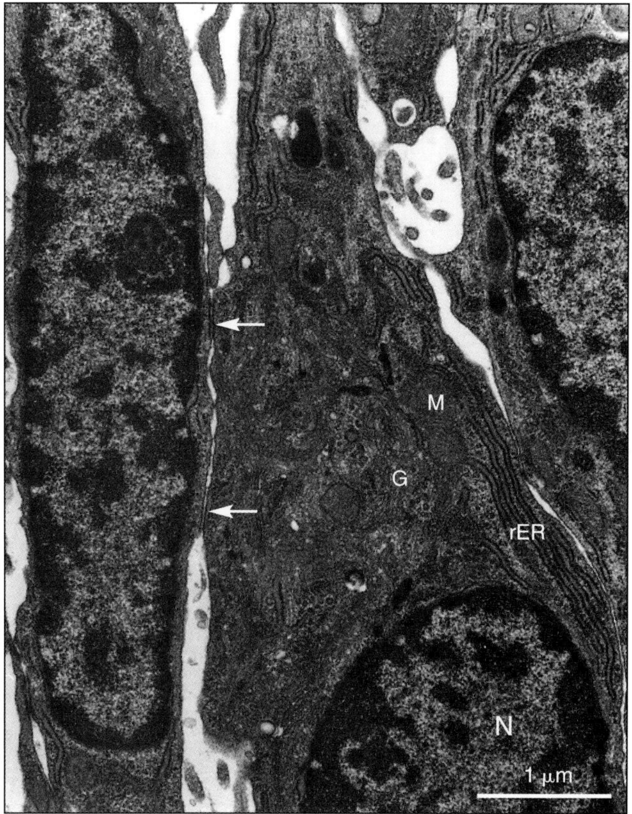

Fig 5-8 Ultrastructure of odontoblast cell body (rat molar). N, nucleus; G, Golgi complex; M, mitochondria; rER, rough endoplasmic reticulum; *arrows*, cell-cell junctions.

The cytoplasmic feature of the odontoblast cell body varies according to the cell's functional activity.[92-95] Actively synthesizing odontoblasts exhibit all characteristics of matrix-synthesizing cells. They display prominent organelles consisting of an extensive rough endoplasmic reticulum, a well-developed Golgi complex, numerous mitochondria, and numerous vesicles (Fig 5-8). A large oval nucleus is eccentrically located in the basal part of the cell body. This nucleus contains up to four nucleoli and is surrounded by a nuclear envelope. A particularly well-developed rough endoplasmic reticulum is found throughout the entire cell body, closely associated with numerous mitochondria. The rough endoplasmic reticulum consists of closely stacked cisternae that are usually aligned parallel to the long axis of the cell body. Numerous ribosomes are associated with the membranes of the cisternae. A well-developed Golgi complex composed of several stacks of saccules is centrally located in the supranuclear region. Numerous transport vesicles are accumulated at the immature face of the Golgi complex, and secretory granules of various sizes are found at the mature face. Autoradiographic studies using a radioactive collagen precursor (^{3}H-proline) as a tracer revealed that the synthesis, migration, and

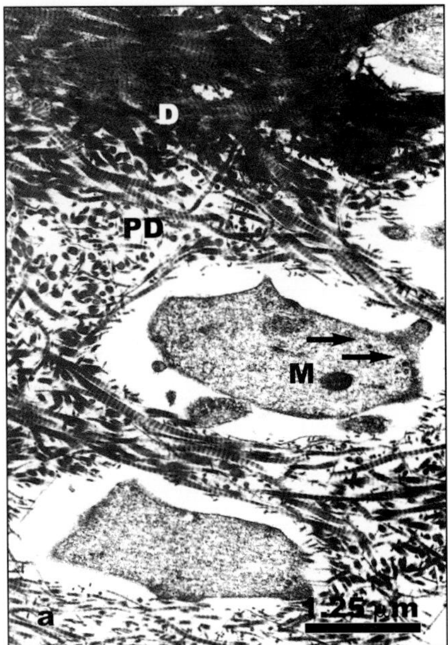

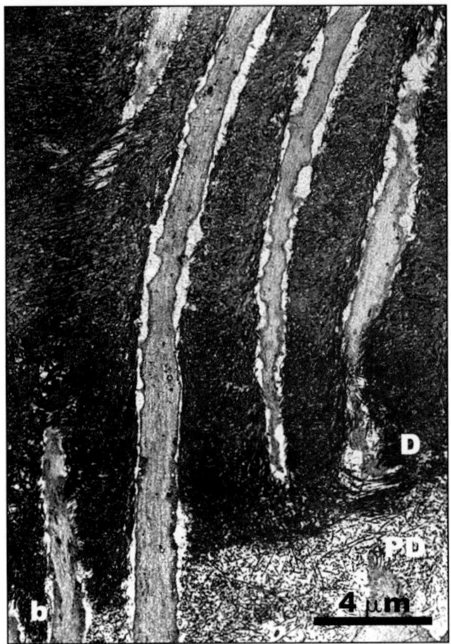

Fig 5-9 Ultrastructure of odontoblast process (rat molar). D, dentin; PD, predentin. *(a)* Cross section of processes in predentin showing mitochondria (M) and vesicles *(arrows)*. *(b)* Longitudinal section of processes situated in predentin and dentin showing parallel alignment of microtubules and filaments.

release of collagen precursors in odontoblasts follow the classical pathway for secretion of extracellular proteins. The isotope was rapidly incorporated in the rough endoplasmic reticulum and transported to the Golgi apparatus, where it was packed into secretory vesicles. The vesicles then migrated to the base of the cellular process, where the labeled vesicles fused with the cell membrane and the contents were released into the predentin matrix.[91,96] Numerous mitochondria are evenly distributed throughout the cell body. Besides being the major site of adenosine triphosphate (ATP) production, mitochondria in odontoblasts may also serve as sites for intracellular storage and regulation of calcium.[91] Numerous filaments and microtubules are located among the organelles described above. This cytoskeleton contributes to cell shape and polarity.

Quiescent odontoblasts are shorter and less polarized than actively synthesizing cells and show a reduction in number and size of the endoplasmic reticulum, Golgi complex, and mitochondria.[93-95] When the cells are in the transitional stage between active synthesis and quiescence, these organelles tend to show perinuclear distribution. Autophagic vacuoles can be seen within the cytoplasm, and thus an autophagic process may mediate the reduction of organelles. At the final stage of the cell's life cycle, these organelles are located only within the infranuclear region; the supranuclear region is devoid of organelles except for large lipid-filled vacuoles.[94]

Odontoblast process

The odontoblast process is a direct extension of the cell body and occupies most of the space within the dentinal tubules (Fig 5-9). Its diameter is 3 to 4 µm at the pulp-predentin border and gradually narrows as it passes within the dentinal tubules. The process has numerous side branches that may contact the branches of other odontoblasts. In contrast to the main cell body, the process is virtually devoid of major organelles for synthetic activity. A few cisternae of the endoplasmic reticulum, sparsely occurring mitochondria, and occasional ribosome-like granules are seen, mostly at the level of the predentin. However, the process displays a well-developed cytoskeleton as its principal component, filled with numerous microfilaments and microtubules oriented parallel to its long axis.[92,95,97–101] The process also contains numerous secretory vesicles and coated vesicles of various sizes and shapes.

Cavity or crown preparation may disturb odontoblast processes, leading to irreversibly damage odontoblasts. Thus information on the extent or length of odontoblast processes is important to clinicians because it allows for better estimation of the impact of tooth cutting on the pulpodentin complex. There is, however, controversy regarding the extent of the odontoblast process. It was long believed that the process occupies the full length of dentinal tubules. Several scanning and transmission electron microscopic studies, however, demonstrated that the process is present only in the inner third of the dentin.[97,99,102–106] However, the possibility that this finding is the result of shrinkage of the odontoblast processes during tissue preparation cannot be ruled out. On the other hand, other investigations using scanning electron microscopy (SEM) described the presence of odontoblast process-like structures in the periphery of dentin, even at the dentinoenamel junction.[107–110] It has been pointed out, however, that the images do not show actual processes but display an organic sheet-like structure, the so-called lamina limitans, which lines the inner peritubular dentin throughout the length of the tubules.[105,106] In immunohistochemical studies in which antibodies directed against cytoskeletal proteins (tubulin, actin, and vimentin) were employed, immunoreactivity was observed in the full thickness of the dentin, which suggests that the processes extend to the very periphery of the dentin.[110–112] However, a recent study employing fluorescent carbocyanine dye and confocal laser scanning microscopy also demonstrated that the processes in rat molars do not extend to the outer dentin except during the early stage of tooth development.[113] It seems obvious that this controversy is not yet resolved.

Odontoblast junctions

Several types of cell-cell junctions occur between adjacent odontoblasts. Desmosome-like junctions, which do not contain the intercellular disks found in typical epithelial desmosomes, occur along the lateral surfaces of the odontoblasts.[93,114–116] This type of junctional contact may promote cell-cell adhesion and play a role in maintaining the polarity of the odontoblasts. Gap junctions have also been described between the lateral surfaces of the odontoblasts.[115,116] These specialized junctions may provide pathways for intercellular transfer of ions and small water-soluble metabolites and thus may play a role in controlling cytodifferentiation of the odontoblasts and mineralization of dentin. From this perspective, gap junctions help to coordinate intercellular responses. The most prominent contact between odontoblasts is in the border region between the cell body and the process. This region contains the connecting apparatus, terminal bar–terminal web structures, which consists mostly of small-gap and tight junctions.[115,116] The tight junctions are seen exclusively in this region and may prevent passage of material between the odontoblasts. It is still unclear whether they completely encircle the odontoblasts (ie, as zonular tight junctions) or whether they are macular or "leaky." It is known that some small nerve fibers[2] and collagen fibers[7,8] pass through the interodontoblastic space and reach the predentin. This observation may indicate that the junctional complex in odontoblasts does not completely encircle the cell body. However, when the permeability of the junctions was tested by perfusion of intercellular tracers, no penetration of the tracers occurred beyond the tight junctions,[117–119] which may mean that the odontoblast layer acts as a physiologic barrier. One of the tracer experiments also demonstrated that the tracer penetrated into predentin and dentin following cavity preparation.[118] Such perturbation of the barrier suggests an increased outward dentinal

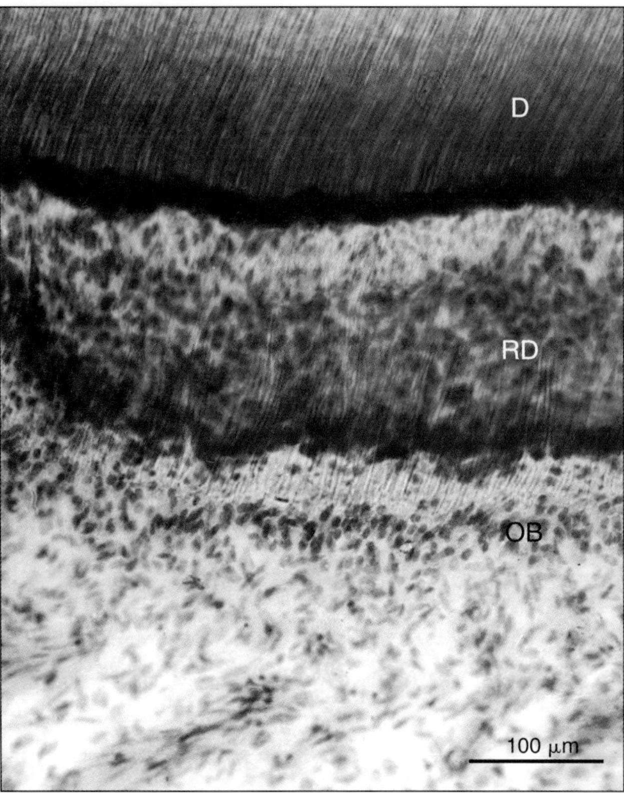

Fig 5-10 Reparative dentin (RD) formed in response to caries in a human third molar, showing more irregular, less mineralized, and less tubular structure than found in primary dentin (D). Odontoblasts (OB) are cuboidal.

fluid. This phenomenon may contribute to reparative processes, for it may transfer reparative compounds and ions to the site of injury and prevent inward diffusion of external noxious substances.

Responses of odontoblasts to injury

The pulpodentin complex has a unique kind of defense and repair reaction not seen in most other connective tissues. This reaction involves the formation of new mineralized tissue in response to injury (see also chapter 3). Either the odontoblasts already exist in the pulp (primary odontoblasts) or newly generated mineralized tissue-forming cells may elaborate the new mineralized tissue.

Under physiologic conditions, primary odontoblasts in the adult tooth produce new dentin (secondary dentin) at a very slow rate. Once the primary odontoblasts are injured, the dentin production may be accelerated as a defense/repair reaction. Depending on the nature, magnitude, and duration of the injury, the primary odontoblasts may be reversibly damaged or they may actually die. In the latter situation, the dead cells may be replaced by secondary (replacement) odontoblasts that produce new dentin matrix. For example, cavity preparation and/or desiccation of exposed dentin surface sometimes cause a particular type of irreversible injury to odontoblasts, termed *odontoblast aspiration*. In this reaction, the cell bodies of odontoblasts are sucked into the dentinal tubules, presumably by a rapid outward movement of fluids in the tubules. Such displacement results in the autolysis of odontoblasts. However, new dentin may eventually be laid down on the dentinal wall corresponding to the site of injury by the action of newly recruited secondary odontoblasts. The new dentin produced in response to the injury is called *tertiary dentin*. Some researchers define *reactionary dentin* as the new dentin secreted by surviving primary odontoblasts, in contrast to *reparative dentin*, which is produced by newly recruited secondary odontoblasts (see also chapter 3).[120]

The quality of tertiary (reparative and reactionary) dentin is quite variable. In general, it is more irregular, less mineralized, and contains fewer dentinal tubules than either primary or secondary dentin (Fig 5-10). Severe injury (eg, deep cavity preparation and deep caries) may cause the formation of better organized tertiary dentin, whereas mild injury may lead to the formation of tertiary dentin that resembles the structural integrity of primary dentin.[121] Tertiary dentin increases the thickness of the hard tissue barrier overlying the pulp. Moreover, the dentinal tubules are usually discontinuous between primary and tertiary dentin. Hence, tertiary dentin physically attenuates external stimuli to the pulp derived from dentinal tubules, and thus its formation may be regarded as a defense reaction.

Although controversy still surrounds the origin of secondary odontoblasts, undifferentiated mesenchymal cells in the pulp proper and/or differentiated pulpal cells that dedifferentiate into undifferentiated cells and then redifferentiate into odontoblasts have been implicated as likely sources.[122-124] Although variable in morphology, secondary odontoblasts may be less columnar and more sparsely arranged than primary odontoblasts. However, secondary odontoblasts seem to share several phenotypic and functional properties with primary odontoblasts. A study of reparative dentinogenesis in rats demonstrated that secondary odontoblasts express mRNA for type I but not type III collagen and that they are immunopositive for dentin sialoprotein, a dentin-specific protein that marks the odontoblast phenotype.[47]

Fibroblasts of the pulp

Fibroblasts are the most numerous connective tissue cells with the capacity to synthesize and maintain connective tissue matrix (Fig 5-11; see also Fig 5-5a). They are widely distributed throughout the connective tissue of the pulp and are found in high densities in the cell-rich zone of the coronal pulp. Synthesis of collagens type I and type III is a main function of fibroblasts in the pulp, as in fibroblasts elsewhere in the body. They are also responsible for the synthesis and secretion of a wide range of noncollagenous extracellular matrix components, such as proteoglycans and fibronectin.

The morphology of pulp fibroblasts varies according to their functional state, which is in common with fibroblasts in other parts of the body. Intensely synthetic cells have several irregularly branched cytoplasmic processes with a nucleus located at one end of the cell. They are rich in rough endoplasmic reticulum, and the Golgi complex is well developed. This type of cell is particularly common in the young pulp. However, quiescent cells, frequently seen in older pulp, are smaller than the active cells and tend to be spindle-shaped with fewer processes. The amount of rough endoplasmic reticulum in these cells is also smaller. When the quiescent cells are adequately stimulated, their synthetic activity may be reactivated. Mitotic activity of fibroblasts is quite low in adult connective tissues, but active cell division occurs when the tissue is damaged.

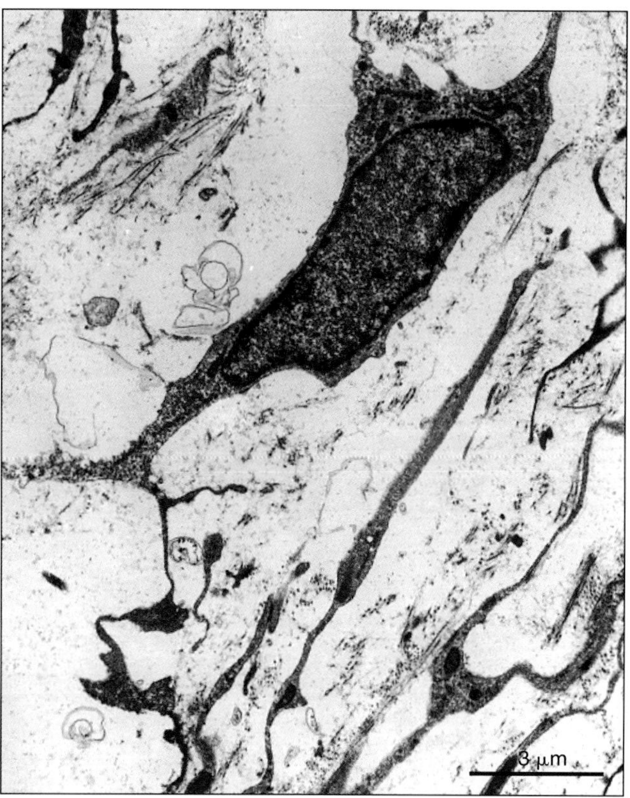

Fig 5-11 TEM of a fibroblast in the coronal pulp of a rat molar. This cell has several long cytoplasmic processes and relatively well-developed organelles.

In addition to synthetic activity, fibroblasts are implicated in the degradation of extracellular matrix components and thus are essential in the remodeling of connective tissues. Fibroblasts are able to phagocytose collagen fibrils and digest them intracellularly by lysosomal enzymes. Moreover, these cells are a source of a group of zinc enzymes called matrix metalloproteinases (collagenase, gelatinase, stromelysin, etc) that degrade matrix macromolecules such as collagens and proteoglycans. In vitro studies demonstrated that matrix metalloproteinase production from cultured pulp fibroblasts showed an increase following stimulation with cytokines and/or bacterial components.[58-60] These findings suggest that fibroblasts stimulated by inflammatory cytokines and bacterial byproducts play a role in the degradation of pulpal connective tissue during pulp inflammation.

Undifferentiated mesenchymal cells

Undifferentiated mesenchymal cells are distributed throughout the cell-rich zone and the pulp core, frequently occupying the perivascular area. These cells appear as stellate-shaped cells with a relatively high nucleus-to-cytoplasmic ratio. However, they are usually difficult to distinguish from fibroblasts under light microscopy. After receiving appropriate stimuli, they may undergo terminal differentiation and give rise either to fibroblasts or to odontoblasts. In older pulps, the number of undifferentiated mesenchymal cells may diminish, which may also reduce the regenerative potential of the pulp.

Immunocompetent cells

The ability of connective tissue to generate and support local inflammatory and immune reactions makes it an active participant in host defense. A considerable part of this capacity depends on immunocompetent cells resident in the tissue. These cells are recruited from the bloodstream, where they reside as somewhat transient inhabitants. Once foreign antigens gain entry into connective tissue, these cells interact to create mechanisms that help defend the tissue from antigenic invasion.

Lymphocytes

The specificity of immune responses is due to lymphocytes, for they are the only cells in the body capable of specifically recognizing different antigens. They are broadly divided into B lymphocytes and T lymphocytes, which are quite different in phenotype and function. B lymphocytes differentiate into antibody-secreting cells (ie, plasma cells) and thus play a major role in humoral immunity. They carry membrane-bound forms of antibodies by which they can recognize antigens. T lymphocytes play a central role in specific immune responses to protein antigens. They are subdivided into helper ($CD4^+$) and cytotoxic ($CD8^+$) types. The main function of cytotoxic T lymphocytes is to cause lysis of other cells that carry foreign antigens, such as cells infected by intracellular microbes (viruses, etc). Thus, cytotoxic T lymphocytes are predominantly involved in cell-mediated immunity. Helper T lymphocytes play a crucial role in orchestrating both humoral and cell-mediated immune responses through production of cytokines, a group of bioactive molecules that regulates the intensity and/or duration of the immune response by either stimulating or inhibiting the action of various target cells. Following activation, helper T lymphocytes secrete several cytokines. According to the profile of cytokine production, these cells are further classified into Th1 and Th2 cells.[125] Th1 cells predominantly produce interleukin (IL) -2 and interferon-gamma (IFN-γ) and are primarily involved in activation of macrophages. Th2 cells predominantly produce IL-4, IL-5, and IL-6 and stimulate proliferation and differentiation of B lymphocytes.

Mechanism of T-lymphocyte activation: Role of antigen-presenting cells. The T-lymphocyte response to protein antigens requires the participation of antigen-presenting cells. These cells uptake protein antigens, convert them to peptide fragments, assemble the peptides with proteins encoded for the MHC, and then express the assembly on their surface. T lymphocytes are able to recognize not the antigens themselves but the assembly. Class I and Class II MHC molecules bind to CD8 and CD4 molecules on T lymphocytes, respectively, and are involved in the T-lymphocyte response. Class I MHC molecules, designated as human leukocyte antigen (HLA) -A, -B, and -C in humans, are expressed on almost all cells of the body and are involved in the activation of $CD8^+$ T lymphocytes. Class II MHC molecules (HLA-DR, -DP, and -DQ in humans) are expressed on limited types of cells; dendritic cells and B lymphocytes constitutively express these molecules, whereas macrophages, endothelial cells, and some other types of cells can be induced to express them. The interaction between antigen-presenting cells and $CD4^+$ T lymphocytes involves contact between the Class II MHC molecule-associated peptide and the T-cell receptor, the first signal required for T lymphocytes to become activated. Binding of several co-stimulatory molecules on antigen-presenting cells to their ligands on T lymphocytes is also necessary for the activation. Throughout this chapter, the term *antigen-presenting cells* will be used to denote cells that are involved in the class II-restricted antigen recognition, although it seems appropriate that target cells of $CD8^+$ T lymphocytes should be included in antigen-presenting cells as well.

Lymphocytes of the pulp. The composition of lymphocytes in the pulp resembles that seen in other connective tissues, such as the dermis of the skin. T lymphocytes are recognized as normal residents of human and rat dental pulp (Fig 5-12). These cells are scattered predominantly along the blood vessels in the pulp proper, although numerically fewer among pulpal cellular elements. Several immunohistochemical studies have demonstrated that $CD8^+$ T lymphocytes outnumber $CD4^+$ T lymphocytes.[126-129] In normal human pulp, T lymphocytes usually express CD45RO, a marker for memory T lymphocytes.[127,128] Thus they are predominantly composed of memory T lymphocytes. However, cells expressing phenotypic markers for activated T lymphocytes, such as CD25 (interleukin-2 receptor), are rarely found. As will be described later, T lymphocytes may be involved in the initial immunodefense of the pulp following interaction with Class II MHC molecule-expressing cells.

B lymphocytes and plasma cells, the terminally differentiated B lymphocytes with a specialized capacity for antibody synthesis, are rarely encountered in normal human pulp.[126,127,129-131] In studies of rat molar pulp, a few plasma cells were occasionally detected in the coronal pulp.[132,133] At present, it seems difficult to identify a significant role for B lymphocytes in the normal pulp.

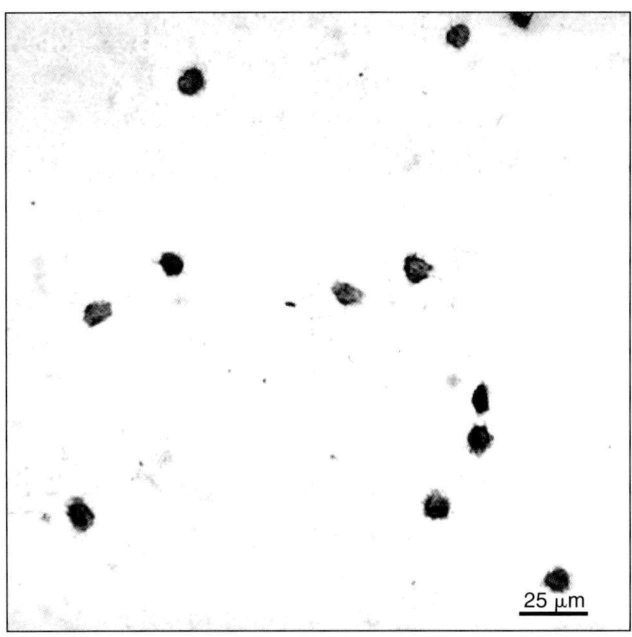

Fig 5-12 T lymphocytes in the coronal pulp of a human third molar visualized by immunoperoxidase staining using a monoclonal CD3 antibody (reactive to all T lymphocytes). Small, round cells are scattered in the connective tissue of the pulp.

Macrophages

Macrophages are constituents of the mononuclear phagocyte system, which consists of heterogeneous populations of bone marrow-derived cells whose primary function is phagocytosis. They primarily act as scavenger cells that phagocytose and digest foreign particles (eg, microbes) as well as self-tissues and cells that are injured or dead. Macrophages are activated by a variety of stimuli and acquire several properties that contribute to the defense and repair of connective tissues. For example, activated macrophages show an elevated production of various bioactive substances such as bactericidal enzymes, reactive oxygen species, cytokines, and growth factors. Upon expression of Class II MHC molecules on their cell surface, macrophages acquire the capac-

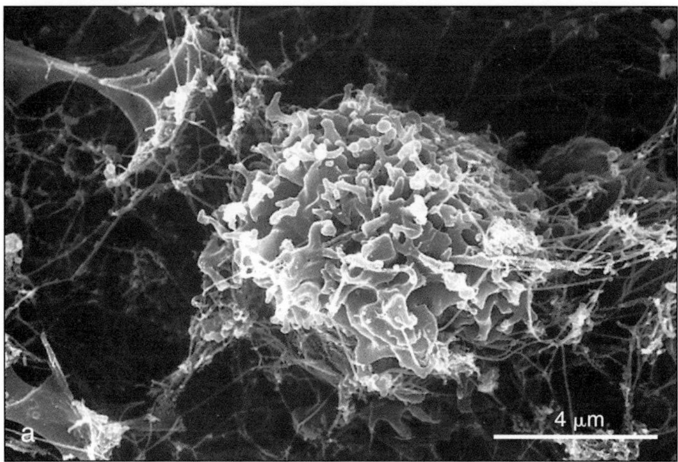

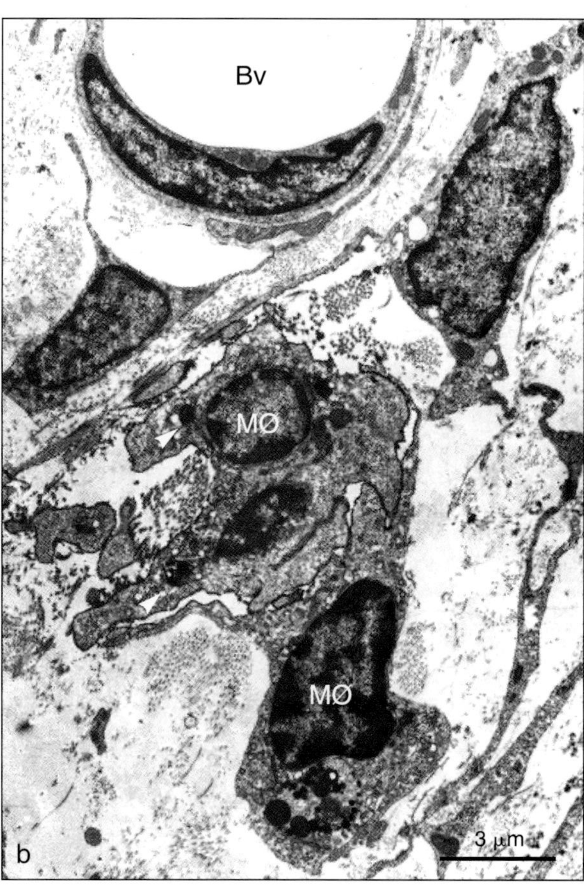

Fig 5-13 Ultrastructure of macrophages (coronal pulp of rat molars). *(a)* SEM of a macrophage with numerous microvilli on its surface. *(b)* TEM of two macrophages (MØ) in the central portion of the coronal pulp. Immunoperoxidase staining using a monoclonal antibody against rat Class II MHC molecules (OX6) was used. One of the macrophages *(upper cell)* shows OX6-immunoreactivity on its cytoplasmic membrane. *Arrowheads*, phagosomes; Bv, blood vessel. (Courtesy of Dr T. Kaneko, Tokyo Medical and Dental University.)

ity of antigen presentation and thus play a role in T-lymphocyte activation.

Macrophages show diversity in terms of morphology, phenotype, and function. This heterogeneity mostly reflects local microenvironmental conditions and the resulting difference in the state of differentiation and activation.[134] Morphology of macrophages varies according to the state of activation and differentiation, but it is generally characterized by an irregular surface with protrusions and indentations, a well-developed Golgi complex, many lysosomes, and a prominent rough endoplasmic reticulum (Fig 5-13).

Macrophages of the pulp. Macrophages are classically described as histiocytes predominantly located in the vicinity of blood vessels. Recent immunohistochemical studies have demonstrated that there is a remarkably high number of cells expressing macrophage-associated antigens throughout the pulpal connective tissue (Fig 5-14).[132,133,135] These cells are particularly rich in the perivascular area of the inner pulp. The morphologic appearance of these cells is diverse, but cells with long, slender, branching processes are predominant. Typically, the ultrastructural appearance of these cells is characterized by an irregularly indented cell surface and the presence of relatively well-developed lysosomal structures within the cytoplasm.

Macrophages of the pulp have several phenotypes. They express varying combinations of several macrophage-associated antigens, such as CD14, CD68, coagulation factor XIIIa, and HLA-DR in humans.[135] In the rat, the majority of cells immunoreactive to the monoclonal antibody ED1 (a general macrophage marker that recognizes an intracytoplasmic CD68-like antigen) coexpress immunoreactivity to ED2 (a monoclonal antibody exclusively reactive with tissue-resident macrophages [see Fig 5-14]). This expression indicates that macrophages of the pulp are predominantly composed of typical resident-type cells, as in most other connective tissues. Moreover, part of these macrophages coexpress Class II MHC molecules (see Fig 5-13b) and thus may have a capacity for antigen presentation to T lymphocytes. In rat molars, approximately 30% of the $ED1^+$ cells in the coronal pulp and 15% of cells in the root pulp coexpress Class II MHC molecules.[132] This ratio may be higher in human pulp because it has been reported that 86.9% of $CD68^+$ cells coexpress HLA-DR.[135] As will be described later, a certain proportion of these Class II MHC molecule–expressing cells may represent dendritic cells, although precise discrimination of dendritic cells from macrophages is at present difficult to achieve due to a lack of dendritic cell–specific markers.

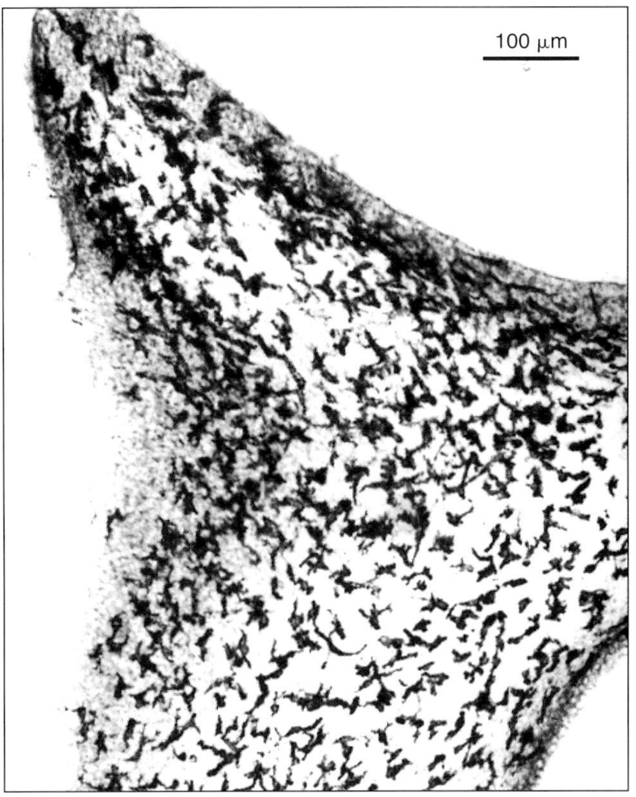

Fig 5-14 Macrophages in the coronal pulp of a rat molar visualized by immunoperoxidase staining using a monoclonal antibody against tissue-resident macrophages (ED2). Cells with diverse profiles are distributed throughout the connective tissue of the pulp.

Dendritic cells

Dendritic cells are discrete populations of hematopoetically derived leukocytes sparsely distributed in almost all tissues and organs of the body. They are characterized by *(1)* peculiar dendritic morphology, *(2)* constitutive expression of a high amount of Class II MHC molecules, *(3)* high motility, *(4)* limited phagocytic activity, and *(5)* potent capacity for antigen presentation to T lymphocytes.[136,137] Dendritic cells generally express several cell-surface molecules, including Class II MHC molecules and various adhesion and co-stimulatory molecules. Expression of myeloid-associated antigens is generally weak or lacking. However, the profile of the expression of those markers varies, mostly due to the difference in the state of maturation and local microenvironmental conditions. Following maturation in the bone marrow and circulation in the bloodstream, dendritic cells populate peripheral nonlymphoid tissues, where they monitor the invasion of antigens and thus act as an immunosurveillance component. During primary immune responses, they are the only cell type able to stimulate naive T lymphocytes (cells that have not previously been exposed to any antigen). Dendritic cells capture invaded antigens and then migrate through afferent lymphatics to lymphoid tissues, where they fully mature and present antigens to resting T lymphocytes. During secondary immune responses, both dendritic cells and Class II MHC molecule–expressing macrophages may present antigens to locally recruited memory T lymphocytes.

Dendritic cells of the pulp. In human pulp, Class II MHC molecule–expressing ($HLA\text{-}DR^+$) cells form a continuous reticular network throughout the entire pulp[126,127,135,138] The majority of these cells co-express coagulation factor XIIIa, a marker for antigen-presenting cells of the der-

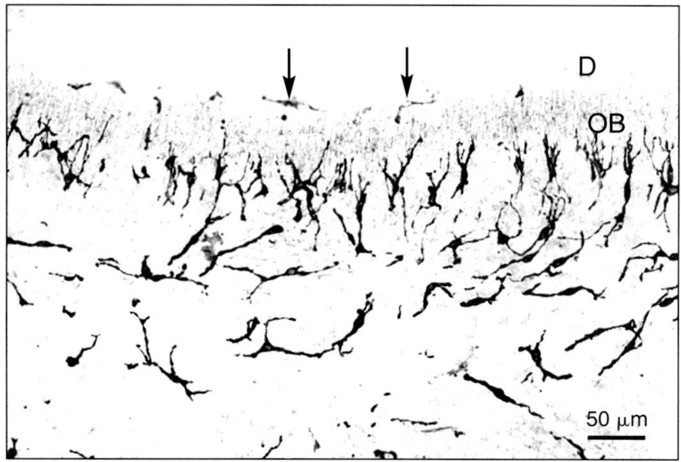

Fig 5-15 Distribution of cells expressing coagulation factor XIIIa (a marker for antigen-presenting cells of the dermis) in the peripheral portion of the coronal pulp (human third molar). Immunoperoxidase staining using an antiserum against factor XIIIa was used. Positively stained cells with a dendritic profile are arranged in and just subjacent to the odontoblast layer (OB). Cells located in the vicinity of the pulp-predentin border *(arrows)* extend their processes into dentinal tubules. D, dentin.

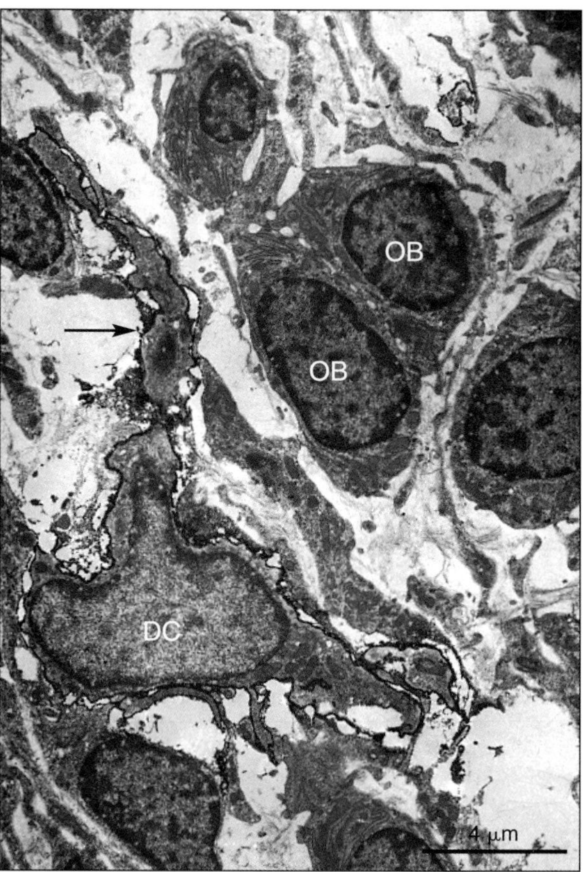

Fig 5-16 TEM showing a dendritic cell (DC) in the odontoblast layer of a rat molar. Immunoperoxidase staining using a monoclonal antibody against rat class II MHC molecules (OX6) was used. Immunoreaction is seen on the cytoplasmic membrane. The positively stained cell has a long cytoplasmic process *(arrow)*. OB, odontoblasts. (Courtesy of Dr T. Kaneko, Tokyo Medical and Dental University.)

mis[135] (Fig 5-15). The HLA-DR$^+$ cells have three or more branched cytoplasmic processes of more than 50 μm in longitudinal length. They are particularly rich in the periphery of the pulp (in and just subjacent to the odontoblast layer), where they compete for space with the odontoblasts and sometimes extend their processes into the dentinal tubules.[127,138] The cells are also rich in the perivascular area, where they are arranged with their longitudinal axes parallel to the endothelial cells.[135] Rat pulp tissue also contains similar types of cells.[132,139]

Class II MHC molecule–expressing cells of the pulp are most likely composed of macrophages and "true" dendritic cells, although it is often difficult to make a clear-cut discrimination solely by means of light microscopic appearances. Transmission electron microscopy has thus been employed, and cells with ultrastructural characteristics comparable to those of dendritic cells in other tissues ("true" dendritic cells) have been identified (Fig 5-16). The "true" dendritic cells are reported to exhibit narrow, tortuous cytoplasmic processes and to contain fine tubulovesicular

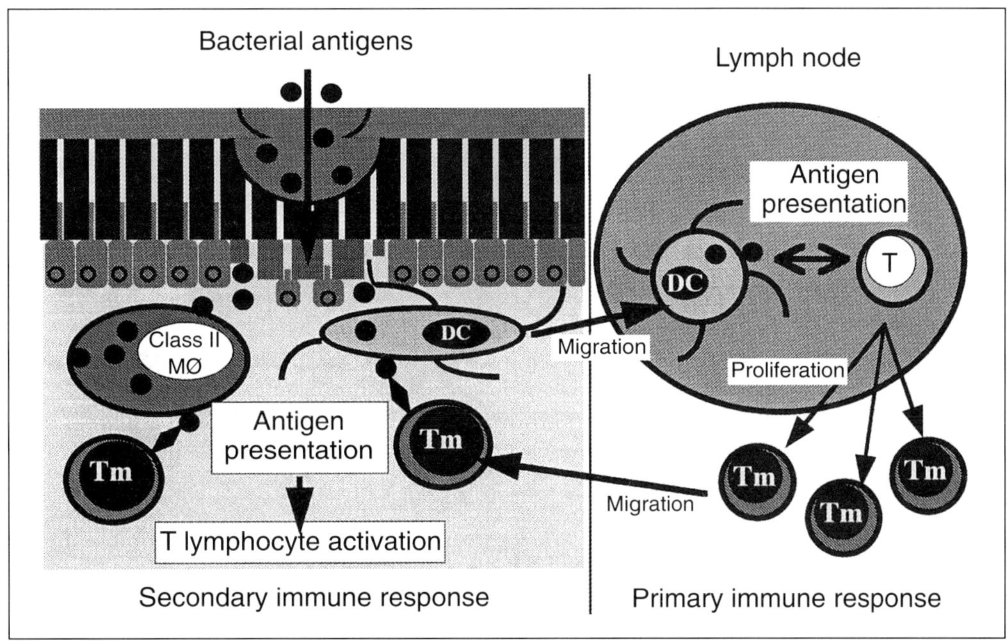

Fig 5-17 Role of Class II MHC molecule–expressing cells in the pulp. Dendritic cells (DC) capture antigens in the pulp and then migrate to regional lymph nodes, where the dendritic cells present antigens to antigen-specific naïve $CD4^+$ T lymphocytes (T) (primary immune responses). The antigen presentation causes clonal expansion and development of antigen-specific memory T lymphocytes (Tm), which leave the lymph nodes and scan peripheral tissues such as the pulp. When the same antigens again challenge the pulp, both dendritic cells and macrophages (MØ) are able to present the antigens directly in the pulp to the memory T lymphocytes (secondary immune responses). The resultant activation of the memory T lymphocytes triggers the effector phase of immune responses.

structures, a moderately developed Golgi apparatus, and poorly developed lysosomal structures within the cytoplasm.[126,138-141] These cells are predominantly located in and just beneath the odontoblast layer of the coronal pulp. Other studies employing double-labeling immunohistochemistry have shown that the pulp contains Class II MHC molecule–expressing cells that lack expression of macrophage markers.[132,135] In human pulp, these cells account for about 13% of HLA-DR^+ nonendothelial cells.[135]

Functions of Class II MHC molecule–expressing cells have been investigated in vitro using enzymatically released pulp cells from rat incisors. The results indicate that *(1)* dendritic cells may correspond to a minor subpopulation of Class II MHC molecule–expressing cells with weak phagocytic capacity,[139] and *(2)* dendritic cells may have a stronger capacity for providing signals to cause proliferation of mitogen-stimulated T lymphocytes than macrophages.[142] The T-lymphocyte proliferation was influenced by neuropeptides (substance P and calcitonin gene-related peptide), suggesting that dendritic cell–T lymphocyte interaction in the pulp may be modulated by these neuropeptides.[28]

In summary, the pulp is equipped with dendritic cells as a minor but distinct subpopulation of Class II MHC molecule–expressing cells. Their primary function may be to monitor invasion of antigens. Following ingestion of invading antigens, they may act in either of two ways (Fig 5-17): *(1)* migrate to regional lymph nodes, where they present antigens to antigen-specific naïve T lymphocytes in order to initiate primary immune responses, or *(2)* locally present antigens to patrolling memory T lymphocytes when the antigens again challenge the pulp (secondary immune responses).[3,4] Class II MHC molecule–expressing macrophages may interact only with memory T lymphocytes and thus may be involved in the initiation of secondary immune responses. Dendritic cells are particularly rich in and just subjacent to the odontoblast layer. This characteristic distribution suggests that dendritic cells are strategically positioned in the area where the opportunity for these cells to encounter exogenous antigens is the greatest.

Effects of Injury on Pulpal Immunocompetent Cells

Immunocompetent cells resident in the connective tissue of the pulp may respond to a number of clinical situations that cause loss of hard tissue integrity, eg, caries, tooth fracture, and cavity preparation. Bacteria and their by-products invading from the oral cavity are the key elements associated with such a response. It should be noted that the response may be initiated even when the pulp is not directly exposed to the oral environment (see also chapters 4 and 12). Studies have revealed that Class II MHC molecule–expressing cells respond promptly and actively to dentinal injuries, presumably by detecting incoming antigens and subsequently initiating immune responses by acting as antigen-presenting cells. The Class II MHC molecule–expressing cells are most likely composed of "true" dendritic cells and macrophages. The two types of cells are collectively termed *pulpal dendritic cells* because complete discrimination of these cells is not always possible.

Response to cavity preparation and restoration

Cavity preparation in rat molars causes a rapid and intense accumulation of pulpal dendritic cells under the freshly exposed dentinal tubules. The accumulation is transient and gradually subsides following initiation of reparative dentinogenesis.[143] In a recent study, responses of pulpal dendritic cells to deep-cavity preparation and immediate restoration with 4-META/MMA-TBB resin were studied.[144] Results demonstrated that the restoration reduced the accumulation of these cells, and subsequently sound reparative dentin was formed, whereas unrestored teeth initially developed an intrapulpal abscess and then exhibited partial pulp necrosis. Findings from these studies[143,144] indicate that pulpal dendritic cells are able to respond to a transdentinal bacterial challenge resulting from acute dentinal exposure. The restoration most likely reduced the bacterial challenge and thereby diminished the response of pulpal dendritic cells. This phenomenon may strongly support the key concept that reduction of transdentinal bacterial challenge by the use of dentin adhesive materials is of utmost importance for vital pulp therapy (see also chapters 4, 13, and 14).

Response to dentinal caries

The kinetics of pulpal dendritic cells was investigated following experimental caries induction in rat molars.[145] The initial pulpal response was characterized by a localized accumulation of these cells beneath the pulpal ends of dentinal tubules communicating with early caries lesions. The accumulation in this position may indicate that these cells respond promptly and actively to incoming bacterial antigens diffusing through the dentinal tubules. On the other hand, the accumulation was not evident following reparative dentin formation, suggesting in that case the influx of bacterial antigens is reduced or inhibited. However, these cells again accumulated markedly when the reparative dentin was invaded by caries. These findings support the view that the intensity of inflammatory/immunologic responses beneath dentinal caries does not necessarily correspond to the depth of the lesion but may be associated with the status and quality of reactive/reparative processes of dentin that influence dentin permeability.

A similar pattern is served in human teeth that have dentinal caries without pulp exposure, in

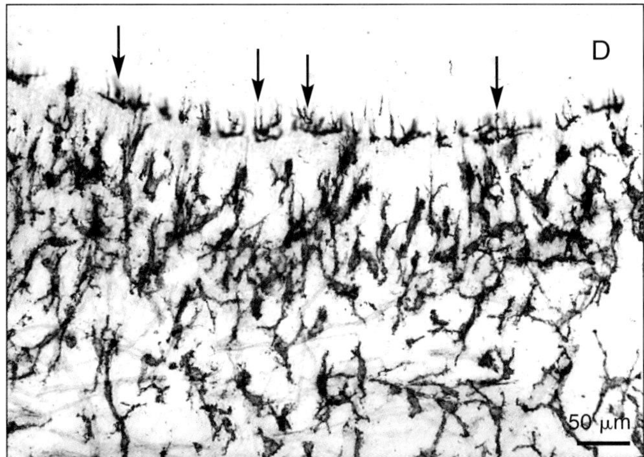

Fig 5-18 Distribution of pulpal dendritic cells in a human third molar with dentinal caries. Peripheral portion of the pulp corresponding to carious dentinal tubules. Immunoperoxidase staining with an anti–HLA-DR monoclonal antibody was used. Note accumulation of immunopositive cells. Many cells located in the vicinity of the pulp-predentin border extend their processes *(arrows)* into dentinal tubules. D, dentin. (Courtesy of Dr K. Sakurai.)

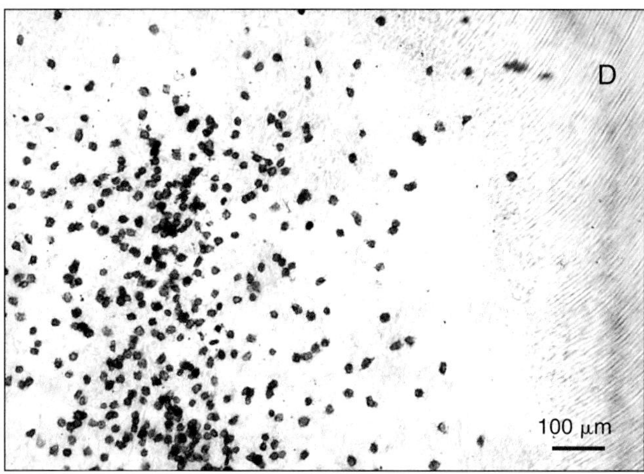

Fig 5-19 Accumulation of T lymphocytes in the peripheral portion of the coronal pulp in a human third molar with dentinal caries. Immunoperoxidase staining using a monoclonal CD3 antibody (reactive to all T lymphocytes). D, dentin. (Courtesy of Dr K. Sakurai.)

which there is a marked localized accumulation of HLA-DR$^+$ pulpal dendritic cells in the para-odontoblast region immediately subjacent to the pulpal end of the carious dentinal tubules (Fig 5-18). Here, numerous dendritic cells extend their cytoplasmic processes into the affected dentinal tubules, probably representing the high motility of these cells.[127,138] This localized accumulation is more evident in teeth without reparative dentin.[127] Studies have also demonstrated that T lymphocytes increase under these conditions (Fig 5-19). This increase is evident even in teeth with relatively shallow carious lesions, whereas increase of B lymphocytes is noticeable only in teeth with deep lesions.[127,128] Thus, T lymphocytes may be more deeply involved in the initial immunologic reactions that take place following caries attack than are B lymphocytes. The majority of T lymphocytes may be memory T lymphocytes expressing CD45RO.[127] Taken together, these findings suggest an early critical role of local interaction between pulpal dendritic cells and memory T lymphocytes in the initial immunodefense of the pulp against dentinal tubule–derived carious antigenic stimuli. It is postulated that the interaction results in the activation of both T lymphocytes and pulpal dendritic cells, which in turn may facilitate the recruitment and activation of several types of effector cells and thus may trigger a cascade of immunopathologic events involved in the process of pulpal pathosis associated with dental caries.

References

1. Kishi Y, Takahashi K. Changes of vascular architecture of dental pulp with growth. In: Inoki R, Kudo T, Olgart LM (eds). Dynamic Aspects of Dental Pulp. London: Chapman and Hall, 1990:97–129.
2. Byers MR. Dynamic plasticity of dental sensory nerve structure and cytochemistry. Arch Oral Biol 1994;39 (suppl):13S–21S.
3. Jontell M, Bergenholtz G. Accessory cells in the immune defense of the dental pulp. Proc Finn Dent Soc 1992;88 (suppl 1):345–355.
4. Jontell M, Okiji T, Dahlgren U, Bergenholtz G. Immune defense mechanisms of the dental pulp. Crit Rev Oral Biol Med 1998;9:179–200.

5. Wigglesworth DJ, Longmore GA, Kuc IM, Murdoch C. Early dentinogenesis in mice: Von Korff fibres and their possible significance. A preliminary study by light and electron microscopy. Acta Anat (Basel)1986;127:151-160.
6. Sogaard-Pedersen B, Boye H, Matthiessen ME. Scanning electron microscope observations on collagen fibers in human dentin and pulp. Scand J Dent Res 1990;98:89-95.
7. Bishop MA, Malhotra M, Yoshida S. Interodontoblastic collagen (von Korff fibers) and circumpulpal dentin formation: An ultrathin serial section study in the cat. Am J Anat 1991;191:67-73.
8. Salomon JP, Septier D, Goldberg M. Ultrastructure of inter-odontoblastic fibres in the rat molar. Arch Oral Biol 1991;36:171-176.
9. Takagi M, Hishikawa H, Hosokawa Y, Kagami A, Rahemtulla F. Immunohistochemical localization of glycosaminoglycans and proteoglycans in predentin and dentin of rat incisors. J Histochem Cytochem 1990;38:319-324.
10. Yoshiba N, Yoshiba K, Iwaku M, Ozawa H. Immunolocalization of the small proteoglycan decorin in human teeth. Arch Oral Biol 1996;41:351-357.
11. Yoshiba N, Yoshiba K, Iwaku M, Nakamura H, Ozawa H. A confocal laser scanning microscopic study of the immunofluorescent localization of fibronectin in the odontoblast layer of human teeth. Arch Oral Biol 1994;39:395-400.
12. Yoshiba N, Yoshiba K, Nakamura H, Iwaku M, Ozawa H. Immunoelectron-microscopic study of the localization of fibronectin in the odontoblast layer of human teeth. Arch Oral Biol 1995;40:83-89.
13. Kim S, Liu M, Simchon S, Dörscher-Kim JE. Effects of selected inflammatory mediators on blood flow and vascular permeability in the dental pulp. Proc Finn Dent Soc 1992;88(suppl 1):387-392.
14. Heyeraas KJ, Berggreen E. Interstitial fluid pressure in normal and inflamed pulp. Crit Rev Oral Biol Med 1999;10:328-336.
15. Bergenholtz G, Lindhe J. Effect of soluble plaque factors on inflammatory reactions in the dental pulp. Scand J Dent Res 1975;83:153-158.
16. Bergenholtz G. Effect of bacterial products on inflammatory reactions in the dental pulp. Scand J Dent Res 1977;85:122-129.
17. Bergenholtz G. Pathogenic mechanisms in pulpal disease. J Endod 1990;16:98-101.
18. Matthews B, Vongsavan N. Interactions between neural and hydrodynamic mechanisms in dentine and pulp. Arch Oral Biol 1994;39(suppl):87S-95S.
19. Pashley DH. Dentine permeability and its role in the pathobiology of dentine sensitivity. Arch Oral Biol 1994;39(suppl):73S-80S.
20. Pashley DH. Dynamics of the pulpo-dentin complex. Crit Rev Oral Biol Med 1996;7:104-133.
21. Heyeraas KJ, Kvinnsland I. Tissue pressure and blood flow in pulpal inflammation. Proc Finn Dent Soc 1992;88(suppl 1):393-401.
22. Olgart L. Neural control of pulpal blood flow. Crit Rev Oral Biol Med 1996;7:159-171.
23. Matthews B, Andrew D, Amess TR, Ikeda H, Vongsavan N. The functional properties of intradental nerves. In: Shimono M, Maeda T, Suda H, Takahashi K (eds). Dentin/Pulp Complex. Tokyo: Quintessence,1996:146-153.
24. Närhi M, Yamamoto H, Ngassapa D. Function of intradental nociceptors in normal and inflamed teeth. In: Shimono M, Maeda T, Suda H, Takahashi K (eds). Dentin/Pulp Complex. Tokyo: Quintessence, 1996:136-140.
25. Akai M, Wakisaka S. The distribution of peptidergic nerves. In: Inoki R, Kudo T, Olgart LM (eds). Dynamic Aspects of Dental Pulp. London: Chapman and Hall, 1990:337-348.
26. Kerezoudis NP, Olgart L, Edwall L. Evans blue extravasation in rat dental pulp and oral tissues induced by electrical stimulation of the inferior alveolar nerve. Arch Oral Biol 1993;38:893-901.
27. Olgart LM, Kerezoudis NP. Nerve-pulp interactions. Arch Oral Biol 1994;39(suppl):47S-54S.
28. Okiji T, Jontell M, Belichenko P, Dahlgren U, Bergenholtz G, Dahlström A. Structural and functional association between substance P- and calcitonin gene-related peptide-immunoreactive nerves and accessory cells in the rat dental pulp. J Dent Res 1997;76:1818-1824.
29. Bongenhielm U, Haegerstrand A, Theodorsson E, Fried K. Effects of neuropeptides on growth of cultivated rat molar pulp fibroblasts. Regul Pept 1995;60:91-98.
30. Trantor IR, Messer HH, Birner R. The effects of neuropeptides (calcitonin gene-related peptide and substance P) on cultured human pulp cells. J Dent Res 1995;74:1066-1071.
31. Jacobsen EB, Heyeraas KJ. Effect of capsaicin treatment or inferior alveolar nerve resection on dentine formation and calcitonin gene-related peptide and substance P-immunoreactive nerve fibres in rat molar pulp. Arch Oral Biol 1996;41:1121-1131.
32. Uitto VJ, Larjava H. Extracellular matrix molecules and their receptors: An overview with special emphasis on periodontal tissues. Crit Rev Oral Biol Med 1991;2:323-354.
33. Van Amerongen JP, Lemmens IG, Tonino GJ. The concentration, extractability and characterization of collagen in human dental pulp. Arch Oral Biol 1983;28:339-345.
34. Uitto VJ, Antila R. Characterization of collagen biosynthesis in rabbit dental pulp in vitro. Acta Odontol Scand 1971;29:609-617.

35. Shuttleworth CA, Ward JL, Hirschmann PN. The presence of type III collagen in the developing tooth. Biochim Biophys Acta 1978;535:348-355.
36. Lechner JH, Kalnitsky G. The presence of large amounts of type III collagen in bovine dental pulp and its significance with regard to the mechanism of dentinogenesis. Arch Oral Biol 1981;26:265-273.
37. Magloire H, Joffre A, Grimaud JA, Herbage D, Couble ML, Chavrier C. Distribution of type III collagen in the pulp parenchyma of the human tooth: Light and electron microscope immunotyping. Histochem 1982; 74:319.
38. Linde A. The extracellular matrix of the dental pulp and dentin. J Dent Res 1985;64:523-529.
39. Tsuzaki M, Yamauchi M, Mechanic GL. Bovine dental pulp collagens: Characterization of types III and V collagen. Arch Oral Biol 1990;35:195-200.
40. Hillmann G, Geurtsen W. Light-microscopical investigation of the distribution of extracellular matrix molecules and calcifications in human dental pulps of various ages. Cell Tissue Res 1997;289:145-154.
41. Shuttleworth CA. Dental pulp matrix: Collagens and proteoglycans. In: Inoki R, Kudo T, Olgart LM (eds). Dynamic Aspects of Dental Pulp. London: Chapman and Hall, 1990:239-287.
42. Karjalainen S, Soderling E, Pelliniemi L, Foidart JM. Immunohistochemical localization of types I and III collagen and fibronectin in the dentine of carious human teeth. Arch Oral Biol 1986;31:801-806.
43. Ruch JV. Odontoblast differentiation and the formation of the odontoblast layer. J Dent Res 1985;64:489-498.
44. Ohsaki Y, Nagata K. Type III collagen is a major component of interodontoblastic fibers of the developing mouse molar root. Anat Rec 1994;240:308-313.
45. Sodek J, Mandell SM. Collagen metabolism in rat incisor predentine in vivo: Synthesis and maturation of type I, alpha 1 (I) trimer, and type V collagens. Biochem 1982; 21:2011-2015.
46. Lukinmaa PL, Waltimo J. Immunohistochemical localization of types I, V, and VI collagen in human permanent teeth and periodontal ligament. J Dent Res 1992;71: 391-397.
47. D'Souza RN, Bachman T, Baumgardner KR, Butler WT, Litz M. Characterization of cellular responses involved in reparative dentinogenesis in rat molars. J Dent Res 1995;74:702-709.
48. Ten Cate AR, Melcher AH, Pudy G, Wagner D. The non-fibrous nature of the von Korff fibres in developing dentine: A light and electron microscope study. Anat Rec 1970;168:491-523.
49. Ten Cate AR. A fine structural study of coronal and root dentinogensis in the mouse: Observations on the so-called "von Korff fibres" and their contribution to mantle dentine. J Anat 1978;125:183-197.
50. Tabata S, Nakayama T, Yasui K, Uemura M. Collagen fibrils in the odontoblast layer in the teeth of the rat and the house shrew, *Suncus murinus*, by scanning electron microscopy using a maceration method. Connect Tissue Res 1995;33:115-121.
51. Shroff B, Thomas HF. Investigation of the role of von Korff fibers during murine dentinogenesis. J Biol Buccale 1992;20:139-144.
52. Lukinmaa PL, Vaahtokari A, Vainio S, Sandberg M, Waltimo J, Thesleff I. Transient expression of type III collagen by odontoblasts: Developmental changes in the distribution of pro-alpha 1(III) and pro-alpha 1(I) collagen mRNAs in dental tissues. Matrix 1993;13:503-515.
53. Shuttleworth CA, Berry L, Kielty CM. Microfibrillar components in dental pulp: Presence of both type VI collagen- and fibrillin-containing microfibrils. Arch Oral Biol 1992;37:1079-1084.
54. Fried K, Risling M, Edwall L, Olgart L. Immuno-electron-microscopic localization of laminin and collagen type IV in normal and denervated tooth pulp of the cat. Cell Tissue Res 1992;270:157-164.
55. Orlowski WA. The turnover of collagen in the dental pulp of rat incisors. J Dent Res 1977;56:437.
56. Morand MA, Schilder H, Blondin J, Stone PJ, Franzblau C. Collagenolytic and elastinolytic activities from diseased human dental pulps. J Endod 1981;7:156-160.
57. Martinez EF, Machado de Souza SO, Corrêa L, Cavalcanti de Araújo V. Immunohistochemical localization of tenascin, fibronectin and type III collagen in human dental pulp. J Endod 2000;26:708-711.
58. Panagakos FS, O'Boskey JF Jr, Rodriguez E. Regulation of pulp cell matrix metalloproteinase production by cytokines and lipopolysaccharides. J Endod 1996;22: 358-361.
59. Tamura M, Nagaoka S, Kawagoe M. Interleukin-1 α stimulates interstitial collagenase gene expression in human dental pulp fibroblast. J Endod 1996;22:240-243.
60. Nakata K, Yamasaki M, Iwata T, Suzuki K, Nakane A, Nakamura H. Anaerobic bacterial extracts influence production of matrix metalloproteinases and their inhibitors by human dental pulp cells. J Endod 2000;26:410-413.
61. Schröder U. Effects of calcium hydroxide-containing pulp-capping agents on pulp cell migration, proliferation, and differentiation. J Dent Res 1985;64:541.
62. Higashi T, Okamoto H. Electron microscopic study on interodontoblastic collagen fibrils in amputated canine dental pulp. J Endod 1996;22:116-119.
63. Kitasako Y, Shibata S, Arakawa M, Cox CF, Tagami J. A light and transmission microscopic study of mechanically exposed monkey pulps: Dynamics of fiber elements during early dentin bridge formation. Oral Surg Oral Med Oral Pathol Oral Radiol Endod 2000;89: 224-230.

64. Bradamante Z, Pecina-Hrncevic A, Ciglar I. Oxytalan fibres in human dental pulp. Experientia 1980;36: 1210–1211.
65. Van Amerongen JP, Lemmens AG, Tonino GJM. Glycosaminoglycans in dental pulp. In: Inoki R, Kudo T, Olgart LM (eds). Dynamic Aspects of Dental Pulp. London: Chapman and Hall, 1990:259–276.
66. Linde A. A study of the dental pulp glycosaminoglycans from permanent human teeth and rat and rabbit incisors. Arch Oral Biol 1973;18:49–59.
67. Embery G. Glycosaminoglycans of human dental pulp. J Biol Buccale 1976;4:229–236.
68. Sakamoto N, Okamoto H, Okuda K. Qualitative and quantitative analysis of bovine, rabbit and human dental pulp glycosaminoglycans. J Dent Res 1979;58: 646–655.
69. Mangkornkarn C, Steiner JC. In vivo and in vitro glycosaminoglycans from human dental pulp. J Endod 1992;18:327–331.
70. Hjerpe A, Engfeldt B. Proteoglycans of dentine and predentine. Calcif Tissue Res 1976;22:173–182.
71. Rahemtulla F, Prince CW, Butler WT. Isolation and partial characterization of proteoglycans from rat incisors. Biochem J 1984;218:877–885.
72. Linde A. Glycosaminoglycan turnover and synthesis in the rat incisor pulp. Scand J Dent Res1973;81:145–154.
73. Bouvier M, Joffre A, Magloire H. In vitro mineralization of a three-dimensional collagen matrix by human dental pulp cells in the presence of chondroitin sulphate. Arch Oral Biol 1990;35:301–309.
74. Tziafas D, Amar S, Staubli A, Meyer JM, Ruch JV. Effects of glycosaminoglycans on in vitro mouse dental cells. Arch Oral Biol 1988;33:735–740.
75. Gaffar A, Coleman EJ, Marcussen HW. Penetration of dental plaque components into gingiva: Sequential topical treatments with hyaluronidase and streptococcal polysaccharide in rats. J Periodontol 1981;52:197–205.
76. Hashioka K, Suzuki K, Yoshida T, Nakane A, Horiba N, Nakamura H. Relationship between clinical symptoms and enzyme-producing bacteria isolated from infected root canals. J Endod 1994;20:75–77.
77. Linde A, Johansson S, Jonsson R, Jontell M. Localization of fibronectin during dentinogenesis in rat incisor. Arch Oral Biol 1982;27:1069–1073.
78. Van Amerongen JP, Lemmens IG, Tonino GJ. Immunofluorescent localization and extractability of fibronectin in human dental pulp. Arch Oral Biol 1984;29:93–99.
79. Lukinmaa PL, Mackie EJ, Thesleff I. Immunohistochemical localization of the matrix glycoproteins—tenascin and the ED-sequence-containing form of cellular fibronectin—in human permanent teeth and periodontal ligament. J Dent Res 1991;70:19–26.
80. Ruch JV, Lesot H, Begue-Kirn C. Odontoblast differentiation. Int J Dev Biol 1995;39:51–68.
81. Ruch JV, Lesot H, Cam Y, Meyer J-M, Bloch-Zupan A, Bègue-Kirn C. Control of odontoblast differentiation: Current hypotheses. In: Shimono M, Maeda T, Suda H, Takahashi K (eds). Dentin/Pulp Complex. Tokyo: Quintessence, 1996:105–111.
82. Lesot H, Fausser JL, Akiyama SK, Staub A, Black D, Kubler MD, Ruch JV. The carboxy-terminal extension of the collagen binding domain of fibronectin mediates interaction with a 165 kDa membrane protein involved in odontoblast differentiation. Differentiation 1992;49: 109–118.
83. Yoshiba K, Yoshiba N, Nakamura H, Iwaku M, Ozawa H. Immunolocalization of fibronectin during reparative dentinogenesis in human teeth after pulp capping with calcium hydroxide. J Dent Res 1996;75:1590–1597.
84. Izumi T, Yamada K, Inoue H, Watanabe K, Nishigawa Y. Fibrinogen/fibrin and fibronectin in the dentin-pulp complex after cavity preparation in rat molars. Oral Surg Oral Med Oral Pathol Oral Radiol Endod 1998;86:587–591.
85. Milam SB, Haskin C, Zardeneta G, Chen D, Magnuson VL, Klebe RJ, Steffenson B. Cell adhesion proteins in oral biology. Crit Rev Oral Biol Med 1991;2:451–491.
86. Zhu Q, Safavi KE, Spångberg LSW. The role of integrin β 1 in human dental pulp cell adhesion on laminin and fibronectin. Oral Surg Oral Med Oral Pathol Oral Radiol Endod 1998;85:314–318.
87. Zhu Q, Safavi KE, Spångberg LSW. Integrin expression in human dental pulp cells and their role in cell attachment on extracellular matrix proteins. J Endod 1998;24:641–644.
88. Sawada T. Expression of basement membrane components in the dental papilla mesenchyme of monkey tooth germs: An immunohistochemical study. Connect Tissue Res 1995;32:55–61.
89. Butler WT, Ritchie H. The nature and functional significance of dentin extracellular matrix proteins. Int J Dev Biol 1995;39:169–179.
90. Linde A. Dentin mineralization and the role of odontoblasts in calcium transport. Connect Tissue Res 1995;33:163–170.
91. Frank RM, Nalbandian J. Development of dentine and pulp. In: Oksche A, Vollrath L (eds). Teeth: Handbook of Microscopic Anatomy, vol 6. New York: Springer, 1989: 73–171.
92. Garant PR, Szabo G, Nalbandian J. The fine structure of the mouse odontoblast. Arch Oral Biol1968;13:857–876.
93. Takuma S, Nagai N. Ultrastructure of rat odontoblasts in various stages of their development and maturation. Arch Oral Biol 1971;16:993–1011.
94. Couve E. Ultrastructural changes during the life cycle of human odontoblasts. Arch Oral Biol 1986;31:643–651.
95. Frank RM, Nalbandian J. Structure and ultrastructure of dentine. In: Oksche A, Vollrath L (eds). Teeth: Handbook of Microscopic Anatomy, vol 6. New York: Springer, 1989:173–247.

96. Weinstock M, Leblond CP. Synthesis, migration and release of precursor collagen by odontoblasts as visualized by autoradiography after ^{3}H-proline administration. J Cell Biol 1974;60:92–127.
97. Garant PR. The organization of microtubules within rat odontoblast processes revealed by perfusion fixation with glutaraldehyde. Arch Oral Biol 1972;17:1047–1058.
98. Holland GR. The dentinal tubule and odontoblast process in the cat. J Anat 1975;120:169–177.
99. Holland GR. The extent of the odontoblast process in the cat. J Anat 1976;121:133–149.
100. Holland GR. The odontoblast process: Form and function. J Dent Res 1985;64:499–514.
101. Frank RM, Steuer P. Transmission electron microscopy of the human odontoblast process in peripheral root dentine. Arch Oral Biol 1988;33:91–98.
102. Frank RM. Ultrastructural relationship between the odontoblast, its process and the nerve fibre. In: Symons NBB (ed). Dentine and Pulp: Structure and Reactions. London: Livingstone, 1968:115–148.
103. Brännström M, Garberoglio R. The dentinal tubules and the odontoblast processes: A scanning electron microscopic study. Acta Odontol Scand 1972;30:291–311.
104. Thomas HF. The extent of the odontoblast process in human dentin. J Dent Res 1979;58:2207–2218.
105. Thomas HF, Carella P. Correlation of scanning and transmission electron microscopy of human dentinal tubules. Arch Oral Biol 1984;29:641–646.
106. Thomas HF. The lamina limitans of human dentinal tubules. J Dent Res 1984;63:1064–1066.
107. Gunji T, Kobayashi S. Distribution and organization of odontoblast processes in human dentin. Arch Histol Jpn 1983;46:213–219.
108. Maniatopoulos C, Smith DC. A scanning electron microscopic study of the odontoblast process in human coronal dentine. Arch Oral Biol 1983;28:701–710.
109. Yamada T, Nakamura K, Iwaku M, Fusayama T. The extent of the odontoblast process in normal and carious human dentin. J Dent Res 1983;62:798–802.
110. Sigal MJ, Pitaru S, Aubin JE, Ten Cate AR. A combined scanning electron microscopy and immunofluorescence study demonstrating that the odontoblast process extends to the dentinoenamel junction in human teeth. Anat Rec 1984;210:453–462.
111. Sigal MJ, Aubin JE, Ten Cate AR. An immunocytochemical study of the human odontoblast process using antibodies against tubulin, actin, and vimentin. J Dent Res 1985;64:1348–1355.
112. Sigal MJ, Aubin JE, Ten Cate AR, Pitaru S. The odontoblast process extends to the dentinoenamel junction: An immunocytochemical study of rat dentine. J Histochem Cytochem 1984;32:872–877.
113. Byers MR, Sugaya A. Odontoblast processes in dentin revealed by fluorescent Di-I. J Histochem Cytochem 1995;43:159–168.
114. Frank RM. Etude au microscope electronique de l'odontoblaste et du canalicule dentinaire humain. Arch Oral Biol 1966;11:179–199.
115. Sasaki T, Nakagawa K, Higashi S. Ultrastructure of odontoblasts in kitten tooth germs as revealed by freeze-fracture. Arch Oral Biol 1982;27:897–904.
116. Calle A. Intercellular junctions between human odontoblasts: A freeze-fracture study after demineralization. Acta Anat 1985;122:138–144.
117. Bishop MA. Evidence for tight junctions between odontoblasts in the rat incisor. Cell Tissue Res 1985; 239:137–140.
118. Turner DF, Marfurt CF, Sattelberg C. Demonstration of physiological barrier between pulpal odontoblasts and its perturbation following routine restorative procedures: A horseradish peroxidase tracing study in the rat. J Dent Res 1989;68:1262–1268.
119. Bishop MA, Yoshida S. A permeability barrier to lanthanum and the presence of collagen between odontoblasts in pig molars. J Anat 1992;181:29–38.
120. Smith AJ, Cassidy N, Perry H, Begue-Kirn C, Ruch JV, Lesot H. Reactionary dentinogenesis. Int J Dev Biol 1995;39:273–280.
121. Trowbridge HO. Pathogenesis of pulpitis resulting from dental caries. J Endod 1981;7:52–60.
122. Fitzgerald M. Cellular mechanics of dentinal bridge repair using ^{3}H-thymidine. J Dent Res 1979;58: 2198–2206.
123. Yamamura T. Differentiation of pulpal cells and inductive influences of various matrices with reference to pulpal wound healing. J Dent Res 1985;64:530–540.
124. Fitzgerald M, Chiego DJ Jr, Heys DR. Autoradiographic analysis of odontoblast replacement following pulp exposure in primate teeth. Arch Oral Biol 1990;35: 707–715.
125. Mosmann TR, Coffman RL. TH1 and TH2 cells: Different patterns of lymphokine secretion lead to different functional properties. Ann Rev Immunol 1989;7: 145–173.
126. Jontell M, Gunraj MN, Bergenholtz G. Immunocompetent cells in the normal dental pulp. J Dent Res 1987; 66:1149–1153.
127. Sakurai K, Okiji T, Suda H. Co-increase of nerve fibers and HLA-DR- and/or factor XIIIa-expressing dendritic cells in dentinal caries-affected region of the human dental pulp: An immunohistochemical study. J Dent Res 1999;78:1596–1608.
128. Izumi T, Kobayashi I, Okamura K, Sakai H. Immunohistochemical study on the immunocompetent cells of the pulp in human non-carious and carious teeth. Arch Oral Biol 1995;40:609–614.
129. Hahn C-L, Falkler WA Jr, Siegel MA. A study of T and B cells in pulpal pathosis. J Endod 1989;15:20–26.
130. Pulver WH, Taubman MA, Smith DJ. Immune components in normal and inflamed human dental pulp. Arch Oral Biol 1977;22:103–111.

131. Pekovíc DD, Fillery ED. Identification of bacteria in immunopathologic mechanisms of human dental pulp. Oral Surg Oral Med Oral Pathol 1984;57:652-661.
132. Okiji T, Kawashima N, Kosaka T, Matsumoto A, Kobayashi C, Suda H. An immunohistochemical study of the distribution of immunocompetent cells, especially macrophages and Ia antigen-expressing cells of heterogeneous populations, in normal rat molar pulp. J Dent Res 1992;71:1196-1202.
133. Okiji T, Kosaka T, Kamal AMM, Kawashima N, Suda H. Age-related changes in the immunoreactivity of the monocyte/macrophage system in rat molar pulp. Arch Oral Biol 1996;41:453-468.
134. Dijkstra CD, Damoiseaux JG. Macrophage heterogeneity established by immunocytochemistry. Prog Histochem Cytochem 1993;27:1-65.
135. Okiji T, Jontell M, Belichenko P, Bergenholtz G, Dahlström A. Perivascular dendritic cells of the human dental pulp. Acta Physiol Scand 1997;159:163-169.
136. Steinman RM. The dendritic cell system and its role in immunogenicity. Ann Rev Immunol 1991;9:271-296.
137. Hart DN. Dendritic cells: Unique leukocyte populations which control the primary immune response. Blood 1997;90:3245-3287.
138. Yoshiba N, Yoshiba K, Nakamura H, Iwaku M, Ozawa H. Immunohistochemical localization of HLA-DR-positive cells in unerupted and erupted normal and carious human teeth. J Dent Res 1996;75:1585-1589.
139. Jontell M, Bergenholtz G, Scheynius A, Ambrose W. Dendritic cells and macrophages expressing class II antigens in the normal rat incisor pulp. J Dent Res 1988; 67:1263-1266.
140. Ohshima H, Kawahara I, Maeda T, Takano Y. The relationship between odontoblasts and immunocompetent cells during dentinogenesis in rat incisors: An immunohistochemical study using OX6-monoclonal antibody. Arch Histol Cytol 1994;57:435-447.
141. Ohshima H, Maeda T, Takano Y. The distribution and ultrastructure of class II MHC-positive cells in human dental pulp. Cell Tissue Res 1999;295:151-158.
142. Jontell M, Eklöf C, Dahlgren U, Bergenholtz G. Difference in capacity between macrophages and dendritic cells from rat incisor pulp to provide signals to concanavalin-A-stimulated T lymphocytes. J Dent Res 1994; 73:1056-1060.
143. Ohshima H, Sato O, Kawahara I, Maeda T, Takano Y. Responses of immunocompetent cells to cavity preparation in rat molars: An immunohistochemical study using OX6-monoclonal antibody. Connect Tissue Res 1995;32:303-311.
144. Kamal AMM, Okiji T, Suda H. Responses of class II molecule-expressing cells and macrophages to cavity preparation and restoration with 4-META/MMA-TBB resin. Int Endod J 2000;33:367-373.
145. Kamal AMM, Okiji T, Kawashima N, Suda H. Defense responses of dentin/pulp complex to experimentally induced caries in rat molars: An immunohistochemical study on kinetics of pulpal Ia antigen-expressing cells and macrophages. J Endod 1997;23:115-120.

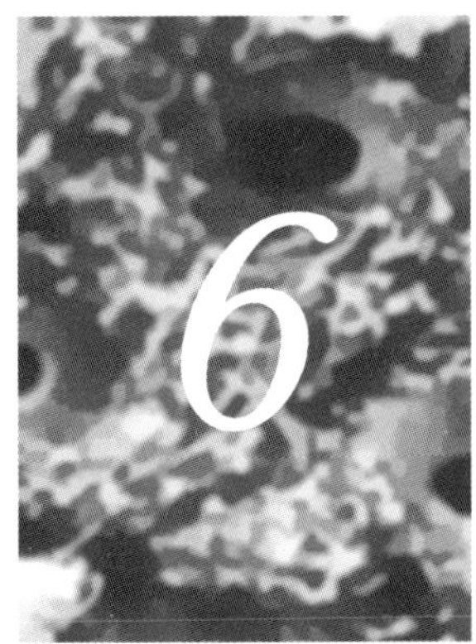

The Circulation of the Pulp

Hideaki Suda, DDS, PhD
Hideharu Ikeda, DDS, PhD

The microcirculatory system of dental pulp serves many essential roles. This system is critically important in maintaining tissue homeostasis and yet is capable of undergoing a dynamic response to injury by altering local capillary filtration rates, initiating immunologic responses to injury and inflammation (via endothelial expression of adhesion molecules[1]), and even sprouting via angiogenesis. This chapter will review the anatomy and physiology of this important system and emphasize its response characteristics following pulpal inflammation caused by dental procedures, infection, or trauma. This information is critical for clinicians so that they can minimize injury to pulp during dental procedures and assess the status of the pulp's microcirculatory system in individual clinical cases.

Organization of Pulpal Vasculature

The dental pulp is a microcirculatory system because it lacks true arteries and veins; the largest vessels are arterioles and venules.[2] Its primary function is to regulate the local interstitial environment of dental pulp via the transport of nutrients, hormones, and gases and the removal of metabolic waste products. However, the pulpal microcirculation is a dynamic system that regulates blood flow in response to nearby metabolic events (including dentinogenesis). It also responds to inflammatory stimuli with a great change in circulatory properties and the endothelial expression of certain proteins, leading to the recruitment of immune cells to the site of tissue injury (see chapters 5, 10, 11, and 17). Clearly, knowledge of this system is essential to an understanding of the dental pulp in health and disease.

Arterioles

The pulp has an extensive vascular supply[3] (Fig 6-1). The organizational structure of dental pulp is presented in Fig 6-2. The arterioles are resistance vessels, measuring approximately 50 μm in diameter, and have several layers of smooth muscle, which regulate vascular tone. The transitional structure between arterioles and capillaries is called the *terminal arteriole*. This segment of

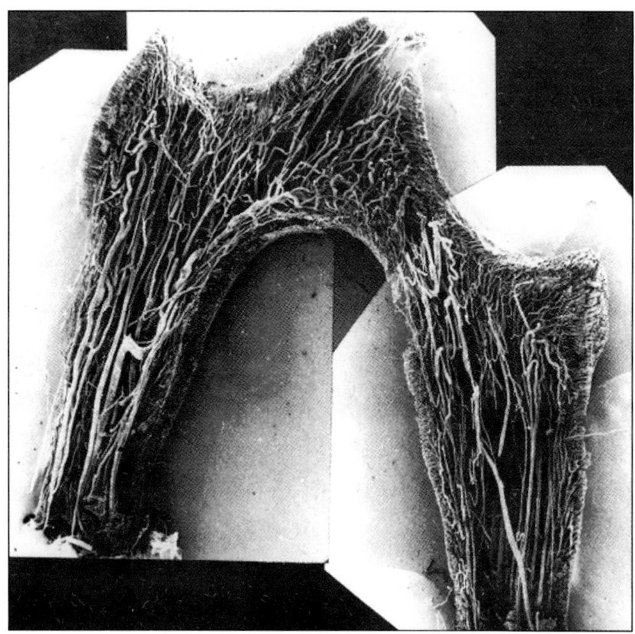

Fig 6-1 Montage of scanning electron micrographs of dental pulp illustrating the extensive vascular network in the dog mandibular first molar. The superficial capillary layer has been removed to better illustrate the organizational features of the pulpal circulatory system. (Reprinted from Kishi and Takahashi[3] with permission.)

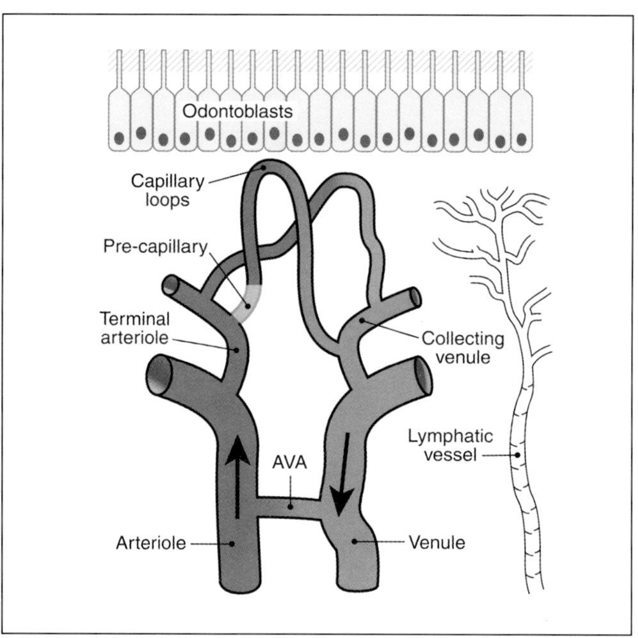

Fig 6-2 Major organizational features of the microcirculatory system of dental pulp. AVA, arteriovenous anastomosis.

the arteriole has the same dimensions as a capillary but is surrounded by a few smooth muscle cells. These smooth muscle cells are organized in a spiral fashion surrounding the endothelial cells. The arterioles then divide into terminal arterioles and then precapillaries. Metarterioles give off capillaries, which are about 8 µm in diameter (Figs 6-3 and 6-4). The arterioles, the capillaries, and the venules form functional units that respond to signals elaborated from the nearby tissue (discussed later in the chapter). This is an important concept, because virtually every cell in the body is within 50 to 100 µm of capillaries. Thus, there is a functional coupling between cellular activity and nearby capillary blood flow.

The branch points of terminal arterioles and capillaries are characterized by the presence of clumps of smooth muscle that serve as precapillary sphincters. These sphincters are under neuronal and local cellular control (via soluble factors) and act to regulate local blood flow through a capillary bed. These functional units permit localized changes in blood flow and capillary filtration, so that adjacent regions of the pulp have substantially different circulatory conditions. Thus, pulpal inflammation can elicit a localized circulatory response restricted to the area of inflammation and does not necessarily produce pulpwide circulatory changes.

Capillaries

Capillaries serve as the workhorse of the circulatory system, because they function as the exchange vessels regulating the transport or diffu-

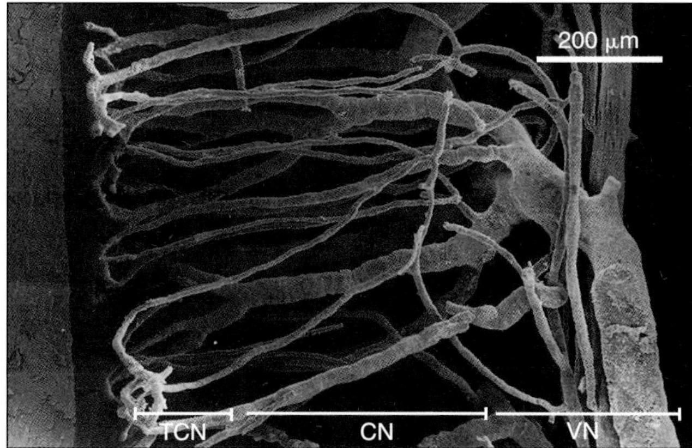

Fig 6-3 Scanning electron micrograph of a resin injection cast of dental pulp vasculature illustrating the extensive arborization of capillaries from the metarterioles. High-magnification view of the superficial three layers of the vascular network: TCN, terminal capillary network; CN, capillary network; VN, venular network. (Reprinted from Kishi and Takahashi[3] with permission.)

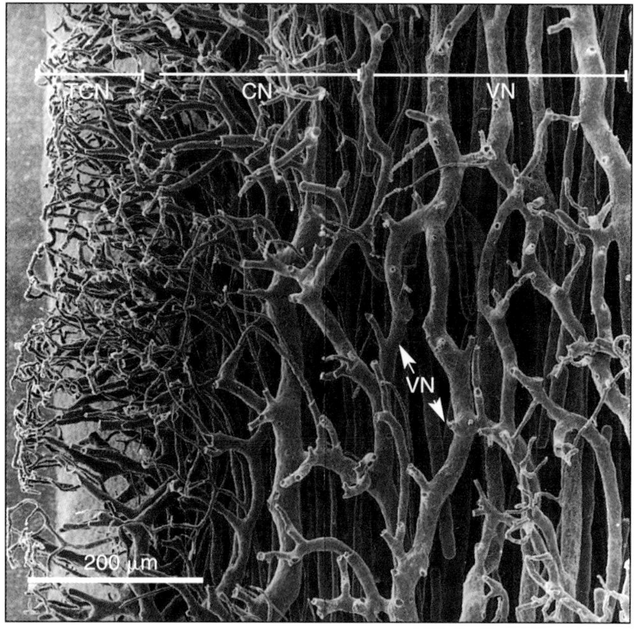

Fig 6-4 The superficial layer of the vascular network from Fig 6-3 has been removed to show the venular network (VN). The terminal capillary network (TCN) is on the far-left side, the capillary network (CN) is in the middle, and the venular network is on the right side. (Reprinted from Kishi and Takahashi[3] with permission.)

sion of substances (gases, fluids, proteins, etc) between blood and local interstitial tissue elements. At any given moment, only about 5% of the blood supply circulates in capillaries, but this is the major site of nutrient and gas exchange with local tissues. Capillaries consist of a single layer of endothelium surrounded by a basement membrane and a loose group of reticular and collagenous fibers. In dental pulp, capillaries often form extensive loops in the subodontoblastic region (see Figs 6-3 and 6-4). The basement membrane is composed of fine reticular filaments embedded in a mucopolysaccharide matrix.

The wall of a capillary is about 0.5 μm thick and serves as a semipermeable membrane. This semipermeable membrane restricts egress of proteins and cells from the vascular compartment under normal conditions, and it is this filtering property that generates a colloidal osmotic pressure within the vascular system. This has important implications for the regulation of capillary filtration under normal and inflamed conditions, as described in detail later in the chapter.

There are several major classes of capillaries that differ dramatically in their properties as semipermeable membranes[4] (Fig 6-5). The first class of capillary is the *fenestrated capillary*. These structures are characterized by endothelium with openings (fenestrations) in the capillary walls. These fenestrations can be open or occluded by a thin diaphragm. Fenestrated capillaries are found in dense networks in dental pulp as well as in the renal glomerulus, the intestinal mucosa, and the sulcular gingiva.[5,6]

The second class is the *continuous (or nonfenestrated) capillary*; these vascular structures

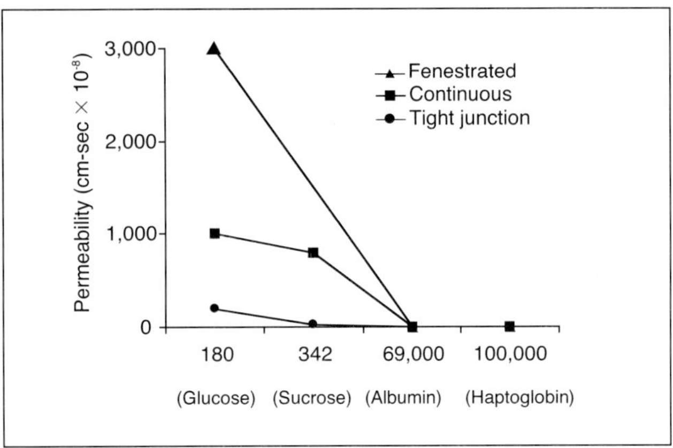

Fig 6-5 Relative permeability of three major classes of capillaries to hydrophilic substances of various molecular weights. Permeability of nonfenestrated capillaries (eg, skin), fenestrated capillaries (eg, gastrointestinal mucosa), and tight-junction capillaries (eg, brain) were compared for glucose (molecular weight = 180), sucrose (molecular weight = 342), albumin (molecular weight = 69,000), and haptoglobin (molecular weight = 100,000). (Redrawn from Renkin[4] with permission.)

are defined by endothelium devoid of fenestrations. Continuous capillaries are found in dental pulp as well as in heart, lung, and muscle.[6] The intercellular space contains gap junctions, which are localized openings with a width of 5 to 10 nm. Continuous capillaries are found near odontoblasts during early tooth development (ie, before dentin is formed). With the active expression of primary dentin, capillaries become fenestrated and form a dense network adjacent to the odontoblastic layer. When dentin formation is nearly complete, the capillary bed switches back to a continuous capillary morphology and retreats to below the odontoblastic layer.[6] Thus, the morphology and location of pulpal capillary beds follow odontoblast activity levels during development (see chapter 2).

The third major class of capillary is the *discontinuous capillary*. These capillaries consist of discontinuous endothelium with wide intercellular spaces of approximately 5 to 10 nm. The basement membrane is also discontinuous. Discontinuous endothelium is found in the spleen, liver, and bone marrow.

The fourth major class of capillary is the *tight-junction capillary*, found in the central nervous system and the retina. The differences in the semipermeable properties of these classes of capillary play an essential role in defining the basal filtration properties of these vessels.

The microcirculatory organization of the subodontoblastic region is divided into three major layers[7] (see Fig 6-4). The terminal capillary network is located in the first layer, also called the *odontoblastic layer*. The second layer, also known as the *capillary network*, contains precapillary and postcapillary vessels organized adjacent to the odontoblastic layer. The third layer consists of a venular network of vessels. During aging, there is a general reduction in pulpal metabolism, and the capillary organization is often simplified and becomes one single layer of capillaries terminating directly into venules.

Venules

The venular organization in dental pulp has several important characteristics. First, the collecting venules receive pulpal blood flow from the capillary bed and transfer it to the venules. As described earlier, these structures are characterized by a spiral organization of smooth muscle. Accordingly, the contractile state of these vessels play an important role in regulating postcapillary hydrostatic pressure. Moreover, arteriovenous anastomosis (AVA) shunts permit regional control of pulpal blood flow via direct shunting of blood from arterioles to venules (Figs 6-2 and 6-6).

Lymphatic vessels

The lymphatic system plays a critical role in tissue homeostasis and response to injury. Because of the semipermeable nature of capillaries, they do not absorb solutes of high molecular weight (eg, proteins such as albumin). Instead, the lymphatic system is the dominant mechanism for removal of high-molecular weight solutes from the interstitial fluid. This reduces the interstitial colloidal osmotic pressure and therefore regulates the development of tissue edema or interstitial pressure. In addition, the lymphatic vessels transport lymph to regional lymph nodes prior to reentry into the vascular compartment. This provides an important immunosurveillance function by direct transport of antigens to nodal collections of immune cells.

Lymphatic vessels are formed from a fine mesh of small, thin-walled lymph capillaries. The lymphatic vessels coalesce to form larger vessels that resemble veins equipped with valves to prevent backflow (see Fig 6-2). An extensive network of lymphatic vessels and ducts carries the tissue fluid back into the vascular system. Lymph from dental pulp (and nearby orofacial tissues) drains into the submaxillary and submental lymph glands and eventually to superficial and deep cervical glands that are distributed along the external and internal jugular veins.

Dental pulp contains lymphatic vessels. This statement was controversial in the older dental literature because early histologic studies had difficulty distinguishing lymphatic vessels from similar-appearing veins or capillaries. The main structural differences between the lymphatic vessels and capillaries are the lack of a basement membrane and the absence of fenestration in the endothelial cells. However, careful observations at the light[8-11] and electron microscopic[9,12,13] levels have provided evidence supportive of the presence of pulpal lymphatic vessels.

Physiologic tracking studies have provided additional evidence demonstrating that lymph capillaries originate as blind openings near the zone of Weil and odontoblastic layer.[14,15] The collecting vessels then pass apically in the pulp, accompanying blood vessels and nerves. The large-caliber lymphatic vessels contain valves, which are not present in similar-sized veins. Multiple collecting lymph vessels exit through the apical foramen to drain into large lymph vessels in the periodontal ligament.

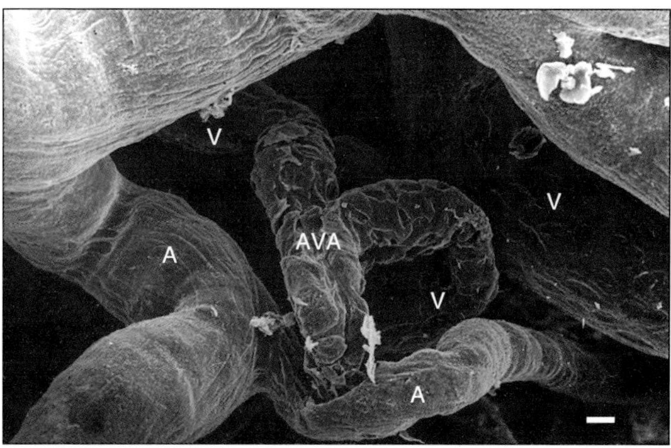

Fig 6-6 Scanning electron micrograph of a resin cast illustrating the presence of a Y-shaped arteriovenous anastomosis (AVA) between an arteriole (A) and a venule (V) using a sample from a dog tongue. Bar = 10 μm. (Reprinted from Kishi and Takahashi[3] with permission.)

More definitive studies have recently confirmed the presence of lymphatic vessels in dental pulp. An enzyme-histochemical double-staining method, which exploits the enzyme activity differences between lymphatic vessels (higher activity of 5'-nucleotidase [5'-Nase]) and blood vessels (higher activity of alkaline phosphatase), is useful for discriminating between the two kinds of vessels.[15-17] Immunohistochemical staining methods with monoclonal antibodies to the human thoracic duct and desmoplakin also can identify lymphatic vessels specifically.[18] In human frozen sections, both enzyme-histochemical and immunohistochemical methods demonstrated that large lymphatic vessels are located in the central part of the pulp, while small lymphatic vessels are found in the periphery of the pulp (Fig 6-7), suggesting that lymphatic drainage of the human dental pulp starts from the periphery of the pulp and collects in the central part of the pulp.[19,20]

Fig 6-7 Serial sections of human dental pulp: B, blood vessels; L, lymphatic vessels. *(a)* Section immunostained with anti-L. The basement membrane reacting with anti-L in blood vessels and lymphatic vessels is shown. It is difficult to discriminate the lymphatic vessel from the blood vessels by the difference in reactivity to anti-L. *(b)* Higher magnification view of the vessels in the sections shown in *(a)*. *(c)* Adjacent section immunostained with mAb-D. A lymphatic vessel is strongly stained, and blood vessels are not stained. *(d)* Higher-magnification view of the vessels in the sections shown in *(c)*. Immunostaining with mAb-D. Reaction products are on the endothelial cells. (Reprinted from Sawa et al[20] with permission.)

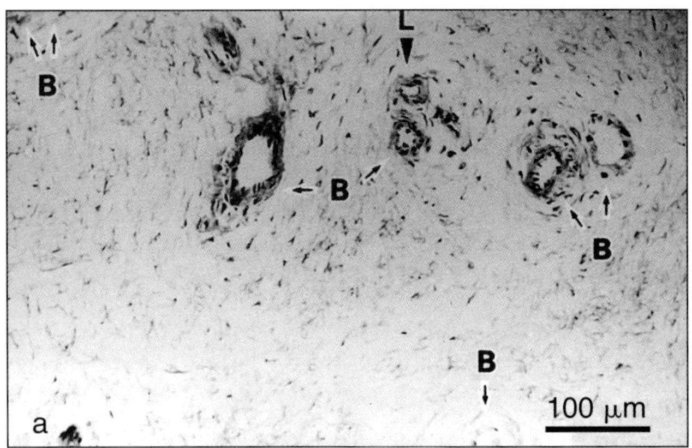

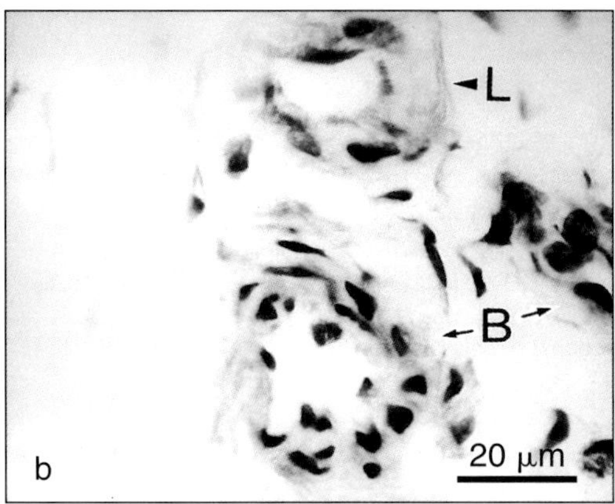

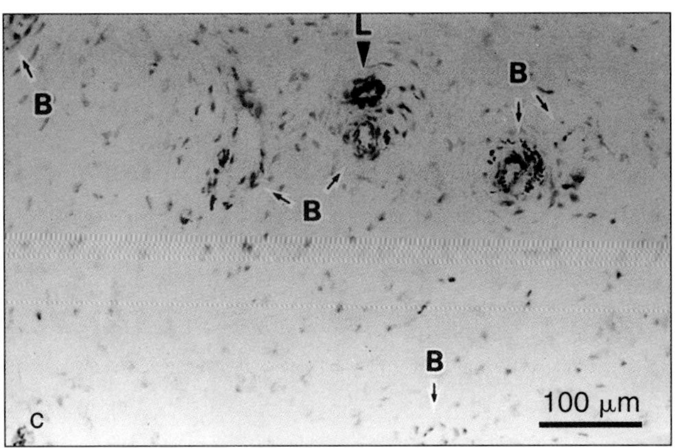

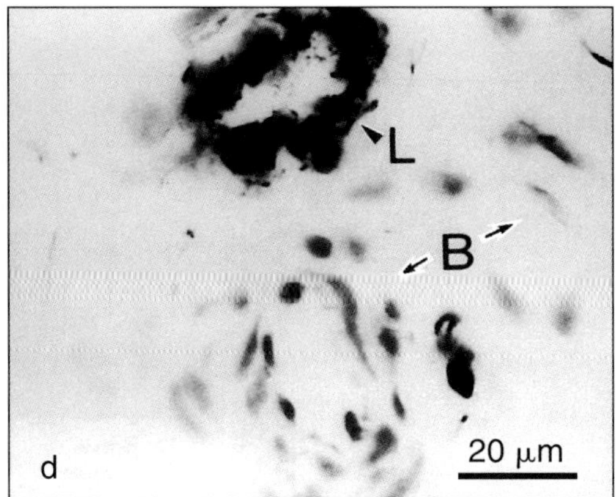

Effect of Microvascular Exchange on Interstitial Pressure

Microcirculation

The exchange of nutrients, hormones, metabolic wastes, and gases between capillaries and the interstitial compartment is controlled by two major determinants. The first determinant is the control of the microcirculation. This process directs capillary blood flow to those local pulpal regions with the greatest metabolic need. Moreover, alterations in capillary blood flow produce changes in capillary hydrostatic pressure (P_c); this, in turn, regulates fluid balance between the vascular and interstitial compartments.

Not all capillaries are continuously perfused, and the proportion of perfused capillaries may range from 10% (during vasoconstriction) to nearly 100%. The terminal arterioles and precapillary sphincters play major roles in the control of capillary perfusion (see Fig 6-2). In contrast, the major sites of blood volume control and postcapillary resistance are the muscular venules. Pulpal blood flow (PBF) is determined by the following relationship:

$$PBF = \frac{(P_A - P_V)}{R_T}$$

where P_A is the arteriolar hydrostatic pressure, P_V is the venular hydrostatic pressure, and R_T is the total resistance. Under normal conditions (ie, no changes in systemic pressure), the major determinant of pulpal blood flow is R_T, which is determined primarily by arteriolar resistance. Thus, interventions that produce vasoconstriction of pulpal arterioles (eg, epinephrine and norepinephrine) reduce pulpal blood flow by increasing resistance (R_T).

Transcapillary exchange

The second major determinant in the exchange of nutrients, wastes, and gases between capillaries and the interstitial space is transcapillary exchange. Several processes regulate the exchange of materials between the vascular compartment and the interstitial space. First is the morphology of the capillary bed. Clearly, fenestrated capillaries possess much higher exchange rates than do nonfenestrated or tight-junction capillaries (see Fig 6-5). The junctional openings in capillary walls permit passage of many low-molecular weight substances while they restrict exchange of larger plasma proteins (eg, albumin). The semipermeable nature of the junctions helps to maintain vascular colloidal pressure. These junctional openings permit passive exchange of solutes and gases by either diffusion (ie, the net movement of molecules such as glucose, O_2, CO_2, and H_2O down their respective concentration gradient) or osmosis (ie, the selective movement of fluid and solutes through a semipermeable membrane). The osmotic-driven exchange of fluid and solutes is termed *capillary filtration*.

A second factor regulating exchange is the composition and concentration gradient of the substance of interest; smaller or more lipophilic substances cross cell membranes relatively easily, whereas larger or more hydrophilic substances require capillary openings or transport mechanisms. A third process is active transport via pinocytosis. Of these three general processes, capillary filtration is a major mechanism for the transcapillary exchange of solutes.

The rate of capillary filtration is defined by the Starling forces, named for the English physiologist who first described them.[21,22] The difference between capillary hydrostatic pressure (P_C) and interstitial hydrostatic pressure (P_I), that is, $P_C - P_I$, generally favors an outward direction of fluid flow (filtration) at the arteriolar end of capillaries. The second Starling force is the difference between capillary colloidal osmotic pressure (COP_C) and interstitial colloidal osmotic pressure (COP_I), or $COP_C - COP_I$; this generally favors an inward direction of fluid flow (absorption) at the venular end of capillaries.

Thus, under normal conditions, there is a net outward flow of fluid (filtration) at the arteriolar end of capillaries, because the filtration pressure gradient exceeds the colloidal osmotic pressure gradient, and a net inward flow of fluid (absorption) at the venular end of capillaries, because colloidal osmotic pressure gradient exceeds the filtration pressure gradient (Fig 6-8). Overall, the amount of fluid movement across the entire capillary system of the body is enormous; it has been estimated that every minute the net capillary filtration rate equals the entire plasma volume, with an equal absorption rate back into capillaries and lymphatics.[23] The clinical significance of the Starling forces is that they are altered during inflammation, giving rise to dramatic increases in localized interstitial pressure (P_I) that may have pathophysiologic significance for injured regions of dental pulp.[22,24]

Pulpal interstitial pressure

Several experimental techniques have been developed to measure pulpal interstitial pressures. Determination of this pressure during homeostasis

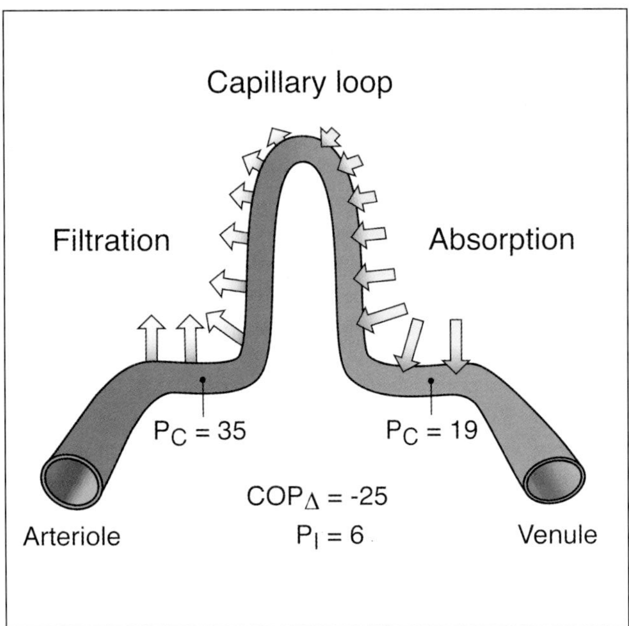

Fig 6-8 Capillary loop in dental pulp. Theoretical values (mm Hg) are given for capillary hydrostatic pressure (P_C) at the arteriole and venule ends of the capillary; interstitial hydrostatic pressure (P_I); and colloidal osmotic pressure gradient (COP_Δ) between the capillary and interstitial space. The negative value for COP_Δ indicates a net inward pressure. The size and direction of the arrows illustrate the relative magnitudes of fluid flow out of (filtration) and into (absorption) the capillaries.

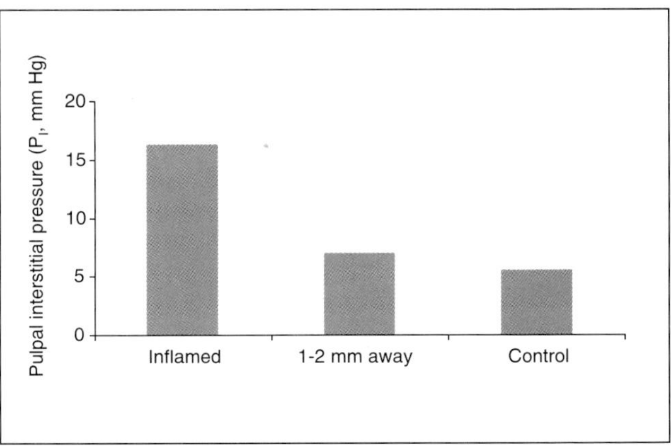

Fig 6-9 Evidence for localized increases in interstitial pressure (P_I) in inflamed versus adjacent dental pulp. Interstitial hydrostatic fluid pressures in cat dental pulp were measured by a server-controlled null micropuncture technique. The P_I was measured under the site of pulpal inflammation and 1 to 2 mm away from the site of pulpal inflammation. The control P_I values were measured in a separate group of teeth. (Redrawn from Tønder and Kvinnsland[28] with permission.)

and during inflammation is critical for understanding vascular responses to pulpal injury. Methods to determine pulpal interstitial pressure include photoelectric methods,[25] pressure transducer systems,[26] tonometric measurements,[27] and micropuncture techniques.[11,22,28,29]

Many of the earlier methods in this area produced relatively large injuries to the pulp, and interstitial pressures of about 16 to 60 mm Hg were recorded.[26,30-32] The micropuncture technique is much less invasive; the pipettes have tip diameters of only 2 to 4 μm.[33] These studies measured pulpal interstitial pressures of about 5 to 6 mm Hg under controlled conditions.[24,28,29,34-36] Using these hydrostatic measurement techniques, Tønder and Naess[33] reported that arteriole pressure is 43 mm Hg, capillary pressure is 35 mm Hg, venule pressure is 19 mm Hg, and pulpal interstitial pressure is 6 mm Hg.

Studies have demonstrated that P_I increases in response to inflammation.[32,37] Tønder and Kvinnsland[28] used glass micropipettes connected to a servocontrolled counter-pressure system to measure not only the pulpal interstitial pressure but also the intravascular pressure of cat teeth. The P_I in cat dental pulp was 16.3 mm Hg at the site of pulpal inflammation and 7.0 mm Hg at a site 1 to 3 mm away (Fig 6-9). The pulpal interstitial pressure in control teeth (ie, in the contralateral arch) was 5.5 mm Hg.

The results of the aforementioned study are important because they demonstrate that the pulpal interstitial pressure response to pulpal inflammation is restricted to the site of injury and is not generalized throughout the pulp. A generalized increase in P_I during pulpal inflammation has been theorized to occur and would lead to a generalized collapse of venules and cessation of blood flow (the pulpal strangulation theory). Studies such as the one by Tønder and Kvinnsland[28] have refuted this concept of pulpal strangulation. Instead, it appears that circulatory responses to pulpal inflammation are localized reactions to release of inflammatory mediators or other factors.[22,29,38,39] This finding is similar to that of other studies demonstrating localized tissue responses to pulpal inflammation (eg, localized sprouting of calcitonin gene-related peptide fibers; see chapter 7).

A number of factors help to restrict the increase in P_I to the site of tissue injury and prevent a generalized pulpwide increase in P_I.[22] First, an increase in P_I will reduce capillary filtration by reducing the Starling hydrostatic pressure gradient (ie, an increase in P_I reduces the difference between capillary and interstitial hydrostatic pressures [P_C-P_I]). Second, an increase in P_I at the site of inflammation may lead to an increase in capillary absorption in nearby uninflamed pulpal tissue. Third, increased lymph outflow will reduce both interstitial tissue fluid volume and interstitial protein concentrations (thereby reducing interstitial colloid osmotic pressure). This is an important function of lymphatic vessels because the lymphatic system is the predominant mechanism for removing osmotically active proteins from the interstitial space. These factors help to restrict increases in P_I to the site of injury under many conditions of pulpal inflammation. However, it is still possible that major insults to the pulp (eg, involving microvascular hemorrhage or extreme capillary permeability) may lead to widespread increases in P_I.

Collectively, studies indicate that numerous factors regulate the interstitial hydrostatic pressure in dental pulp. Changes in the interstitial fluid pressure (ΔP_I) are due to changes in the volume of the interstitial fluid and tissue compliance:

$$\Delta P_I = \Delta V / C_I$$

where ΔV is the change in pulpal tissue volume and C_I is the compliance of dental pulpal tissue. The change in pulpal tissue volume (ΔV) is regulated to a large extent by the capillary filtration rate; increases in filtration rate lead to increased fluid in the interstitial space.

The value for pulpal compliance (C_I) is low because pulp is encased in a hard mineralized structure: dentin. In many tissues in the body, an increase in capillary filtration rate will not necessarily lead to great changes in tissue pressure because the tissue is compliant and can expand to accommodate increased fluid volume. This is not the case in dental pulp, where localized increases in interstitial fluid volume can lead to great localized changes in interstitial pressure.

The following factors lead to increased interstitial fluid volume (ΔV):

1. Arteriolar dilation (increased P_C)
2. Venular constriction (increased P_C)
3. Decreased colloidal osmotic pressure in capillaries
4. Increased colloidal osmotic pressure in interstitial compartment
5. Increased capillary permeability (eg, certain inflammatory mediators)
6. Reduced lymphatic outflow

The first four factors are merely the Starling forces described earlier. Clearly, alteration in these forces will lead to alterations in capillary filtration rate, and a net outpouring of fluid (ie, increased ΔV), leading to increased interstitial fluid pressure (ΔP_I). The fifth factor, increased capillary permeability, occurs after release of certain inflammatory mediators and increases the capillary filtration rate in a dramatic fashion. Increased interstitial fluid volume compensates for the sixth factor, reduced lymphatic outflow. The rest of this chapter will focus on mechanisms regulating pulpal circu-

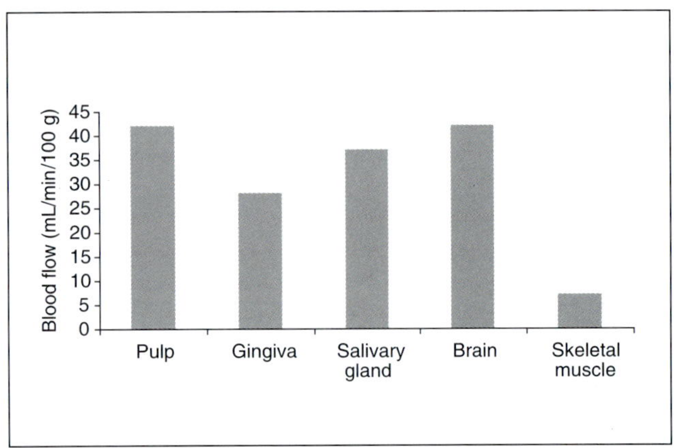

Fig 6-10 Blood flow among various tissues. Blood flow was measured by intravenous injection of 15-µm radiolabeled microspheres in young dogs maintained at a 45% hematocrit. (Redrawn from Kim[47] with permission.)

lation and describe the effects of dental procedures, drugs, injury, and inflammation on pulpal hemodynamics.

Regulation of Pulpal Blood Flow

Measurement of pulpal blood flow

Pulpal blood flow has been measured in animals with a variety of methods: tracer disappearance (eg, potassium [^{42}K], lead [^{86}Pb] iodine [^{131}I], hydrogen [^{2}H], or xenon [^{133}X]); electrical impedance; plethysmography; and other techniques.[39-45] Of these, the ^{42}K, ^{86}PB, and ^{133}X tracer disappearance and the microsphere methods yield the highest and most similar blood flow values: approximately 40 to 50 mL/min per 100 g of pulpal tissue.[46]

Blood flow values for various oral and visceral tissues at a hematocrit of 45% have been compared (Fig 6-10). Blood flow in the pulp is the highest among oral tissues and is similar to levels found in the brain. However, the blood flow per unit weight for kidney, spleen, and other vital organs is about fivefold to tenfold greater than pulpal blood flow. Thus, blood flow seems to reflect the functional activity of an organ.

The anatomic heterogeneity of the vascular network within the pulp is closely related to the heterogenous regional flow distribution.[39,40,46,47] The highest capillary density occurs in the peripheral layer of the coronal region. The central core of the apical region has the lowest density. Overall, about 14% of the volume of dental pulp consists of blood vessels; the mean density of capillaries in cat pulp is 1,402/mm^2.[48] The blood flow of the coronal half of the pulp is about twice that of the apical half of pulp. The average peripheral blood flow in the coronal region is 70 mL/min per 100 g of tissue, whereas the average flow in the central core region of apical dental pulp measures 15 mL/min per 100 g.

Comparisons among flow values, measured with 8-, 9-, and 15-µm microspheres, indicate considerable shunting of 8- and 9-µm spheres in the pulp. The shunting occurs mostly in the apical half of the pulp,[40] suggesting that AVA shunts participate in the regulation of pulpal blood flow. The shunting is facilitated by U-turn loops in the apical half of the pulp as well as the numerous AVA shunts.[49]

Using intravital microscopy, Kim et al[43] found that the fastest mean intravascular flow velocity in a 42-µm arteriole was 2.1 mm/s; the slowest mean intravascular flow velocity (0.11 mm/s) was measured in an 11-µm postcapillary venule. The mean flow velocity sharply decreased with decreasing vessel diameter on the arterial side. On the venous side, a gradual increase in the velocity curve was observed in 24- to 72-µm-diameter vessels. The fastest mean velocity obtained in the venous side was 0.7 mm/s in a 61-µm venule, substantially slower than the fastest mean velocity achieved in a comparable arteriolar vessel.

As described earlier in the chapter, pulpal blood flow is regulated by the arteriolar-venular pressure gradient as well as the total vascular resistance: PBF = $(P_A - P_V)/R_T$. During homeostasis,

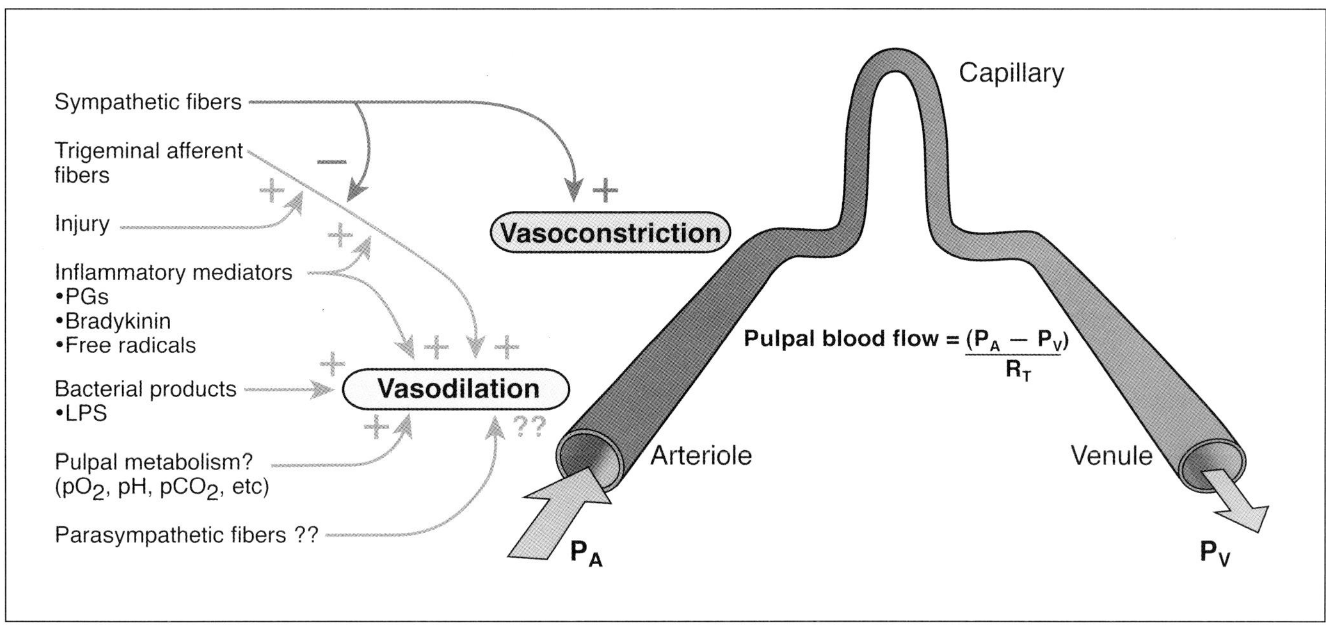

Fig 6-11 Major mechanisms regulating pulpal blood flow: PGs, prostaglandins; LPS, lipopolysaccharide.

the major determinant of pulpal blood flow is R_T, which is determined primarily by arteriolar resistance. Therefore, factors that regulate arteriolar vasoconstriction have major effects on regulating pulpal blood flow. These factors can be divided into three broad classes: metabolic factors, neuronal factors, and paracrine/endocrine factors (Fig 6-11).

Metabolic regulation of pulpal blood flow

In most tissues of the body, the arteriolar vascular tone is regulated by locally released metabolic by-products. This serves as an efficient mechanism to couple local blood flow with increased metabolic activity. The actual by-product that evokes arteriolar vasodilation differs in different tissues. In the heart, interstitial oxygen tension regulates vascular tone. In the brain, interstitial carbon dioxide levels (or pH) regulate vascular tone. In other tissues, such as muscle, more than one by-product appears to regulate vascular tone. These effects are independent of nerves, because these by-products have been shown to have direct vasodilatory effects on vascular smooth muscle.

Comparatively few studies have evaluated the effect of metabolic activity on pulpal blood flow.[44] This is a relatively difficult problem for investigation, because pulpal tissue is not easily accessible, and the pulp is thought to have a relatively low basal metabolic rate. However, studies have suggested that adenosine, low interstitial pO_2 levels, low pH, or elevated pCO_2 levels may increase pulpal blood flow via vasodilatory effects.[44] On the other hand, there is no evidence that transient vascular blockage (20- and 60-second occlusion of the external carotid artery) produces a reactive hyperemia in pulp.[48] Collectively, these studies are consistent with the notion that localized increases in pulpal activity (eg, dentinogenesis) may lead to localized increases in pulpal

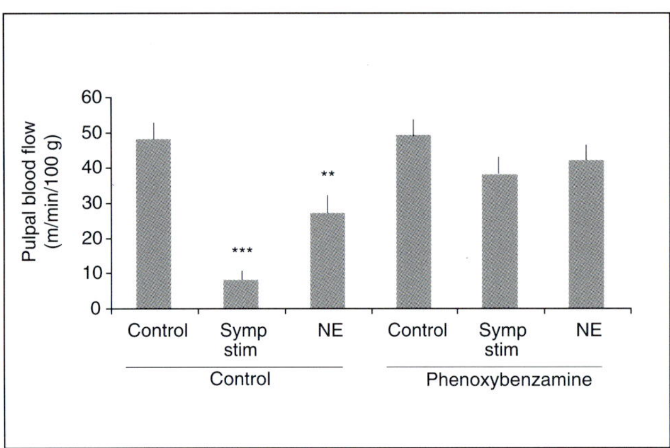

Fig 6-12 Effect of the role of α-adrenergic receptors in regulating pulpal blood flow. Pulpal blood flow was measured with 15-μm microspheres, and blood flow was altered by either electrical stimulation of pulpal sympathetic fiber (by stimulation of the cervical sympathetic nerve; symp stim) or administration of norepinephrine (NE). Phenoxybenzamine pretreatment was used to block α-adrenergic receptors. $^{**}P < .05$; $^{***}P < .001$. (Redrawn from Kim and Dorscher-Kim[39] with permission.)

blood flow. However, the relatively low overall metabolic activity of the pulp suggests that metabolic control of pulpal blood flow may not be a major regulatory mechanism for the entire dental pulp.

Neuronal regulation of pulpal blood flow

In contrast to the relative dearth of studies evaluating metabolic control of pulpal blood flow, numerous investigations have characterized neuronal regulation of pulpal blood flow. Three major neuronal systems are implicated in the regulation of pulpal blood flow: sympathetic fibers, parasympathetic fibers, and afferent (sensory) fibers.

Sympathetic nerves and the regulation of pulpal blood flow

Dental pulp is innervated by the sympathetic nervous system.[42,50,51] The sympathetic fibers terminate as free nerve endings in pulp and innervate predominantly the arterioles, although other vessels also receive some innervation.[2,51-53] Depolarization of sympathetic nerve fibers in pulp from animals or humans leads to the local release of several neurotransmitters, including norepinephrine, neuropeptide Y (NPY), and adenosine triphosphate, which constrict vessels expressing the appropriate receptors. Studies conducted with human dental pulp have confirmed that norepinephrine is present in pulp, is released from local terminal endings in pulpal tissue, and is regulated by several presynaptic receptors.[54-58] The distribution of sympathetic fibers is highest in blood vessels in the pulp horns near the odontoblastic region and is lowest in the apical region of mouse molars.[59]

Activation of the sympathetic nervous system reduces pulpal blood flow. Electrical stimulation of sympathetic efferent nerves reduces pulpal blood flow via local release of neurotransmitters in the pulp.[60] At the resting stage, pulpal vessels are not under the tonic influence of sympathetic nerve discharge. However, electrical stimulation of the cervical sympathetic trunk causes a pronounced reduction of pulpal blood flow in the dog, cat, and rat,[46,61-65] owing to activation of α-adrenergic receptors.[33,39,66,67] Stimulation of pulpal sympathetic fibers reduces pulpal blood flow by more than 80%; this effect is blocked by pretreatment with an α-adrenergic receptor antagonist, phenoxybenzamine (Fig 6-12).

Reflex excitation of the entire sympathetic nervous system by experimental hypotension (nitroprusside infusion and graded hemorrhage) or decrease in systemic oxygen transport (extreme hemodilution and hemoconcentration) also causes pulpal vasoconstriction and a reduction of pulpal blood flow.[42,47] Similar studies have been conducted in human dental pulp; results indicated that systemic alterations of the activity of sympathetic nervous system produce alterations in pulpal blood flow.[67] Thus, activation of the sympathetic fibers innervating dental pulp by either local or reflexive activity produces a profound reduction in pulpal blood flow.

Administration of sympathetically derived neurotransmitters also reduces pulpal blood flow. The catecholamines, such as epinephrine and norepinephrine, exert their physiologic effects on α-adrenergic and β-adrenergic receptors in the blood vessels. The α-adrenergic receptors are responsible for contraction of vascular musculature and produce vasoconstriction. Norepinephrine-induced reduction in pulpal blood flow is mediated by activating α-adrenergic receptors, because pretreatment with an α-adrenergic receptor antagonist blocks the effect (see Fig 6-12).[33,39,66] This general finding has been replicated in numerous studies and several species.[46,47,61,63] In addition, administration of the α_1-adrenergic agonist phenylephrine causes a sharp decrease of pulpal blood flow that is blocked by pretreatment with the α_1-adrenergic antagonist prazosin. Administration of the α_2-adrenergic agonists results in a less pronounced reduction in pulpal blood flow than does α_1-adrenergic receptor activation.[68-70]

In anesthetized dogs, the infiltration injection of 2% lidocaine with 1:100,000 epinephrine produces a significant reduction in pulpal blood flow, whereas 3% mepivacaine without epinephrine increases it (Fig 6-13). The effect of the former is due to the catecholamine component, because injection of plain 2% lidocaine produces a vasodilatory effect. Thus, α_1-adrenergic receptors appear to be primarily responsible for mediating reduced pulpal blood flow by either endogenous catecholamines (eg, stimulation of pulpal sympathetic fibers) or exogenous adrenergic agonists (eg, administration of "vasoconstrictors" in local anesthetics).

Neuropeptide Y (NPY) is another sympathetically derived neurotransmitter that is co-localized in terminals with norepinephrine. Human dental pulp contains NPY in sympathetic fibers, and pulpal blood vessels express the Y_1 class of NPY receptors.[2,72,73] Figure 6-14 illustrates the perivascular distribution of pulpal nerves that express NPY immunoreactivity.[2] Administration of NPY to dental pulp reduces pulpal blood flow via vasoconstriction.[74] Administration of NPY produces a reduction in pulpal blood flow that is similar in magnitude to that produced by electrical stimulation of the sympathetic fibers that innervate the pulp (Fig 6-15).

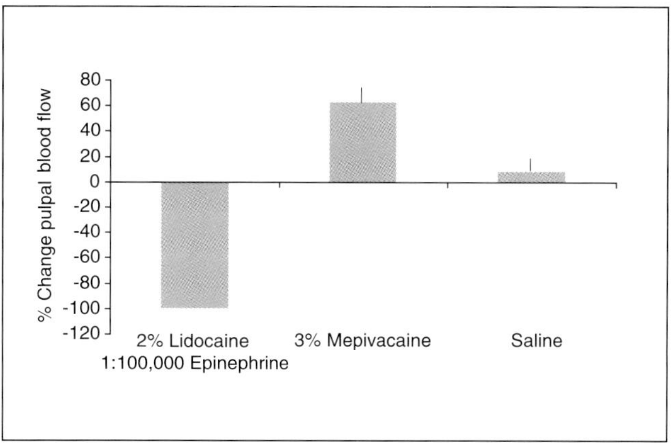

Fig 6-13 Effect of infiltration anesthesia using 2% lidocaine with 1:100,000 epinephrine or 3% mepivacaine on pulpal blood flow in anesthetized dogs. Pulpal blood flow was measured with the microsphere injection method. (Redrawn from Kim[71] with permission.)

Stimulation of β-adrenergic receptors causes a relaxation of the vascular musculature. Pulpal blood vessels respond to β-adrenergic agonists,[75] but the β-adrenergic receptors may be expressed at relatively low levels.[33] The local administration of isoproterenol, a β-adrenergic agonist, to exposed dentinal tubules produces a vasodilatory effect, as measured by dose-related increases in pulpal blood flow.[75,76] In contrast, the injection of systemic (intra-arterial) or larger doses of isoproterenol causes an initial increase and subsequent decrease in pulpal blood flow in dogs.[46,75-77]

Three hypotheses have been advanced to explain this biphasic finding.[39,76] First, the reduction in pulpal blood flow following intra-arterial administration of isoproterenol may result from "stealing" of blood flow by the adjacent tissues, which have a much greater vasodilator response to isoproterenol.[38,77] Second, the effect of systemic isoproterenol may have been due to active

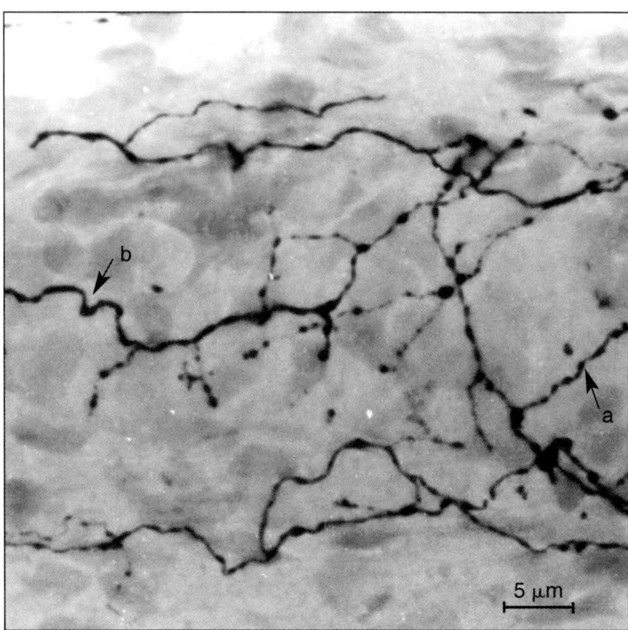

Fig 6-14 Light micrograph showing a perivascular meshwork of neuropeptide Y–immunoreactive (NPY-IR) nerves. The meshwork consists of both fine nerve fibers (a) and medium-sized nerve fibers (b). Terminal varicosities are numerous in the fine fibers, but there are only a few in the medium-sized fibers. The vascular axis is horizontal. (Reprinted from Zhang et al[2] with permission.)

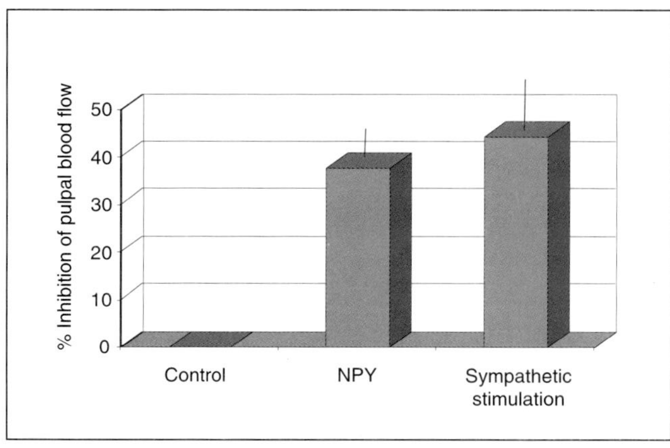

Fig 6-15 Effects of neuropeptide Y (NPY) administration (1.3 to 2.0 mg/kg) and electrical stimulation of the sympathetic fibers that innervate dental pulp on pulpal blood flow in anesthetized cats. (Redrawn from Kim et al[74] with permission.)

AVA shunting, especially in the apical region of the dental pulp. Third, the biphasic effect may have been due to initial vasodilation of pulpal arterioles, leading to an increase in pulpal interstitial pressure. This increase in interstitial pressure then led to a collapse of pulpal venules and reduced pulpal blood flow.[39,46,47] There is strong evidence to support this third potential mechanism, and increased interstitial pressure may serve as an edema-preventing mechanism because it will lead to increased lymphatic outflow.[22,25]

Parasympathetic nerves and the regulation of pulpal blood flow

The parasympathetic nervous system does not appear to have as dominant a role in regulating pulpal blood flow as the sympathetic nervous system, and some investigators have suggested that the former may be a relatively minor player in the regulation of pulpal circulation.[70]

The two major neurotransmitters derived from parasympathetic fibers are acetylcholine and vasoactive intestinal polypeptide (VIP). Histologic studies have suggested the existence of pulpal parasympathetic fibers in dental pulp.[78-81] Acetylcholinesterase (AChE) is a key enzyme in the degradation of acetylcholine and has been found in dental pulp.[50,79] However, the presence of AChE is not a selective marker for parasympathetic fibers. Moreover, at least some species do not possess a parasympathetic (cholinergic) vasodilator mechanism.[33,82] The local administration of acetylcholine to exposed dentinal tubules had been shown to produce an increase in pulpal blood flow, and this effect is blocked by the muscarinic receptor antagonist, atropine.[75,76] Immunoreactive VIP is present in pulp, and the intra-arterial injection of VIP also increases pulpal blood flow.[70,83] However, the existence of neurotransmitters and receptors does not necessarily indicate that they are derived from parasympathetic fibers, and the magnitude of parasympathetic contribution to pulpal blood flow appears low.[70]

Peptidergic afferent fibers and the regulation of pulpal blood flow

Dental pulp is innervated by sensory neurons originating from the trigeminal ganglion. Although these neurons are classified as sensory (ie, afferent), they have major efferent functions because of their release of neuropeptides from their peripheral terminals, innervating tissues such as dental pulp (see chapter 7).[70,84-86] Neuropeptides released from these fibers include substance P and calcitonin gene–related peptide (CGRP).

It has been estimated that about 80% of neuropeptides such as substance P are transported to the peripheral terminals of these afferent fibers rather than to their central terminals.[87] Thus, there is a substantial pool of these neuropeptides in peripheral terminals. This "sensory" system of afferent fibers plays a major role in modulating pulpal circulatory and immune systems via peripheral release of neuropeptides (see chapters 7, 11, and 15). Studies conducted in dental pulp indicate that sensory-derived neuropeptides, such as immunoreactive substance P, CGRP, and neurokinin A, terminate primarily near blood vessels, although some free nerve endings are also observed.[53,81,88-90] Both substance P and CGRP are released from terminals of pulpal nociceptors consisting of certain unmyelinated C[91] and thinly myelinated A-delta[92,93] fibers. Other studies have demonstrated that the appropriate receptors for these neuropeptides are also found in dental pulp.[94,95]

Activation of trigeminal sensory neurons has several effects on the pulpal circulatory system. Antidromic stimulation of sensory nerves induces pulpal vasodilation and increases pulpal blood flow.[24,48,86,96-98] This is a powerful system; stimulation of just a single pulpal C fiber is capable of inducing a detectable increase in pulpal blood flow.[98] In contrast, electrical stimulation of denervated pulp has no effect on pulpal blood flow (Fig 6-16).

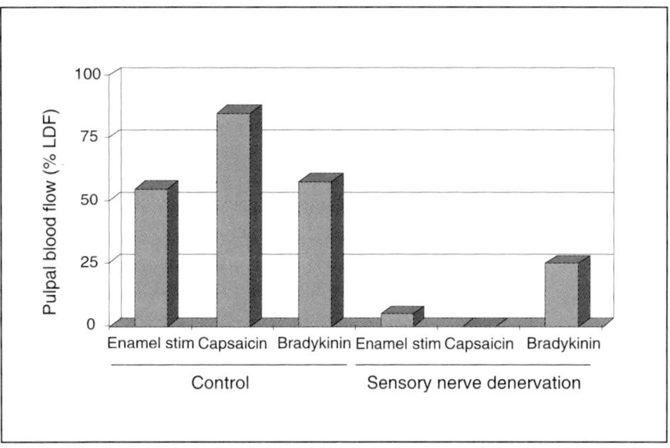

Fig 6-16 Effect of denervation of a sensory nerve on peak pulpal blood flow after electrical stimulation of the enamel (five impulses 2 Hz at 50 μA), application of capsaicin (1 mmol/L), or application of bradykinin (1 mmol/L) to exposed dentinal tubules. Pulpal blood flow was measured with a laser Doppler flowmeter (LDF). Denervation was accomplished by transsection of the inferior alveolar nerve 10 days prior to the experiment. The contralateral nerve was used as the control. (Data from Olgart.[102])

The effect of electrical stimulation is inhibited by pretreatment with antagonists to the receptors for substance P or CGRP, and is greatly diminished after 4 to 5 hours of stimulation.[86,99-101] These studies suggest that finite pools of substance P and CGRP are available for regulation of pulpal blood flow, requiring replenishment via axonal transport from the neuron's cell bodies, located in the trigeminal ganglion.

Activation of capsaicin-sensitive fibers in dental pulp increases pulpal blood flow.[102-105] Capsaicin is an extract of hot chili peppers and causes pain (ie, activates polymodal nociceptors) when eaten or injected, because capsaicin's receptor (VR1) is expressed on a major subclass of

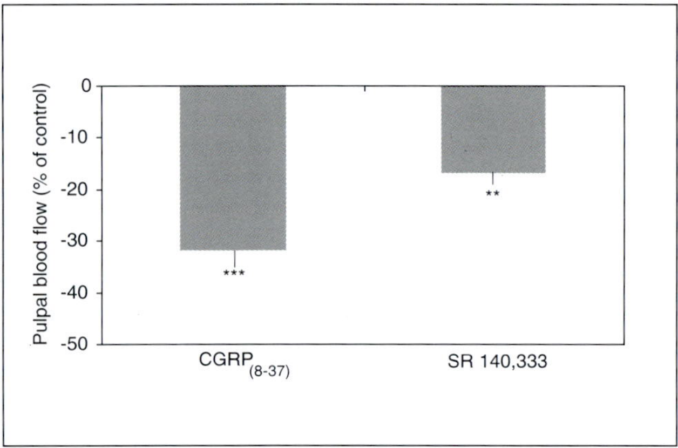

Fig 6-17 Demonstration that tonic release of calcitonin gene–related peptide (CGRP) and substance P regulates basal pulpal blood flow in the ferret. Blood flow was measured with a laser Doppler flowmeter in anesthetized ferrets before and after intra-arterial infusion of an antagonist to the CGRP receptor, $CGRP_{(8\text{-}37)}$ (150 µg/kg), or an antagonist to the neurokinin 1 substance P receptor, SR 140,333 (300 µg/kg). $^{**}P < .05$; $^{***}P < .005$. (Data from Berggreen and Heyeraas.[101])

nociceptors, including unmyelinated C fibers and some lightly myelinated A-delta fibers.[93,106] Activation of pulpal nociceptors with capsaicin evokes the peripheral release of neuropeptides such as substance P and CGRP.[107]

Given these findings, it is not surprising that the application of capsaicin to exposed dentinal tubules increases pulpal blood flow in intact teeth but not teeth that have been previously denervated (see Fig 6-16). Repeated application of capsaicin reduces the vascular response, possibly because of neuropeptide depletion or destruction of the terminals.[93,103] These and other findings[70,86] (see chapter 7) support the conclusion that capsaicin-sensitive fibers represent a major source of the substance P and CGRP that regulates pulpal circulatory responses.

There is evidence that the basal rate of release of CGRP and, to a lesser extent, substance P, regulates resting pulpal blood flow. In the ferret dental pulp, this resting vasodilator tone is due to tonic release of CGRP, substance P, and nitric oxide.[100,101] The intra-arterial infusion of the CGRP receptor antagonist, $CGRP_{(8\text{-}37)}$, results in a 32% reduction in basal pulpal blood flow (Fig 6-17). The administration of the neurokinin 1 substance P receptor antagonist, SR 140,333, produces a 17% decline in basal pulpal blood flow. These results suggest that the basal tonic release of these neuropeptides in dental pulp plays an important role in regulating basal vasodilatory state and therefore pulpal homeostasis.

Studies have indicated that the peripheral release of afferent neuropeptides such as substance P and CGRP has additional effects besides vasodilation. For example, these neuropeptides are known to produce plasma extravasation in other tissues as well as in dental pulp.[107-109] Plasma extravasation increases outflow of fluid from the vascular compartment as well as inflammatory mediators normally sequestered within the vascular compartment (eg, the kinin system). Thus, tissue injury may activate these high-threshold nociceptors, sending signals back to the brain as well as initiating neurogenic inflammatory responses (see chapter 7).[85,86] Moreover, prolonged sensory nerve stimulation leads to an accumulation of immune cells in dental pulp.[86]

The administration of neurotransmitters derived from trigeminal sensory neurons also evokes major effects on pulpal circulation. Administration of exogenous substance P and CGRP induces vasodilation in pulpal vasculature.[76,109-113] The direct application of substance P to exposed dentinal tubules leads to vasodilation, whereas the intra-arterial injection of substance P has been reported to produce biphasic effects (an initial vasodilation followed by a vasoconstriction).[76,111] It is unclear whether these contrasting effects are the results of differences in dose, route of injection, methods of measurement, physiologic responses, or species studied. However, substance P–induced vasodilation is a consistent observation.

Both CGRP and substance P exert their effect predominantly on precapillary vessels, whereas nitric oxide acts predominantly on postcapillary vessels.[100] In the mature rat molar pulp, the main targets for substance P acting through the neurokinin 1 receptors are blood vessels in the odontoblastic and subodontoblastic layer.[94]

Given the importance of the trigeminal sensory neurons in regulating basal and stimulated pulpal blood flow, it is not surprising that other systems act to modulate the release of these neuropeptides. There is strong evidence that sympathetic fibers act to inhibit the release of substance P or CGRP via presynaptic actions (see Fig 6-11).[108,114,115] Evidence supports both an adrenergic and NPY mechanism for inhibiting these fibers.[108,114,115] Other studies have shown that bradykinin and prostaglandins enhance release of CGRP from dental pulp terminals[116] and that the ability of bradykinin to increase pulpal blood flow is significantly reduced in denervated animals[102] (see Fig 6-16). Thus, the peripheral release of substance P and CGRP can be presynaptically modulated, resulting in either reduced or enhanced release.[107]

Paracrine/endocrine regulation of pulpal blood flow

Another group of factors that regulates pulpal blood flow is substances of paracrine or endocrine origin. Paracrine factors are locally produced or released at their site of action and do not circulate in the bloodstream. Endocrine factors are released from a distant gland and circulate in the bloodstream to modify the activity of the target cell. An example of hormones thought to participate in regulation of pulpal blood flow include circulating epinephrine and norepinephrine, although the magnitude of this effect may be relatively small.

There are several examples of paracrine factors that regulate pulpal blood flow. One factor is bradykinin. Bradykinin is locally produced at a site of inflammation via plasma extravasation of its precursor (kininogen) and releasing enzyme (kallikrein) that normally circulate in the bloodstream.[117] Bradykinin levels are elevated in irreversible pulpitis,[118] and the application of bradykinin increases pulpal blood flow.[76,102] About one half of bradykinin's effect is lost in denervated pulp, suggesting that this paracrine factor acts partly by activating sensory neuron release of neuropeptides and partly by a direct action on pulpal vasculature (see Figs 6-11 and 6-16).

Bradykinin has been shown to evoke prostaglandin release from a number of tissues, and the two inflammatory mediators can produce additive or synergistic effects when coadministered to pulp.[116] The coadministration of indomethacin, a cyclooxygenase inhibitor, with bradykinin significantly reduces the effect on pulpal blood flow compared to that produced by bradykinin alone.[76] Microsphere studies have indicated that bradykinin can produce a biphasic effect on pulpal blood flow similar to that induced by other substances.[119] One interpretation of the biphasic flow response is related to the low-compliance environment of the tooth, in which active arteriolar vasodilation increases interstitial hydrostatic pressure, which in turn could increase flow resistance by compression of venules, thereby causing a reduction in pulpal blood flow.

A second example of a paracrine factor is the prostaglandins. As mentioned, prostaglandins enhance the effect of bradykinin on increasing pulpal blood flow,[76] and prostaglandin levels are elevated in samples of dental pulp with the clinical diagnosis of irreversible pulpitis.[120] Administration of prostaglandin E_2 increases pulpal blood flow by more than 60% over basal levels and induces a moderate degree of plasma extravasation.[119,121]

A third example of a paracrine factor is histamine. Histamine increases pulpal blood flow to a moderate extent but produces a profound increase in plasma extavasation.[76,119] Histamine's effect on blood flow is reduced by pretreatment with diphenhydramine, a histamine receptor antagonist.[76] The effect of histamine on plasma extravasation is also reduced by pretreatment with ciproxifan or BP 2-94, antagonists to the H_3 histamine receptor.[122] Compared to administration of histamine alone, administration of the combination of histamine with prostaglandin E_2 produces relatively little change in pulpal blood flow but evokes nearly 50% greater plasma extravasation.[119]

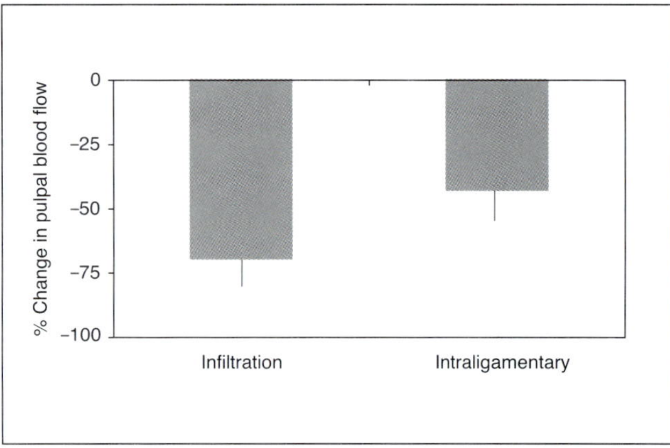

Fig 6-18 Effect of infiltration injection and intraligamentary injection of 2% lidocaine with 1:100,000 epinephrine on pulpal blood flow in canine teeth of anesthetized dogs (N = 5 or 6 per group). The same local anesthetic was used for the two routes of injection, but the injection volume differed. (Data from Kim[71] and Kim et al.[124])

Circulatory Responses to Dental Procedures, Inflammation, and Drugs

Effect of local anesthetics on pulpal circulation

Vasoconstrictors are added to local anesthetic agents for the purpose of prolonging the anesthetic state and for obtaining a deeper anesthesia. This effect is the result of arteriolar vasoconstriction, which reduces pulpal blood flow primarily by increasing vascular resistance (see Fig 6-11). Several studies have characterized the reduction in pulpal blood flow that occurs following local anesthetic injection with various vasoconstrictors such as epinephrine.[123,124] At doses of epinephrine exceeding 10^{-8} mol/L, the pulpal vessels collapse and total ischemia of the pulp results.[125]

Fortunately, dental pulp recovers from these periods of reduced pulpal blood flow. Langeland's classic study[126] demonstrated that human dental pulp is not damaged permanently by injections of local anesthetic agents. Others have shown that the metabolic activity of rat pulps after 2 to 5 hours of ischemia is not significantly different from that of control pulps.[127] These investigators concluded that the anaerobic metabolic activity of the dental pulp would enable it to survive the vasoconstrictive action of the local anesthetic. In clinical usage, the vasoconstricting effect of epinephrine may be reduced by some local anesthetics, such as lidocaine, which possesses a vasodilating effect.

Both infiltration and intraligamentary routes of injection of local anesthetic with vasoconstrictor produce a profound reduction in pulpal blood flow (Fig 6-18). Although both routes of injection were made with the same local anesthetic (2% lidocaine with 1:100,000 epinephrine), the infiltration route of injection produced about a 50% greater reduction in pulpal blood flow than did the intraligamentary route of injection.[71,124] This difference is most likely due to the difference in the injection volume (ie, dose) used in infiltration and intraligamentary techniques.

The reduction in pulpal blood flow is due to the presence of the vasoconstrictor, because injection of lidocaine alone actually causes an increase in pulpal blood flow and has limited success in obtaining anesthesia.[71] Similar results have been found in clinical trials, in which epinephrine (1:80,000) increases the duration of 2% lidocaine anesthesia from 25 to 100 minutes after infiltration injection.[128] Although the vasoconstrictor is necessary for successful anesthesia through these routes of injection,[128,129] there is no significant difference between intraligamental injection of 2% lidocaine with 1:100,000 epinephrine and 2% lidocaine without 1:100,000 epinephrine in onset of anesthesia in the cat.[130]

Effect of dental procedures on pulpal circulation

Restorative or prosthetic dental procedures

Dental procedures alter pulpal microcirculation via two major routes: thermal stimulation when handpieces or certain techniques are used and

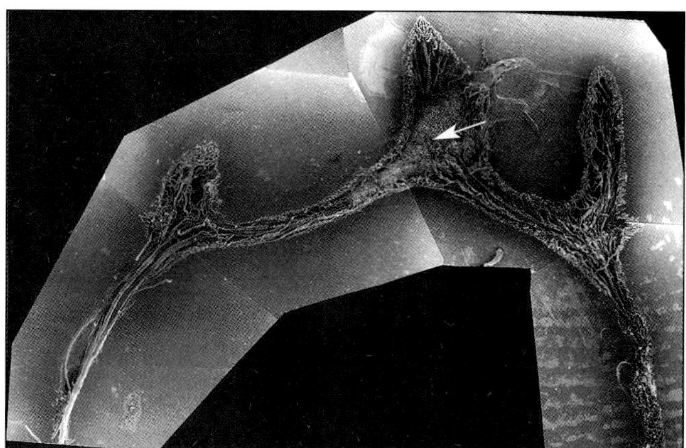

Fig 6-19a Vascular cast of a first molar 4 hours after cavity preparation with a carbide bur in a high-speed handpiece without water spray. Presence of extensive plasma extravasation *(arrow)*, as indicated by leakage of resin into the interstitial space. The terminal capillary network on the superficial layer of pulp never showed any particular changes. (Reprinted from Takahashi[131] with permission.)

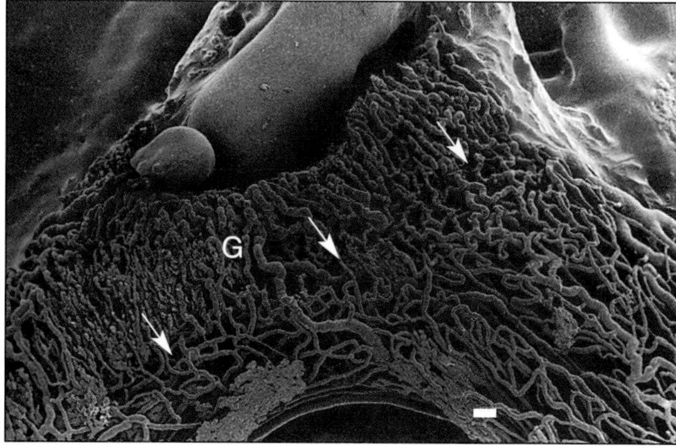

Fig 6-19b High-magnification view of a vascular cast of a mandibular premolar 1 week after cavity preparation. Furrows *(arrows)* located between the glomerulus-like network (G) and normal network. Bar = 100 μm. (Reprinted from Takahashi[131] with permission.)

the effect of dental treatment, including restorative materials. The effects of restorative materials (see chapters 4, 14, and 15) and thermal stimulation (see chapter 16) on dental pulp are discussed elsewhere in this text. This chapter will focus on circulatory responses to dental procedures.

It is critical that clinicians use water spray to control heat buildup when performing restorative or prosthetic dental procedures. Heat generated by tooth preparation can cause major changes in the pulpal microcirculation, including extensive plasma extravasation. Figures 6-19a and 6-19b show a vascular cast of a dog molar 4 hours and 1 week, respectively, after cavity preparation without water spray.[131] The development of plasma extravasation is indicated by the extensive leakage of resin near the site of the cavity preparation.

Other studies have replicated the finding that water spray minimizes the development of pulpal inflammatory changes after restorative procedures. Figure 6-20 illustrates the effect of water spray on pulpal blood flow after crown preparation.[132] Crown preparation without water spray causes about a 95% reduction in pulpal blood flow by 1 hour after preparation. In contrast, the use of water spray virtually eradicates any alteration in pulpal blood flow. The reduction in coronal pulp blood flow is the result of an increase in blood flow through the apically positioned AVA shunts and a redistribution of blood flow from the drilled side to the opposite side of the pulp.[43,119]

What physiologic system mediates this large response in blood flow in coronal pulp? Of the several potential factors known to regulate pulpal blood flow (see Fig 6-11), the trigeminal sensory nerves appear to mediate pulpal circulatory responses to cavity preparation. This was demonstrated in an elegant study in which cavity preparations were performed in control and denervated teeth (Fig 6-21). Denervation of the inferior alveolar nerve reduces the peak pulpal blood flow responses by about 75% in shallow dentinal prepa-

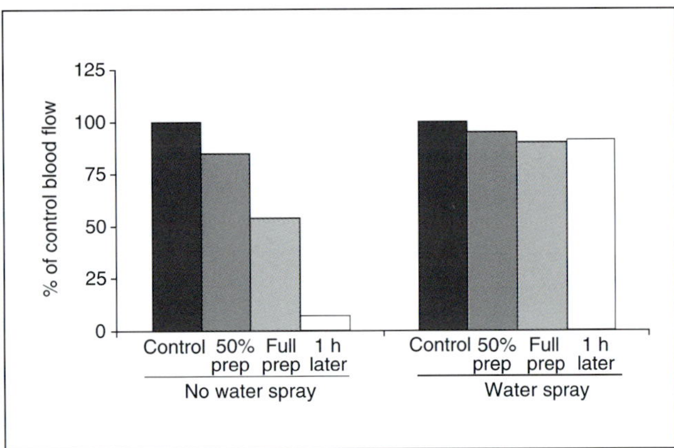

Fig 6-20 Effect of crown preparation with and without the use of water spray on pulpal blood flow. Pulpal blood flow was measured at a control period, at one-half completion of crown preparation (50% prep), at the completion of the crown preparation (Full prep), and 1 hour after completion of the preparation. (Redrawn from Kim et al[132] with permission.)

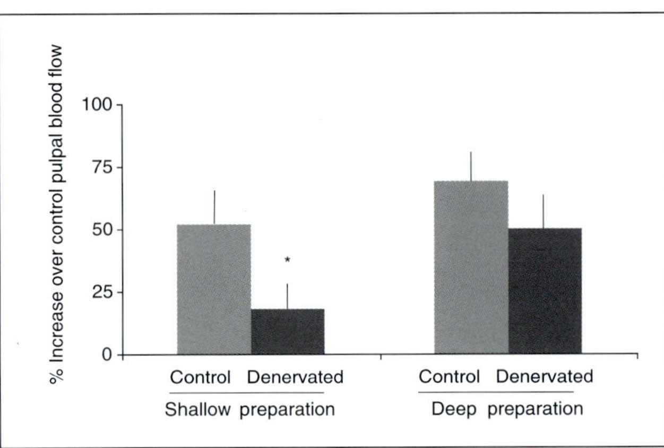

Fig 6-21 Effect of dentin grinding on pulpal blood flow in control teeth and inferior alveolar nerve–denervated teeth. Flow was measured with a laser Doppler flowmeter. Dentin was stimulated by grinding with a low-speed handpiece (1.5-mm round diamond) three times, each time for 1 second. $^{*}P < .05$. Shallow preparations were in outer dentin. Deep preparations were in inner dentin. (Redrawn from Olgart et al[133] with permission.)

rations.[133] Collectively, these studies indicate that water spray plays a critical role in reducing pulpal inflammatory responses to dental preparation procedures and that the absence of water spray induces a circulatory response that is mediated primarily by activation of trigeminal sensory nerves in tooth pulp.

A systematic evaluation of changes in microcirculatory dynamics following various dental procedures and materials currently used in dentistry has obvious clinical importance in minimizing pathophysiologic pulpal responses. The placement of zinc phosphate cement at the base of a Class V preparation results in a biphasic response to pulpal blood flow; an initial 33% increase is followed by a subsequent 33% decrease in blood flow after the cement hardens.[134] Acid etching of rat incisors with 36% phosphoric acid produces a minimal effect when done over 15 to 20 seconds but produces a profound vasoconstriction when continued for longer periods (eg, 60 seconds), with up to 40% of tested pulps showing stasis of blood flow.[135]

Longer-term effects following restorative dental procedures can also occur. Many of these changes are mediated via diffusion of substances through exposed dentinal tubules (see chapters 4, 14, and 15). For example, the application of zinc phosphate base to shallow cavity preparations results in a 40% to 50% elevation of pulpal blood 1 week and 1 month after completion of treatment.[136]

Mechanical, chemical, and microbiologic irritation of dentin under a provisional restoration could cause severe hyperemia when there is no adhesive lining. It is of vital importance that the freshly exposed dentin surface be covered securely. Application of adhesive resins to coat freshly exposed dentin seems to provide a new technique for minimizing pulpal irritation for indirect restoration.[137]

Endodontic therapy

If the pulp is partially extirpated during endodontic therapy, a profuse hemorrhage may result because of the rupture of wide-diameter vessels in the central part of the pulp. There would be less hemorrhage if the pulp were extirpated closer to the apex of the tooth. Therefore, excessive bleeding during instrumentation of the canal may indicate that some pulpal tissue remains in the apical portion of the root canal. The apex locator is useful for detecting the position of the apical foramen in such cases.[138,139]

Kishi et al[140] reported that a flat and dense vascular network is newly formed 1 week after pulpotomy in dog molars. Eight weeks after pulpotomy, the vascular network just beneath the thick dentin bridge consists of three normal layers. Unfortunately, because of the location of the remaining pulpal tissue, neither electrical nor thermal testing can determine the vitality, and hence the presence of circulation, in the apical portion of the pulp.[141]

Orthodontic therapy

Orthodontic treatment has substantial effects on the microcirculatory system of the dental pulp. Following localized tooth movement, a steady and significant increase in blood flow can be observed not only in the periodontal tissues but also in the pulp.[142] At later time points, orthodontic movement stimulates a large and coordinated sprouting in pulpal nerve terminals and blood vessels.[143] This has raised the hypothesis that orthodontic movement leads to an increase in pulpal concentrations of angiogenic growth factors. Indeed, extracts of human pulp taken after orthodontic movement have increased concentrations of angiogenic factors and show increased growth of blood vessels even when cultured in vitro.[144,145] Other studies have shown that growth factors, including vascular endothelial growth factor, are embedded in dentin and are released from the matrix following injury (see chapter 3).[146] Thus, it is possible that dental procedures that lead to release of these growth factors from the dentin matrix may result in enhanced angiogenesis.

Orthognathic surgery

Occlusal abnormalities may be corrected by maxillary or mandibular segmental osteotomies. Attempts have been made to determine the effects of such procedures on the blood flow to the oral mucosa, bone, and dental pulp. Techniques that have been used for this purpose include microangiography,[147] isotope fractionization and particle distribution,[148] hydrogen washout technique,[149] and laser Doppler flowmetry (LDF).[150] Of all the tissues, pulpal blood flow was most severely decreased (by 82%) immediately after surgery.[149] However, blood flow has been reported to be reestablished at later time points.

More recent studies using a laser Doppler flowmeter have reported that, although pulpal blood flow is detectable 6 months after a Le Fort I procedure, it is still significantly lower than preoperative levels.[151] Early studies have claimed that tooth pulp responses to thermal and electrical stimuli return to normal in more than 90% of patients,[152,153] although recovery of pulpal sensitivity may take days or weeks.[154] Thus, preemptive endodontic therapy or extraction is not warranted in patients undergoing these types of surgeries unless there is evidence of periradicular pathoses.[155]

Inflammation

A number of inflammatory mediators that are released after pulpal injury may have direct effects, or indirect effects via modulation of trigeminal sensory nerve fibers, on pulpal vasculature (see Fig 6-11). Previous sections of this chapter have already reviewed several of these mediators, including bradykinin, prostaglandins, and histamine.

The two major actions of mediators of acute inflammation are alterations in pulpal blood flow and increases in capillary permeability, leading to plasma extravasation. The increased permeability of the vessels permits the escape of plasma proteins and leukocytes from the capillaries into the inflamed area to carry out neutralization, dilution, and phagocytosis of the irritant. In the acute pulpitis stage following cavity preparation without water coolant, increased permeability of blood vessels is seen not in the superficial, terminal capillaries just beneath the cavity but in the venular and capillary networks. In the inflamed pulp, vascular loops, AVA shunts, increased blood flow, and increased lymphatic outflow may represent protective changes against inflammation.[22,24,29,131]

The introduction of bacterial plaque into dental pulp or the administration of bacterial lipopolysaccharide induces profound alterations in pulpal blood flow. Pulpal blood flow can increase up to 40% over control levels in dental pulp moderately inflamed with bacterial plaque.[119] As pulp becomes partially necrotic, there is a reduction in blood flow.[119] In other studies, application of bacterial lipopolysaccharide to pulp has resulted in a large increase in pulpal prostaglandins, leukotrienes, and plasma extravasation.[28,119,156] Thus, bacteria and their by-products produce profound circulatory responses in dental pulp.

During chronic inflammation, pulpal tissue pressure is elevated, although not as greatly as it is during acute inflammation.[28,37] The muscular elements in the microcirculation reestablish control over capillary pressure. Capillary permeability is gradually decreased as repair occurs.

In severe inflammation, the lymphatic vessels are closed, resulting in persistently increased fluid and pulpal pressure. The final result may be pulpal necrosis. Care must be taken, however, to assess the vital pulp restricted to the apical portion of the root in teeth with coronal necrosis.[141] In addition, histologic and physiologic changes, including pulpal tissue pressure,[34,38] could take place at the site of inflammation, while the neighboring region shows no sign of inflammation.[4] Thus, total pulpal necrosis represents the gradual accumulation of local necrosis.

Detection of Pulpal Circulation As a Diagnostic Test

Given the essential role of the pulpal microcirculation in maintaining the health of this tissue, it is not surprising that the circulatory status of dental pulp has been proposed by clinicians to assess the vitality of this tissue. Several general methods have been used to clinically evaluate pulpal circulation, including LDF, pulse oximetry, and transmitted-light photoplethysmography.

Laser Doppler flowmeters are based on the principle that reflected light from blood flow will demonstrate a Doppler (frequency shifting) effect, depending on the relative velocity of the blood flow compared to the probe. Several studies have suggested a reliability of greater than 80% to 90% for LDF assessment of vitality.[157-166] However, others have observed lower levels of reliability or technical difficulties, including the potential confounding factor that up to 80% of the signals measured by LDF originate from the periodontal tissue.[151,166-169] The use of a dual-probe LDF system has been suggested to increase the reliability of this method, as has the use of a 633-nm laser source placed 2 to 3 mm above the gingival margin.[158,164] The method is contraindicated in heavily restored teeth and teeth with apical viability (because LDF probes detect only coronal pulpal blood flow).[165]

The use of a pulse oximeter is a clinically accepted technique for evaluating oxygen saturation of tissues. Pulse oximeters are often configured as finger or ear probes. Pulse oximeters have been used to assess pulpal vitality; some studies have reported greater success[166,167] than others.[168] Although the pulse oximetry approach is promising, additional developmental research should be conducted before this method is considered clinically acceptable.

Transmitted-light photoplethysmography[169,170] may be useful for vitality testing of young permanent teeth.[163,171] Validation studies have reported that 565 nm gives a peak intensity of signal when transmitted-light photoplethysmography is used on extracted teeth.[170]

Although promising, these current techniques suffer from concerns about sensitivity, specificity, and ease of use. However, given the central importance of their approach (assessment of pulpal microcirculation as a measure of pulpal vitality), it is hoped that future research and development will lead to the introduction of methods that are reliable, valid, and easy to apply.

References

1. Sawa Y, Yoshida S, Shibata KI, Suzuki M, Mukaida A. Vascular endothelium of human dental pulp expresses diverse adhesion molecules for leukocyte emigration. Tissue Cell 1998;30:281–291.
2. Zhang JQ, Nagata K, Iijima T. Scanning electron microscopy and immunohistochemical observations of the vascular nerve plexuses in the dental pulp of rat incisor. Anat Rec 1998;251:214–220.
3. Kishi Y, Takahashi K. Change of vascular architecture of dental pulp with growth. In: Inoki R, Kudo T, Olgart L (eds). Dynamic Aspects of Dental Pulp. London: Chapman and Hall, 1995:97–129.
4. Renkin EM. Multiple pathways of capillary permeability. Circ Res 1997;41:735–743.
5. Corpron RE, Avery JK, Lee SD. Ultrastructure of capillaries in the odontoblastic layer. J Dent Res 1973;52:393.
6. Yoshida S. Changes in the vasculature during tooth eruption of the rat molar. Jpn J Oral Biol 1984;26:94–115.
7. Kishi Y, Shimozono N, Takahashi K. Vascular architecture of cat pulp using corrosive resin cast under scanning electron microscope. J Endod 1989;15:478–483.
8. Ruben MP, Prieto-Hernandez JR, Gott FK, Kramer GM, Bloom AA. Visualization of lymphatic microcirculation of oral tissues. II. Vital retrograde lymphography. J Periodontol 1971;42:774–784.
9. Bishop M, Mahorta M. An investigation of lymphatic vessels in the feline dental pulp. Am J Anat 1990;187:247–253.
10. Marchetti C. Weibel-Palade bodies and lympathic endothelium: Observations in the lympathic vessels of normal and inflamed human dental pulps. Vasa 1996;25:337–340.
11. Matthews B, Andrew D. Microvascular architecture and exchange in teeth. Microcirculation 1995;2:305–313.
12. Kukletová M. An electron-microscopic study of the lymphatic vessels in the dental pulp in the calf. Arch Oral Biol 1970;15:1117–1124.
13. Dahl E, Mjör IA. The fine structure of the vessels in the human dental pulp. Acta Odontol Scand 1973;31:223–230.
14. Bernick S, Patek PR. Lymphatic vessels of the dental pulp in dogs. J Dent Res 1969;48:959–964
15. Bernick S. Morphological changes to lymphatic vessels in pulpal inflammation. J Dent Res 1977;56:70–77.
16. Vetter W. Alkaline Phosphatasen in Mastzallen, Blut- und Lymphgefässen der Rattenzunge: 5'-Nucleotidase-unspezifische alkaline phosphatase- und Polyphosphatase- (ATP'ase) Aktivität under besondere Berücksichtigung des pH. Z Anat Entwicklungsgesch 1970;130:153.
17. Kato S. Histochemical localization of 5'-nucleotidase in the lymphatic endothelium. Acta Histochem Cytochem 1990;23:613–620.
18. Sawa Y, Shibata KI, Braithwaite MW, Suzuki M, Yoshida S. Expression of immunoglobulin superfamily members on the lymphatic endothelium of inflamed human small intestine. Microvasc Res 1999;57:100–106.
19. Matsumoto Y, Kato S, Miura M, Yanagisawa S, Shimizu M. Fine structure and distribution of lymphatic vessels in the human dental pulp: A study using an enzyme-histochemical method. Cell Tissue Res 1997;288:79–85.
20. Sawa Y, Yoshida S, Ashikaga Y, Kim T, Yamaoka Y, Suzuki M. Immunohistochemical demonstration of lymphatic vessels in human dental pulp. Tissue Cell 1998;30:510–516.
21. Starling E. On the absorption of fluids from the connective tissue spaces. J Physiol Lond 1896;19:312–326.
22. Heyeraas KJ, Berggreen E. Interstitial fluid pressure in normal and inflamed pulp. Crit Rev Oral Biol Med 1999:10:328–336.
23. Ganong W. Review of Medical Physiology, ed 20. New York, McGraw-Hill, 2001:chap 30.
24. Heyeraas KJ, Kvinnsland I. Tissue pressure and blood flow in pulpal inflammation. Proc Finn Dent Soc 1992;88(suppl 1):393–401.
25. Upthegrove D, Bishop J, Dorman H. Indirect determination of the blood pressure in the dental pulp. Arch Oral Biol 1968;13:929–932.
26. Brown AC, Yankowitz D. Tooth pulp pressure and hydraulic permeability. Circ Res 1964;15:42–50.
27. Christiansen R, Meyer M, Visscher M. Tonometric measurement of dental pulpal and mandibular marrow blood pressures. J Dent Res 1977;56:635–639.
28. Tønder KJ, Kvinnsland I. Micropuncture measurements of interstitial fluid pressure in normal and inflamed dental pulp in cats. J Endod 1983;9:105–109.
29. Heyeraas KJ. Pulpal hemodynamics and interstitial fluid pressure: Balance of transmicrovascular fluid transport. J Endod 1989;15:468–472.
30. Brown A, Beveridge E. The relation between tooth pulp pressure and systemic arteriolar pressure. Arch Oral Biol 1966;11:1181–1186.
31. Van Hassel HJ, Brown AC. Effect of temperature changes on intrapulpal pressure and hydraulic permeability in dogs. Arch Oral Biol 1969;14:301–315.
32. Stenvik A, Iverson J, Mjör IA. Tissue pressure and histology of normal and inflamed tooth pulps in macaque monkeys. Arch Oral Biol 1972;17:1501–1511.
33. Tønder KH, Naess G. Nervous control of blood flow in the dental pulps of dogs. Acta Physiol Scand 1978;104:13–23.
34. Heyeraas KJ. Interstitial fluid pressure and transmicrovascular fluid flow. In: Inoki R, Kudo T, Olgart L (eds). Dynamic Aspects of Dental Pulp. London: Chapman and Hall, 1990:189–198.

35. Heyeraas KJ, Kim S, Raab WH-R, Byers MR, Liu M. Effect of electrical tooth stimulation on blood flow and interstitial fluid pressure and substance P and CGRP-immunoreactive nerve fibers in the low compliant cat dental pulp. Microvasc Res 1994;47:329–343.

36. Jacobsen E, Heyeraas K. Pulp interstitial fluid pressure and blood flow after denervation and electrical tooth stimulation in the ferret. Arch Oral Biol 1997;42:407–415.

37. Van Hassel HJ. Physiology of the human dental pulp. In: Siskin M (ed). The Biology of the Human Dental Pulp. St Louis: Mosby, 1973:16.

38. Heyeraas KJ. Pulpal microvascular and tissue pressure. J Dent Res 1985;64(special issue):585–589.

39. Kim S, Dorsher-Kim J. Haemodynamic regulation of the dental pulp. In: Inoki R, Kudo T, Olgart L (eds). Dynamic Aspects of Dental Pulp. London: Chapman and Hall, 1990:167–188.

40. Meyer MW, Path MG. Blood flow in the dental pulp of dogs determined by hydrogen polarography and radioactive microsphere methods. Arch Oral Biol 1979;24:601–605.

41. Meyer MW. Symposium. 5. Methodologies for studying pulpal hemodynamics. J Endod 1980;6:466–472.

42. Kim S, Fan F, Chen R, Simchon S, Schuesser G, Chien S. Symposium. 3. Effects of changes in systemic hemodynamic parameters on pulpal hemodynamics. J Endod 1980;6:394–397.

43. Kim S, Schuessler G, Chien S. Measurement of blood flow in the dental pulp of dogs with the 133xenon washout method. Arch Oral Biol 1983;28:501–505.

44. Okabe E, Todoki K, Ito H. Microcirculation: Function and regulation in microvasculatorure. In: Inoki R, Kudo T, Olgart L (eds). Dynamic Aspects of Dental Pulp. London: Chapman and Hall, 1990:151–166.

45. Kim S, Dorsher-Kim J, Kim S. Contribution of the low compliance environment to the pathophysiology of the pulp. In: Shimono M, Maeda T, Suda H, Takahashi K (eds). Dentin/Pulp Complex. Tokyo: Quintessence, 1996:154–157.

46. Kim S. Microcirculation of the dental pulp in health and disease. J Endod 1985;11:465–471.

47. Kim S. Regulation of pulpal blood flow. J Dent Res 1985;64(special issue): 590–596.

48. Vongsavan N, Matthews B. Changes in pulpal blood flow and in fluid flow through dentine produced by autonomic and sensory nerve stimulation in the cat. Proc Finn Dent Soc 1992;88(suppl 1):491–497.

49. Takahashi K. A scanning electron microscope study of the blood vessels of dog pulp using corrosion resin casts. J Endod 1982;8:131–135.

50. Pohto M, Antila R. Innervation of blood vessels in the dental pulp. Int Dent J 1972;22:228–239.

51. Okamura K, Kobayashi I, Matsuo K, Taniguchi K, Ishibashi Y, Izumi T, et al. An immunohistochemical and ultrastructural study of vasomotor nerves in the microvasculature of human dental pulp. Arch Oral Biol 1995;40:47–53.

52. Okamura K, Kobayashi I, Matsuo K, Taniguchi K, Ishibashi Y, Izumi T, et al. Ultrastructure of the neuromuscular junction of vasomotor nerves in the microvasculature of human dental pulp. Arch Oral Biol 1994;39:171–176.

53. Tabata S, Ozaki HS, Nakashima M, Uemura M, Iwamoto H. Innervation of blood vessels in the rat incisor pulp: a scanning electron microscopic and immunoelectron microscopic study. Anat Rec 1998;251:384–391.

54. Casasco A, Frattini P, Casasco M, Santagostino G, Springall DR, Kuhn DM, Polak JM. Catecholamines in human dental pulp. A combined immunohistochemical and chromatographic study. Eur J Histochem 1995;39:133–140.

55. Schachmann MA, Rosenberg PA, Linke HA. Quantitation of catecholamines in uninflamed human dental pulp tissues by high-performance liquid chromatography. Oral Surg Oral Med Oral Pathol Oral Radiol Endod 1995;80:83–86.

56. Parker DA, Marino V, Ivar PM, de la Lande IS. Modulation by presynaptic β-adrenoceptors of noradrenaline release from sympathetic nerves in human dental pulp. Arch Oral Biol 1998;43:949–954.

57. Parker DA, Marino V, Zisimopoulos S, de la Lande IS. Evidence for presynaptic cholinergic receptors in sympathetic nerves in human dental pulp. Arch Oral Biol 1998;43:197–204.

58. Parker DA, de la Lande IS, Marino V, Ivar PM. Presynaptic control of noradrenaline release from sympathetic nerves in human dental pulp. Arch Oral Biol 1994;39:35–41.

59. Avery JK, Cox CF, Chiego DJ Jr. Presence and location of adrenergic nerve endings in the dental pulps of mouse molars. Anat Rec 1980;198:59–71.

60. Weiss R, Tansy M, Chaffee R. Functional control of intrapulpal vasculature. I. Relationship of tooth pulp and lateral nasal artery pressures. J Dent Res 1970;49(6, suppl):1407–1413.

61. Edwall L, Kindlovà M. The effect of sympathetic nerve stimulation on the rate of disappearance of tracers from various oral tissues. Acta Physiol Scand 1971;29:387–400.

62. Scott D Jr, Scheinin A, Karjalainen S, Edwall L. Influence of sympathetic nerve stimulation on flow velocity in pulpal vessels. Acta Odontol Scand 1972;30:277–287.

63. Tønder KH. The effects of variations in arterial blood pressure and baroreceptor reflexes on blood flow in dogs. Arch Oral Biol 1975;20:345–349.

64. Kerezoudis NP, Olgart L, Edwall L, Gazelius B, Nomikos GG. Activation of sympathetic fibers in the pulp by electrical stimulation of rat incisor teeth. Arch Oral Biol 1992;37:1013–1019.
65. Taylor AD. Microscopic observation of the living tooth pulp. Science 1950;3:40–46.
66. Forssell-Ahlberg KF, Edwall L. Influence of local insults on sympathetic vasoconstrictor control in the feline dental pulp. Acta Odontol Scand 1977;35:103–110.
67. Aars H, Gazelius B, Edwall L, Olgart L. Effects of autonomic reflexes on tooth pulp blood flow in man. Acta Physiol Scand 1992;146:423–429.
68. Dorscher-Kim J, Kim S. The adrenergic system and dental pulp. In: Inoki R, Kudo T, Olgart L (eds). Dynamic Aspects of Dental Pulp. London: Chapman and Hall, 1990:283–296.
69. Ibricevic H, Heyeraas KH, Pasic JE, Hamamdzic M, Djordjevic N, Krnic J. Identification of α-2 adrenoceptors in the blood vessels of the dental pulp. Int Endod J 1991;24:279–289.
70. Olgart L. Neural control of pulpal blood flow. Crit Rev Oral Biol 1996;7:159–171.
71. Kim S. Ligamental injection: A physiological explanation of its efficacy. J Endod 1986;12:486–491.
72. Uddman R, Kato J, Cantera L, Edvinsson L. Localization of neuropeptide Y Y1 receptor mRNA in human tooth pulp. Arch Oral Biol 1998;43:389–394.
73. Luthman J, Luthman D, Hokfelt T. Occurrence and distribution of different neurochemical markers in the human dental pulp. Arch Oral Biol 1992;37:193–208.
74. Kim SK, Ang L, Hsu YY, Dorscher-Kim J, Kim S. Antagonistic effect of D-myo-inositol-1,2,6-trisphosphate (PP56) on neuropeptide Y-induced vasoconstriction in the feline dental pulp. Arch Oral Biol 1996;41: 791–798.
75. Liu M, Kim S, Park D, Moskowitz K, Bilotto G, Dorscher-Kim J. Comparison of the effects of intra-arterial and locally applied vasoactive agents on pulpal blood flow in dog canine teeth determined by laser Doppler velocimetry. Arch Oral Biol 1983;35:405–410.
76. Okabe E, Todoki K, Ito H. Direct pharmacological action of vasoactive substances on pulp blood flow. An analysis and critique. J Endod 1989;15:473–477.
77. Tønder KH. Effect of vasodilating drugs on external carotid and pulpal blood flow in dogs: "Stealing" of dental perfusion pressure. Acta Physiol Scand 1976;97: 75–87.
78. Chiego DJ Jr, Cox CF, Avery JK. H3-HRP analysis of the nerve supply to primate teeth. J Dent Res 1980;59: 736–744.
79. Avery JK, Chiego DJ Jr. The cholinergic system and the dental pulp. In: Inoki R, Kudo T, Olgart L (eds). Dynamic Aspects of Dental Pulp. London: Chapman and Hall, 1990:297–331.
80. Segade L, Quintanilla D, Nunez J. The postganglionic parasympathetic fibers originating in the oticganglion are distributed in several branches of the trigeminal mandibular nerve: An HRP study in the guinea pig. Brain Res 1987;411:386–390.
81. Wakisaka S, Akai M. Immunohistochemical observation on neuropeptides around the blood vessel in feline dental pulp. J Endod 1989;15:413–416.
82. Sasano T, Shiji N, Sanjo D, Izumi H, Karita K. Absence of parasympathetic vasodilation in cat dental pulp. J Dent Res 1995;74:1665–1670.
83. Uddman R, Bjorlin G, Moller B, Sundler F. Occurrence of VIP nerves in mammalian dental pulps. Acta Odontol Scand 1980;38:325–328.
84. Hargreaves, KM, Roszkowski M, Jackson DL, Swift JQ. Orofacial pain: Peripheral mechanisms. In: Fricton J, Dubner R (eds). Advances in Pain Research and Therapy. Vol 21: Orofacial pain and temporomandibular disorders. New York: Raven Press, 1955:33–42.
85. Hargreaves, KM. Neurochemical factors in injury and inflammation in orofacial tissues. In: Lavigne G, Lund J, Sessle B, Dubner R (eds). Orofacial Pain: Basic Science to Clinical Management. Chicago: Quintessence, 2001.
86. Fristad I. Dental innervation: Functions and plasticity after peripheral injury. Acta Odontol Scand 1997;55: 236–254.
87. Brimijoin S, Lundberg J, Brodin E, Hokfelt T, Nilsson G. Axonal transport of substance P in the vagus and sciatic nerves of the guinea pig. Brain Res 1980;191: 443–457.
88. Uddman R, Grundithz T, Sundler F. Calcitonin gene-related peptide: A sensory transmitter in dental pulps? Scand J Dent Res 1986;94:219–224.
89. Jacobsen EB, Fristad I, Heyeraas KJ. Nerve fibers immunoreactive to calcitonin gene-related peptide, substance P, neuropeptide Y, and dopamine β-hydroxylase in innervated and denervated oral tissues in ferrets. Acta Odontol Scand 1998;56:220–228.
90. Sato O, Takeuchi-Maeno H, Maeda T, Takano Y. Immunoelectron microscopic observation of calcitonin gene-related (CGRP) -positive nerves in the dental pulp of rat molars. Arch Histol Cytol 1992;55:561–568.
91. Närhi M, Jyvasjarvi E, Virtanen A, Huopaniemi T, Ngassapa D, Hirvonen T. Role of intradental A- and C-type nerve fibers in dental pain mechanisms. Proc Finn Dent Soc 1992;88(suppl 1):507–516.
92. Ikeda H, Sunakawa M, Suda H. Three groups of afferent pulpal feline nerve fibres show different electrophysiological response properties. Arch Oral Biol 1995;40:895–904.
93. Ikeda H, Tokita Y, Suda H. Capsaicin sensitive Ad fibers in cat tooth pulp. J Dent Res 1997;76:1341–1349
94. Fristad I, Vandevska-Radunovic V, Kvinnsland IH. Neurokinin-1 receptor expression in the mature dental pulp of rats. Arch Oral Biol 1999;44:191–195.

95. Uddman R, Kato J, Lindgren P, Sunderl F, Edvinsson L. Expression of calcitonin gene-related peptide-1 receptor mRNA in human tooth pulp and trigeminal ganglion. Arch Oral Biol 1999;44:1-6.
96. Gazelius B, Olgart L. Vasodilation in the dental pulp produced by electrical stimulation of the inferior alveolar nerve in the cat. Acta Physiol Scand 1980;108: 181-186.
97. Brodin E, Gazelius B, Olgart L, Nilsson G. Tissue concentration and release of substance P-like immunoreactivity in the dental pulp. Acta Physiol Scand 1981;111: 141-149.
98. Andrew D, Matthews B. Some properties of vasodilatory nerves innervating tooth pulp in the cat. In: Shimono M, Maeda T, Suda H, Takahashi K (eds). Dentin/ Pulp Complex. Tokyo: Quintessence, 1996:254-257.
99. Kerezoudis NP, Fried K, Olgart L. Haemodynamic and immunohistochemical studies of rat incisor pulp after denervation and subsequent re-innervation. Arch Oral Biol 1995;40:815-823.
100. Bergreen E, Heyeraas K. The role of sensory neuropeptides and nitric oxide on pulpal blood flow and tissue pressure in the ferret. J Dent Res 1999;78: 1535-1543.
101. Berggreen E, Heyeraas K. Effect of neuropeptides antagonists h-CGRP(8-37) and SR 140.33 on pulpal and gingival blood flow in ferrets. Arch Oral Biol 2000;45: 537-542.
102. Olgart L. Involvement of sensory nerves in hemodynamic reactions. Proc Finn Dent Soc 1992,88:(suppl 1):403-410.
103. Liu M, Pertl C, Markowitz K, Dorscher-Kim J, Kim S. The effects of capsaicin on pulpal blood flow. Proc Finn Dent Soc 1992;88(suppl 1):463-467.
104. Pertl C, Liu MT, Markowitz K, Kim S. Effects of capsaicin on KCl-induced blood flow and sensory nerve activity changes in the tooth pulp. Pain 1993;52: 351-358.
105. Raab WH, Magerl W, Muller H. Changes in dental blood flow following electrical tooth pulp stimulation—Influences of capsaicin and guanethidine. Agents Actions 1988;25:237-239.
106. Caterina MJ, Schumacher M, Tominaga M, Rosen T, Levine J, Julius D. The capsaicin receptor: A heat-activated ion channel in the pain pathway. Nature 1997; 389:816-824.
107. Hargreaves KM, Swift JQ, Roszkowski MT, Bowles WR, Garry MG, Jackson DL. Pharmacology of peripheral neuropeptide and inflammatory mediator release. Oral Surg Oral Med Oral Pathol 1994;78:503-510.
108. Kerezoudis NP, Olgart L, Funato A, Edwall L. Inhibitory influence of sympathetic nerves on afferent nerve-induced extravasation in the rat incisor pulp upon direct electrical stimulation of the tooth. Arch Oral Biol 1993;38:483-490.
109. Ohkubo T, Shibata M, Yamada Y, Kaya H, Takahashi H. Role of substance P in neurogenic inflammation in the rat incisor pulp and the lower lip. Arch Oral Biol 1993; 38:151-158.
110. Skrabanek P, Powell D. Substance P, vol 1. Montreal: Eden Press, 1977.
111. Kim S, Dorscher-Kim J, Liu MT, Trowbridge HO. Biphasic pulp blood-flow response to substance P in the dog as measured with a radiolabelled, microsphere injection method. Arch Oral Biol 1988;33:305-309.
112. Gazelius B, Olgart L, Edwall L, Trowbridge HO. Effects of substance P on sensory nerves and blood flow in the feline dental pulp. In: Anderson DJ, Matthews B (eds). Pain in the Trigeminal Region. Amsterdam: Elsevier/ North Holland Biomedical Press, 1977:95-101.
113. Gazelius B, Edwall B, Olgart L, Lundberg J, Hokfelt T, Fisher J. Vasodilatory effects of coexistence of CGRP and substance P in sensory nerves of cat dental pulp. Acta Physiol Scand 1987;130:33-40.
114. Kerezoudis NP, Funato A, Edwall L, Olgart L. Activation of sympathetic nerves exerts an inhibitory influence on afferent nerve-induced vasodilation unrelated to vasoconstriction in rat dental pulp. Acta Physiol Scand 1993;147:27-35.
115. Gibbs JL, Flores CM, Poon A, Wagner L, Garcia N, Hargreaves KM. Evaluation of NPY Y1 agonist effects on exocytotic activity from central and peripheral terminals of capsaicin-sensitive nociceptors. Abstracts Soc Neurosci 2000;26:935.
116. Goodis HE, Bowles W, Hargreaves KM. Prostaglandin E2 enhances bradykinin-evoked iCGRP release in bovine dental pulp. J Dent Res 2000;79:1604-1607.
117. Hargreaves KM, Costello A. Glucocorticoids suppress release of immunoreactive bradykinin from inflamed tissue as evaluated by microdialysis probes. Clin Pharmacol Ther 1990;48:168-178.
118. Lepinski A, Hargreaves KM, Goodis H, Bowles W. Bradykinin levels in dental pulp by microdialysis. J Endod 2000;26:744-747.
119. Kim S, Liu M, Simchon S, Dorscher-Kim JE. Effects of selected inflammatory mediators on blood flow and vascular permeability in the dental pulp. Proc Finn Dent Soc 1992;88(suppl 1):387-392.
120. Nakanishi T, Matsuo T, Ebisu S. Quantitiative analysis of immunoglobulins and inflammatory factors in human pulpal blood from exposed pulps. J Endod 1995;21:131-136.
121. Okiji T, Morita I, Sunada I, Murota S. Involvement of arachidonic acid metabolites in increases in vascular permeability in experimental dental pulp inflammation in the rat. Arch Oral Biol 1989;34:523-528.
122. Boucher Y, Hofman S, Joulin Y, Azerad J. Effects of BP 2-94, a selective H(3) receptor agonist, on blood flow and vascular permeability of the rat mandibular incisor pulp. Arch Oral Biol 2001:46:83-92.

123. Olgart L, Gazelius B. Effects of adrenaline and felypressin (octapressin) on blood flow and sensory nerve activity in teeth. Acta Odontol Scand 1977;35:69–75.
124. Kim S, Edwall L, Trowbridge H, Chien S. Effects of local anesthetic on pulpal blood flow in dogs. J Dent Res 1984;63:650–652.
125. Simard-Savoie S, Lemay H, Taleb L. The effect of epinephrine on pulpal microcirculation. J Dent Res 1979;58:2074–2079.
126. Langeland K. Effects of local anesthetics on pulp tissue. Dent Prog 1962;3:13–18.
127. Röckert HOE, Örtendal T. Recovery of aerobic respiratory activity of the dental pulp after anoxic periods of two to five hours. IRCS Med Sci 1980;8:99.
128. Pitt Ford TR, Seare MA, McDonald F. Action of adrenaline on the effect of dental local anaesthetic solutions. Endod Dent Traumatol 1993;9:31–35.
129. Odor TM, Pitt Ford TR, McDonald F. Adrenaline in local anaesthesia: The effect of concentration on dental pulpal circulation and anaesthesia. Endod Dent Traumatol 1994;10:167–173.
130. Suda H, Sunakawa M, Ikeda H, Yamamoto H. Neurophysiological evaluation of intraligamentary anesthesia. Dent Jpn 1994;31:46–50.
131. Takahashi K. Pulpal vascular changes in inflammation. Proc Finn Dent Soc 1992;88(special issue):381–385.
132. Kim S, Dörscher-Kim J, Liu M, Grayson A. Functional alterations in pulpal microcirculation in response to various dental procedures and materials. Proc Finn Dent Soc 1992:88(suppl 1):65–71.
133. Olgart L, Edwall L, Gazelius B. Involvement of afferent nerves in pulpal blood flow reactions in response to clinical and experimental procedures in the cat. Arch Oral Biol 1991;36:575–581.
134. Kim S, Trowbridge H, Suda H. Pulpal reactions to caries and dental procedures. In: Cohen S, Burns R (eds). Pathways of the Pulp, ed 8. St Louis: Mosby, 2002:573–600.
135. Ivanyi I, Kispelyi B, Fazekas A, Rosivall L, Nyarasdy I. The effect of acid etching on vascular diameter of pulp-vessels in rat incisor (vital microscopic study). Oper Dent 2001;26:248–252.
136. Kim S, Dorsher-Kim J, Baek S. Effects of tooth preparation and dental materials on pulpal microcirculation: Shunting of 9- and 10-mm microspheres. In: Shimono M, Maeda T, Suda H, Takahashi K (eds). Dentin/Pulp Complex. Tokyo: Quintessence, 1996:58–61.
137. Inokoshi S, Fujitani M, Otsuki M, Sonoda H, Ketasako Y, Shimada Y, Tagami J. Monkey pulpal response to conventional and adhesive luting cements. Oper Dent 1998;23:21–29.
138. Sunada I. New method for measuring the length of the root canal. J Dent Res 1962;41:375–387.
139. Kobayashi C, Suda H. New electronic canal measuring device based on the ratio method. J Endod 1994;20: 111–114.
140. Kishi Y, Shimozono N, Takahashi K. Vascularization after pulpotomy. Proc Finn Dent Soc 1992;88(suppl 1):487–490.
141. Ikeda H, Suda H. Subjective sensation and objective neural discharges recorded from clinically nonvital and intact teeth. J Endod 1998;24:552–556.
142. Vandevska-Radunovic V, Kristiansen AB, Heyeraas KJ, Kvinsland S. Changes in blood circulation in teeth and supporting tissues incident to experimental tooth movement. Eur J Orthod 1994;16:361–369.
143. Vandevska-Radunovic V, Kvinsland S, Kvinsland IH. Effect of experimental tooth movement on nerve fibers immunoreactive to calcitonin gene-related peptide, protein gene product 9.5, and blood vessel density and distribution in rats. Eur J Orthod 1997;19:517–529.
144. Derringer KA, Jaggers DC, Linden RW. Angiogenesis in human dental pulp following orthodontic tooth movement. J Dent Res 1996;75:1761–1766.
145. Derringer KA, Linden RW. Enhanced angiogenesis induced by diffusible angiogenic growth factors released from human dental pulp explants of orthodontically moved teeth. Eur J Orthod 1998;20:357–367.
146. Roberts-Clark DJ, Smith AJ. Angiogenic growth factors in human dentine matrix. Arch Oral Biol 2000;45: 1013–1016.
147. Bell W. Bone healing and revascularization after total maxillary osteotomy. J Oral Surg 1975;33:253–257.
148. Meyer M, Cavanaugh G. Blood flow changes after orthognathic surgery: Maxillary and mandibular subapical osteotomies. J Oral Surg 1976;34:495–499.
149. Indresano AT, Lundell MI. Blood flow changes in the rabbit maxilla following an anterior osteotomy. J Dent Res 1983;62:743–745.
150. Emshoff R, Kranewitter R, Gerhard S, Norer B, Hell B. Effect of segmental Le Fort I osteotomy on maxillary tooth type-related pulpal blood-flow characteristics. Oral Surg Oral Med Oral Pathol Oral Radiol Endod 2000;89:749–752.
151. Buckley JG, Jones ML, Hill M, Sugar AW. An evaluation of the changes in maxillary pulpal blood flow associated with orthognathic surgery. Br J Orthod 1999;26: 39–45.
152. Pepersack W. Tooth vitality after alveolar segmental osteotomy. J Maxillofac Surg 1973;1:85–90.
153. Theisen F, Gurnsey L. Postoperative sequelae after anterior segmental osteotomies. Oral Surg Oral Med Oral Pathol Oral Radiol Endod 1976;41:139–144.
154. Okada Y. The evaluation of the process of recovery of the dental pulp after Le Fort I osteotomy. J Stomatol Soc Jpn (in press).
155. Casey DM, Aguirre A. Dental blood supply in the segmentally resected mandible. J Endod 1999:25: 629–632.
156. Okiji T, Morita I, Suda H, Murota S. Pathophysiological roles of arachidonic acid metabolites in rat dental pulp. Proc Finn Den Soc 1992;88(suppl 1):433–438.

157. Ingolfsson AR, Tronstad L, Hersh EV, Riva CE. Efficacy of laser Doppler flowmetry in determining pulp vitality of human teeth. Endod Dental Traumatol 1994;10: 83–87.
158. Roebuck EM, Evans DJ, Stirrups D, Strang R. The effect of wavelength, bandwidth, and probe design and position on assessing the vitality of anterior teeth with laser Doppler flowmetry. Int J Paediatr Dent 2000;10: 213–220.
159. Ebihara A, Tokita Y, Izawa T, Suda H. Pulpal blood flow assessed by laser Doppler flowmetry in a tooth with a horizontal root fracture. Oral Surg Oral Med Oral Pathol 1996;81:229–233.
160. Wilder-Smith PEEB. A new method for the non-invasive measurement of pulpal blood flow. Int Endod J 1988;21:307–312.
161. Evans D, Reid J, Strang R, Stirrups D. A comparison of laser Doppler flowmetry with other methods of assessing the vitality of traumatized anterior teeth. Endod Dent Traumatol 1999;15:284–290.
162. Hartman A, Azerad J, Boucher Y. Environmental effects on laser Doppler pulpal blood-flow measurements in man. Arch Oral Biol 1996;41: 333–339.
163. Sasano T, Nakajima I, Shoji N, Kuriwada S, Sanjo D, Ogino H, Miyahara T. Possible application of transmitted laser light for the assessment of human pulpal vitality. Endod Dent Traumatol 1997;13:88–91.
164. Roeykens H, Van Maele G, De Moor R, Martens I. Reliability of laser Doppler flowmetry in a 2-probe assessment of pulpal blood flow. Oral Surg Oral Med Oral Pathol Oral Radiol Endod 1999;87:742–748.
165. Edwall B, Gazelius B, Berg JO, Edwall L, Hellander K, Olgart L. Blood flow changes in the dental pulp of the cat and rat measured simultaneously by laser Doppler flowmetry and local 125I clearance. Acta Physiol Scand 1987;131:81–91.
166. Schnettler JM, Wallace JA. Pulse oximetry as a diagnostic tool of pulpal vitality. J Endod 1991;17:488–490.
167. Goho C. Pulse oximetry evaluation of vitality in primary and immature permanent teeth. Pediatr Dent 1999; 21:125–127.
168. Kahan RS, Gulabivala K, Snook M, Setchell DJ. Evaluation of a pulse oximeter and customized probe for pulp vitality testing. J Endod 1996;22:105–109.
169. Schmitt JM, Webber RL, Walker EC. Optical determination of dental pulp vitality. IEEE Trans Biomed Eng 1991;38:346–352.
170. Ikawa M, Horiuchi H, Ikawa K. Optical characteristics of human extracted teeth and the possible application of photoplethysmography to the human pulp. Arch Oral Biol 1994;39:821–827.
171. Miwa Z, Ikawa M, Iijima H, Saito M, Takagi Y. Application of transmitted-light photoplethysmography to the vitality test for young permanent teeth. Jpn J Pediatr Dent 1999;37:991–999.

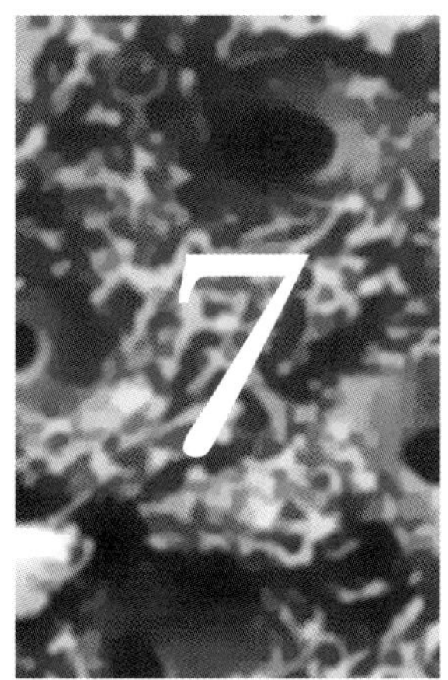

Nerve Supply of the Pulpodentin Complex and Responses to Injury

Margaret R. Byers, PhD; Matti V. O. Närhi, DDS, PhD

The pulpodentin complex is among the most densely innervated tissues in the body, yet we rarely perceive sensations from this structure unless a tooth is injured or inflamed. Many questions have arisen about this tissue. Why is there so much innervation? Where do those fibers end and how are they activated? Why do we just feel pain from teeth? What are those nerve fibers doing when our teeth are not hurting? Why do so many dentinal tubules contain nerve fibers? How do nerve fibers react to injury, and what do they contribute to healing? What (if anything) do odontoblasts or other pulpal cells contribute to tooth pain? Conversely, what do nerve fibers contribute to pulpal, dentinal, odontoblastic, inflammatory, and immune functions? Questions such as these have been asked about dental innervation for more than a century.[1-28] Our improved understanding over the past several decades has depended on development of additional techniques for visualizing pulpal innervation and for testing sensory functions. Highlights from the extensive literature in this field, first related to structural issues and then to physiology, are cited in this chapter. Other chapters in this text cover the related topics of central mechanisms of pain (chapter 8), pharmacologic management of pain (chapter 9), and differential diagnosis of odontogenic and nonodontogenic dental pain (chapter 20).

Preservation of enamel over many decades requires healthy dentin and pulp, and sensory nerve fibers have important interactions with other pulpal cells, such as odontoblasts, fibroblasts, blood vessels, and immunocompetent cells, that contribute to pulpal survival.[16-28] For example, the profuse innervation of pulp and dentin contains many neuropeptide-rich fibers that can release those peptides when stimulated. The timing, concentration, and location of secreted neuropeptides act as important signals for other pulpal cells about the status of the tooth (see also chapter 8). Neural agents are an important signal for neurogenic inflammation, for stimulation of repair, and for assisting with the everyday "housekeeping" functions in the dentin-pulp border area. Similarly, pulpal fibroblasts make neurotrophin growth factors such as nerve growth factor (NGF). They alter their expression of those factors after injury, and those changes are detected by odontoblasts, immune cells, and nerve fibers that express the high affinity receptor for NGF.[29,30]

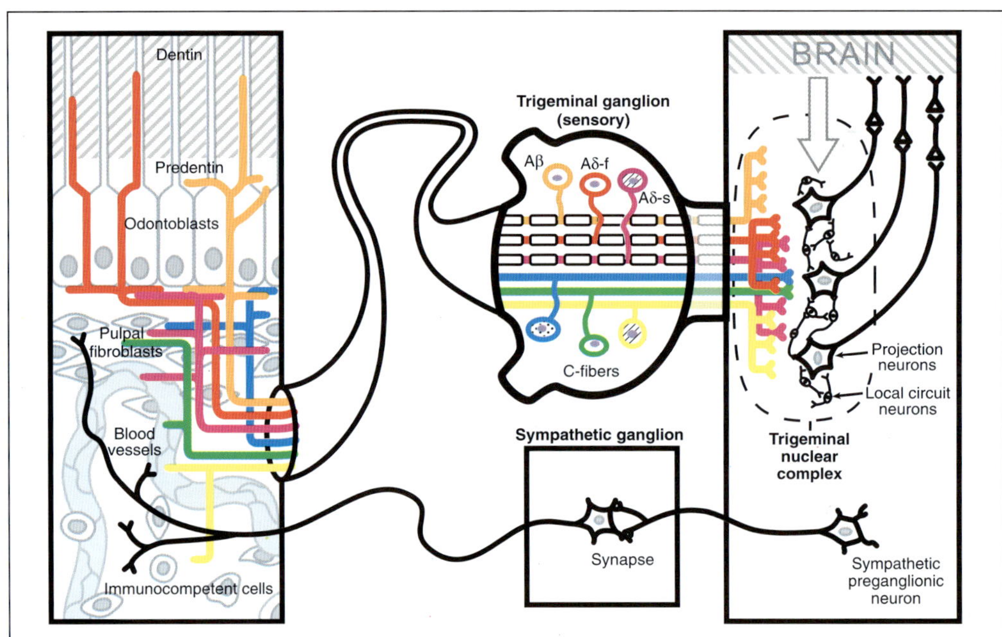

Fig 7-1 Review of the key regions in sensory neurons compared to sympathetic neurons. There are at least six different types of sensory neurons that innervate teeth: A-beta (Aβ, *orange*), A-delta-fast (Aδ-f, *red*), A-delta-slow polymodal (Aδ-s, *pink*), nociceptive C-fibers *(blue)*, glial-derived neurotrophic factor–regulated C-fibers *(green)*, and polymodal nociceptive C-fibers *(yellow)*. Each sensory neuron has a cell body in the trigeminal ganglion, numerous central synaptic endings, and a long peripheral axon that travels in a nerve to the target tissue, where the axon makes receptive endings. Approximate distribution sites for Aβ, Aδ-f, Aδ-s, and C-fibers are shown in relation to tooth morphology. In addition, a sympathetic neuron *(black)* is shown originating in a sympathetic ganglion and ending near dental blood vessels and central pulpal cells. At the central endings, there are synaptic connections with local circuit neurons and projection neurons, as well as descending modulation from the brain *(open arrow)*.

During different phases of injury and healing, the nerve fibers (and other cells) adjust their responses either to enhance their defense and tissue repair phenotypes or to begin returning to the normal resting condition, depending on the homeostatic needs of the pulp.

Cells in the dental pulp respond directly to endocrine, paracrine, and autocrine signals. Nerve fibers, however, have their control center (ie, cell body) located far away in the trigeminal ganglion for sensory neurons, and in the cervical sympathetic ganglia for sympathetic fibers (Fig 7-1). Thus, retrograde axonal transport is required to bring many of the tissue factors to the neuronal cell body, and then new neuropeptides, receptors, or ion channels are sent back out to the endings via anterograde transport.[31] These sequential axonal transport signals alter neuronal gene expression and phenotype, but the round trip to and from the cell body requires at least several hours and can take up to several days (Fig 7-2a). The electrophysiologic signals also contribute to tooth protection, of course, when they trigger pain and defensive reflexes via action potential signaling (Fig 7-2b).[32] The distinction between very rapid signals via action potentials that travel along nerve membranes and the much slower chemical signals carried by axonal transport is

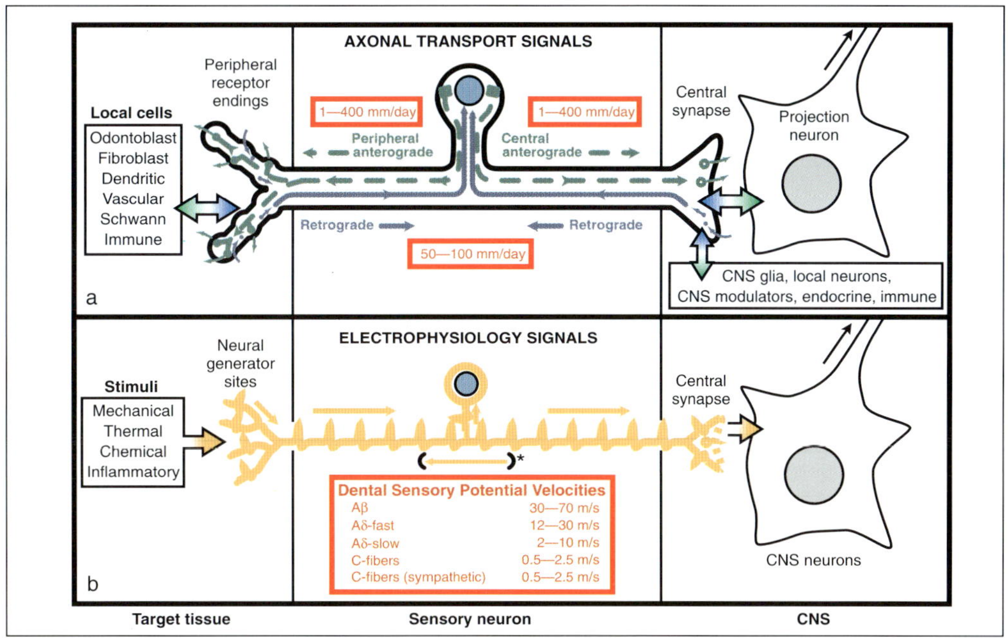

Figs 7-2a and 7-2b The two main information systems for neurons: axonal transport *(a)* and electrophysiologically conducted action potentials *(b)*. For axonal transport, specific molecules in vesicles or cytoplasm can go in the retrograde direction, from the endings (receptive or central synaptic endings) to the cell body, or in the anterograde direction, from the cell body out to the endings. The rates of axonal transport vary from 1 to 400 mm/day for the anterograde, and from 50 to 100 mm/day for the retrograde system, both of which are much slower than the conducted action potentials. Local cells, such as odontoblasts, fibroblasts, dendritic cells, blood vessels, smooth muscle cells, and immune cells, modulate the activity of sensory receptive endings of somatosensory neurons. At the central endings there are modulatory interactions with glia, local neurons, axons from higher centers, endocrine, and immune signals. The receptive generator sites in the nerve endings detect tissue stimuli such as mechanical, thermal, chemical, and inflammatory signals. Their conducted action potentials usually travel from periphery to central endings, where they trigger synaptic communication with central neurons. The signals in some cases *(*)*, such as axon reflex, travel in the opposite direction out to the peripheral endings, where they stimulate the secretion of neuropeptides and other neural agents.

important to the understanding of the functions of sensory nerves in teeth, their interactions with pulp, and their injury responses. Additional interactions of nerve fibers with pulp involve endocrine, paracrine, and autocrine responses in the nerve endings, as well as efferent action potentials that backfire the sensory nerve endings and cause release of neuropeptides. The variety of nerve-pulp interactive systems and the high density of sensory innervation in teeth indicate a powerful role for dental innervation in pulpal biology and dental injury reactions.

Normal Anatomy of Dental Innervation

Types of innervation and terminal locations

The nerve fibers in pulp and dentin are components of a larger peripheral nervous system that also includes sensory innervation of the gingiva, junctional epithelium, periodontal ligament, tongue, lips, mastication muscles, and temporo-

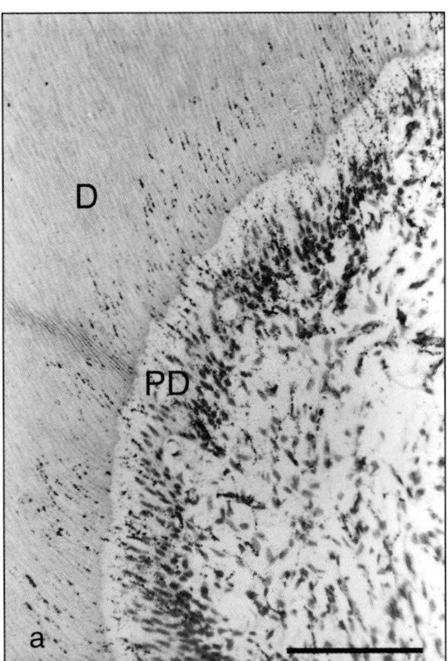

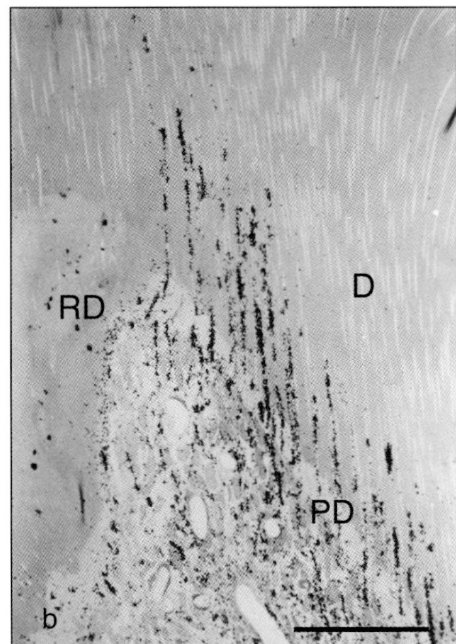

Fig 7-3 Light microscopic autoradiography of nerve endings in dentin. *(a)* About half of tubules in the inner dentin (D) of this monkey canine tooth have autoradiographic label indicating the location of trigeminal nerve endings. PD, predentin. Bar = 0.1 mm. (Modified from Byers et al[42] with permission.) *(b)* Autoradiographically labeled trigeminal nerve endings in an adult rat molar are concentrated in the tubular dentin (D), while avoiding the reparative dentin (RD). The predentin (PD) is wider at the innervated regions than it is for other crown dentin. Bar = 0.065 mm. (Modified from Byers et al[43] with permission.)

mandibular joint. Each part of the system contributes different kinds of somatosensory information that is needed for tooth use and preservation. For example, from the gingiva we perceive sensations of touch, pressure, and temperature via activation of special mechanoreceptors or thermoreceptors. The junctional epithelium is richly innervated by sensory fibers that release neuropeptides to regulate vasodilation and transmigration of leukocytes across the epithelium into the oral cavity for defense against oral pathogens. The periodontal ligament contains many Ruffini mechanoreceptors from the trigeminal ganglion or mesencephalic nucleus. These mechanoreceptors give us our sensations of tooth touch and occlusal plane during chewing, speech, and swallowing.[33-41] Some part of the sensory information from the periodontal mechanoreceptors may remain unconscious and subserve automatic responses needed for the regulation of the masticatory functions. All the orofacial tissues also have specific and polymodal nociceptive nerve fibers (eg, silent nociceptors and autonomic nerve fibers) that initiate acute pain sensation if there is damage or inflammation. Together, the multiple nerve fiber systems of these regions provide an integrated regulatory system acting on teeth and their supporting tissues.

The sensory innervation of teeth terminates primarily in the coronal odontoblast layer, predentin, and inner dentin (Figs 7-3 and 7-4), and morphologically it is made up of at least six different kinds of nerve fiber, each of which has a preferred location (see Fig 7-1).[3,11,20,41-48] A small proportion is medium-sized (A-beta) myelinated fibers. They innervate mainly dentin and the dentin-pulp border near the pulp horn tip and lack the receptors for the low-affinity NGF receptor.[41] They are the most sensitive fibers to mechanical (hydrodynamic) stimulation of dentin.[13,14] The A-beta fibers form some of the large endings that make close appositions with odontoblasts (Fig

7-5), and they probably comprise the endings that have been shown by Gunji to form a series of large endings near neighboring odontoblast processes.[45]

About 25% to 50% of dental nerve fibers are small myelinated (A-delta) fibers that contain the neuropeptide calcitonin gene-related peptide (CGRP) and express receptors for NGF. Most of these innervate dentin, predentin, and the odontoblast layer in the coronal regions underlying enamel (see Figs 7-4 and 7-5).[16-20,53-58] The dentinal endings occur close to the odontoblast processes and may form some type of association with them, or they may simply be located nearby. No synaptic or gap junctions have been found for nerve-odontoblast associations, but a paracrine signaling mechanism would be facilitated by close association. Most of the A-delta innervation is concentrated in dentin near the pulp horn tip; it is progressively less frequent toward the cervical region and least prevalent in the root dentin. Thus, there are focal regions of dense innervation of dentin and specific gradients of innervation. There are also a few slow-conducting thin A-delta fibers that have capsaicin sensitivity and that may end primarily in pulp.[56]

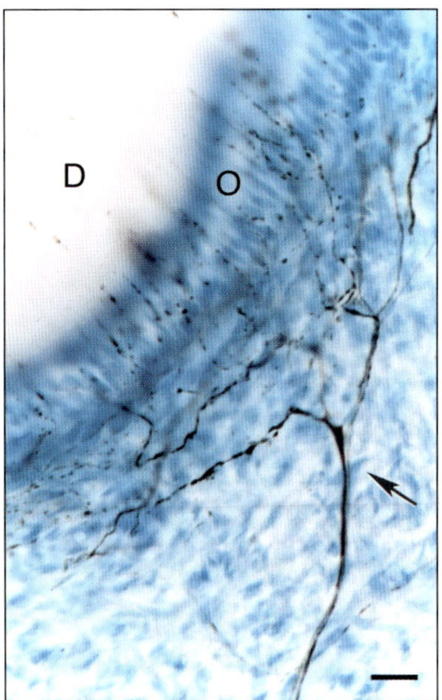

Fig 7-4 Section showing a portion of the terminal arborization of a single calcitonin gene-related peptide (CGRP) -immunoreactive nerve fiber. Its branches *(arrow)* spread out parallel to the dentin-pulp border in the subodontoblast plexus region and send many terminal branches into the odontoblast layer (O) and dentin (D). These endings originated from a myelinated axon that had a diameter of 4 mm in the root nerve (counterstained with methylene blue). Bar = 10 mm. (Modified from Byers[44] with permission.)

The majority of nerve fibers in teeth are unmyelinated, slowly conducting C-fibers. Most are regulated by NGF in the adult, and about half require NGF during development, while others utilize brain-derived neurotrophic factor (BDNF) or glial-derived neurotrophic factor (GDNF).[29,30,57-61] In spite of varying morphology and terminal distribution, most of the C-fibers of the pulp seem functionally to be quite uniform. They are polymodal and responsive to capsaicin and to inflammatory mediators such as histamine and bradykinin. C-fibers express NGF-receptors and neuropeptides such as substance P, CGRP, or neurokinin A.[16,41,57-61] They terminate in peripheral pulp or along blood vessels, and they are mostly activated by pulpal damage (see below). The C-fiber sensory population in other tissues such as skin can be subdivided into at least three groups: specific, polymodal, and silent. While some dental C-fibers respond to intense heat or cold, it is not clear that they differ from the polymodal receptors, as described below. The axon caliber of nerves entering teeth range from C to A-beta sizes that then branch and become progressively narrower in cervical and crown levels until virtually all preterminal and terminal fibers are unmyelinated in the cell-rich, cell-free, odontoblast and dentinal regions (Fig 7-6).

Finer details about anatomic and chemical subspecializations within the categories of A-beta, A-delta, and C sensory fibers are still being discovered; therefore, a full picture of dentinal sensory subtypes cannot yet be given. It has been recognized for some time that these nerve fibers are dynamic and continually adjusting their association with pulpal cells and dentin.[9,11,17-20,62] That ability has been further explained by recent studies showing growth-associated protein-43 in dental nerve fibers and endings.[63]

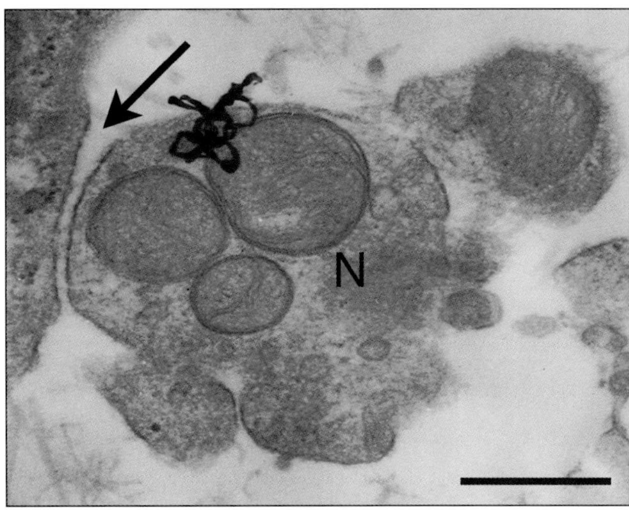

Fig 7-5a An autoradiographically labeled trigeminal fiber (N) is separated by a small, uniform space *(arrow)* from an odontoblast, as well as from other nerve-like fibers, in a rat molar. Bar = 0.5 μm. (Modified from Byers[49] with permission.)

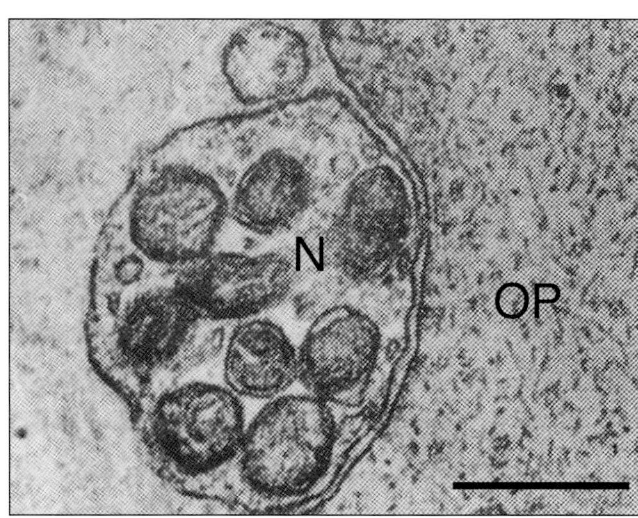

Fig 7-5b This nerve-like fiber (N) in a human tooth maintains a separation from the adjacent odontoblast process (OP). Bar = 0.5 μm. (Modified from Frank[50] with permission.)

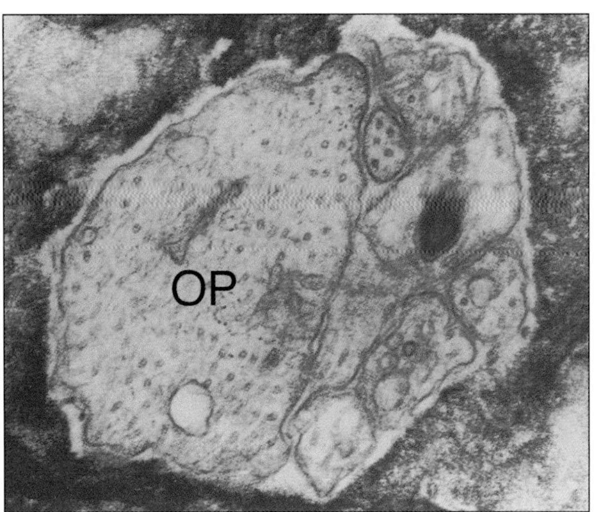

Fig 7-5c The large odontoblast process (OP) is close to many small fibers in a dentinal tubule of a cat canine (original magnification ×32,000). (Modified from Holland[51] with permission.)

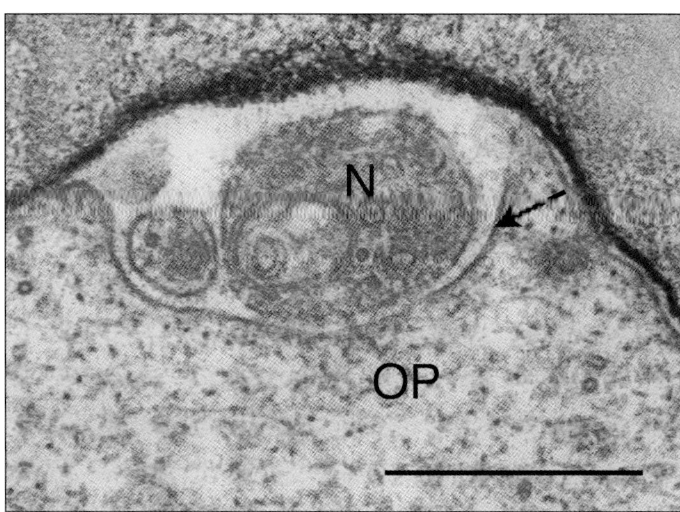

Fig 7-5d This dentinal tubule from a human tooth contains two nerve-like processes (N) that maintain their separation *(arrow)* from the odontoblast process (OP) in that region of the terminal fiber. Bar = 0.5 μm. (Modified from Byers et al[52] with permission.)

A great many other cytochemical features of dental nerve fiber subgroups have been identified, such as calcium-binding proteins or receptors for nociceptor modulating agents such as opioid peptides, somatostatin, cannabinoids, excitatory amino acids, and adenosine triphosphate (ATP) (Box 7-1; see also chapter 8).[64-66] Recent studies indicate that some of the dental innervation is regulated by NGF and GDNF during development and possibly in mature teeth.[60] An interesting aspect of tooth innervation is that some intradental fibers are branches from larger, faster-conducting "parent"

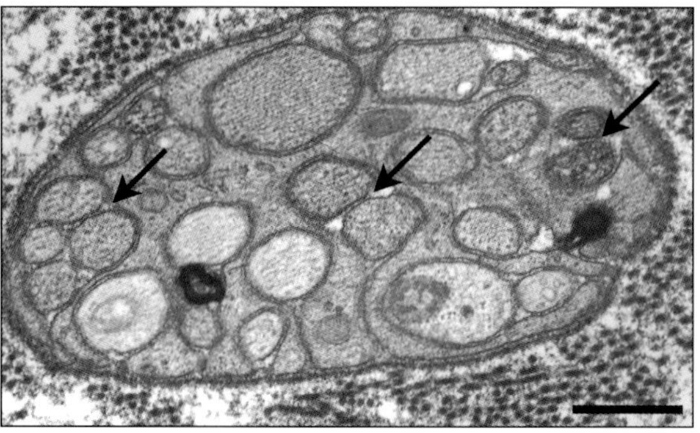

Fig 7-6a Preterminal axons in the plexus of Raschkow from a human tooth. All have lost myelin and some are close to each other *(arrows)* without a Schwann cell sheath. Bar = 1.0 μm. (Modified from Byers et al[46] with permission.)

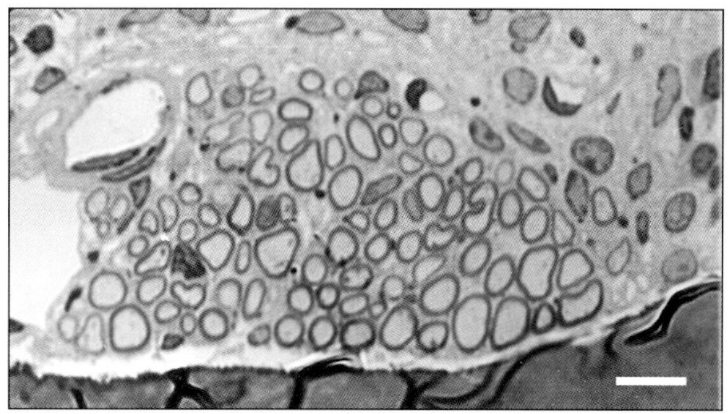

Fig 7-6b Various sizes of myelinated axon, including A-beta and A-delta sizes, in a mouse molar root. Bar = 10 mm.

Box 7-1 Some agents involved in neuropulpal interactions*

Neural agents that affect pulpal cells and blood vessels

- Sensory neuropeptides: CGRP, substance P, neurokinin A, somatostatin, galanin
- Sensory neurotransmitters: glutamate, acetylcholine
- Autonomic factors: norepinephrine, peptide histidine isoleucine, acetylcholine, neuropeptide Y
- Schwann cell factors: NGF, GDNF, neurotrophin receptors

Dentinal, pulpal, vascular, or immune agents that affect dental nerve function

- Odontoblast-specific molecules†
- Neurotrophic factors: NGF, BDNF, GDNF
- Inflammatory mediators: serotonin, histamine, bradykinin, prostanoids, cytokines
- Cellular breakdown products: ATP, cyclooxygenase, oxidative radicals
- Altered pH and its excitation or inhibition of molecular functions
- Heat shock proteins
- Somatostatin and endocrine factors
- Antinociceptive agents (eg, opioid peptides, cannabinoids, adenosine)
- Extracellular matrix factors (eg, laminin and metalloproteinases)
- Ionic environment
- Oxygen tension and interstitial fluid pressures

"Neural" factors expressed by pulp

- Neurotensin, nestin, protein gene product (PGP) 9.5
- Tachykinin-precursor and receptor
- Neurotrophin receptors: tyrosine kinase A (TrkA), p75
- Neurotrophins: NGF, BDNF, GDNF
- Nitric oxide

*This list is partial. There is still much to learn about cell signaling in teeth.
†At least 130 odontoblast-specific genes, some of which would affect neural function, have been identified.[67]

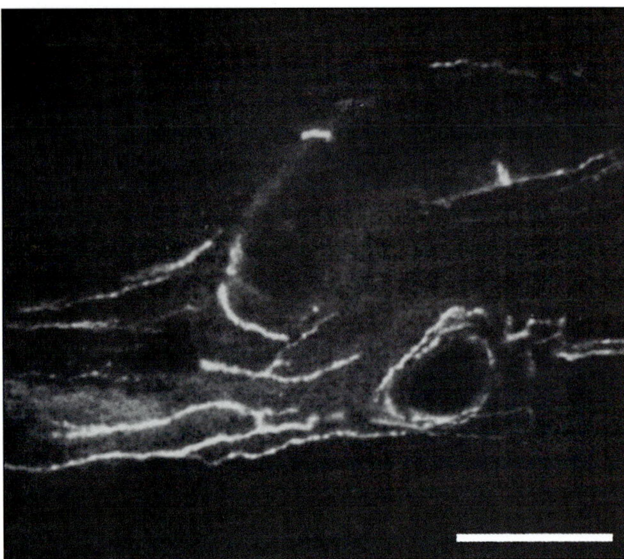

Fig 7-7a Cholinergic fibers associated with blood vessels in the pulp of a monkey tooth are shown by fluorescence immunocytochemistry. Bar = 0.1 mm. (Reprinted from Pohto and Antila[71] with permission.)

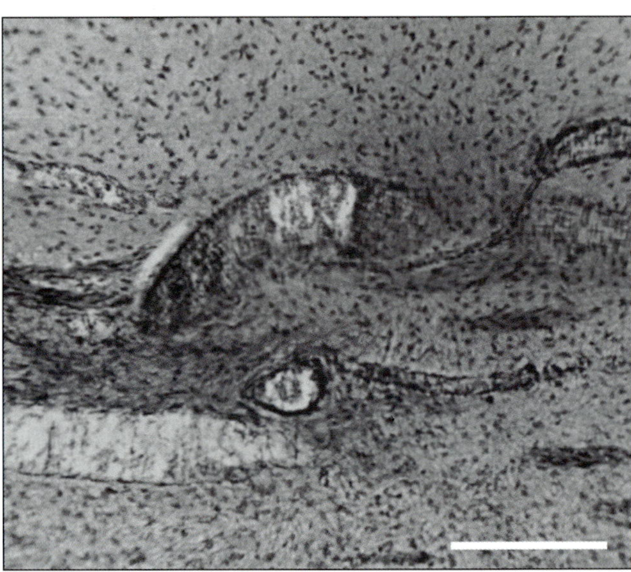

Fig 7-7b Bright field microscopy of the section in Fig 7-7a shows the vascular structure of that region. Bar = 0.1 mm. (Reprinted from Pohto and Antila[71] with permission.)

axons located outside.[68] Although the conduction velocities and size spectra increase in main trigeminal nerves compared to pulpal nerves, there are also A-beta fibers in pulpal nerves (see Fig 7-6).[13,20]

The key feature of all of the nerve fibers described above is that they have specific membrane receptors for chemical signaling with their neighboring cells. Ultrastructural and immunocytochemical data show a close association of nerve fibers with odontoblasts (see Fig 7-5), fibroblasts, blood vessels, and immunocompetent cells.[6,8,9,11,17,21,24-28,41,45-47,51,69] In research that uses specific labeling of sensory nerve fibers (eg, axonally transported protein), such associated cells are simply close neighbors without the specific junctions or the specialized structural features found in synapses. It may be important that there are similar associations between unmyelinated axons and Schwann cells in preterminal pulpal nerve bundles (see Fig 7-6), where paracrine signaling would be enhanced. Specific synaptic or gap junctional connections between pulpal cells and clearly identified nerve fibers do not occur.[9,20] However, the dental sensory fibers can interact with pulpal cells via paracrine signaling. Those interactions can be complex; for example, NGF is made by pulpal fibroblasts for signaling to odontoblasts, dendritic cells, and nerve fibers, as well as to the fibroblasts.[29,30,60,61,70] Some of the neural responses to NGF involve axonal retrograde transport back to the trigeminal ganglion for induction of altered gene expression.

Sympathetic and parasympathetic innervation of teeth

The vasodilatory functions of sensory innervation in teeth are opposed by vasoconstriction by the sympathetic fibers (see Figs 7-1 and 6-11), as described below.[8,18,21,25,28] The sympathetic fibers are much less numerous than are sensory fibers, although there are species differences in those relative proportions (Fig 7-7).[71-73] Sympathetic fiber distribution also differs from that of sensory fibers in that they are located mainly in deeper pulp and along blood vessels.[71] Parasympathetic activity can affect blood flow in teeth, but it is not clear whether that is from intradental or periodontal sites; in any case, the relative importance of parasympathetic activity is much less than that

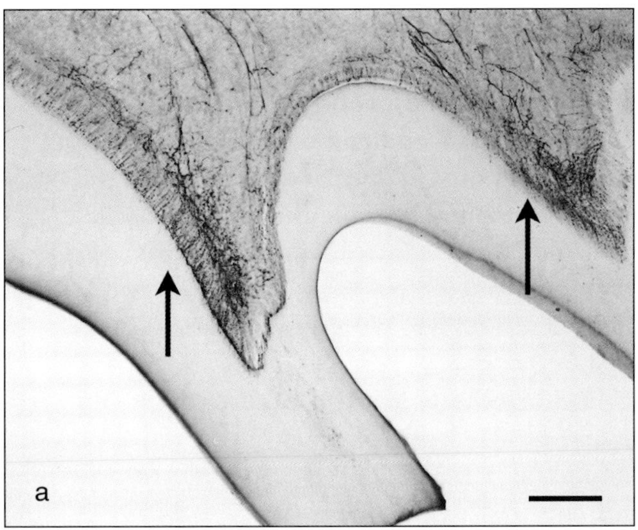

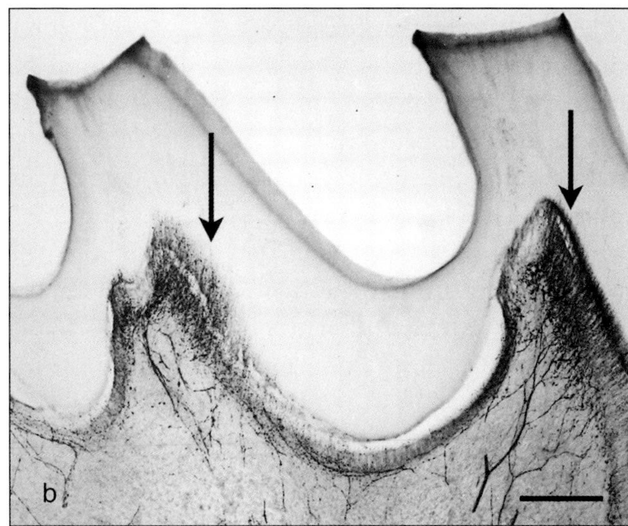

Figs 7-8a and 7-8b Asymmetric innervation *(arrows)* of developing rat molar dentin occurs on opposite sides of the maxillary *(a)* and mandibular cusps *(b)*, as shown by immunocytochemistry for CGRP. The maxillary cusps of rat molars are tilted posteriorly and the mandibular cusps tilt anteriorly when newly erupted. Thus, the first nerve fibers that enter dentin during development target the side of each cusp that is oriented closest to the occlusal plane. Bar = 0.2 mm. (Modified from Byers et al[76] with permission.)

of the sympathetic activity.[18,74,75] These neuronal classes are discussed in detail in chapter 6.

Developing and primary teeth

During tooth development, the innervation enters the pulp during the crown stage and makes branches near the pulp horn odontoblasts (see also chapter 2). There is a rapid increase in nerve fiber entry into dentin when eruption starts, and then innervation density continues to increase during maturation of the tooth.[11,52,57,61,76,77] During maturation and aging, the pulp becomes progressively narrower and usually acquires regions with tertiary dentin or dead tracks. Those areas, as well as reparative regions, generally lose most of their dentinal innervation.[9,11,20,52,78] The sensory innervation adjusts its location to maintain its greatest association with the surviving primary odontoblasts close to the pulp horn tip (Fig 7-8). Its associations with blood vessels are also maintained during the progressive maturation of pulp. With increasing loss of primary dentin, tooth innervation decreases and its cytochemistry changes to have reduced expression of neuropep-

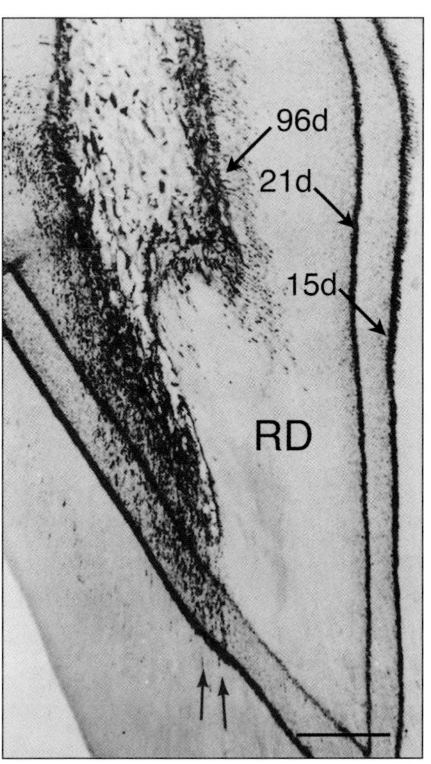

Fig 7-8c This sample has radioactive growth lines that were made in dentin by systemic injections of tritiated proline at postnatal days 15 and 21. Those lines indicate that the initial innervation of this tooth maintained its position, with the nerve endings *(double arrow)* still in the early dentin at 96 days later, when they were mapped by radioactive axonal transport. RD, reparative dentin. Bar = 0.2 mm. (Modified from Byers et al[76] with permission.)

tides and neurotrophin receptors.[79,80] The location of innervation is approximately the same for primary and permanent teeth, and the number of fibers increases for larger teeth.[80,81] In most mature teeth, regardless of size and dental type, there is some innervation at the most occlusal 0.5 to 1.0 mm of a pulp horn that extends into the neighboring tubular dentin for up to 0.1 to 0.2 mm.[9,11,17,20] An exception to this is found in continuously erupting teeth, such as rodent incisors, where innervation of dentin is sparse or absent.[20] The development of crown innervation complexity can proceed even when tooth buds are transplanted to the anterior chamber of the eye or to other tissues, or when osteopetrotic overgrowth of bone prevents tooth eruption.[82-84]

Interactions Between Sensory Fibers and Pulp

All peripheral nerve fibers have a definable set of interactions with local cells that are specific for different functional subtypes. For example, mechanoreceptors that end in cutaneous epithelia are associated with Merkel cells, a special kind of neuroendocrine cell that secretes an array of neuroactive substances that are essential to the location and function of the nerve endings. Pacinian corpuscles are completely encapsulated mechanoreceptors with their terminal support cells also inside, while Ruffini mechanoreceptors are partly covered but also have direct contacts with the ligament fibers. By contrast, nociceptive endings throughout the body are more exposed to tissue factors because they have only a basal lamina covering in addition to partial Schwann cell support.[85,86] Each of these types of somatosensory nerve fibers contains the sensory transducer in its peripheral endings and does not associate with special receptor cells.

Although some have proposed that odontoblasts are special receptor cells, there are no synaptic or gap junctions connecting them with the nerve terminals (see Fig 7-6).[6,8,11,20,46] All other somatosensory receptors and nociceptors have the sensory transduction function (ie, the ability to convert tissue events into neural signals) in their peripheral ending, so it is unlikely that pulpal nerve fibers use a special system. The nerve endings that extend into the dentin-pulp border zone and into dentin are especially exposed to tissue factors because they have little or no covering by Schwann cells or basal lamina after leaving the cell-free zone.

Odontoblasts are the predominant non-neuronal cells in peripheral pulp, predentin, and dentin; as a result, any special support functions for the free nerve fibers would have to be supplied by them. Several interesting studies on odontoblasts have detected calcium currents that are thought to regulate primarily dentin matrix production and calcification.[87,88] However, it is possible that nearby sensory fibers can detect and respond to current fluctuations in odontoblasts, in addition to their ability to respond to hydrodynamic movement of dentinal tubule contents.[7]

The new knowledge about paracrine interactions of cells in pulp, including the dentinal nerve fiber, supports the hypothesis that dental nerve fibers and odontoblasts may have a profound influence on each other's activity levels. Demonstrations of neuropeptide and neurotrophin receptors on odontoblasts are consistent with this proposal.[30,89] Indeed, the main contribution of odontoblasts to sensory functions in teeth may be their production of a permissive interactive environment. This idea is supported by the following observations: *(1)* the nerve fibers prefer dentinal tubules with coronal primary odontoblasts, *(2)* they avoid tertiary dentin or odontoblast-free tubules, and *(3)* they prefer the special odontoblasts that make the dentin that lies directly under enamel.[20,43,51,78,90]

Pulpal cells and pain mechanisms

The current hypothesis is that pulpal cells do not act as special sensory receptors analogous to the photoreceptors in the eye or to hair cells of the inner ear. Instead, the pulpal cells provide the environment in which the nerve fibers function. The odontoblasts may well assume some Schwann-like functions since Schwann cells are rare in peripheral pulp and dentin. In addition, some neuroendocrine activity is suggested by the demonstration of neurotensin-like immunoreactivity in odontoblasts.[91] Recent work has identified at least 130 odontoblast-specific genes, demonstrating that there is great capacity for important paracrine signaling that might affect nerve fibers as well as other neighboring cells.[67]

It has been suggested that odontoblastic ion currents, which are related to dentinal matrix production and calcification, might also alter the ionic environment for the nearby nerves.[51,87,88] The resident pulpal cells, along with the invading immune cells, provide signals that regulate sensory phenotype (see Box 7-1) and thus have important effects on the functional activity of peripheral neurons, including nociceptive transmission. Conditions such as hypersensitive dentin may have a central component caused by altered signal processing in the central nervous system (see chapter 8), but they also include a peripheral component caused by altered pulpal conditions that affect nerve activity. For example, many enzymes and membrane receptors acquire different functional levels in inflamed or acidic conditions. Thus, there may be important but indirect roles for pulpal cells in dental pain, related to their effects on the local environment and the functional phenotype of the sensory fibers. A partial list of pulpal agents that affect dental nerve fibers and neural agents that affect pulp can be found in Box 7-1.

Neuroanatomic Responses to Tooth Injury and Infection

Injury to the pulpodentin complex produces numerous neuronal responses. The nerve fibers not only send rapid electrophysiologic signals to the ganglion and central pain pathways, but they also release neuropeptides from their peripheral terminals that regulate vasodilation and leukocyte invasion of the injury site.[12,18,24,26-28] Thus, if the sensory innervation has been removed prior to injury, the pulp is less able to defend itself, promote neurogenic inflammation, or heal after pulpal exposure.[20,54,77,92]

Nerve sprouting and cytochemical changes

The dental sensory fibers also react to tooth injury by extensive anatomic and cytochemical changes in their preterminal branches and endings. In rat models of dental injury, there is an initial depletion of neuropeptides that are released into the pulp tissue, followed by increased neuropeptide content and sprouting of the terminal fibers within 1 day after injury. Those responses differ in intensity and duration depending on the severity of the injury.[19,20,26,28,29,54,77,79,90,92-96] Innocuous stimuli such as cold, heat, and vibration may cause nerve fibers to be activated at levels sufficient to cause changes in neurally regulated pulpal blood flow and interstitial fluid pressure (see also chapter 6). Gentle or superficial stimuli do not usually injure dentin or pulp, but they can cause sufficient dentinal fluid movement to induce some pain.[1,7,13,14,97-100] Low-intensity electrical stimulation is able to induce similar pulpal responses and also evoke nonpainful (prepain) sensations.[97-100]

Stimuli that injure the pulpodentin complex have been classified at four different levels (Table 7-1).[19,20] Type I injuries are least damaging. They cause a transient change in pulp, and the dentinal damage can be easily fixed by reactive dentinogenesis (the original odontoblasts survive and are not replaced by reparative cells). There is extensive sprouting of neuropeptide-rich nerve fiber endings near the injury that return to normal within a few days to a few weeks. Those changes have been correlated with local production of NGF by the fibroblasts near the injury site.[29] Under these conditions, there is little or no invasion of leukocytes, and the local defense mechanisms are sufficient. Examples of this type of

Table 7-1 Characteristics of different types of tooth injury

Type of injury	Tissue reactions	Outcome
Type I Superficial injury to dentin	Transient inflammation Local infection control Little or no pulp loss Nerve sprouting for a few days Reactive dentinogenesis	Heals within days to weeks
Type II Deep dentin cavity	Prolonged acute inflammation Leukocyte influx Focal pulp loss Abscess sealed off by dense scar Nerve sprouting at acute inflammation Reparative dentinal formation	Heals within a few months
Type III Large pulpal exposures or damage	Irreversible pulpitis Advancing pulpal necrosis Retreating vital pulp Persistent acute inflammation in vital pulp Persistent nerve sprouting in vital pulp Failure to repair dentin or heal the pulp	Persists until treated
Type IV Pulpal and periodontal involvement	Tooth loss	Persists until treated

injury are shallow cavity preparation, shallow scaling of cervical dentin, minor occlusal trauma, strong orthodontic force, transient heat, or moderate hydrodynamic dentinal injury.[20,95]

Type II injuries have more extensive dentinal injury with some loss of pulpal tissue and focal inflammation. There is invasion of leukocytes and local vascular responses, but the pulp can repair itself and form reparative dentin. For these lesions, there is extensive sprouting of sensory fibers that have enhanced neuropeptide contents such as CGRP and substance P. Examples of this type of injury include deep dentinal cavities, small pulpal exposures, and heat stimulation of long duration and/or high intensity. For these intermediate injuries, the sprouting and CGRP up-regulation continue as long as there is active inflammation that has not been walled off by scar formation (Figs 7-9a and 7-9b). Once an effective scar and dentin repair are underway, the sensory sprouting decreases and neuropeptide levels return to normal range or are subnormal (Fig 7-9c).[19,20,92-96] During aging of teeth, the pulp narrows, the innervation is reduced, the nerve fibers contain fewer neuropeptides, and much of the tubular primary dentin that nerve fibers prefer to innervate is replaced by reparative dentin. While those changes may alter the ability of teeth to defend against injuries and to heal effectively, a study of dentinal cavity injury in old rats found essentially the same ability for sprouting responses as in the younger teeth.[101] If infection is pre-

Figs 7-9a to 7-9c Different patterns of nerve fibers in rat molars detected by immunocytochemistry for CGRP.

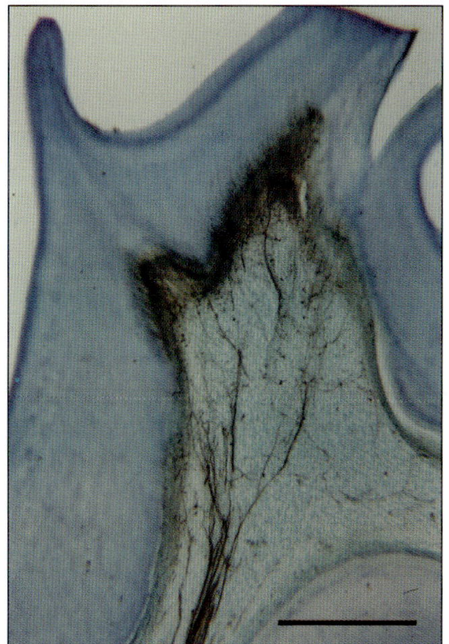

Fig 7-9a Pattern in normal molars. Bar = 0.2 mm. (Modified from Kimberly and Byers[54] with permission.)

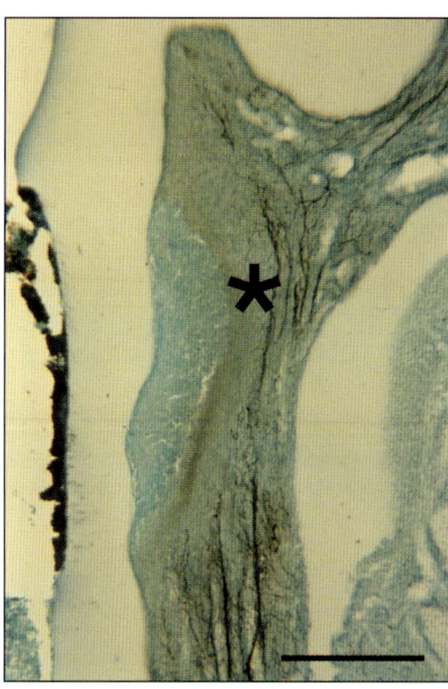

Fig 7-9b Pattern 4 days after inducing a large abscess (*) near a cervical dentinal cavity. Bar = 0.2 mm. (Modified from Taylor and Byers[96] with permission.)

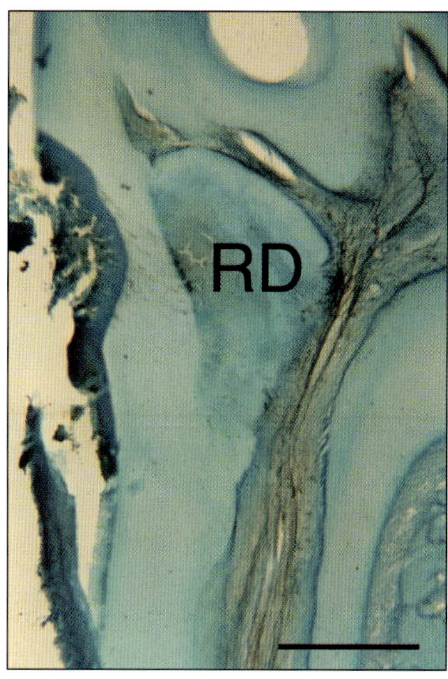

Fig 7-9c Pattern after 3 weeks of healing and reparative dentin (RD) formation at an injury site that was similar to Fig 7-9b. Bar = 0.2 mm. (Modified from Taylor and Byers[96] with permission.)

vented, then much larger injuries can have a successful repair outcome.[102]

When injuries reach the Type III level, there is enough pulpal damage or infection that local repair is not possible, and irreversible pulpitis ensues.[54] If a tooth has been denervated prior to injury, the extent of damage is greater and the progression to necrosis proceeds more quickly (Fig 7-10).[92] Some of the conditions that lead to irreversible pulpitis are large infected pulpal exposures, bacterial invasion at failed restorations, deep infected caries, failure of pulp to make a scar barrier around an abscess, and coronal pulp destruction by heat or other excessive stimulation. In some cases a Type II injury (eg, one occurring at a crack in enamel and dentin) can persist a long time (Fig 7-11), or can shift to Type III level if pulpal defense mechanisms are overwhelmed. An increased intensity of sensory nerve sprouting in the surviving pulp near the lesion correlates with elevated pulpal cell expression of NGF after dentinal injury (Fig 7-12); in contrast, both the NGF expression and sensory sprouting are low at sites of healing (see Fig 7-9c).[20,54,93,94,96]

Type IV injuries involve other tissues in addition to dentin and pulp. These complex situations occur when pulpal infections expand out of the tooth into the periradicular tissues to affect ligament and bone (Fig 7-13) (see also chapter 17). Periodontal tissues are also involved at the time of initial injury in a variety of dental fractures. In addition, tooth extractions damage the ligament extensively, and pulpotomy can cause long-term nerve reactions in the periradicular tissue.[103]

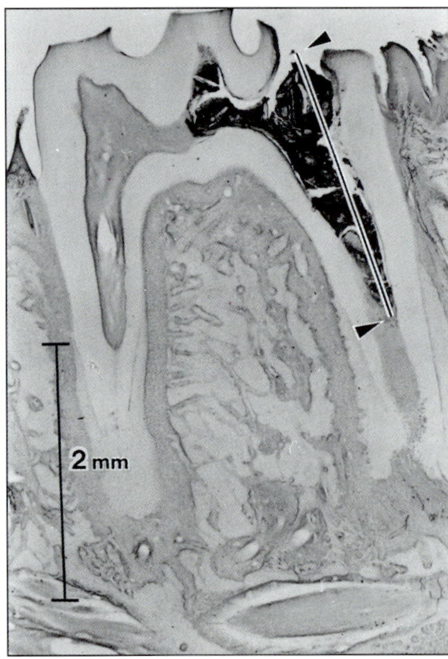

Fig 7-10a If rat molars are denervated several days before a small pulpal exposure, the pulpal damage and necrosis are severe *(arrowheads and bar)* at 6 days after the injury. (Reprinted from Byers and Taylor[92] with permission.)

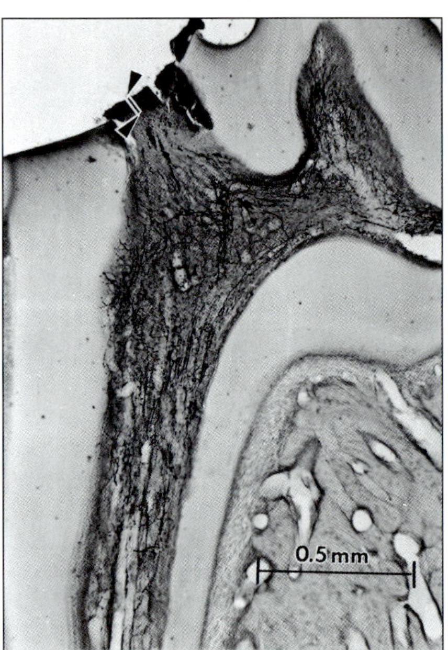

Fig 7-10b The innervated contralateral teeth with many sprouting nerve fibers had only small loss of pulp *(arrowheads and bar)*. The sprouting nerve fibers showed immunoreactivity for CGRP. (Reprinted from Byers and Taylor[92] with permission.)

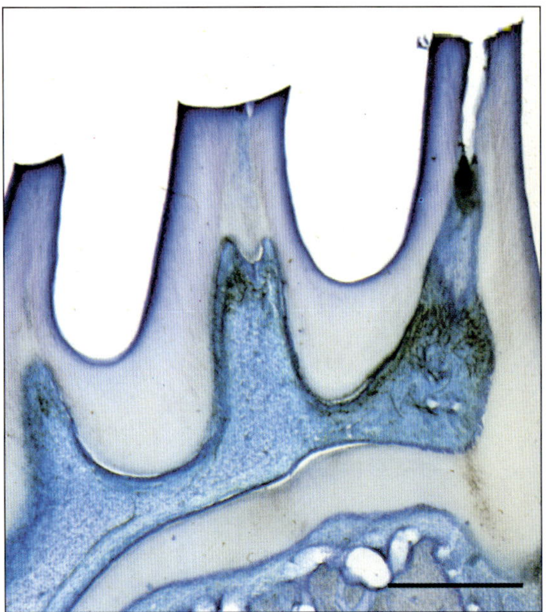

Fig 7-11a Persistent sprouting of nerve fibers that are immunoreactive for CGRP occurred in vital pulp near a long-term crack in dentin of a rat molar *(counterstained with methylene blue)*. Bar = 0.5 mm. (Courtesy of Dr Inger H. Kvinnsland, University of Bergen, Norway).

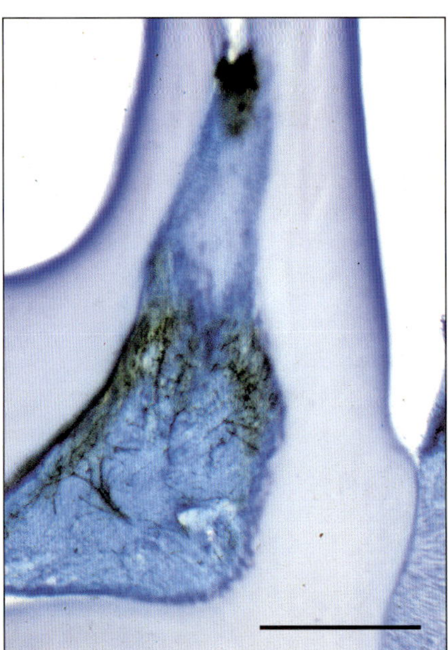

Fig 7-11b Higher magnification of Fig 7-11a *(counterstained with methylene blue)*. Bar = 0.25 mm. (Courtesy of Dr Inger H. Kvinnsland, University of Bergen, Norway.)

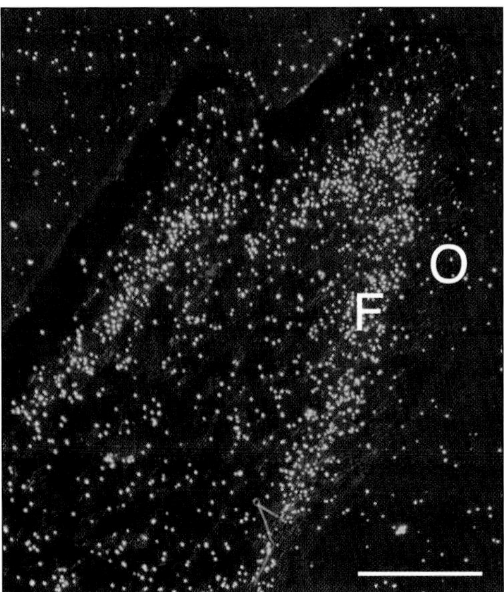

Fig 7-12a Expression of nerve growth factor occurs in fibroblast-like pulpal cells (F) below the odontoblast layer (O) of normal adult rat molars, as demonstrated by in situ hybridization. Dark-field microscopy was used to detect autoradiographic signal (counterstained with methylene blue). Bar = 100 μm. See Byers et al[29] for further details.

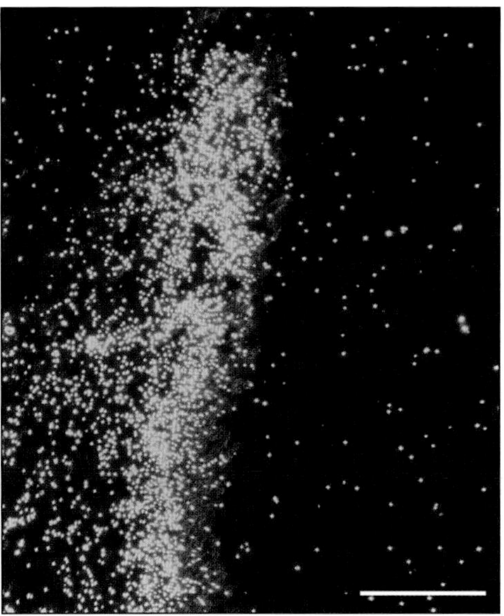

Fig 7-12b Six hours after cavity preparation in crown dentin of a rat molar, the mRNA expression had increased to five to eight times the normal amount. Bar = 100 μm. See Byers et al[29] for further details.

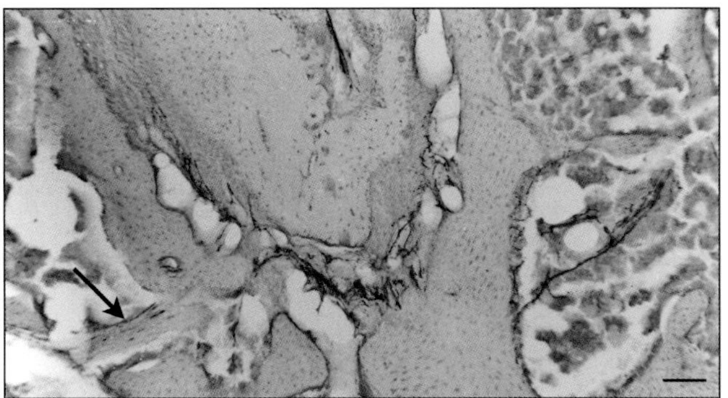

Fig 7-13a This normal periapical region of a rat molar was immunoreacted for CGRP and shows sparse innervation of the periodontal ligament. The arrow indicates the adjoining periapical nerve. Bar = 0.1 mm. (Reprinted from Kimberly and Byers[54] with permission.)

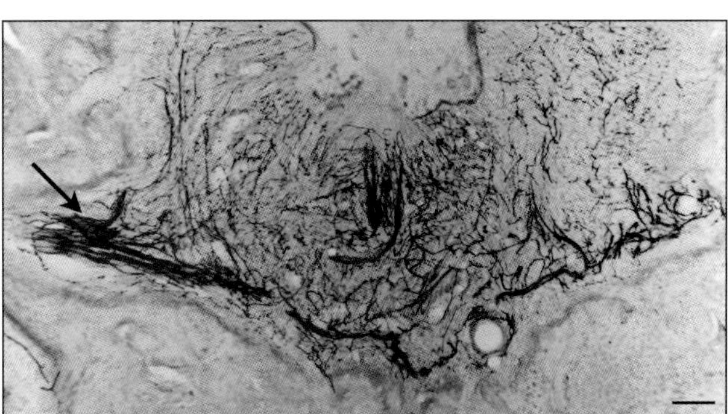

Fig 7-13b Periapical changes and sprouting nerve fibers appeared 3 to 5 weeks following establishment of irreversible pulpitis subsequent to pulpal exposure lesions. The nerve fiber immunoreactivity for CGRP was also enhanced in the adjoining periapical nerve *(arrow)* compared to Fig 7-13a. Bar = 0.1 mm. (Reprinted from Kimberly and Byers[54] with permission.)

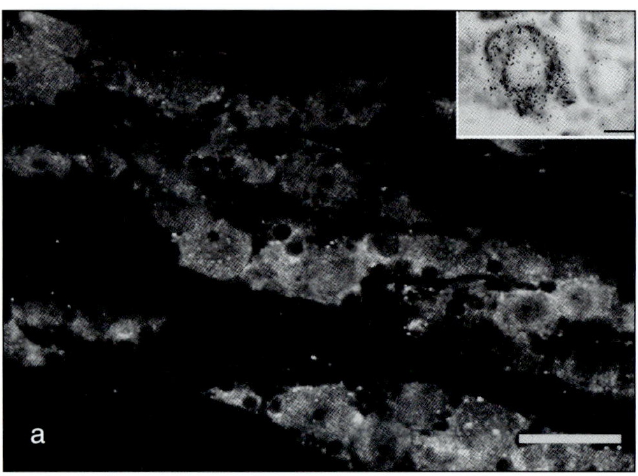

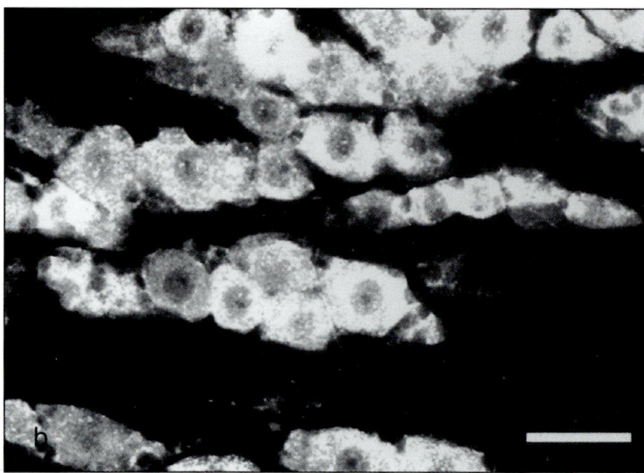

Figs 7-14a and 7-14b The normal immunoreactivity patterns for PQ-type voltage-gated calcium channels are shown in trigeminal cell bodies in the region that supplies innervation for maxillary teeth for normal ganglia *(a)* and at 8 days after making pulpal exposure lesions in the right maxillary molars *(b)*. By 8 days after tooth injury, the calcium channel expression was greatly enhanced. Bar = 50 mm. (Modified from Westenbroek and Byers[104] with permission.) *(inset)* When radioactive NGF is implanted into rat molars, it transports retrogradely to large and medium cell bodies in the trigeminal ganglion within 15 hours. Bar = 20 μm. (Inset photo courtesy of Dr C. Von Bartheld, University of Reno, Nevada. Modified from Wheeler et al[70] with permission.)

Distant plasticity in the trigeminal ganglion and central endings after tooth injury

The discussion so far has focused on dental sensory reactions in the terminal branches within the tooth. These neurons also have extensive changes in their alveolar branches (see Fig 7-13), at their cell bodies in the trigeminal ganglion (Fig 7-14), at their sensory endings in the brain stem, and in the second-order neurons within the CNS (Fig 7-15). The responses at the ganglion are generally similar to those shown for spinal nerves responding to tissue inflammation, including increased expression of neurotrophin receptors, neuropeptides, and voltage gated ion channels by the neurons and increased expression of injury proteins by the satellite cells.[20,70,77,104-106] Those changes can have profound effects on central pain pathways. For example, tooth injuries can cause persistent expression of the c-Fos transcription factor by central neurons (see Fig 7-15), which may indicate altered central pain pathway functions.[107-109] Further discussion of the extraordinary functional and cytochemical plasticity of sensory neurons, as well as that of central neurons responding to the input of sensory neurons, is found in the next chapter.

Neurophysiology of Pulpal Nociceptors and Dentinal Sensitivity

As described earlier, distinct groups of pulpal afferent nerve fibers can be classified based on their morphologic characteristics and conduction velocities. A number of recent studies indicate that these neuronal classes are functionally different and their activation may mediate different types of prepain and pain sensations.[110] Generally, these studies indicate that firing of pulpal afferents in human teeth induces mostly, if not entirely, painful sensations.[97-99] However, the type of pain may vary according to the type of stimulus applied, the type of neuronal fiber activated, or the condition of the pulp.

Tissue injury and inflammation can sensitize and activate certain pulpal neurons. In previous experimental studies on animals, pulpal inflammation has been associated with reduced thresholds to external stimulation and spontaneous discharges of pulpal nerve fibers.[111,112] These changes are probably due to synthesis or release of a number of inflammatory mediators, which have been shown to activate pulpal nerves and sensitize them to external stimuli (see also chapter 8).[12,110,112-114]

Application of a cold stimulus to hypersensitive dentin in human subjects induces pain that, in many cases, can reach a very high intensity.[110,115,116] Moreover, patients experiencing acute pulpitis often report moderate to severe pain.[117,118] However, this is not invariable: Pulpitis may proceed to a total pulpal necrosis with only minor symptoms or without any symptoms at all.[117,118] Considering the exceptionally rich nociceptive innervation of the pulp, such asymptomatic cases ("silent pulpitis") are puzzling. However, recent studies indicate that pulpal nociceptor activation may be abolished by local inhibitory mediators (eg, local opioids, cannabinoids, or somatostatin),[18,64,112,114,119] or by loss of functional terminals of these fibers (eg, via apoptosis or secondary to liquefaction necrosis). In addition to these peripheral factors, other central neural mechanisms may have a significant impact in the development of dental pain conditions (see chapter 8).[15,120-122]

Collectively, these studies indicate that there is a poor correlation between clinical pain symptoms and the histopathologic status of the pulp.[117,118,123,124] This is not surprising considering that hyperalgesia is a perceptual event mediated by peripheral and central pain mechanisms at the molecular level; these mechanisms are not necessarily discernible with microscopes evaluating biopsies of human dental pulp. In the following sections, the function of the pulpal neurons in healthy teeth and their responses to tissue injury and inflammation will be described. The role of different pulpal nerve fiber groups in the mediation of pulpal and dentinal pain under normal and pathologic conditions will be discussed in the next two chapters (chapters 8 and 9).

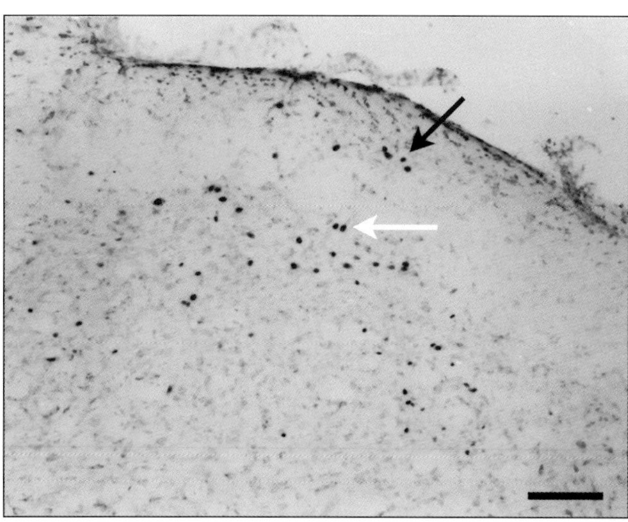

Fig 7-15 Two weeks after untreated pulpal exposure lesions were made in rat molars, persisting expression of the c-Fos transcription factor occurred in the superficial neurons of the trigeminal subnucleus caudalis *(white arrow)* and paratrigeminal nucleus *(black arrow)*. This central plasticity, which was still present 4 weeks after similar injuries in other rats, did not occur for shallow filled dentinal cavity lesions. Bar = 0.1 mm. (Modified from Byers et al[107] with permission.)

Sensory functions of pulpal nerves under normal conditions

A major part of our knowledge regarding the function of dental nerves is based on electrophysiologic recordings performed on animals (eg, cats, dogs, and monkeys). In such experiments, single intradental nerve fibers are identified and their responses to various stimuli are recorded (Figs 7-16 and 7-17). These electrophysiologic responses to various external stimuli have been compared to the perceptual responses induced by the same stimuli applied to human teeth. Such comparisons have shed light on how different pulpal nerve fiber groups contribute to different pain responses under normal and pathologic conditions. The morphologic similarity of the intradental innerva-

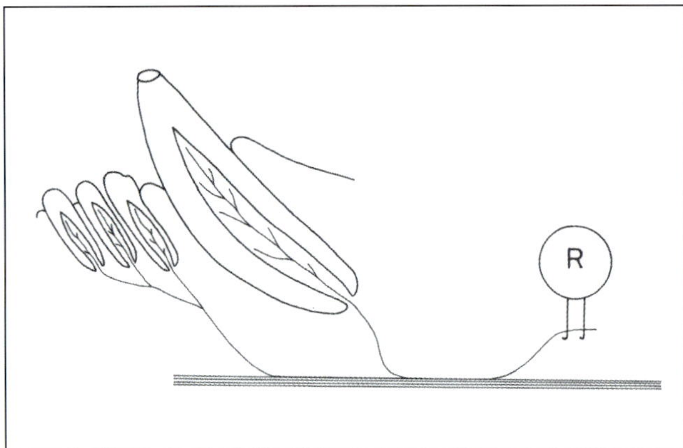

Fig 7-16 Schematic presentation of the setup for electrophysiologic recording of single intradental nerve fibers. The inferior alveolar nerve is exposed and the nerve filaments dissected from the nerve trunk. Single fibers innervating the canine or incisor teeth are recorded using metal wire electrodes (R). The nerve fibers are identified using electrical stimulation applied to the tooth crown. (Reprinted from Närhi and Hirvonen[125] with permission.)

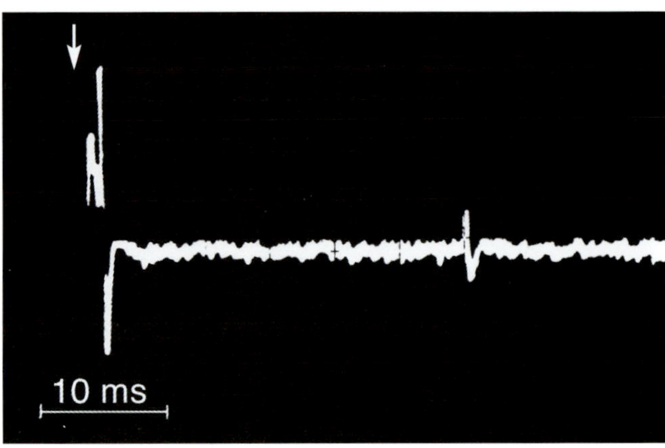

Fig 7-17 Nerve recording from a nerve filament containing one A- and one C-fiber. The action potential of the A-fiber shows after a latency of only about 2 milliseconds after the electrical stimulus artifact on the left *(arrow)*. The C-fiber action potential on the right is delayed by about 30 milliseconds because of slow conduction along the axon. By dividing the conduction distance (the length of the nerve fiber) by the conduction delay, the conduction velocity of the recorded fiber can be calculated.

tion of animals and humans serves as a good basis for such comparisons (see above).

The classification of the pulpal primary afferents as A- and C-fibers is based on their conduction velocities measured in single-nerve-fiber recording experiments (see Figs 7-16 and 7-17).[68,126–128] These two classes correspond to the myelinated and unmyelinated fibers found in morphologic studies.[11,129–131] According to the results of electrophysiologic recordings, the A- and C-fibers are functionally different.[14,56,110,126,127,132,133] In addition, the A-fiber group is not uniform because some slow-conducting (small) A-fibers seem to be sensitive to capsaicin, whereas most of the faster-conducting fibers respond to hydrodynamic stimulation but are not activated by capsaicin.[14,56,110,112,128,132–135] The results of the electrophysiologic studies also indicate that C-fibers do not respond to dentinal hydrodynamic stimulation. Instead, the sensitivity of dentin is entirely based on the function of intradental A-fibers.[14,115,133] Comparison of the sensory responses from stimulated human teeth to the electrophysiologic responses from animal studies reveals functional differences between these two fiber groups in response to tissue injury.[12,100,110,133,136]

As described above, pain and prepain are the only sensations that can be evoked by intradental nerve stimulation in human subjects. However, the quality of the pain can vary depending on the type of stimuli applied and can range from sharp, stabbing pain to dull, aching, throbbing pain sensations.[100,116,127,136,137] The variation is caused by activation of different nerve fiber types and differences in the nerve firing patterns (temporal summation) evoked by various stimuli.[14,110,127,136]

The application of low-intensity electric stimulation of human teeth can produce a nonpainful sensation.[97–99,118] It has been proposed that intradental low-threshold and fast-conducting A-beta type afferents mediate such prepain sensations.[97,98] A-beta fibers do have low electric thresholds. However, the thresholds of A-beta and A-delta fibers overlap considerably (Fig 7-18) and, accordingly, both fiber groups may be involved in the mediation of prepain sensations.[110,126] It is also important to note that painful sensations can be induced by increasing the stimulation frequency at prepain intensities,[99,110] a procedure that produces temporal summation of the nerve activity at the level of the trigeminal nuclei. Collectively, these findings suggest that prepain and pain sensations are mediated by the same afferent fibers.

On the basis of the single-fiber recordings (see Fig 7-18), it can be concluded that activation of only a small number of pulpal afferents is needed to evoke prepain or pain sensations.[110,126] This is clinically important because it suggests that pulp testing may produce a false-positive response, even in teeth with extensive pulpal necrosis, as long as at least some pulpal axons are still responsive. This could explain the clinical observation of a positive pulpal response in a tooth with a periradicular radiolucency (see also chapter 17).

It has been suggested that non-noxious mechanical (tactile) stimulation of the intact tooth crown activates pulpal A-beta fibers.[13,138–140] On the basis of such findings, those fibers were regarded as a discrete functional group that would be involved with the regulation of masticatory functions and the sensation of food texture between the teeth. However, A-beta and A-delta fibers show similar responses to various external stimuli and to inflammatory mediators,[110,125,127,128,134] and the results suggest that the fibers belong to the same functional group.

Taken together, the results of human and animal experiments indicate that a hydrodynamic mechanism mediates intradental nerve activation in response to several different stimuli (see also chapters 8 and 9).[1,117,133,141–144] The responding fibers consist of the A-delta and A-beta classes of neurons (Fig 7-19). Considering the tissue distortion and injury in the dentin-pulp border related to their activation,[145] the responding receptors can be classified as high-threshold mechanoreceptors or mechanical nociceptors.[146,147]

The pulpal C-fibers are polymodal because they respond to several different modes of stimulation and have high thresholds for activation.[126,127,132]

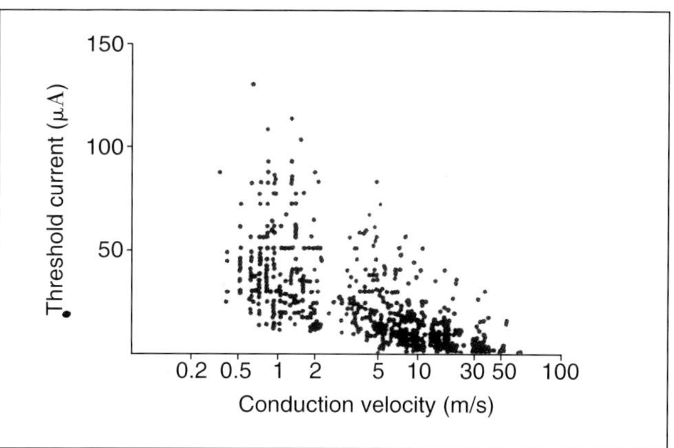

Fig 7-18 Electrical thresholds of intradental nerve fibers of the cat canine teeth plotted against their conduction velocities. The figure shows that the thresholds of many A-fibers are extremely low; in addition, a considerable overlap in the thresholds between A-fibers of different conduction velocities is obvious. (Reprinted from Närhi et al[110] with permission.)

They are activated only if stimuli reach their terminal endings inside the pulp. In an intact tooth, given the insulating enamel and dentinal layers, rather intense thermal stimuli are needed for their activation. The insensitivity of pulpal C-fibers to dentinal (hydrodynamic) stimulation[110,132,148] is consistent with the location of their endings and receptive fields deep in the pulp.[14,127,132] They also respond to histamine and bradykinin (Fig 7-20) applied to the exposed pulp,[14,110] which indicates that this fiber group also may be activated in connection with pulpal inflammatory reactions. Thus, the dull pain induced by pulpitis may be evoked by C-fiber activation. C-fibers also respond to capsaicin, which is a selective irritant of small nociceptive- and neuropeptide-containing afferents.[14,56,110,149]

The application of intense heating or cooling to human teeth produces a sharp pain sensation with a short latency, typically within a few seconds.[127,137] If the stimulation is continued, a dull, radiating pain response follows.[127,137] Corre-

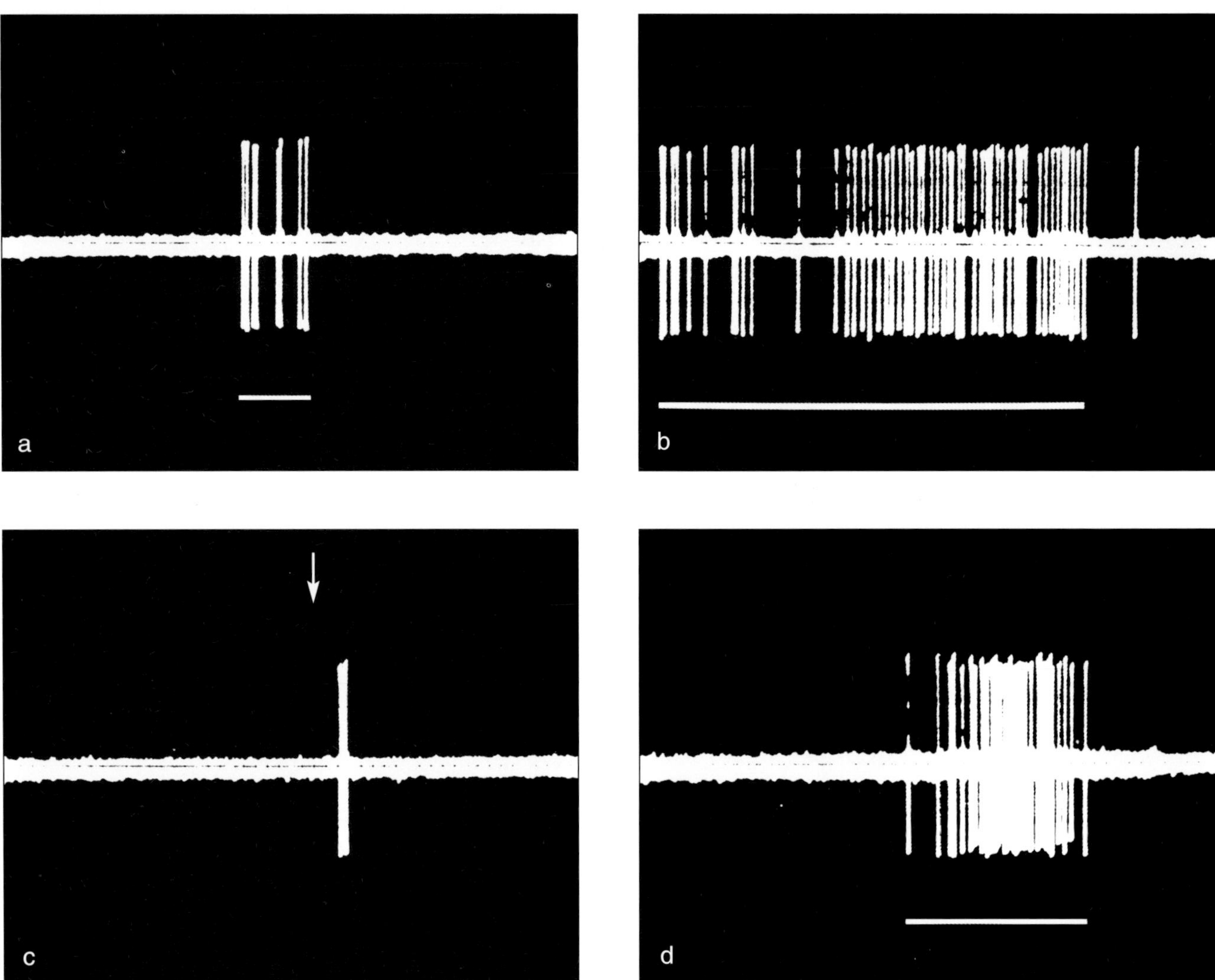

Fig 7-19 Responses of a single intradental A-fiber to *(a)* probing; *(b)* air blast; *(c)* hypertonic, 4.9 mol/L calcium chloride applied to dentin; and *(d)* drilling of dentin. The approximate timing of the stimulus application is indicated by the horizontal lines in Figs 7-19a, 7-19b, and 7-19d, and by the arrow in Fig 7-19c. 1 second = 54 mm. (Reprinted from Närhi et al[134] with permission.)

spondingly, biphasic responses to thermal stimuli are observed in cat teeth (Fig 7-21). The first response is an immediate or short-latency firing of intradental A-fibers, followed by a delayed C-fiber activation.[14,110,127] The initial A-fiber responses are supposedly induced by the dentinal fluid flow resulting from the rapid temperature changes.[117,141] The delayed C-fiber activation is probably induced by a direct effect of heat and cold on the nerve endings in the pulp.[110,127,132]

The results of these thermal stimulation studies strongly indicate that intradental A- and C-fibers may mediate different perceptual qualities of dental pain, ie, sharp and dull, respectively. In addition, certain other stimuli, such as air drying of exposed dentin and bradykinin applied to the exposed pulp, which are known to activate selectively pulpal A- or C-fibers, are also able to induce either sharp or dull pain, respectively, in human experiments.[116,136]

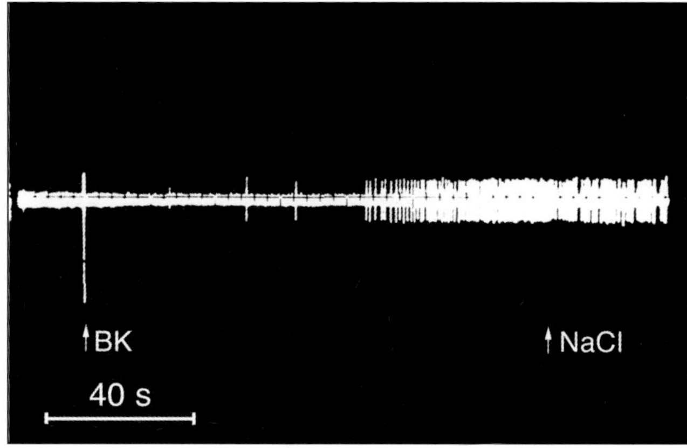

Fig 7-20 Responses of a single intradental C-fiber (small action potential) in the exposed pulp of a cat canine tooth to bradykinin application (BK) and after washing with physiologic saline (NaCl). The A-fiber (large action potential) in the same nerve filament only shows firing of a single action potential at the time of the bradykinin application, probably because of a mechanical effect. (Reprinted from Närhi[14] with permission.)

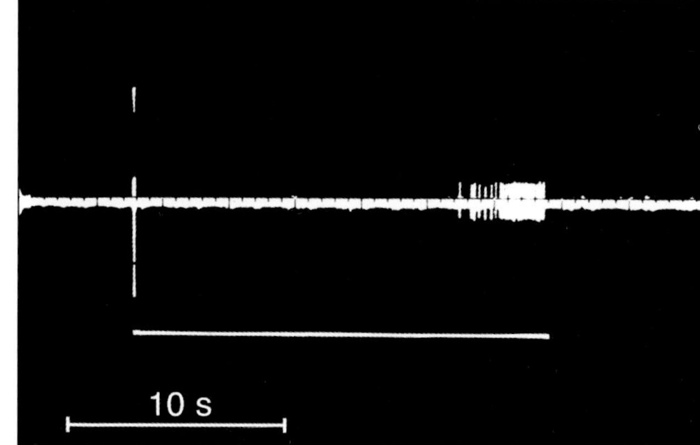

Fig 7-21 Responses of intradental nerve fibers to intense heating of an intact cat canine tooth. The timing of the stimulus application is indicated by the horizontal line. The A-fiber (large action potential) in the filament gives an immediate response at the beginning of stimulation. In contrast, activation of the C-fiber (small action potential) is much delayed. (Reprinted from Närhi[14] with permission.)

Neurophysiologic mechanisms of dentinal sensitivity

Numerous published studies indicate that the nociceptors in the dentin-pulp border area are activated by hydrodynamic fluid flow in response to dentinal stimulation (the hydrodynamic mechanism).[1,117,141] The fluid flow in turn stimulates the nerve endings in the dentin-pulp border area and causes their activation (Fig 7-22). Movement of dentinal fluid can also be induced in unexposed dentin, but in such cases the capillary forces are not activated and the effect of the stimulus is much weaker.

The results supporting the hydrodynamic mechanism of pulpal nerve activation are based both on in vivo studies on human subjects and experimental animals and in vitro experiments performed on extracted teeth. The results of the human experiments uniformly confirm that patency of the dentinal tubules is a prerequisite for the sensitivity of exposed dentin.[115,141,150-152] The relationship between the dentinal tubular condition and dentinal sensitivity was further confirmed in experiments showing a significant positive correlation between the degree of the dentinal sensitivity and the density of open dentinal tubules counted in exposed cervical dentinal surfaces in a scanning electron microscopic replica study on human teeth.[153] In vitro measurements have also shown that opening or blocking of the tubules determines the hydraulic conductance of dentin[154,155] and, accordingly, the fluid flow in the dentinal tubules (see also chapter 4).

Several electrophysiologic studies performed on cats and dogs have shown that acid etching of drilled dentin significantly increases the responsiveness of intradental nerves to air blasts, probing, and hyperosmotic solutions.[128,134,148,156,157] The increased sensitivity is strongly related to the patency of the dentinal tubules.[143] The sensitizing effect of acid etching can be abolished almost completely by blocking the tubules (eg, with oxalates or composite resins).[143] Similar studies conducted in human teeth indicate that acid etching increases dentinal sensitivity.[117,141]

According to the hydrodynamic theory, rapid dentinal fluid flow serves as the final stimulus acti-

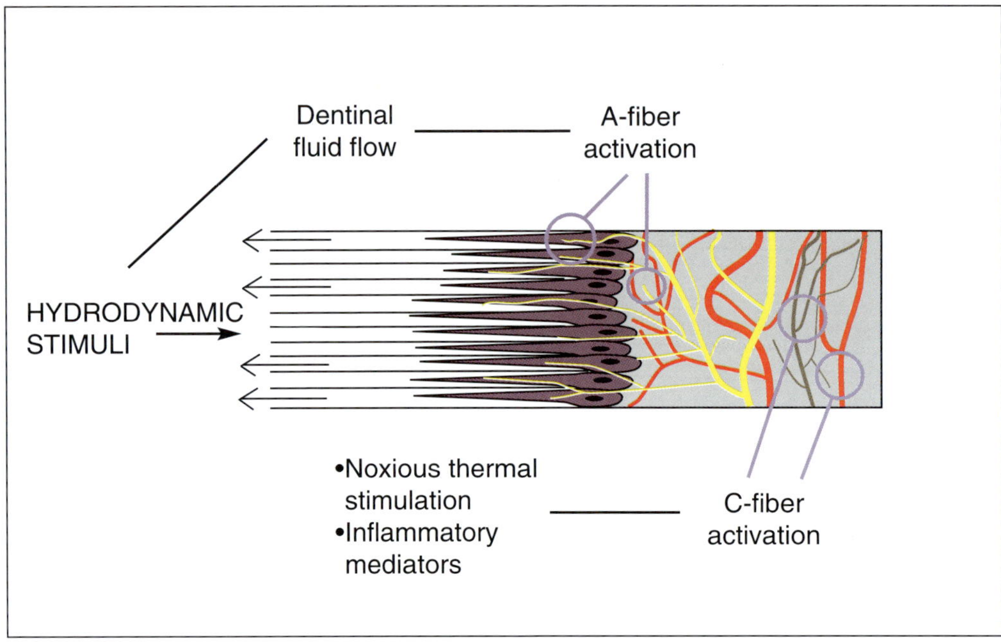

Fig 7-22 Activation mechanisms of intradental nerve fibers. A-fibers in the dentin-pulp border area respond to stimulus-induced fluid flow in the dentinal tubules and consequent deformation of the peripheral pulpal tissues containing the nerve endings (hydrodynamic mechanism). For C-fiber activation the applied stimuli must reach the nerve endings, which are mostly located deeper in the pulp. C-fibers also respond to certain inflammatory mediators.

vating intradental nociceptors for many different types of stimuli. In support of this hypothesis, single intradental A-fibers respond to a number of different hydrodynamic stimuli including dentinal probing, air blasts, and hyperosmotic solutions (see Fig 7-19).[14,110,115,125,128,133,134] Studies conducted in vitro demonstrate that all these stimuli induce fluid flow in the dentinal tubules.[117,141,142,158] It is the osmotic strength of solutions and not their chemical composition that elicit pain responses in human teeth, nerve responses in experimental animals, and fluid flow responses in dentinal tubules.[115,125,158-161] Finally, recent electrophysiologic recordings performed on cat canine teeth indicate that a direct relationship exists between the dentinal fluid flow and intradental nerve activation.[144] However, inflammation may develop, leading to sensitization of the intradental nerves.[115] Such changes may result in poor responses to treatment of hypersensitive dentin and may be significant in cases with open dentinal tubules that have been exposed for a long time.[115]

Sensory functions of pulpal nerves under conditions of pulpal inflammation

As is discussed in chapter 8, the two major mechanisms of pulpal pain are related to dentinal sensitivity and pulpal inflammation. Injury to the pulp can alter both of these pain mechanisms. Intense hydrodynamic stimulation may induce tissue injury in the dentin-pulp border area, including disruption of the odontoblast layer with aspiration of the cells into the dentinal tubules.[117,141,145,162] The nerve endings may also be injured.[163,164] The inflammation-induced elaboration of growth factors can lead to subsequent morphologic and phenotypic changes in the nociceptive nerve endings, including sprouting and increased neuropeptide expression[92,164,165]; these changes may contribute to long-term functional changes in the pulpal afferents.[20,112] For example, the local changes in the density of the innervation in the dentin and pulp might result in changes in the regional sensitivity of the affected tooth. However, our current knowledge about the possible functional correlates of the morphologic changes is limited.

The effect of various inflammatory mediators on pulpal nerve function has been studied in cat and dog teeth. They activate intradental nociceptors and/or sensitize them to subsequent stimuli (ie, they reduce the threshold for firing).[14,110] For example, serotonin activates A-fibers and sensitizes them to external stimulation (eg, hydrodynamic stimuli).[110,113,166] Intense, repeated heating sensitizes intradental nerves in cat canine teeth, and prostaglandins seem to mediate this response.[10] As stated earlier, pulpal C-fiber responses are activated by histamine and bradykinin, which may be significant for the development of pain in pulpitis.[14,110] Thus, the injury-induced inflammatory cascade probably signals pulpitis pain and acts to amplify dentinal hypersensitivity.

According to single-fiber recordings, the faster-conducting pulpal afferents primarily respond to hydrodynamic stimulation of dentin, although certain small-diameter myelinated afferents may also be activated.[110,115,128,134] Hydrodynamic stimulation also affects the pulpal blood flow, indicating that the nerve fibers activated by such stimulation are able to induce neurogenic vascular effects.[18,114]

Pulpal A-fibers comprise functionally distinct classes of sensory neurons. Although most of the intradental A-fibers are activated by hydrodynamic stimulation, there exists a rather high number of relatively slowly conducting pulpal A-delta fibers that are not sensitive to hydrodynamic stimulation of the coronal dentin of healthy teeth.[110,112,115,167-169] This class of "silent" A-fibers can be activated only by intense heat or cold that reaches the pulp proper, and their mechanical receptive fields are located deep in the pulp.[168,169] However, the sensitivity of these silent A-delta fibers is enhanced in pulpal inflammation, when they significantly increase their responsiveness to dentinal stimulation.[112]

Studies to date suggest that there is a functional significance to the sprouting of sensory terminals that occurs during inflammation. For example, experiments on dog teeth indicate that nerve sprouting may be reflected in the size of the receptive fields of pulpal afferents responsive to hydrodynamic stimulation of dentin.[20,112] In healthy teeth, gentle probing of the exposed dentinal surface revealed small receptive fields that were most often composed of a single small spot in the exposed dentin.[112,169] In contrast, gentle probing of exposed dentin in inflamed teeth revealed a dramatic change, with emergence of wide receptive fields, sometimes covering the whole dentinal surface at the crown tip in inflamed incisors.[112] This increase in the size of the receptive field could be caused by sprouting as well as activation of normally "silent" terminals of branched axons. An increase in the size of receptive fields would result in an increased overlap of receptive fields and, accordingly, would enhance spatial summation of peripheral nerve activity with resulting increased pain intensity in response to dentinal stimulation.

Inflammation may also increase the regional sensitivity of dentin in various parts of the tooth. In normal dog teeth, the nerve fibers innervating the cervical dentin are far less responsive to hydrodynamic dentinal stimulation compared to those innervating dentin in the crown tip.[168,169] However, in inflamed teeth the sensitivity of cervical dentin can increase to the same level as that of the crown tip.[168,169]

Although most inflammatory mediators activate or sensitize peripheral neurons, some mediators released in pulp after injury, including endogenous opioids and somatostatin, appear to be inhibitory. In experiments performed on inflamed dog teeth, the local application of a somatostatin antagonist increases firing of intradental nerves, suggesting that the release of endogenous somatostatin reduces firing during injury.[112,119] In other preliminary experiments, administration of the opioid antagonist naloxone produced a similar effect.[112] In addition, local application of morphine in deep cavities completely abolished the pulpal nerve responses to mustard oil, a substance that induces inflammation and activates nociceptive afferents. These results suggest that in pulpal inflammation both somatostatin and endogenous opioids effectively reduce or abolish intradental nerve activity, despite the presence of other inflammatory mediators that have a stimulatory effect. These data suggest that one possible mechanism for the frequently reported lack of clinical symptoms in teeth with pulpal inflammation may be based, in part, on the release of local inhibitory mediators in the inflamed tissue.

Conclusions

Research conducted over the last two decades has greatly increased our understanding of dentinal innervation and sensitivity, efferent signals from sensory nerve fibers that affect pulp cells (and vice versa), the neurophysiology of pulpal nociceptors, neuroanatomic and functional responses to injury, pulpal neuroinflammatory interactions, and the relationship of all these different features to dental pain. However, there is still much to be determined about types of nerve fibers in teeth and their different functional states and injury responses, neuropulpal interactions (especially nerve-odontoblast interactions), and the mechanisms and treatment of hypersensitive teeth. The pace of discovery in this field suggests that new answers and clinical insights concerning the peripheral mechanisms of dental pain will be developed rapidly.

References

1. Gysi A. An attempt to explain the sensitiveness of dentin. Brit J Dent Soc 1900;43:865–868.
2. Bender IB. Pulp pain diagnosis—A review. J Endod 2000;26:175–179.
3. Fearnhead RW. The neurohistology of human teeth. Proc R Soc Med Br 1961;54:267–277.
4. Bernick S. Innervation of teeth. In: Finn SB (ed). Biology of the Dental Pulp. Birmingham: University of Alabama Press, 1968:285–308.
5. Anderson DJ, Hannam AG, Matthews B. Sensory mechanisms in mammalian teeth and their supporting structures. Physiol Rev 1970;50:171–195.
6. Frank RM, Sauvage C, Frank P. Morphological basis for dental sensitivity. Int Dent J 1972;22:1–19.
7. Brännström M, Åström A. The hydrodynamics of the dentine; Its possible relationship to dentinal pain. Int Dent J 1972;22:219–227.
8. Arwill T, Edwall L, Lilja J, Olgart LM, Svensson SE. Ultrastructure of nerves in the dentinal pulp border zone after sensory and autonomic transection in the cat. Acta Odontol Scand 1973;31:273–281.
9. Byers MR, Kish SJ. Delineation of somatic nerve endings in rat teeth by autoradiography of axon-transported protein. J Dent Res 1976;55:419–426.
10. Ahlberg KF. Dose-dependent inhibition of sensory nerve activity in the feline dental pulp by anti-inflammatory drugs. Acta Physiol Scand 1978;102:434–440.
11. Byers MR. Dental sensory receptors. Int Rev Neurobiol 1984;25:39–94.
12. Olgart LM. The role of local factors in dentin and pulp in intradental pain mechanisms. J Dent Res 1985;64:572–578.
13. Dong WK, Chudler EH, Martin RF. Physiological properties of intradental mechanoreceptors. Brain Res 1985;334:389–394.
14. Närhi MVO. The characteristics of intradental sensory units and their responses to stimulation. J Dent Res 1985;64:564–571.
15. Sessle BJ. Acute and chronic craniofacial pain: Brainstem mechanisms of nociceptive transmission and neuroplasticity and their clinical correlates. Crit Rev Oral Biol Med 2000;11:576–591.
16. Silverman J, Kruger L. An interpretation of dental innervation based on the pattern of calcitonin gene-related peptide (CGRP) -immunoreactive thin sensory axons. Somatosens Res 1987;5:157–175.
17. Hildebrand C, Fried K, Tuisku F, Johansson CS. Teeth and tooth nerves. Prog Neurobiol 1995;45:165–222.
18. Olgart LM. Neural control of pulpal blood flow. Crit Rev Oral Biol Med 1996;7:159–171.
19. Byers MR, Taylor PE, Khayat BG, Kimberly CL. Effects of injury and inflammation on pulpal and periapical nerves. J Endod 1990;16:78–84.
20. Byers MR, Narhi MVO. Dental injury models: Experimental tools for understanding neuro-inflammatory interactions and polymodal nociceptor functions. Crit Rev Oral Biol Med 1999;10:4–39.

21. Vongsavan N, Matthews B. Changes in pulpal blood flow and in fluid flow through dentine produced by autonomic and sensory stimulation in the cat. Proc Finn Dent Soc 1992;88(suppl 1):491-497.
22. Bongenhielm U, Haegerstrand A, Theodorsson E, Fried K. Effects of neuropeptides on growth of cultivated rat molar pulp fibroblasts. Regul Pept 1995;60:91-98.
23. Pashley DH. Dynamics of the pulp-dentin complex. Crit Rev Oral Biol Med 1996;7:104-133.
24. Jontell M, Okiji T, Dahlgren U, Bergenholtz G. Immune defense mechanisms of the dental pulp. Crit Rev Oral Biol Med 1998;9:179-200.
25. Berggreen E, Heyeraas KJ. Effect of the sensory neuropeptide antagonists h-CGRP (8-37) and SR 140.33 on pulpal and gingival blood flow in ferrets. Arch Oral Biol 2000;45:537-542.
26. Fristad I, Kvinnsland IH, Jonsson R, Heyeraas KJ. Effect of intermittent long-lasting electrical tooth stimulation on pulpal blood flow and immunocompetent cells: A hemodynamic and immunohistochemical study in young rat molars. Exp Neurol 1997;146:230-239.
27. Corporon RE, Avery JK. The ultrastructure of intradental nerves in developing mouse molars. Anat Rec 1973; 175:585-606.
28. Heyeraas KJ, Kim S, Raab WH-M, Byers MR, Liu M. Effect of electrical tooth stimulation on blood flow, interstitial fluid pressure and substance P and CGRP-immunoreactive nerve fiber reactions in the low compliant cat dental pulp. Microvasc Res 1994;47:329-343.
29. Byers MR, Wheeler EF, Bothwell M. Altered expression of NGF and p75-NGF receptor mRNA by fibroblasts of injured teeth precedes sensory nerve sprouting. Growth Factors 1992;6:41-52.
30. Woodnutt DA, Wager-Miller J, O'Neill PC, Bothwell M, Byers MR. Neurotrophin receptors and nerve growth factor are differentially expressed in adjacent non-neuronal cells of normal and injured tooth pulp. Cell Tissue Res 2000;299:225-236.
31. Brady S, Colman DR, Brophy P. Subcellular organization of the nervous system: Organelles and their functions. In: Zigmond MJ, Bloom FD, Landis SC, Roberts JL, Squire LR (eds). Fundamental Neuroscience. New York: Academic Press, 1999:71-106.
32. McCormick DA. Membrane potential and action potential. In: Zigmond MJ, Bloom FD, Landis SC, Roberts JL, Squire LR (eds). Fundamental Neuroscience. New York: Academic Press, 1999:129-154.
33. Byers MR. Sensory innervation of periodontal ligment of rat molars consists of unencapsulated Ruffini-like mechanoreceptors and free nerve endings. J Comp Neurol 1985;231:500-518.
34. Byers MR, O'Connor TA, Martin RF, Dong WK. Mesencephalic trigeminal sensory neurons of cat: Axon pathways and structure of mechanoreceptive endings in periodontal ligament. J Comp Neurol 1986;250: 181-191.
35. Maeda T. Sensory innervation of the periodontal ligament in the incisor and molar of the monkey, *Macaca fuscata*. An immunohistochemical study for neurofilament protein and glia-specific S-100 protein. Arch Histol Jpn 1987;50:437-454.
36. Maeda T, Sato O, Kannari K, Takagi H, Iwanaga T. Immunohistochemical localization of laminin in the periodontal Ruffini endings of rat incisors: A possible function for terminal Schwann cells. Histol Cytol 1991; 54:339-348.
37. Kannari K, Sato O, Maeda T, Iwanaga T, Fujita T. A possible mechanism of mechanoreception in Ruffini endings in the periodontal ligament of hamster incisors. J Comp Neurol 1991;313:368-376
38. Nakakura-Ohshima K, Maeda T, Ohshima H, Noda T, Takano Y. Postnatal development of periodontal Ruffini endings in rat incisors: An immunoelectron microscopic study using protein gene product 9.5 (PGP 9.5) antibody. J Comp Neurol 1995;362:551-564.
39. Byers MR, Maeda T. Periodontal innervation: Regional specializations, ultrastructure, cytochemistry and tissue interactions. Acta Med Dent Helv 1997;2:116-133.
40. Maeda T, Ochi K, Nakakura-Ohshima K, Youn SH, Wakisaka S. The Ruffini ending as the primary mechanoreceptor in the periodontal ligament: Its morphology, cytochemical features, regeneration and development. Crit Rev Oral Biol Med 1999;10:307-327.
41. Byers MR. Segregation of NGF receptor in sensory receptors, nerves and local cells of teeth and periodontium demonstrated by EM immunocytochemistry. J Neurocytol 1990;19:765-777.
42. Byers MR, Närhi MV, Dong WK. Sensory innervation of pulp and dentin in adult dog teeth as demonstrated by autoradiography. Anat Rec 1987;218:207-215.
43. Byers MR, Narhi MV, Mecifi KB. Acute and chronic reactions of dental sensory nerve fibers to cavities and desiccation in rat molars. Anat Rec 1988;221:872-883.
44. Byers MR. Dynamic plasticity of dental sensory nerve structure and cytochemistry. Arch Oral Biol 1994;39 (suppl):13S-21S.
45. Gunji T. Morphological work on the sensitivity of dentin. Arch Histol Jpn 1982;45:45-67.
46. Byers MR, Neuhaus SJ, Gehrig JD. Dental sensory receptor structure in human teeth. Pain 1982;13:221-235.
47. Maeda T, Iwanaga T, Fujita T, Kobayashi S. Immunohistochemical demonstration of nerves in the predentin and dentin of human third molars with the use of an antiserum against neurofilament protein (NFP). Cell Tissue Res 1986;243:13-23.

48. Arwill T. Studies on the ultrastructure of dental tissues. II. The predentine-pulpal border. Odontol Rev 1967;18:191–208.
49. Byers MR. Fine structure of trigeminal receptors in rat molars. In: Anderson DL, Matthews B (eds). Pain in the Trigeminal Region [Proceedings of a symposium held in the Department of Physiology, University of Bristol, 25–27 July, 1977, England]. Amsterdam: Elsevier/North-Holland Biomedical, 1977:13–24.
50. Frank RM. Etude au microscope electronique de l'odontoblaste et du canalicule dentainaire humain. Arch Oral Biol 1966;11:179–199.
51. Holland GR. Morphological features of dentine and pulp related to dentine sensitivity. Arch Oral Biol 1994;39(suppl):3S–11S.
52. Byers MR, Gerlach RS, Berger RL. Development of sensory receptor structure and function in rat molars. In: Matthews B, Hill RG (eds). Anatomical, Physiological and Pharmacological Aspects of Trigeminal Pain. Amsterdam: Elsevier, 1982:15–26.
53. Wakisaka S, Ichikawa H, Hishikawa S, Matsuo S, Takano Y, Akai M. The distribution and origin of calcitonin gene-related peptide containing nerve fibers in the feline dental pulp. Histochemistry 1987;86:585–589.
54. Kimberly CL, Byers MR. Inflammation of rat molar pulp and periodontium causes increased calcitonin gene-related peptide and axonal sprouting. Anat Rec 1988;222:289–300.
55. Casasco A, Calligaro A, Casasco M, Springall DR, Polak JM, Poggi P. Peptidergic nerves in human dental pulp. Histochemistry 1990;95:115–121.
56. Ikeda H, Tokita Y, Suda H. Capsaicin-sensitive A-delta fibers in cat tooth pulp. J Dent Res 1997;76:1341–1349.
57. Fristad I, Heyeraas KJ, Kvinnsland I. Nerve fibres and cells immunoreactive to neurochemical narkers in developing rat molars and supporting tissues. Arch Oral Biol 1994;39:633–646.
58. Wakisaka S. Neuropeptides in the dental pulp: Distribution, origins and correlation. J Endod 1990;16:67–69.
59. Qian XB, Naftel JP. Effects of neonatal exposure to anti-nerve growth factor on the number and size distribution of trigeminal neurones projecting to the molar dental pulp in rats. Arch Oral Biol 1996;41:359–367.
60. Pan M, Naftel JP, Wheeler EF. Effects of deprivation of neonatal nerve growth factor on the expression of neurotrophin receptors and brain-derived neurotrophic factor by dental pulp afferents of the adult rat. Arch Oral Biol 2000;45:387–399.
61. Fried K, Nosrat CA, Lillesaar C, Hildebrand C. Molecular signalling and pulpal nerve development. Crit Rev Oral Biol Med 2000;11:318–332.
62. Hattyasy D. Continuous regeneration of dental nerve endings. Nature 1961;189:72–74.
63. Maeda T, Byers MR. Different localizations of growth-associated protein (GAP-43) in mechanoreceptors and free nerve endings of adult rat periodontal ligament, dental pulp and skin. Arch Histol Cytol 1996;59:291–304.
64. Taddese A, Nah S-Y, McClesky EW. Selective opioid inhibition of small nociceptive neurons. Science 1995;270:1366–1369.
65. Ichikawa H, Hidaka H, Sugimoto T. Neurocalcin-immunoreactive primary sensory neurons in the trigeminal ganglion provide myelinated innervation to the tooth pulp and periodontal ligament. Brain Res 2000;864:152–156.
66. Cook SP, Vulchanova L, Hargreaves KM, Elde R, McCleskey EW. Distinct ATP receptors on pain-sensing and stretch-sensing neurons. Nature 1997;387:505–508.
67. Buchaille R, Couble ML, Magloire H, Bleicher F. A subtractive PCR-based cDNA library from human odontoblast cells: Identification of novel genes expressed in tooth forming cells. Matrix Biol 2000;19:421–430.
68. Cadden SW, Lisney SJW, Matthews B. Thresholds to electrical stimulation of nerves in cat canine tooth pulp with A-beta, A-delta, and C-fiber conduction velocities. Brain Res 1983;261:31–41.
69. Ibuki T, Kido MA, Kiyoshima T, Terada Y, Tanaka T. An ultrastructural study of the relationship between sensory trigeminal nerves and odontoblasts in rat dentin/pulp as demonstrated by the anterograde transport of wheat germ agglutinin-horseradish peroxidase (WGA-HRP). J Dent Res 1996;75:1963–1970.
70. Wheeler EF, Naftel JP, Pan M, Von Bartheld CS, Byers MR. Neurotrophin receptor expression is induced in a subpopulation of trigeminal neurons that label by retrograde transport of NGF or fluoro-gold following tooth injury. Brain Res Mol Brain Res 1998;61:23–38.
71. Pohto P, Antila R. Innervation of blood vessels in the dental pulp. Int Dent J 1972;22:228–239.
72. Fried K, Aldskogius H, Hildebrand C. Proportion of unmyelinated axons in rat molar and incisor tooth pulps following neonatal capsaicin treatment and/or sympathectomy. Brain Res 1988;463:118–123.
73. Qian XB, Naftel JP. The effects of anti-nerve growth factor on retrograde labeling of superior cervical ganglion neurones projecting to the molar pulp in the rat. Arch Oral Biol 1994;39:1041–1047.
74. Sasano T, Shoji N, Kuriwada S, Sanjo D, Izumi H, Karita KK. Absence of parasympathetic vasodilatation in cat dental pulp. J Dent Res 1995;74:1665–1670.
75. Aars H, Brodin P, Andersen E. A study of cholinergic and beta-adrenergic commponents in the regulation of blood blow in the tooth pulp and gingivae in man. Acta Physiol Scand 1993;148:441–447.

76. Byers MR, Mecifi KB, Iadarola MJ. Focal c-Fos expression in developing rat molars: Correlations with susequet intradental and epithelial sensory innervation. Int J Dev Biol 1995;39:181-189.
77. Fristad I. Dental innervation: Functions and plasticity after peripheral injury. Acta Odontol Scand 1997;55: 236-254.
78. Byers MR, Dong WK. Autoradiographic location of sensory nerve endings in dentin of monkey teeth. Anat Rec 1983;205:441-454.
79. Fried K. Development, degeneration and regeneration of nerve fibres in the feline inferior alveolar nerve and mandibular incisor pulps. Light and electron microscopic studies. Acta Physiol Scand Suppl 1982;504:1-28.
80. Fried K. Changes in pulpal nerves with aging. Proc Finn Dent Soc 1992;88(suppl 1):517-528.
81. Egan CA, Hector MP, Bishop MA. On the pulpal nerve supply in primary human teeth: Evidence for the innervation of primary dentine. Int J Paediatr Dent 1999;9: 57-66.
82. Granholm AC. Histology, innervation and radiographic appearance of fetal rat tooth germs developing in occulo. Scand J Dent Res 1984;92:381-390.
83. Erdelyi G, Fried K, Hildebrand C. Nerve growth to tooth buds after homotopic or heterotopic autotransplantation. Brain Res 1987;430:39-47.
84. Nagahama SI, Cunningham ML, Lee MY, Byers MR. Normal development of dental innervation and nerve-tissue interactions in the colony-stimulating factor-1 deficient osteopetrotic mouse. Dev Dyn 1998;211:52-59.
85. Andres KH, von During M. Morphology of cutaneous receptors. In: Iggo A (ed). Handbook of Sensory Physiology. Vol 2. Somatosensory System. Berlin: Springer-Verlag, 1974:3-28.
86. Byers MR, Yeh Y. Fine structure of subepithelial "free" and corpuscular trigeminal nerve endings in anterior hard palate of the rat. Somatosens Res 1984;1:265-279.
87. Davidson RM, Guo L. Calcium channel current in rat dental pulp cells. J Membr Biol 2000;178:21-30.
88. Allen B, Couble ML, Magloire H, Bleicher F. Characterization and gene expression of high conductance calcium-activated potassium channels displaying mechanosensitivity in human odontoblasts. J Biol Chem 2000; 275:25556-25561.
89. Fristad I, Vandevska-Radunovic V, Kvinnsland IH. Neurokinin-1 receptor in the mature dental pulp of rats. Arch Oral Biol 1999;44:191-195.
90. Byers MR, Sugaya A. Odontoblast processes in dentin revealed by fluorescent Di-I. J Histochem Cytochem 1995;43:159-168
91. Bhatnagar M, Cintra A, Tinner B, Agnati LF, Kerezoudis N, Edwall L, Fuxe K. Neurotensin-like immunoreactivity in odontoblasts and their processes in rat maxillary molar teeth and the effect of pulpotomy. Regul Pept 1995;58:141-147.
92. Byers MR, Taylor PE. Effect of sensory denervation on the response of rat molar pulp to exposure injury. J Dent Res 1993;72:613-618.
93. Taylor PE, Byers MR, Redd PE. Sprouting of CGRP nerve fibers in response to dentin injury in rat molars. Brain Res 1988;461:371-376.
94. Khayat BG, Byers MR, Taylor PE, Mecifi KB, Kimberly CL. Responses of nerve fibers to pulpal inflammation and periapical lesions in rat molars demonstrated by CGRP-immunocytochemistry. J Endod 1988;4:577-587.
95. Kvinnsland I, Heyeraas KJ. Effect of traumatic occlusion on CGRP and SP immunoreactive nerve morphology in rat molar pulp and periodontium. Histochem 1997;92: 111-120.
96. Taylor PE, Byers MR. An immunocytochemical study of the response of nerves containing calcitonin gene-related peptide to microabscess formation and healing in rat molars. Arch Oral Biol 1990;33:629-638.
97. Mumford JM, Bowsher D. Pain and protopathic sensibility. A review with particular reference to teeth. Pain 1976;2:223-243.
98. McGrath PA, Gracely RH, Dubner R, Heft MW. Non-pain and pain sensation evoked by tooth pulp stimulation. Pain 1983;15:377-388.
99. Virtanen ASJ, Huopaniemi T, Narhi MVO, Pertovaara A, Wallgren K. The effect of temporal parameters on subjective sensations evoked by electrical tooth stimulation. Pain 1987;30:361-371.
100. Ahlquist ML, Edwall L, Franzen O, Haegerstam G. Perception of pain as a function of intradental nerve activity. Pain 1984;19:353-366.
101. Swift ML, Byers MR. Effect of aging on responses of nerve fibers to pulpal inflammation in rat molars analyzed by quantitative immunocytochemistry. Arch Oral Biol 1992;37:901-912.
102. Inoue T, Shimono M. Repair dentinogenesis following transplantation into normal and germ-free animals. Proc Finn Dent Soc 1992;88(suppl 1):183-194.
103. Holland GR. Periapical innervation of the ferret canine one year after pulpotomy. J Dent Res 1992;71:470-474.
104. Westenbroek RE, Byers MR. Up-regulation of class A Ca+ channels in trigeminal ganglion after pulp exposure. Neuroreport 1999;10:381-385.
105. Fried K, Arvidsson J, Roberson B, Pfaller K. Anterograde HRP tracing and immunohistochemistry of trigeminal ganglion tooth pulp neurons after dental nerve lesions in the rat. Neuroscience 1991;43:269-278.
106. Stephenson JL, Byers MR. GFAP immunoreactivity in trigeminal ganglion satellite cells after tooth injury in rats. Exp Neurol 1995;131:11-22.
107. Byers MR, Chudler EH, Iadarola MJ. Chronic tooth pulp inflammation causes transient and persistent expression of Fos in dynorphin-rich regions of rat brain stem. Brain Res 2000;861:191-207.

108. Iwata K, Takahashi O, Tsuboi Y, Ochiai H, Hibiya J, Sakaki T, et al. Fos protein induction in the medullary dorsal horn and first segment of the spinal cord by tooth-pulp stimulation in cats. Pain 1998;75:27-36.
109. Dubner R, Ruda MA. Activity-dependent neuronal plasticity following tissue injury and inflammation. Trends Neurosci 1992;15:96-103.
110. Närhi M, Jyväsjärvi E, Virtanen A, Huopaniemi T, Ngassapa D, Hirvonen T. Role of intradental A- and C-type nerve fibres in dental pain mechanisms. Proc Finn Dent Soc 1992;88(suppl 1):507-516.
111. Ahlberg KF. Influence of local noxious heat stimulation on sensory nerve activity in the feline dental pulp. Acta Physiol Scand 1978;103:71-80.
112. Närhi M, Yamamoto H, Ngassapa D. Function of intradental nociceptors in normal and inflamed teeth. In: Shimono M, Maeda T, Suda H, Takahashi K (eds). Dentin/Pulp Complex. Tokyo: Quintessence, 1996: 136-140.
113. Olgart L. Excitation of intradental sensory units by pharmacological agents. Acta Physiol Scand 1974; 92:48-55.
114. Olgart L. Neurogenic components of pulp inflammation. In: Shimono M, Maeda T, Suda H, Takahashi K (eds). Dentin/Pulp Complex. Tokyo: Quintessence, 1996: 169-175.
115. Närhi M, Kontturi-Närhi V, Hirvonen T, Ngassapa D. Neurophysiological mechanisms of dentin hypersensitivity. Proc Finn Dent Soc 1992;88(suppl 1):15-22.
116. Kontturi-Närhi V, Närhi M. Testing sensitive dentin in man. Int Endod J 1993;26:4.
117. Brännström M. Dentin and Pulp in Restorative Dentistry. London: Wolfe Medical, 1981.
118. Mumford JM. Orofacial Pain: Aetiology, Diagnosis and Treatment, ed 3. Edinburgh: Churchill Livingstone, 1982.
119. Hirvonen T, Hippi P, Närhi M. The effect of an opioid antagonist and a somatostatin antagonist on the nerve function in normal and inflamed dental pulps [abstract]. J Dent Res 1998;77:1329.
120. Sessle BJ. Oral-facial pain: Old puzzles, new postulates. Int Dent J 1978;28:28-42.
121. Sessle BJ. The neurobiology of facial and dental pain: Present knowledge, future directions. J Dent Res 1987; 66:962-981.
122. Sigursson A, Maixner W. Effects of experimental clinical noxious counterirritants on pain perception. Pain 1994;57:265-275.
123. Seltzer S, Bender IB, Ziontz M. The dynamics of pulp inflammation: Correlations between diagnostic data and actual histopathological findings in the pulp. Oral Surg 1963;16:969-977.
124. Seltzer S, Bender IB, Nazimov H. Differential diagnosis of pulp conditions. Oral Surg 1965;19:383-391.
125. Närhi MVO, Hirvonen T. The response of dog intradental nerves to hypertonic solutions of $CaCl_2$ and NaCl, and other stimuli, applied to exposed dentine. Arch Oral Biol 1987;32:781-786.
126. Närhi M, Virtanen A, Huopaniemi T, Hirvonen T. Conduction velocities of single pulp nerve fibre units in the cat. Acta Physiol Scand 1982;116:209-213.
127. Jyväsjärvi E, Kniffki K-D. Cold stimulation of teeth: A comparison between the responses of cat intradental A delta and C fibres and human sensation. J Physiol 1987; 391:193-207.
128. Närhi MVO, Hirvonen TJ, Hakumäki MOK. Responses of intradental nerve fibres to stimulation of dentine and pulp. Acta Physiol Scand 1982;115:173-178.
129. Beasley WL, Holland GR. A quantitative analysis of the innervation of the pulp of cat's canine tooth. J Comp Neurol 1978;178:487-494.
130. Reader A, Foreman DW. An ultrastructural quantitative investigation of human intradental innervation. J Endod 1981;7:493-499.
131. Holland GR, Robinson PP. The number and size of axons at the apex of the cat's canine tooth. Anat Rec 1983;205:215-222.
132. Närhi M, Jyväsjärvi E, Hirvonen T, Huopaniemi T. Activation of heat-sensitive nerve fibres in the dental pulp of the cat. Pain 1982;14:317-326.
133. Närhi MVO. Dentin sensitivity: A review. J Biol Buccale 1985;13:75-96.
134. Närhi MVO, Hirvonen TJ, Hakumäki MOK. Activation on intradental nerves in the dog to some stimuli applied to the dentine. Arch Oral Biol 1982;27:1053-1058.
135. Hirvonen T, Ngassapa D, Närhi M. Relation of dentin sensitivity to histological changes in dog teeth with exposed and stimulated dentin. Proc Finn Dent Soc 1992;88(suppl 1):133-141.
136. Ahlquist ML, Franzen OG, Edwall LGA, Forss UG, Haegerstam GAT. Quality of pain sensations following local application of algogenic agents on the exposed human tooth pulp: A psychophysiological and electrophysiological study. In: Fields HL (ed). Advances in Pain Research and Therapy, vol 9. New York: Raven Press, 1985:351-359.
137. Hensel H, Mann G. Temperaturschmerz und Wärmeleitung im menschlichen Zahn. Stoma 1956;9:76-85.
138. Dong WK, Shiwaku T, Kawakami Y, Chulder EH. Static and dynamic responses of periodontal ligament mechanoreceptors and intradental mechanoreceptors. J Neurophysiol 1993;69:1567-1582.
139. Paphangkorakit J, Osborn JW. The effect of pressure on a maximum incisal bite force in man. Arch Oral Biol 1997;42:11-17.
140. Paphangkorakit J, Osborn JW. Effects on human maximum bite force of biting on a softer or harder object. Arch Oral Biol 1998;43:833-839.

141. Brännstöm M. A hydrodynamic mechanism in the transmission of pain-producing stimuli through the dentine. In: Anderson DJ (ed). Sensory Mechanisms in Dentine. Oxford: Pergamon Press, 1963:73–79
142. Brännström M, Johnson G. Movements of the dentine and pulp liquids on application of thermal stimuli. An *in vitro* study. Acta Odontol Scand 1970;28:59–70.
143. Hirvonen TJ, Närhi MVO, Hakumäki MOK. The excitability of dog pulp nerves in relation to the condition of the dentin surface. J Endod 1984;10:294–298.
144. Vongsavan N, Matthews B. The relationship between fluid flow in dentine and the discharge of intradental nerves. Arch Oral Biol 1994;39(suppl):140S.
145. Hirvonen T, Närhi M. The effect of dentinal stimulation on pulp nerve function and pulp morphology in the dog. J Dent Res 1986;65:1290–1293.
146. Burgess PR, Perl ER. Myelinated afferent fibers responding specifically to noxious stimulation of the skin. J Physiol 1967;190:541–562.
147. Georgopoulos AP. Functional properties of primary afferent units probably related to pain mechanisms in primate glabrous skin. J Neurophysiol 1976;39:71–83.
148. Närhi M, Haegerstam G. Intradental nerve activity induced by reduced pressure applied to exposed dentine in the cat. Acta Physiol Scand 1983;119:381–386.
149. Kenins P. Responses of single nerve fibres to capsaicin applied to the skin. Neurosci Lett 1982;29:83–88.
150. Brännström M. Observations on exposed dentine and the corresponding pulp tissue. A preliminary study with replica and routine histology. Odont Rev 1962;13: 235–245.
151. Brännström M. The surface of sensitive dentine. Odont Rev 1965;16:293–299.
152. Absi EG, Addy M, Adams D. Dentine hypersensitivity. A study of the patency of dentinal tubules in sensitive and non-sensitive cervical dentine. J Clin Periodontol 1987;14:280–284.
153. Närhi M, Kontturi-Närhi V. Sensitivity and surface condition of dentin—A SEM-replica study [abstract]. J Dent Res 1994;73:122.
154. Pashley DH. Mechanisms of dentin sensitivity. Dent Clin North Am 1990;34:449–473.
155. Pashley DH. Dentin permeability and dentin sensitivity. Proc Finn Dent Soc 1992;88(suppl 1):31–37.
156. Panopoulos P, Gazelius B, Olgart L. Responses of feline intradental sensory nerves to hyperosmotic stimulation of dentine. Acta Odontol Scand 1983;41:369–375.
157. Panopoulos P, Mejare B, Edwall L. Effects of ammonia and organic acids on the intradental sensory nerve activity. Acta Odontol Scand 1983;41:209–215.
158. Horiuchi H, Matthews B. Evidence on the origin of impulses recorded from dentine in the cat. J Physiol 1974;243:797–829.
159. Anderson DJ. Chemical and osmotic excitants of pain in human dentine. In: Anderson DJ (ed). Sensory Mechanisms in Dentine. Oxford: Pergamon, 1963:88–93.
160. Anderson DJ, Matthews B. Osmotic stimulation of human dentine and the distribution of dental pain thresholds. Arch Oral Biol 1967;12:417–426.
161. Anderson DJ, Matthews B, Shelton LE. Variations in the sensitivity to osmotic stimulation of human dentine. Arch Oral Biol 1967;12:43–47.
162. Lilja J, Nordenvall K-J, Brännström M. Dentine sensitivity, odontoblasts and nerves under dessicated or infected experimental cavities. Swed Dent J 1982;6:93–103.
163. Närhi M, Byers MR, Hirvonen T, Dong WK. The effect of external irritation on the morphology and function of pulpal and dentinal nerves. In: Thylstrup A, Leach SA, Qvist V (eds). Dentine and Dentine Reactions in the Oral Cavity [Proceedings of a workshop, 24–28 Feb 1987]. Oxford: IRL Press, 1987:77–84.
164. Byers MR. Effect of inflammation on dental sensory nerves and vice versa. Proc Finn Dent Soc 1992;88 (suppl 1):459–506.
165. Byers MR. Neuropeptide immunoreactivity in dental sensory nerves: Variation related to primary odontoblast function and survival. In: Shimono M, Maeda T, Suda H, Takahashi K (eds). Dentin/Pulp Complex. Tokyo: Quintessence, 1996:124–129.
166. Ngassapa D, Närhi M, Hirvonen T. Effect of serotonin (5-HT) and calcitonin gene-related peptide (CGRP) on the function of intradental nerves in the dog. Proc Finn Dent Soc 1992;88(suppl 1):143–148.
167. Matthews B. Responses of intradental nerves to electrical and thermal stimulation of teeth in dogs. J Physiol 1977;264:461–664.
168. Närhi M, Yamamoto H, Ngassapa M, Hirvonen T. The neurophysiological basis and the role of inflammatory reactions in dentine hypersensitivity. Arch Oral Biol 1994;39(suppl):23S–30S.
169. Yamamoto H, Närhi M. Function of nerve fibers innervating different parts of dentine. Arch Oral Biol 1994; 39(suppl):141S.

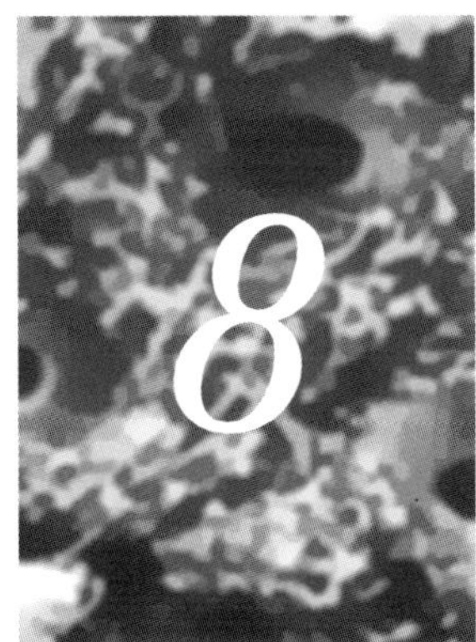

Pain Mechanisms of the Pulpodentin Complex

Kenneth M. Hargreaves, DDS, PhD

The diagnosis and management of pain are foundation skills in clinical dentistry.[1] Although the subject of pain is of considerable significance to all health care providers, the simple reality is that many patients consider *pain* and *dentistry* to be synonymous. This association is even stronger between dental pulp and pain; to many patients, it comes as no surprise that dental pulp is innervated predominantly by pain receptors. Accordingly, this textbook provides an extensive review of mechanisms of pulpal inflammation (see chapters 5, 10, 11, and 12), neuroanatomy and neurophysiology of the dental pulp (see chapter 7), and effective pharmacologic and nonpharmacologic strategies for managing dental pain (see chapter 9). The present chapter contributes to the development of this foundation skill in dental pain therapeutics by reviewing mechanisms of dental pain that arise from dentinal hypersensitivity and pulpal inflammation. This knowledge base should help clinicians to make more accurate diagnoses and to design more effective pain control plans for their patients.

Orofacial pain is one of the most common types of pain, and odontalgia is the most prevalent form of orofacial pain, occurring in nearly 12% to 14% of the population.[2,3] Broadly stated, there are three steps to the perception of acute pain: detection, processing, and perception (Fig 8-1). *Detection* is a primary function of peripheral sensory (afferent) neurons; *processing* is thought to occur largely in the medullary and spinal dorsal horns; and *perception* is the result of activity in more rostral brain regions such as the cerebral cortex. The clinician interacts with all three levels in diagnosing and treating odontalgia.

Transmission of Nociceptive Information to the Central Nervous System

Odontogenic pain is usually caused by either noxious physical stimuli or the release of inflammatory mediators that stimulate receptors located on terminal endings of nociceptive (pain-detecting) afferent nerve fibers (see chapter 7).[4-10] Physical stimuli, via their effect on dentinal fluid flow, can activate the nociceptors that innervate dentinal tubules, leading to the perception of dentinal pain (Fig 8-2). Inflammatory

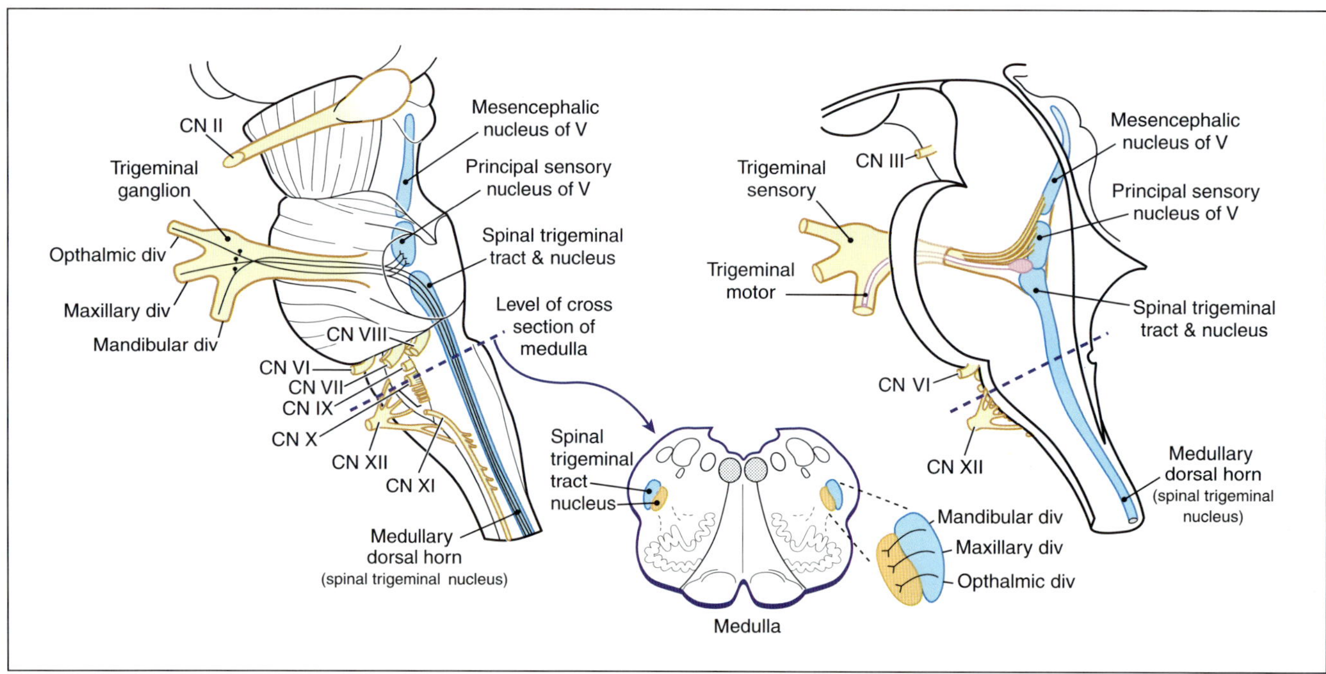

Fig 8-1 General steps in pain transmission in the orofacial region. Detection of noxious injury occurs via primary afferent nociceptors that travel in one of the three divisions of the trigeminal nerve (ophthalmic, maxillary, and mandibular). (In certain chronic pain conditions, detection also may occur by other afferent fibers such as the A-beta fibers.) Processing occurs primarily in the medullary dorsal horn. Nociceptive signaling may be increased by central mechanisms of hyperalgesia or allodynia. Nociceptive signaling may also be reduced by endogenous analgesic systems. The output from the medullary dorsal horn is conveyed predominantly along the trigeminothalamic tract. Perception occurs primarily in the cerebral cortex. Other sensory nerves are also responsible for additional craniofacial signaling (eg, cranial nerves [CN] VII, IX, X, and XII as well as afferent fibers from the cervical spinal cord).

mediators, via activation of their respective receptors, can sensitize or depolarize the nociceptors that innervate pulpal tissue. These topics are discussed in detail later in the chapter. Activation of dental pulp nerves by these physiologic (eg, thermal, mechanical, or chemical) stimuli results in a pure sensation of pain, although experimental studies using certain electrical stimuli can elicit a "prepain" sensation.[10]

Following activation, the C and A-delta fibers from orofacial tissue such as dental pulp transmit nociceptive signals, primarily via trigeminal nerves, to the trigeminal nuclear complex located in the medulla[6,7,11–13] (see Fig 8-1). The trigeminal spinal tract nuclear complex includes the nucleus oralis, nucleus interpolaris, and nucleus caudalis. Trigeminal sensory neurons provide input to all three of these nuclei and to other regions, such as the cervical dorsal spinal cord, reticular formation, and solitary tract nucleus.[13] The nucleus caudalis is an important, but not exclusive, site for processing orofacial nociceptive input.[12–15] It is not exclusive because the more rostral regions of the trigeminal spinal tract do receive some input from dental pulp nociceptors.[16]

The nucleus caudalis has been termed the *medullary dorsal horn* because its anatomic organization is similar to that of the spinal dorsal horn and its caudal extent merges with the cervical extent of the spinal dorsal horn. The medullary dorsal horn is not simply a relay station where nociceptive signals are passively transferred to higher brain regions. Rather, this site plays an important role in processing nociceptive signals, and the output to higher brain regions can be increased (ie, hyperalgesia), decreased (ie, analge-

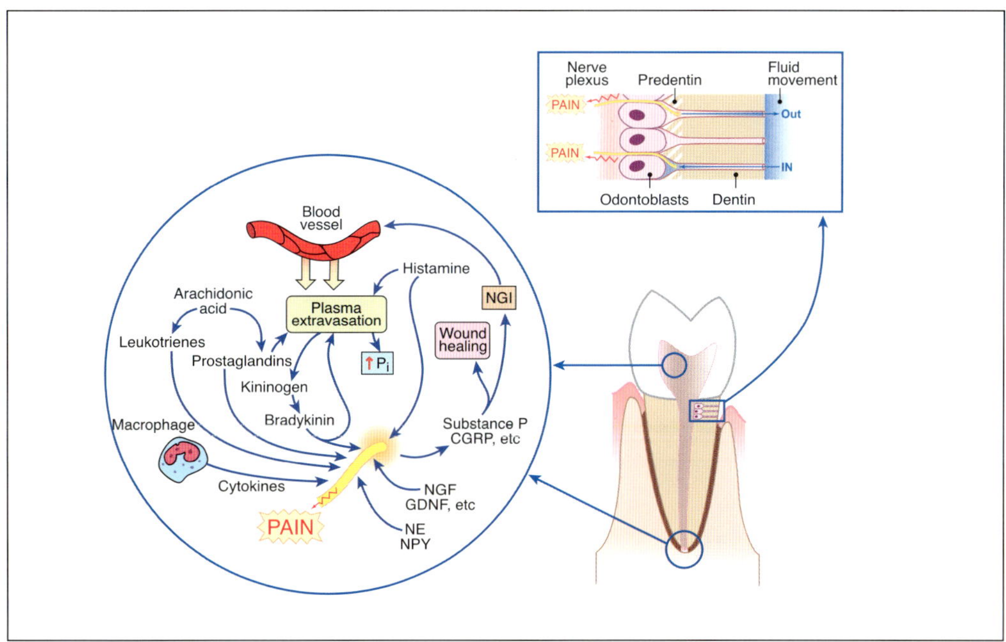

Fig 8-2 Two mechanisms for the peripheral stimulation of nociceptive nerve fibers in tooth pulp. *Acute dentinal pain*: According to the hydrodynamic theory, stimuli that cause fluid movement in exposed dentinal tubules result in the stimulation of nociceptive nerve fibers. *Pain with inflammation*: Inflammation is associated with the synthesis or release of mediators, including prostaglandins, bradykinin, substance P, and histamine (as well as other mediators not shown). The interrelationships of these inflammatory mediators form a positive feedback loop, allowing inflammation to persist far beyond cessation of the dental procedure. NGI, neurogenic inflammation.

sia) or misinterpreted (ie, referred pain) from the incoming activity of the relevant C and A-delta fibers. These three general patterns of processing of nociceptive input (ie, hyperalgesia, analgesia, and referred pain) will be reviewed in this chapter as well as in chapters 7, 9, and 20.

As viewed from a functional perspective, the medullary dorsal horn has five major components related to the processing of nociceptive signals: central terminals of afferent fibers, local circuit interneurons, projection neurons, glia, and terminals from descending neurons. The first component, primary nociceptive afferents (ie, C and A-delta nociceptors), enter the medullary dorsal horn via the trigeminal tract (Figs 8-1 and 8-3). The central terminals of these C and A-delta fibers end primarily in the outer layers of the medullary dorsal horn.

These sensory fibers transmit information by releasing excitatory amino acids such as glutamate or neuropeptides (eg, substance P or calcitonin gene–related peptide [CGRP]). The administration of receptor antagonists to glutamate and substance P in particular, and to CGRP to a lesser extent, reduces hyperalgesia or nociceptive transmission in animal studies.[17-20] Evidence to date strongly implicates antagonists to the glutamate NMDA receptor as being particularly effective in reducing hyperalgesia in animal studies, as will be discussed later. Antagonists to the NMDA and AMPA classes of glutamate receptors are likely to serve as prototypes for future classes of analgesic drugs, and early clinical results in dental pain studies are promising.[4,21] Although animal studies indicate that antagonists to the neurokinin 1 (NK1) class of substance P receptors block

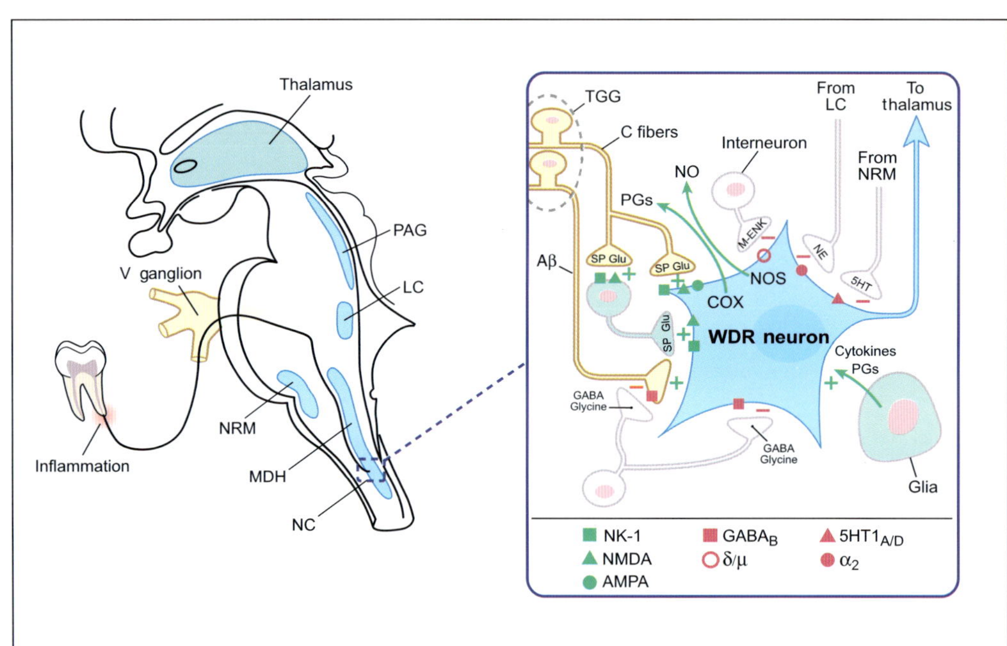

Fig 8-3 Functional processing of nociceptive input in the nucleus caudalis of the medullary dorsal horn (MDH). In this example, activation of pulpal C nociceptive fibers leads to the release of glutamate (Glu) and substance P (SP), which are conveyed across a synapse to a wide-dynamic range (WDR) projection neuron. This projection neuron projects to the thalamus; the information is then relayed to the cortex. Glutamate binds and activates either NMDA or AMPA receptors, while substance P binds and activates the neurokinin 1 (NK-1) receptors. The sensory fibers can directly activate the WDR neuron or indirectly activate it via contacts onto excitatory interneurons. Several signal transduction pathways have been implicated in modulating the responsiveness of projection neurons, including the protein kinase A (PKA) and protein kinase C (PKC) pathways. Projection neurons can themselves modulate nearby cells by synthesis and release of prostaglandins (PGs) via cyclooxygenase (COX) and nitric oxide (NO) via nitric oxide synthase (NOS). Glia can modulate nociceptive processing by release of cytokines (interleukin 1β and tumor necrosis factor) and prostaglandins. Descending terminals of fibers originating in regions such as the nucleus raphe magnus (NRM) or locus coeruleus (LC) can release serotonin (5HT) or norepinephrine (NE). Also depicted are the major proposed receptors for these neurotransmitters. Drugs that alter these receptors or neurotransmitters have potential as analgesics. GABA, γ-aminobutyric acid; PAG, periaquaductal gray.

hyperalgesia, the results from clinical trials have been equivocal, and few studies have shown them to have significant effects on dental pain.[22,23]

Local circuit interneurons are a second component of the dorsal horn, and they regulate transmission of nociceptive signals from the primary afferent fibers to projection neurons.[5,6,13] Interneurons comprise a diverse class of neurons and, depending on their neurotransmitter systems and anatomic connections, can enhance or suppress nociceptive processing (see Fig 8-3).

The third processing component of the dorsal horn is the projection neurons; the cell bodies of these neurons are within the medullary dorsal horn, and their axons comprise the output system for sending orofacial pain information to more rostral brain regions. Three major classes of projection neurons have been described.[5,6] Nociceptive-specific projection neurons receive sensory input from nociceptive afferent fibers. Low-threshold mechanoreceptive projection neurons receive input from non-nociceptors (eg, A-beta fibers). Wide dynamic range (WDR) projection neurons receive input from both nociceptors and non-nociceptors.

A large body of evidence has focused on the role of WDR and nociceptive-specific neurons in encoding orofacial pain, hyperalgesia, and allodynia.[4,7,13,14,15,17] Evidence has accumulated about the receptors and signal transduction pathways in these projection neurons that lead to increased or reduced activity.[24,25] In particular, activation of intracellular protein kinases (eg, protein kinases A and C) and elevation of intracellular calcium levels are thought to lead to facilitated responses to nociceptive input. These projection neurons are also thought to modulate the activity of nearby cells via release of prostaglandins and nitric oxide gas[25] (see Fig 8-3).

A major output pathway for the WDR, nociceptive-specific, and low-threshold mechanoreceptive projection neurons is the trigeminothalamic tract. This tract crosses to the contralateral side of the medulla and ascends to the thalamus (see Figs 8-1 and 8-3). From the thalamus, additional neurons relay this information to the cerebral cortex via a thalamocortical tract.

The perception of pain is thought to occur primarily within the cerebral cortex. The classic clinical studies by Penfield and Rasmussen[26] indicated that a disproportionately large area of the cerebral cortex receives input from orofacial regions (Fig 8-4). Thus, dental procedures that stimulate orofacial structures (eg, lip retraction with a rubber dam) or inflammation of orofacial structures (eg, pulpitis or postoperative inflammation) may activate relatively broad regions of the cerebral cortex.

The glia constitute the fourth component of the medullary dorsal horn involved in pain processing. Although glia have been viewed as merely supportive cells, recent studies strongly implicate their active participation in processing nociceptive input.[27] In the dorsal horn, glia respond to nociceptive input and facilitate the activity of projection neurons by release of cytokines such as interleukin 1β or tumor necrosis factor. Indeed, antagonists to these cytokines have been shown to have central analgesic actions.[28] In peripheral tissues, glia have also been implicated in modulating nociception.[29]

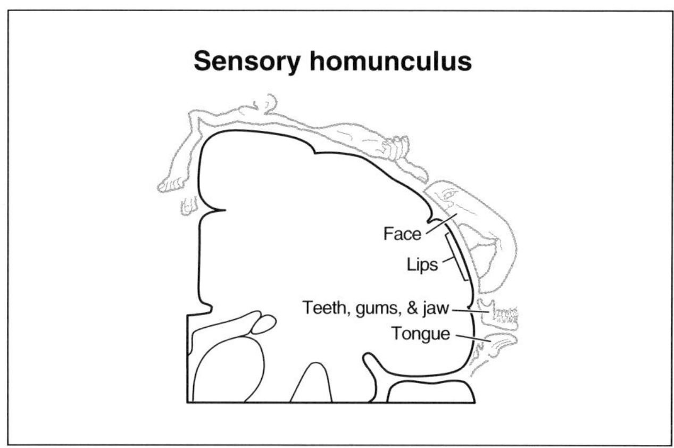

Fig 8-4 Sensory homunculus drawn over a sagittal section of the central gyrus of the cerebral cortex. (Redrawn from Penfield and Rasmussen[26] with permission.)

The fifth component of the medullary dorsal horn consists of the terminal endings of descending neurons (see Fig 8-3). These terminals modulate (inhibit or facilitate) the transmission of nociceptive information. An important component of this endogenous analgesic system is the endogenous opioid peptides (EOPs). The EOPs are a family of peptides that possess many of the properties of exogenous opioids, such as morphine and codeine. The EOP family includes the enkephalins, dynorphins , and β-endorphin–related peptides.

Endogenous opioid peptides are found at several levels of the pain suppression system. This fact underlies the analgesic efficacy of endogenous and exogenous opioids, because their administration conceivably activates opioid receptors located at all levels of the neuraxis. The EOPs are probably released during dental procedures, because blockade of the actions of endogenous opioids by administration of the antagonist nalox-

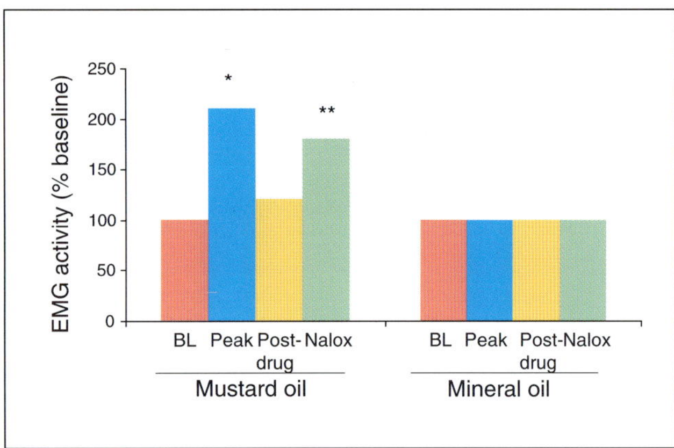

Fig 8-5 Effect of stimulation of dental pulp nociceptors on masseter muscle electromyographic (EMG) activity in anesthetized rats. Either mustard oil or its vehicle was injected into maxillary first molars. EMG data are presented as a percentage of baseline (BL) activity. Data were collected at 30 minutes after drug administration (postdrug), and then both groups of animals were administered naloxone (nalox), an opiate receptor antagonist (1.2 mg/kg, intravenously). $^*P < .05$ (ANOVA) versus baseline. $^{**}P < .05$ versus mustard oil. (Data from Sunakawa et al.[33])

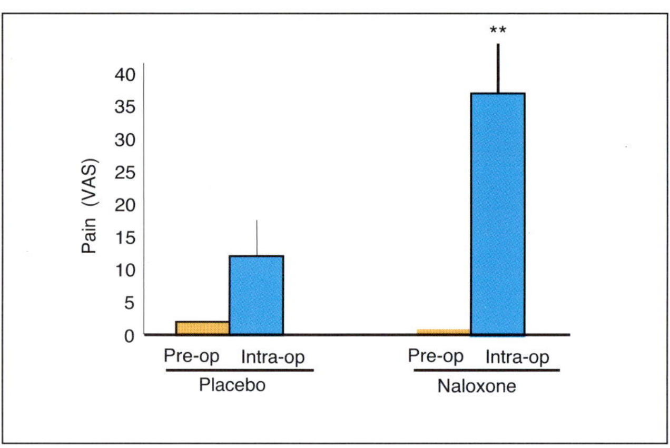

Fig 8-6 Effect of naloxone administration versus placebo on intraoperative pain levels in dental patients undergoing surgical removal of impacted third molars. Patients were anesthetized with local anesthetic and, 10 minutes into surgery, were given an intravenous injection of either naloxone (10 mg) or placebo on a double-blinded randomized basis. $^{**}P < .01$ (ANOVA). VAS, visual analog scale (0 to 100). (Data from Hargreaves et al.[30])

one can significantly increase the perception of dental pain.[30-32] In animal studies, application of mustard oil to dental pulp produces a profound increase in muscle activity, and this effect is enhanced by naloxone[33] (Fig 8-5). In humans, administration of naloxone significantly increases pain perception during dental procedures[30] (Fig 8-6). Collectively, these studies indicate that orofacial pain activates an endogenous analgesic system involving the release of opioids and that blockade of this system by naloxone increases pain perception.

Another example is the endogenous cannabinoid system that inhibits central terminals of C fibers; hypoactivity of this system may mediate some forms of chronic pain.[34,35] Cannabinoids may have profound effects for modulating pain because there are about 10 times more cannabinoid receptors than opioid receptors in the central nervous system. Additional studies have demonstrated cannabinoid receptors on sensory neurons and dental pulp, where they may act to inhibit peripheral terminals of unmyelinated nociceptors.[36-38]

These studies indicate that pain is not simply the result of a noxious stimulus applied to a tooth. Instead, the stimulus must be detected and transmitted to the medullary dorsal horn, where significant processing occurs. In addition, the pattern of peripheral input plays an important role in mediating and modulating pain perception.[8] According to the classic "gate control" theory of pain, activity of larger-diameter low-threshold mechanoreceptors is thought to reduce pain perception, and this is the basis for therapeutic approaches such as transcutaneous electrical nerve stimulation (TENS).[13] However, double-blind randomized clinical trials have indicated that TENS has only a minor effect on altering pulpal pain thresholds[39] (Fig 8-7). Furthermore, systematic reviews of the literature regarding TENS suggest that this effect is not observed consistently in well-controlled trials.[39,40] Thus, TENS may not provide substantial control of dental pain.

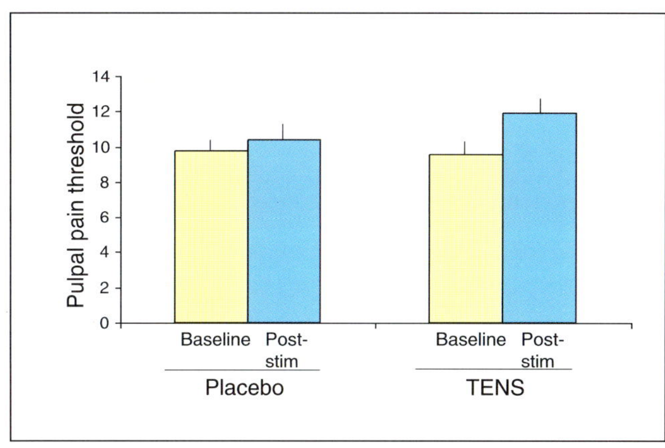

Fig 8-7 Lack of a significant effect of active transcutaneous electrical stimulation (TENS) versus placebo TENS on pulpal pain thresholds in 107 noncarious maxillary first premolars. Teeth were stimulated with an electrical pulp tester (DP2000; 10-millisecond rectangular pulses at 6 Hz with a 3.61-mm^2 contact surface applied to the incisal edge; scale 0 to 32). On a double-blind, randomized basis, patients received placebo TENS or active TENS stimulation (extraoral monopolar 250-millisecond rectangular waves at 160 Hz with pads placed at apices of premolars just inferior to the zygoma). Teeth were then tested 15 minutes later. Error bars represent standard error of the mean. (Redrawn from Schafer et al[39] with permission.)

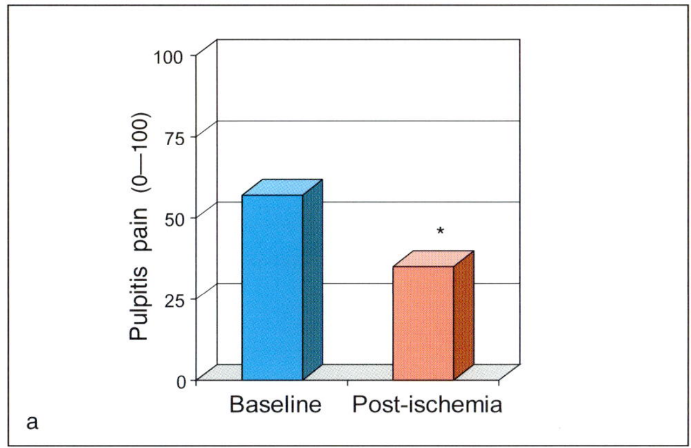

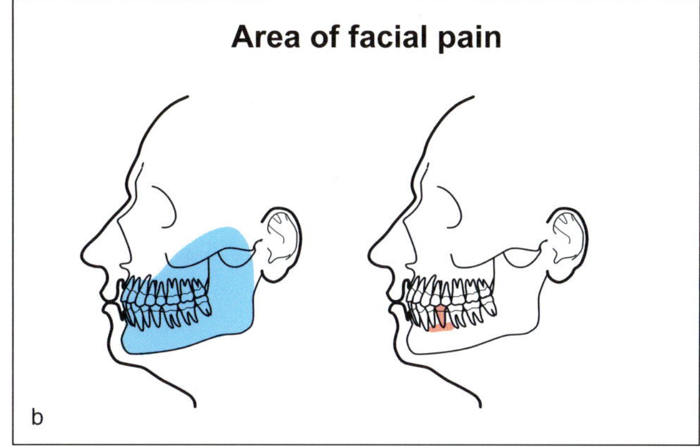

Fig 8-8 Effect of activation of nociceptors from a distant body region on magnitude and area of referred pain in patients with irreversible pulpitis (N = 10). *(a)* Patients with a clinical diagnosis of irreversible pulpitis reported the magnitude of their perceived pain (0 to 100 scale) at baseline and 5 minutes after exercise-induced ischemic pain tolerance (tourniquet applied to forearm prior to exercise). *$P < .05$ (*t* test). *(b)* Drawings of pain referred onto face from one patient at baseline and 5 minutes after ischemic pain test. (Redrawn from Sigurdsson and Maixner[41] with permission.)

Other studies have evaluated whether noxious stimulation of distant body sites can reduce pain perception in other parts of the body. The concept that "pain suppresses pain" or, more formally, of diffuse noxious inhibitory control, has considerable support from animal studies.[13] Clinical studies have provided support for this concept as well. For example, in one study, ischemic muscle pain (application of a tourniquet to a forearm during exercise) significantly reduced pain from irreversible pulpitis[41] (Fig 8-8). Not only was the magnitude of pain reduced, but the area of referred pain was also substantially reduced. These data indicate that the pain arising from pulpitis can be modulated by concurrent input from nociceptors that innervate distant parts of the body.

However, similar studies conducted in patients with temporomandibular pain indicate that ischemic forearm muscle pain does not reduce their temporomandibular pain.[42] Thus, the central modulatory system regulating pulpitis pain is different from the systems regulating temporomandibular pain.[42]

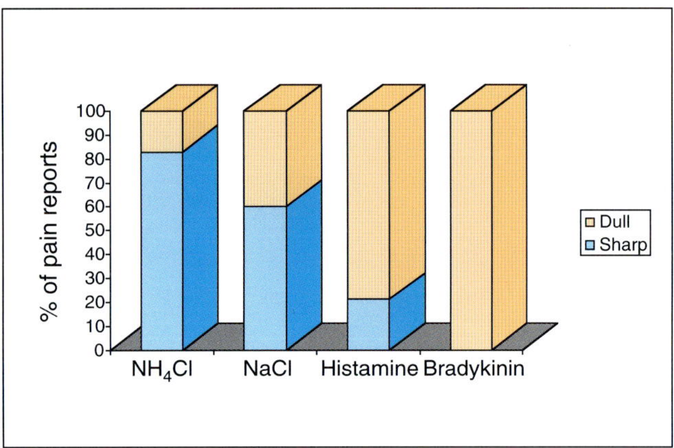

Fig 8-9 Effect of application of inorganic ions or inflammatory mediators to exposed human dental pulp. Volunteers received mepivacaine anesthesia and had their pulp exposed via a Class V cavity preparation. After recovery from anesthesia, the cavity preparations (N = 16) were dried, and test solutions of ammonium chloride (NH_4Cl; 0.77 mol/L), sodium chloride (NaCl; 0.77 mol/L), histamine (10 mg/mL), or bradykinin (10 μg/mL) were placed on the surface of the pulp. The stimulus period was less than 3 minutes, and the interstimulus interval was 5 minutes. The quality of the evoked pain was recorded after application of the test agent. (Redrawn from Ahlquist et al[46] with permission.)

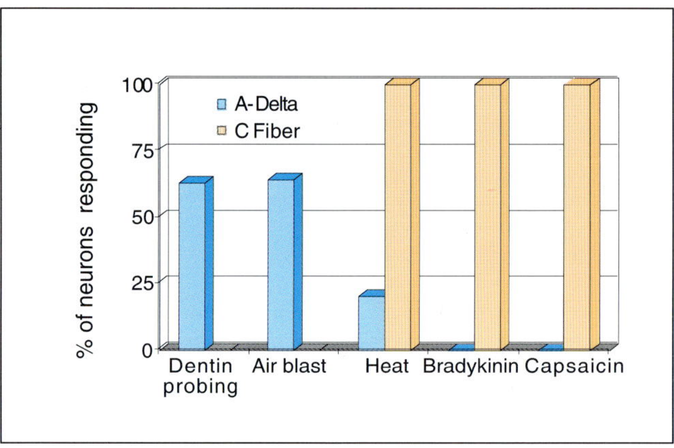

Fig 8-10 Responsiveness of pulpal A-delta afferent neurons and pulpal C afferent neurons to different stimuli applied to deep dentinal cavity preparations in anesthetized cats. (Reprinted from Närhi et al[47] with permission.)

Mechanisms of Dental Pain Caused by Inflammation

Pulpal C nociceptors are thought to have a predominant role in encoding inflammatory pain arising from dental pulp and periradicular tissue. This hypothesis is supported by the distribution of C fibers in dental pulp, their responsiveness to inflammatory mediators, and the strikingly similar perceptual qualities of pain associated with C fiber activation and pulpitis (ie, dull, aching pain).[43-45] Figure 8-9 illustrates the perceptual pain response reported by volunteers in whom inorganic ions or inflammatory mediators were administered to exposed dental pulp.[46] Application of histamine and bradykinin primarily produced reports of dull, aching pain.

Similar results have been observed in electrophysiologic studies evaluating the responsiveness of A-delta and C afferent neurons to stimuli applied to deep cavity preparations[47] (Fig 8-10). The A-delta fibers respond to stimulation of dentinal tubules (eg, air blast), whereas pulpal C fibers respond to bradykinin or capsaicin.[47] Collectively, these and other studies have implicated pulpal A-delta fibers in mediating dentinal sensitivity and pulpal C afferent fibers in mediating pulpal inflammation (see Fig 8-2).

The response to tissue inflammation or infection is complex and involves the coordinated release of multiple classes of inflammatory mediators that display distinct profiles of substance concentration over time (see chapters 10 and 11).[48] In the inflamed dental pulp, the terminals of nociceptive primary afferents detect the presence of inflammatory mediators with receptors that are synthesized in the afferent fiber's cell body and then transported to the periphery. If the mediator reaches a concentration in the inflamed tissue sufficient to activate the receptor, the nociceptive neuron could become activated (ie, the membrane would be depolarized and the signal would be conducted to the central nervous system or sensitized (see Fig 8-2). A sensitized nociceptor displays spontaneous depolarization, reduced threshold for depolarization, and increased after-discharges to suprathreshold stimuli.

Some inflammatory mediators activate these terminals (eg, bradykinin), while others potentiate the effects of inflammatory mediators (eg, prostaglandins). For example, prostaglandin E_2 substantially increases the stimulatory effect of bradykinin[49] (Fig 8-11). Therefore, the combination of mediators present is probably more important than the presence of any one mediator in determining the physiologic response to inflammation. Other inflammatory mediators may produce persistent effects. For example, nerve growth factor is expressed in inflamed dental pulp (see chapter 7), and a single injection of nerve growth factor to humans can evoke pain and allodynia that last up to 1 month.[50,51] This process of nociceptor sensitization has important clinical implications, because it contributes to the altered pain states of hyperalgesia and allodynia.[4,52]

Signal transduction studies have revealed some of the fundamental mechanisms mediating the actions of inflammatory mediators and drugs on sensory neurons.[24,25,53–55] For example, inflammatory mediators whose receptors couple to the G_q guanosine triphosphate binding protein, leading to activation of the protein kinase C pathway of second messengers, activate nociceptors. This includes bradykinin. On the other hand, inflammatory mediators whose receptors couple to the G_s guanosine triphosphate binding protein, leading to activation of the protein kinase A pathway of second messengers, sensitize nociceptors. This includes the prostaglandins. Finally, drugs that activate receptors coupled to the G_i guanosine triphosphate protein tend to be analgesics. This includes opiates, cannabinoids, and adrenergic agonists. This is a simplification of a very active research front that is likely to lead to fundamental advances in the knowledge of pain mechanisms and in the development of new classes of analgesic drugs.

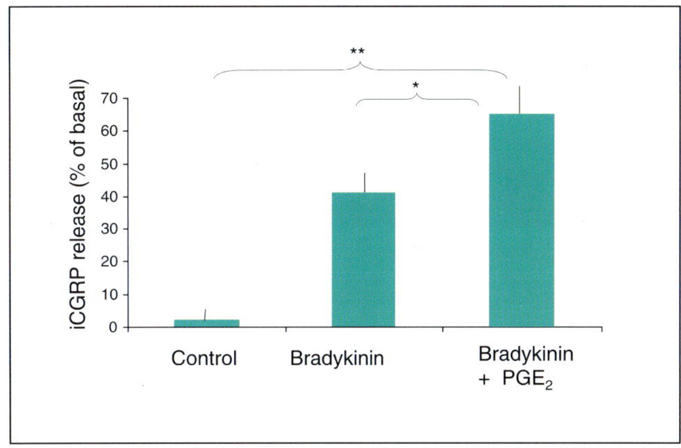

Fig 8-11 Effect of bradykinin alone and with prostaglandin E_2 (PGE_2) on release of immunoreactive calcitonin gene–related peptide (iCGRP) from isolated superfused bovine dental pulp slices. Tissue was pretreated with bradykinin alone or with bradykinin and PGE_2, and released levels of iCGRP were measured by a radioimmunoassay. $^*P < .05$ (ANOVA); $^{**}P < .01$ (ANOVA). (Redrawn from Goodis et al[49] with permission.)

Allodynia and hyperalgesia

The pain system can undergo dramatic changes in response to certain peripheral stimuli, leading to the development of allodynia and hyperalgesia.[19,5,13,20,56,57] These changes do not necessarily take weeks to develop but under certain conditions can occur within a few seconds or minutes after an appropriate stimulus. For example, extensive hyperalgesia and allodynia occur in humans a few minutes after stimulation of cutaneous C nociceptors by injection of capsaicin.[58]

Hyperalgesia is defined as an increase in the perceived magnitude of a painful stimulus and *allodynia* is defined as a reduction in pain threshold so that previously non-noxious stimuli are perceived as painful. Many persons have experienced

Table 8-1 Evaluation of hyperalgesia and allodynia in endodontic diagnostic tests*

Sign of hyperalgesia or allodynia	Related diagnostic test or symptom
Spontaneous pain	Spontaneous pain
Reduced pain threshold	Percussion test; palpation test; throbbing pain
Increased response to painful stimuli	Increased response to pulp test (electrical or thermal pulp test)

*Reprinted from Hargreaves et al[59] with permission.

these altered pain states; common examples include a sunburn or a thermal injury. In the example of a sunburn, the pain experienced when a T-shirt is worn is allodynia (ie, reduced pain threshold), whereas the increased pain responsiveness experienced when someone slaps the burned skin is hyperalgesia (ie, increased pain perception).

Allodynia or hyperalgesia can occur during inflammation of pulpal or periradicular tissue. The outcome of endodontic diagnostic tests and a patient's symptoms can be used to determine the presence of allodynia or hyperalgesia[59] (Table 8-1). Put another way, the systematic evaluation of allodynia or hyperalgesia represents the biologic rationale for endodontic diagnostic tests.

In many cases, endodontic pain occurs as a triad of spontaneous pain, hyperalgesia, and allodynia. For example, percussion of a tooth with a mirror handle (or pain on mastication) tests for the presence of allodynia: a reduction in the mechanical nociceptive thresholds of neurons innervating the periodontal ligament. Under normal conditions, this innocuous stimulation does not elicit pain. However, under conditions of acute inflammation, the mechanical pain threshold is reduced to the point at which tapping with a mirror handle is now perceived as tender or painful.

Similarly, studies in cats have shown that pulpal inflammation lowers the mechanical threshold of pulpal fibers to the level at which increases in systolic blood pressure can activate pulpal neurons. The synchrony of firing of pulpal fibers in response to the heartbeat is thought to mediate the "throbbing" pain of pulpitis.[43,50] Additional studies have shown that the thermal threshold of nociceptors can be reduced to the point at which normal physiologic temperature (ie, 37°C) can activate these peripheral neurons. This may explain why some patients use ice water to relieve pain from severe, irreversible pulpitis, because the neurons would be expected to stop firing when the tissue is cooled. Accordingly, the study of mechanisms and management of allodynia and hyperalgesia are important issues in managing dental pain.

Peripheral mechanisms of allodynia and hyperalgesia

Hyperalgesia is due to both peripheral and central mechanisms.[4,5,7,8,13,14] Several mechanisms have been proposed to contribute to peripheral hyperalgesia (Box 8-1). As mentioned, the concentration and composition of various inflammatory mediators are important and can lead to activation or sensitization of nociceptors (see Fig 8-2). The concentration of the inflammatory mediator is important because tissue levels must be sufficiently high to permit binding and activation of the receptor. For example, prostaglandin E_2 levels are more than 100-fold greater in pulp samples collected from teeth with irreversible pulpitis than they are in normal control teeth[73] (Fig 8-12).

Moreover, heat-induced inflammation in pulp sensitizes pulpal afferent fibers by local release of prostaglandins, because this effect is blocked by pretreatment with nonsteroidal anti-inflammatory drugs such as indomethacin, naproxen, or diclofenac[74] (Fig 8-13). Heat-induced inflammatory changes can occur clinically from tooth preparation procedures performed with insufficient water spray (additional pulpal responses are dis-

Box 8-1 Peripheral mechanisms contributing to allodynia and hyperalgesia*

- Composition and concentration of inflammatory mediators[49,53–55,59]
- Changes in afferent fiber: activation and sensitization[43,58,60–62]
- Changes in afferent fiber: sprouting[63–66]
- Changes in afferent fiber: proteins[4,63–65]
- Tissue pressure[43,47]
- Tissue temperature[67]
- Sympathetic-primary afferent fiber interactions[68–70]
- A-beta fiber plasticity[20,71]

*Modified from Hargreaves et al[72] with permission.

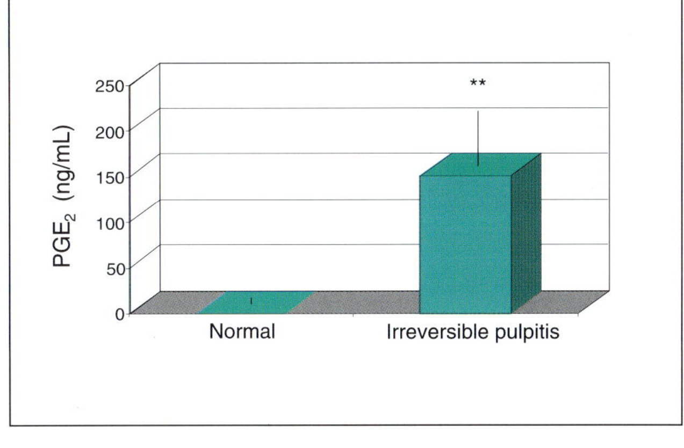

Fig 8-12 Pulpal levels of prostaglandin E_2 (PGE_2) in specimens taken from control pulps (normal diagnosis) (N = 21) and those with irreversible pulpitis (N = 21). Specimens were collected on a nylon pellet, and pulpal levels of immunoreactive PGE_2 were measured by enzyme immunoassay. $^{**}P < .01$ (Mann-Whitney *U* test). (Redrawn from Nakanishi et al[73] with permission.)

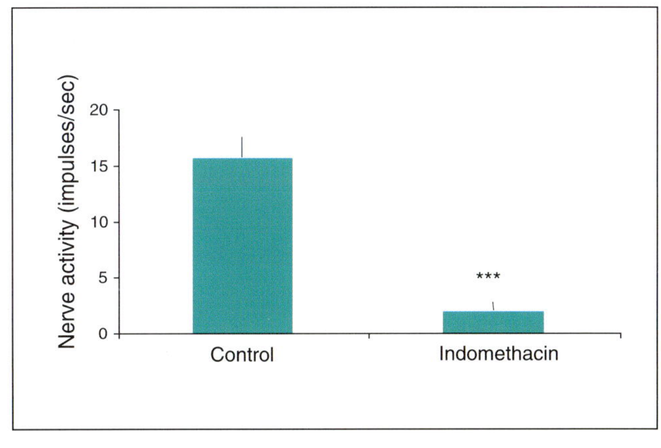

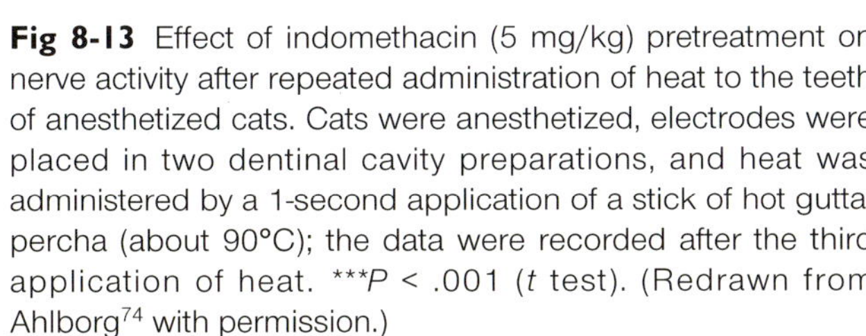

Fig 8-13 Effect of indomethacin (5 mg/kg) pretreatment on nerve activity after repeated administration of heat to the teeth of anesthetized cats. Cats were anesthetized, electrodes were placed in two dentinal cavity preparations, and heat was administered by a 1-second application of a stick of hot gutta-percha (about 90°C); the data were recorded after the third application of heat. $^{***}P < .001$ (*t* test). (Redrawn from Ahlborg[74] with permission.)

cussed in detail in chapters 6 and 13). From a clinical perspective, these studies support the use of the nonsteroidal class of analgesics to treat pulpitis (see chapter 9).

Dental procedures such as the incision and drainage of an abscess or a pulpectomy may reduce pain by reducing concentrations of mediators as well as by lowering tissue pressure. Many inflammatory mediators found in inflamed pulp or periradicular tissue (see chapters 10 and 11) can either activate or sensitize nociceptors and evoke pain when administered to human volunteers. Considerable research is being directed toward clarifying the mechanisms of sensitization of nociceptors in the hope that this information will lead to the development of new classes of analgesic drugs.[75,76]

In addition to activation and sensitization, the peripheral afferent fiber responds to mediators such as nerve growth factor by increasing protein synthesis of substance P and CGRP and by sprouting terminal fibers in the inflamed tissue (see chapter 7).[50,63–65] Similar increases in neuropeptides are seen in human pulp infected by caries.[77] Sprouting increases the density of innervation in inflamed tissue and may contribute to

Box 8-2 Central mechanisms contributing to allodynia and hyperalgesia*

- Increased neurotransmitter release from primary afferent fibers[87]
- Changes in postsynaptic receptors[88]
- Changes in second messenger systems[24,89,90]
- Changes in proto-oncogenes[91,92]
- Changes in endogenous opioids or cannabinoids[30,31,34,91]
- Central sensitization[4,20,93,94]
- Reduced presynaptic inhibition[20,24]
- Reduced postsynaptic inhibition[20,24]
- Windup[20]
- Dark neurons[95]
- Activation of glia[27,28]

*Modified from Hargreaves et al[72] with permission.

increased pain sensitivity in chronic pulpal or periradicular inflammation.[50,63]

Certain afferent fibers also respond to inflammatory mediators by synthesizing other proteins, such as tetrodotoxin (TTX) -resistant sodium channels.[75,78,79] These ion channels are synthesized by a major class of nociceptors and undergo activation by inflammatory mediators.[80-82] Unlike the typical class of TTX-sensitive sodium channels found on sensory neurons, TTX-resistant sodium channels are poorly blocked by local anesthetics. Indeed, it takes about four times more lidocaine to block TTX-resistant channels as it takes to block the typical class of TTX-sensitive ion channels.[83] Given this disparity in lidocaine potency, the synthesis of new types of ion channels on sensory neurons may well contribute to difficulty in obtaining local anesthesia in certain cases of endodontic pain. Indeed, interventions that block the expression of one member of the class of TTX-resistant sodium channels (ie, the PN_3 channel) have a significant effect in reducing nociception in rat models of inflammatory and neuropathic pain.[84]

Several other peripheral mechanisms may contribute to allodynia or hyperalgesia. For example, A-beta fibers are normally thought to be low-threshold mechanoreceptors that do not convey nociceptive signals. However, under certain inflammatory conditions, A-beta fibers begin to express substance P and develop new central terminations in the dorsal spinal cord, now innervating regions that contain nociceptive neurons.[71,85] Thus, it is possible that certain pain conditions may have an allodynic component because of nociceptive transmission by A-beta fibers. Other studies have implicated sympathetic fibers in the activation of C nociceptive afferent fibers after certain forms of tissue injury.[70] Taken together, several peripheral mechanisms contribute to the development of allodynia and hyperalgesia. However, not all of these mechanisms are necessarily equally active in all acute and chronic pain states, and this has led to the concept of developing mechanistically based pain diagnoses.[59,86]

Central mechanisms of allodynia and hyperalgesia

In addition to these peripheral mechanisms, several central mechanisms of hyperalgesia have also been proposed[4,19,20,56,72] (Box 8-2). Central sensitization is the increased excitability of central neurons and is thought to be a major mechanism of hyperalgesia.[20] Central sensitization results from a barrage of impulses from C nociceptors. This results in the central release of glutamate and substance P (as well as other neurotransmitters), leading to activation of central receptors for glutamate (eg, NMDA and AMPA receptors) and for substance P (eg, NK1 receptor) (see Fig 8-3). Under these conditions, stimulation of the normally low-threshold A-beta fibers now produces a much larger response, and this may provide a central mechanism of allodynia.

Several other mechanisms for central sensitization have been proposed and are included in Box 8-2. The concept of central sensitization is important because it implies a dynamic responsiveness of the central nervous system to peripheral input. Put another way, the same stimulus does not always produce the same response.

Activation of pulpal neurons produces a central sensitization.[13,17,33] Application of mustard oil to the pulp of a rat maxillary molar activates pulp-

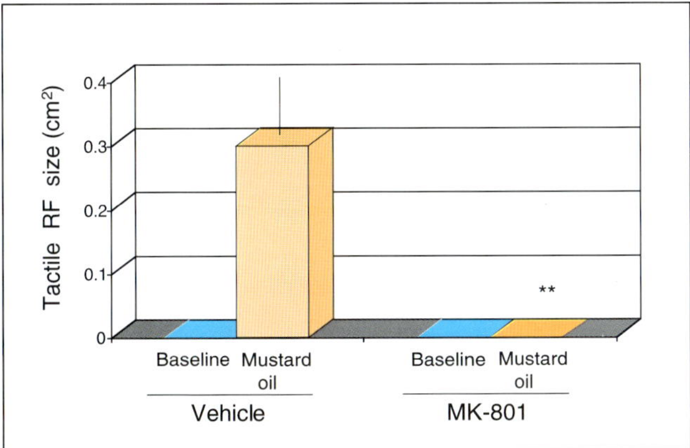

Fig 8-14 Effect of application of mustard oil on pulpal neurons in the rat. Application induces a central sensitization via glutamate release. Anesthetized rats had mustard oil applied to the pulp of a maxillary first molar with simultaneous recordings from nociceptive-specific neurons in the nucleus caudalis. The area of the maxillary skin that activated the nociceptive-specific neurons after light tactile stimulation was recorded as the tactile receptive field (RF) size. Animals were pretreated with either vehicle or an antagonist to the glutamate NMDA receptor (MK-801) before mustard oil was administered to the pulp. $^{**}P < .01$ (ANOVA) versus vehicle treatment. (Redrawn from Chiang et al[17] with permission.)

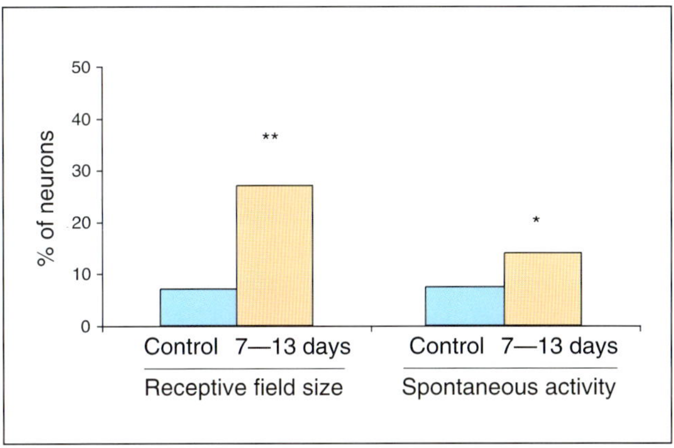

Fig 8-15 Effects of pulpotomy in rat mandibular molar on mechanoreceptive field and spontaneous activity of central neurons located in the trigeminal subnucleus oralis under control conditions and 7 to 13 days after pulpotomy. $^{*}P < .05$ (chi-square test); $^{**}P < .01$ (chi-square test). (Redrawn from Kwan et al[96] with permission.)

al neurons and evokes more than a five-fold increase in the discharge rate of nociceptive-specific neurons located in the nucleus caudalis.[17] This barrage of pulpal C fibers is sufficient to produce a central sensitization, because 20 minutes later there is an enhanced response to light tactile stimuli applied to the maxillary skin (Fig 8-14). This central sensitization is mediated by release of glutamate, because pretreatment with an antagonist to the glutamate NMDA receptor (MK-801) abolishes this effect. Thus, activation of pulpal nociceptors can induce central sensitization via central release of glutamate, and this effect is sufficient to produce an allodynic-like response over the maxillary skin region.[17]

Pulpotomy can also evoke a central sensitization, as measured by both an expansion of receptive field sizes and an increase in spontaneous activity in the nucleus oralis[96,97] (Fig 8-15). In addition, central terminals of afferent fibers continue to exhibit increased release of CGRP, even after removal from the animal.[87] Thus, even in the absence of peripheral input, central mechanisms of hyperalgesia or allodynia can persist for some time.

Because at least some components of allodynia or hyperalgesia can persist even without continued sensory input from inflamed tissue, it is not surprising that up to 80% of patients experiencing pain before endodontic treatment continue to report pain after treatment.[98,99] Thus, even if the endodontic treatment has removed all peripheral factors contributing to hyperalgesia, the central mechanisms can still persist for some time. Indeed, the presence of preoperative hyperalgesia (operationally measured as preoperative pain or allodynia) is a risk factor for the occurrence of postendodontic pain[100] (Fig 8-16). Patients with moderate or severe preoperative pain tended to report greater pain levels for 3 days

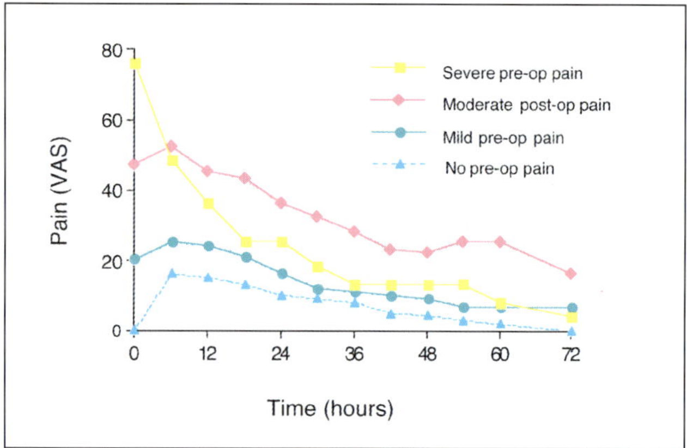

Fig 8-16 Time-response curves for postendodontic pain in patients given a placebo analgesic. Patients were subdivided into four groups based on the magnitude of their preoperative pain. Patients with moderate or severe preoperative pain tended to report greater levels of pain throughout the postendodontic (cleaning and shaping) treatment. VAS, visual analog scale (0 to 100). (Redrawn from Torabinejad et al[100] with permission.)

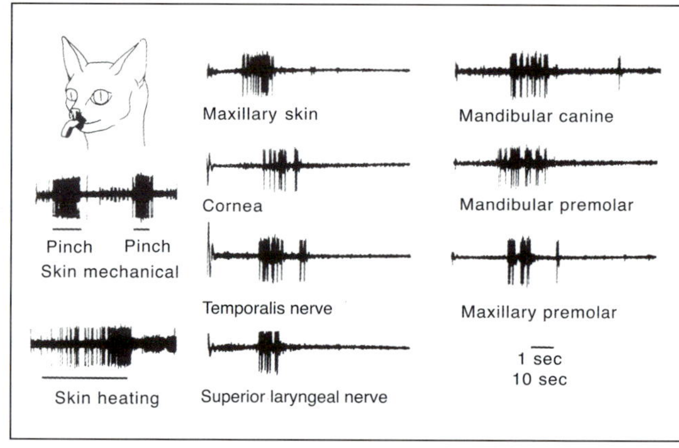

Fig 8-17 Example of convergence of multiple sensory neurons onto the same central neuron in the nucleus caudalis of an anesthetized cat. The receptive field (RF) for the neuron was in the maxillary region. The figure shows the depolarizations of the neuron in the nucleus caudalis to stimulation in various orofacial regions. (Reprinted from Sessle et al[102] with permission.)

after endodontic cleaning and shaping than did patients reporting either no or mild preoperative pain.[48] The presentation of this risk factor should alert the clinician to adjust the pain management strategy for higher levels of pain control (see chapter 9).[48] It is apparent that the mechanisms of allodynia and hyperalgesia are clinically significant factors in understanding strategies for diagnosing and managing endodontic pain.

Referred pain

Referred pain is the condition in which pain is perceived to be localized in one region but is caused by nociception originating from another area. In referred pain, the region of the body where pain is perceived to occur is not the same as the region where the pain originates. Clearly, referred pain represents a diagnostic challenge to the clinician because effective treatment must be directed to the site where pain originates (see also chapter 20).

Suda and colleagues[101] have nicely summarized peripheral and central mechanisms of referred pain. Peripheral mechanisms include branching axons that innervate different structures and axonal reflexes. Central mechanisms include muscle contractions, central sensitization, memory, and convergence of primary afferents. These hypotheses are not mutually exclusive and may contribute to various cases of referred pain. For example, there is good experimental evidence that central sensitization and convergence of primary afferents may mediate many cases of referred pain.

Evidence exists that the central terminals of trigeminal afferent fibers converge onto the same projection neurons. For example, nociceptors in the maxillary sinus and maxillary molars may stimulate the same neuron located in the nucleus caudalis.[12,13,102] About 50% of neurons in the nucleus caudalis exhibit convergence of sensory input from cutaneous and visceral structures.[12] In one example, a single neuron in the nucleus caudalis received input from sensory neurons innervating the maxillary skin, cornea, a mandibular canine, a mandibular premolar, and a maxillary premolar[102] (Fig 8-17). Thus, the clinical problem of referred pain has a biologic basis in the convergence of sensory neurons onto the same central projection neuron.

The theory of convergence has been used to explain the clinical observation of a patient who complains of pain that originates from an inflamed mandibular molar and radiates to the preauricular region or of pain that originates in inflamed maxillary sinuses and radiates to the maxillary posterior teeth. Thus, pain can originate from the dental pulp and be referred to distant regions or, conversely, can originate from distant regions and be referred back to the dental pulp (see also chapter 20).

The latter has been demonstrated in patients with chronic orofacial pain. In patients with trigger points in the superior belly of the masseter, pain can be referred to maxillary posterior teeth[103] (Fig 8-18). Conversely, in patients with trigger points in the inferior border of the masseter muscle, pain can be referred to the mandibular posterior teeth. Thus, it is important to consider multiple diagnostic tests to determine the origin of the patient's pain.

The convergence theory forms the basis for the diagnostic use of local anesthetics in establishing the origin of pain in patients who present with diagnostic challenges. For example, Okeson[104] described the selective injection of local anesthetics as a clinical test to distinguish the site of pain origin from the area of pain referral.

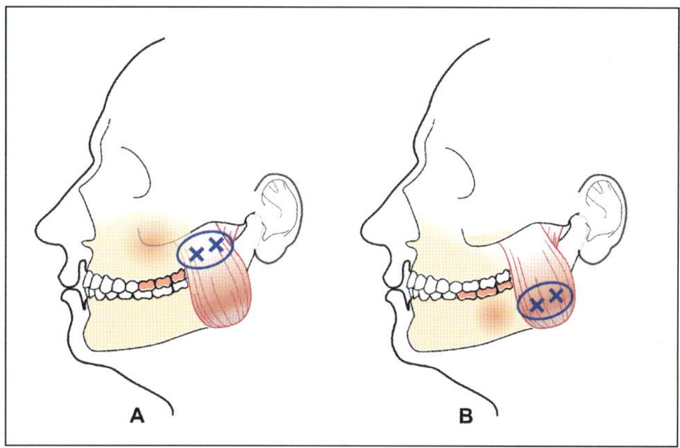

Fig 8-18 Referral patterns in patients with chronic orofacial pain. *(A)* Patients with trigger zones in the superior belly of the masseter have pain referred to regions including the maxillary posterior teeth. *(B)* Patients with trigger zones in the inferior belly of the masseter have pain referred to regions including the mandibular posterior teeth. (Redrawn from Travell and Simons[103] with permission.)

Mechanisms of Dentinal Hypersensitivity

Hydrodynamic theory of dentinal hypersensitivity

Dentinal sensitivity is characterized as a sharp pain that occurs soon after a provoking stimulus.[105] Dentinal tubules are well innervated near the pulp horns (see chapter 7). In this region, up to 74% of the tubules contain nerve fibers, and these fibers can extend up to 200 μm into the tubule (see Fig 8-2). At the midcrown level of the pulp, fewer tubules are innervated, and the intratubule extension of the fibers is shorter. In contrast, root dentin is poorly innervated.

For all innervated tubules, the nerve fibers are in close proximity to odontoblasts, although direct connections are not evident.[50] However, the proximity of these two cell types is consistent with the hypothesis that odontoblasts and afferent terminal endings may have biochemical connections (eg, via expression of receptors and paracrine release of soluble factors) and thereby participate in the sensory transduction of noxious stimuli.

This anatomic relationship between nerve fibers and odontoblasts may be the physiologic basis for the hydrodynamic theory of dentinal pain. This theory, which has strong experimental support, postulates that movement of fluid through the dentinal tubules results in pain.[106–109] Stimuli, including air blasts, cold, and hypertonic sugars ("sweets"), can produce movement of the dentinal fluid. Movement of this fluid results in

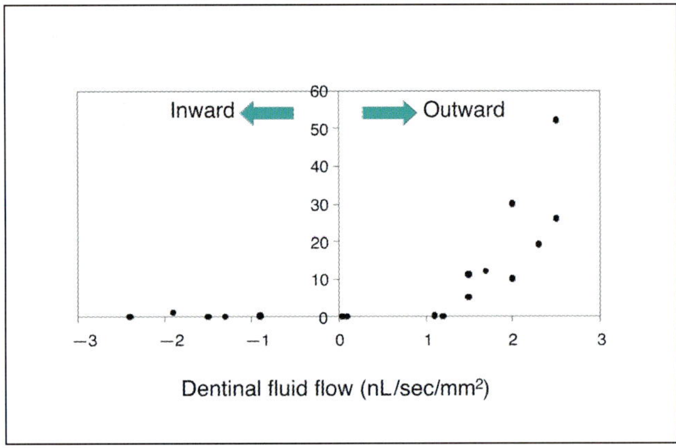

Fig 8-19 Effect of velocity of dentinal fluid flow on the responses of an A-delta fiber that innervates dentin in the anesthetized cat. (Redrawn from Matthews et al[111] with permission.)

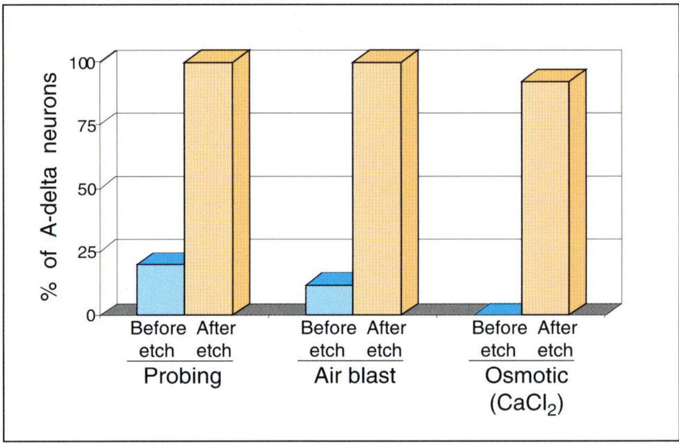

Fig 8-20 Effect of acid etching on the responsiveness of A-delta afferent fibers to stimuli applied to exposed dentin in anesthetized dogs. N = 23 to 25. (Reprinted from Närhi et al[114] with permission.)

stimulation of nociceptive nerve fibers located on the pulpal side of the dentinal tubules[110,111] (Fig 8-19). The fluid movement is thought to serve as a fluid transducer, signaling the presence of stimuli at the outer opening of the dentinal tubules. Indeed, removal of dentinal fluid abolishes the ability to detect these stimuli; sensitivity returns when the fluid is replenished.[112]

It is not known how nerve fibers detect fluid movement. However, the sharp quality of the resulting pain suggests activation of A-delta nociceptive fibers[43,47,105] (see Figs 8-9 and 8-10).

Dentinal sensitivity appears to recede with age or after chronic irritation. The increase in secondary or reparative dentin during these processes is thought to diminish the flow of fluid through the tubules.[113]

Following exposure of dentin, either by loss of enamel or by loss of cementum and gingiva, dentinal sensitivity can develop. Researchers have reported that there is a large increase in A-delta fiber's responsiveness to dentinal stimulation after an acid-etching procedure is performed on exposed dentin[114] (Fig 8-20). The responsiveness to mechanical (eg, probing), drying (eg, air blast), and osmotic stimuli is increased. The buccal surfaces of canines and premolars are common sites of dentinal exposure, probably because of their susceptibility to toothbrush-induced abrasion.[115]

Effects of pulpal inflammation on dentinal sensitivity

Dentinal sensitivity is not an invariant sensation. The responsiveness to dentinal stimulation increases not only with exposure of dentinal tubules (see Fig 8-20) but also in the presence of inflammatory mediators. For example, the administration of the inflammatory mediator leukotriene B4 to deep dentinal preparations increases the responsiveness to osmotic stimuli[61] (Fig 8-21). In an actual model of pulpal inflammation, there is a three-fold increase in the receptive field size of A-delta fibers innervating inflamed dog teeth[43,47,50,66,116] (Fig 8-22). This may result from the sprouting of A-delta fibers and the resultant increase in the area of innervated dentinal tubules. Thus, pulpal inflammation may predispose a tooth to enhanced dentinal sensitivity by reducing the threshold for activation and by increasing the area of innervated dentinal tubules.

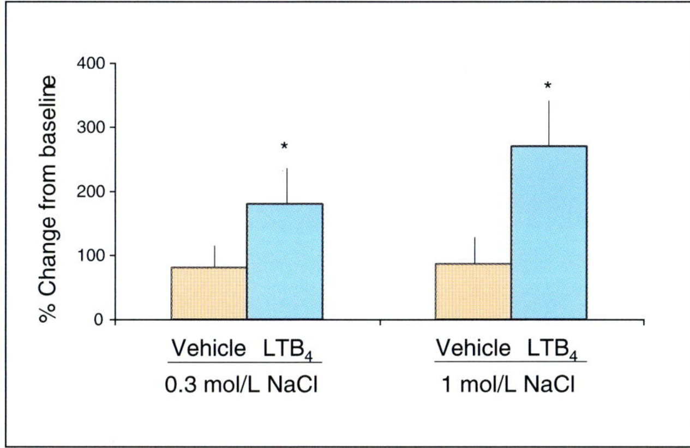

Fig 8-21 Effect of administration of leukotriene B_4 (LTB_4) or vehicle on dentinal sensitivity to osmotic stimuli. LTB_4 (25 mg/mL) or vehicle was applied to exposed dentin in anesthetized cats; electrodes were placed in cavities for intradentinal recordings. Administration of LTB_4 significantly enhanced responsiveness to osmotic stimuli (0.3 and 1.0 mol/L of sodium chloride [NaCl]) applied to the exposed dentin. $*P < .05$ (ANOVA) versus vehicle. (Redrawn from Madison et al[61] with permission.)

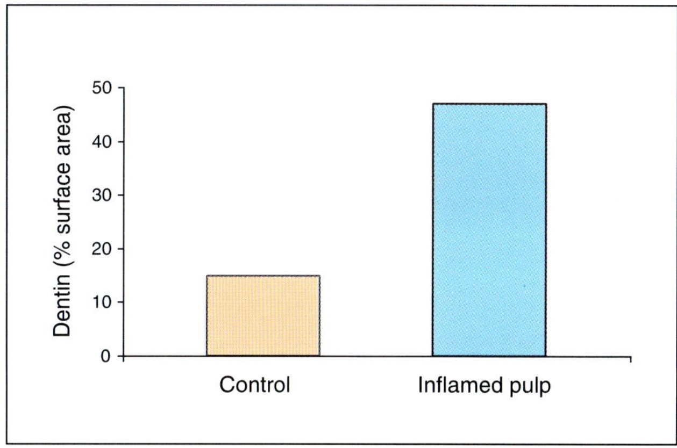

Fig 8-22 Effect of pulpal inflammation on the receptive field size of A-delta fibers innervating the dentin of dog teeth. The teeth underwent resection of the coronal portion of the crown 1 week before the experiment. On the day of the experiment, dogs were anesthetized, single units were isolated, and the exposed dentin was probed to determine the area of innervated dentin. (Redrawn from Närhi et al[66] with permission.)

Pulpal Vitality Testing

One aspect of the diagnosis of pain is the determination of pulpal vitality. The importance of assessing vascular integrity to establish pulpal vitality was discussed in chapter 6. However, methods for assessing vascular integrity are generally not well validated or amenable to all clinical applications. Accordingly, responsiveness to various pulpal stimuli has been used as a surrogate measure of pulpal vitality.[117] In general, this involves the use of electrical or thermal testing or preparation of a test cavity; the patient's response is an outcome measure.

Accepted techniques, such as the use of control teeth interspersed with the suspected tooth, have been described in clinical texts, and the reader is encouraged to review this material.[118] This section will review factors that modify outcomes in electrical and thermal testing and will review studies on sensitivity and specificity.

A common method for assessing pulpal responsiveness is the use of electrical stimuli.[118,119] Under certain conditions, electrical stimuli can elicit a "prepain" sensation that is distinct from pain.[10] The primary factors that affect the electrical pulpal responsiveness test include electrode design (monopolar versus bipolar), electrode surface area, pulse duration, pulse strength (current and voltage), pulse frequency, electrode position (eg, incisal versus gingival), restorative status of the test teeth, and patient health. In general, the amount of current required to activate pulpal A-delta afferent fibers is only about 25% of that required to activate C fibers[120]; most clinical testing activates only A-delta fibers.

Although most commercially available electrical pulp testers are monopolar (ie, cathode on tooth and anode often on the lip), studies have shown that bipolar electrodes (ie, cathode and anode placed on tooth) provide more consistent effects.[120-122] For example, the coefficient of vari-

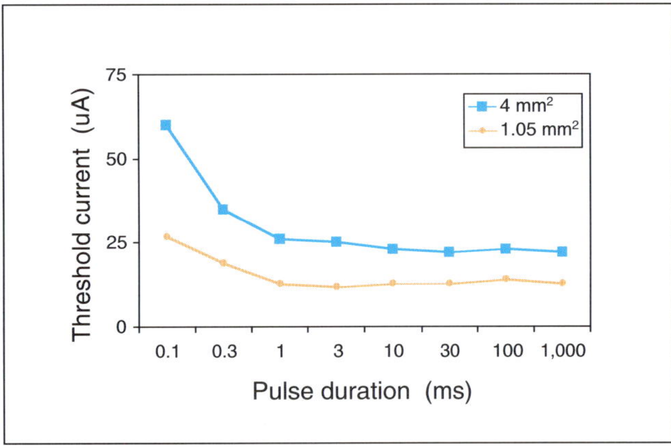

Fig 8-23 Effect of monopolar electrode and stimulation parameters on the threshold for pain perception in humans. Electrodes (1.05-mm^2 or 4-mm^2 surface area) were placed on exposed dentin, and the parameters were evaluated to determine if they caused positive test responses (ie, pain perception threshold of electrical stimulus). (Redrawn from Mumford and Newton[123] with permission.)

ation (a measure of the noise-signal ratio) for bipolar electrode stimulation of A-delta fibers is about 35% less than that for monopolar stimulation of the same units.[121]

The density of the electrical current also plays an important role in this test. Increasing surface area of electrodes requires greater current to produce a detectable sensation, and, at any given electrode area, shorter pulse widths require greater current to produce a sensation[123] (Fig 8-23). This is an important concept because the density of the current is the result of these parameters as well as the pulpal anatomy.

When results in different types of teeth or results from younger patients and older patients (with smaller pulp chambers) are compared, the current delivered cannot be directly compared, because the pulpal anatomy differs. Studies have indicated that electrical testing produces the most consistent effects when the electrode is placed on the incisal or cuspal edge of the tooth.[124,125] In a study of more than 7,000 posterior teeth, electrical testing of the mesiobuccal cusp of mandibular molars gave the lowest response threshold, and, in general, electrical thresholds increased with patient age.[126] Other factors that influence electrical testing include the restorative status of the tooth (eg, porcelain is an insulator) and even the patient's health (hypertensive patients have significantly, although modestly, higher thresholds for electrical testing).[127]

Alternative testing methods include the application of cold or hot stimuli to the tooth.[44,105,128–131] Commonly used cold stimuli include ethyl chloride spray, dichlorodifluoromethane, dry ice (ie, frozen carbon dioxide), and wet ice (ie, frozen water). In general, the response to application of cold stimuli is measured as a positive or negative reaction. This technique is probably used more often than application of hot stimuli.

Commonly used hot stimuli include heated gutta-percha (applied to a lubricated tooth surface) and electrical heat sources (Touch 'N Heat, System B, etc). The initial response to heat is a sharp sensation; if the stimulus is maintained for a sufficient period of time, a dull, aching sensation is perceived. These sensations appear to be mediated by A-delta and C fibers, respectively.

All clinical tests are subject to false-positive (ie, a positive response from a necrotic pulp) and false-negative (ie, a negative response from a vital pulp) results.[132,133] A recent study compared the cold test (ethyl chloride) to an electrical pulp test (Analytic Technology Pulp Tester) to the "gold standard" (endodontic access and clinical verification of vitality) in 59 teeth of unknown pulpal status.[133] The probability that a negative test meant a true necrotic pulp was similar for the cold and electrical tests (89% versus 88%); the hot gutta-percha test was much lower in its ability to detect a true negative (48%). In addition, the probability that a positive test represented a true vital pulp was similar for the cold, electrical, and hot gutta-percha tests (90%, 84%, and 83%, respectively). Overall, the cold and electrical tests had similar accuracy values (86% versus 81%), and both were more accurate than the heat test (71%).

Other studies have reported that the cold test is more accurate (80%) in testing human teeth (N = 50) than the electrical test (64% for monopolar electrodes).[134] In one study of more than 1,000 teeth, two different electrical testers each produced significantly more false-positive results than did the cold test (about five-fold higher). Even when gingival controls were employed, one commercial electrical tester produced about two-fold greater false positives than the cold test.[135]

Conclusions

A review of the mechanisms of pulpodentinal pain has numerous clinical implications. First, dentinal pain is primarily due to myelinated fibers innervating dentinal tubules where fluid movement is detected and signaled back to the brain. Therapeutic reduction of dentinal fluid movement or neuronal activation can reduce dentinal hypersensitivity. Second, inflammation is detected by receptors expressed on pulpal nociceptors; the binding of inflammatory mediators onto these receptors can activate or sensitize these nociceptors. Drugs that reduce tissue levels of inflammatory mediators (eg, NSAIDs) relieve pain by reducing activation of these receptors. Third, hyperalgesia and allodynia can occur during pulpal and periradicular inflammation. Evaluation of the presence of these altered pain states provdes the biologic basis for endodontic diagnostic tests. Fourth, hyperalgesia and allodynia can occur by both peripheral and central mechanisms, and may persist beyond the dental appointment. Thus, patients with preoperative pain have an increased risk of experiencing postoperative pain. Fifth, referred pain is due, in part, to convergence of multiple sensory fibers onto the same central projection neuron. Sixth, pulp testing, using either electrical or thermal stimuli, requires an appreciation of the mechanisms involved for proper interpretation of tooth and patient conditions, and for minimization of potential confusion due to false positive or false negative results.

References

1. Bender IB. Pulpal pain diagnosis—A review. J Endod 2000;26:175–179.
2. Lipton J, Ship J, Larach-Robinson D. Estimated prevalence and distribution of reported orofacial pain in the United States. J Am Dent Assoc 1993;124:115–121.
3. Locker D, Grushka M. Prevalence or oral and facial pain and discomfort: Preliminary results of a mail survey. Community Dent Oral Epidemiol 1987;15:169–172.
4. Woolf C. Transcriptional and posttranslational plasticity and the generation of inflammatory pain. Proc Natl Acad Sci USA 1999;96:7723–7730.
5. Willis W. The Pain System: The Neural Basis of Nociceptive Transmission in the Mammalian Nervous System. Basel: Karger, 1985.
6. Light AR. The Initial Processing of Pain and its Descending Control: Spinal and Trigeminal Systems. Basel: Karger, 1992.
7. Hargreaves KM, Milam S. Mechanisms of pain and analgesia. In: Dionne R, Phero J (eds). Management of Pain and Anxiety in Dental Practice. New York: Elsevier, 2001:18–40.
8. Hargreaves KM. Peripheral mechanisms of inflammatory pain, In: Sessle B, Dubner R, Lavigne G (eds). Orofacial Pain: From Basic Science to Clinical Management. Chicago: Quintessence, 2001:59–66.
9. Lund J, Lavigne G, Dubner R, Sessle B (eds). Orofacial Pain: From Basic Science to Clinical Management. Chicago: Quintessence, 2001.
10. Brown A, Beeler W, Kloka A, Fields R. Spatial summation of pre-pain and pain in human teeth. Pain 1985;21: 1-16
11. Sessle B. Neurophysiology of orofacial pain. Dent Clin North Am 1987;31:595–613.
12. Sessle BJ. Recent developments in pain research: Central mechanisms of orofacial pain and its control. J Endod 1986;12:435–444.
13. Sessle BJ. Acute and chronic craniofacial pain: Brainstem mechanisms of nociceptive transmission and neuroplasticity, and their clinical correlates. Crit Rev Oral Biol Med 2000;11:57–91.
14. Dubner R, Bennett G. Spinal and trigeminal mechanisms of nociception. Ann Rev Neurosci 1983;6: 381–418.
15. Maixner W, Dubner R, Kenshalo DR, Bushnell MC, Oliveras JL. Responses of monkey medullary dorsal horn neurons during the detection of noxious heat stimuli. J Neurophysiol 1989;62:437–439.
16. Dallel R, Clavelou P, Woda A. Effects of tractotomy on nociceptive reactions induced by tooth pulp stimulation in the rat. Exp Neurol 1989;106:78–84.
17. Chiang C, Park S, Kwan C, Hu J, Sessle B. NMDA receptor mechanisms contribute to neuroplasticity induced in caudalis nociceptive neurons by tooth pulp stimulation. J Neurophysiol 1998;80:2621–2631.

18. Ren K, Iadarola M, Dubner R. An isobolographic analysis of the effects of N-methyl-D-aspartate and NK1 tachykinin receptor antagonists on inflammatory hyperalgesia in the rat. Br J Pharmacol 1996;117:196–202.
19. Dubner R, Basbaum AI. Spinal dorsal horn plasticity following tissue or nerve injury. In: Wall PD, Melzack R (eds). Textbook of Pain. Edinburgh: Churchill-Livingston, 1996:225–241.
20. Woolf C. Windup and central sensitization are not equivalent. Pain 1996;66:105–108.
21. Gilron I, Max M, Lee G, Booher S, Sang C, Chappell A, et al. Effects of the 2-amino-3-hydroxy-5-methyl-4-isoxazole-proprionic acid/dainate antagonist LY293558 on spontaneous and evoked postoperative pain. Clin Pharmacol Ther 2000;68:320–327.
22. Hill R. NK1 (substance P) receptor antagonists—Why are they not analgesic in humans? Trends Pharmacol Sci 2000;21:244–246.
23. Dionne RA, Max MB, Gordon SM, Parada S, Sang C, Gracely RH, et al. The substance P receptor antagonist CP-99,994 reduces acute postoperative pain. Clin Pharmacol Ther 1998;64:562–568.
24. Wilcox G, Seybold V. Pharmacology of spinal afferent processing. In: Yaksh T, Maze M, Lynch C, Biebuyck J, Zapol W, Saidman L (eds). Anesthesia: Biologic Foundations. Philadelphia: Lippincott, 1997:557–576.
25. Yaksh T, Malmberg A. Central pharmacology of nociceptive transmission. In: Wall P, Melzack R (eds). Textbook of Pain, ed 3. London: Churchill-Livingston, 1994: 165–200.
26. Penfield W, Rasmussen G. The Cerebral Cortex of Man. New York: MacMillan, 1950.
27. Watkins LR, Milligan ED, Maier SF. Glial activation: A driving force for pathological pain. Trends Neurosci 2001;24:450–455.
28. Sweitzer SM, Schubert P, DeLeo JA. Propentofylline, a glial modulating agent, exhibits antiallodynic properties in a rat model of neuropathic pain. J Pharmacol Exp Ther 2001;297:1210–1217.
29. Pomonis JD, Rogers SD, Peters CM, Ghilardi JR, Mantyh PW. Expression and localization of endothelin receptors: Implications for the involvement of peripheral glia in nociception. J Neurosci 2001;21:999–1006.
30. Hargreaves KM, Dionne R, Goldstein D, Mueller G, Dubner R. Naloxone, fentanyl and diazepam modify plasma beta-endorphin levels during surgery. Clin Pharmacol Ther 1986;40:165–171.
31. Gracely R, Dubner R, Wolskee P, Deeter, W. Placebo and naloxone can alter post-surgical pain by separate mechanisms. Nature 1983;306:264–265.
32. Levine J, Gordon N, Fields H. The mechanism of placebo analgesia. Lancet 1978;2:654–657.
33. Sunakawa M, Chiang C, Sessle BJ. Jaw electromyographic activity induced by the application of algesic chemicals to the rat tooth pulp. Pain 1999;80:493–501.
34. Richardson JD, Aanonsen L, Hargreaves KM. Hypoactivity of the spinal cannabinoid system results in an NMDA-dependent hyperalgesia. J Neurosci 1998;18:451–457.
35. Richardson JD, Aanonsen L, Hargreaves KM. Antihyperalgesic effect of spinal cannabinoids. Eur J Pharmacol 1998;345:145–153.
36. Hohmann AG, Herkenham M. Cannabinoid receptors undergo axonal flow in sensory nerves. Neuroscience 1999;92:1171–1175.
37. Wurm C, Richardson JD, Bowles W, Hargreaves KM. Evaluation of functional G-protein receptors in dental pulp. J Dent Res 1998;77:160.
38. Richardson JD, Kilo S, Hargreaves KM. Cannabinoids reduce hyperalgesia and inflammation via interaction with peripheral CB1 receptors. Pain 1998;75:111–119.
39. Schafer E, Finkensiep H, Kaup M. Effect of transcutaneous electrical nerve stimulation on pain perception threshold of human teeth: A double-blind, placebo-controlled study. Clin Oral Invest 2000;4:81–86.
40. McQuay H, Moore R. An Evidence-Based Resource for Pain. Oxford, England: Oxford University Press, 1998: 172–178.
41. Sigurdsson A, Maixner W. Effects of experimental and clinical noxious counterirritants on pain perception. Pain 1994;57:265–275.
42. Maixner W, Sigurdsson A, Fillingham R, Lundeen T, Booker D. Regulation of acute and chronic orofacial pain. In: Fricton J, Dubner R (eds). Orofacial Pain and Temporomandibular Disorders. Seattle: IASP Press, 1995:85–102.
43. Närhi M. The characteristics of intradental sensory units and their responses to stimulation. J Dent Res 1985;64:564–571.
44. Ahlquist ML, Franzen OG. Inflammation and dental pain in man. Endod Dent Traumatol 1994:10:201–209.
45. Mumford J, Bowsher D. Pain and protopathic sensibility: A review with particular relevance to teeth. Pain 1975;2:223–243.
46. Ahlquist M, Franzen O, Edwall L, Fors U, Haegerstam G. Quality of pain sensations following local application of algogenic agents on the exposed human tooth pulp: A pyschophysical and electrophysiological study. In: Fields H (ed). Advances in Pain Research and Therapy, vol 9. New York: Raven Press, 1985:351–359.
47. Närhi M, Jyvasjarv E, Virtanen A, Huopaniemi T, Ngassapa D, Hirvonen T. Role of intradental A and C type nerve fibers in dental pain mechanisms. Proc Finn Dent Soc 1992;88:(suppl 1):507–516.
48. Hargreaves, KM, Hutter JW. Endodontic pharmacology. In: Cohen S, Burns R (eds). Pathways of the Pulp, ed 8. St Louis: Mosby, 2002:665–682.
49. Goodis H, Bowles W, Hargreaves KM. Prostaglandin E_2 enhances bradykinin-evoked iCGRP release in bovine dental pulp. J Dent Res 2000;79:1604–1607.

50. Byers MR, Närhi MVO. Dental injury models: Experimental tools for understanding neuroinflammatory nociceptor functions. Crit Rev Oral Biol 1999;10:4-39.
51. Petty B, Cornblath D, Flexner C, Wachsman M, Sinicropi D, Burton L, et al. The effect of systemically administered recombinant human nerve growth factor in healthy human subjects. Ann Neurol 1994;36:244-246.
52. Lewin G, Rueff A, Mendell L. Peripheral and central mechanisms of NGF-induced hyperalgesia. Eur J Neurosci 1994;6:1903-1912.
53. Julius D, Basbaum AI. Molecular mechanisms of nociception. Nature 2001;413:203-210.
54. Dray A. Inflammatory mediators of pain. Br J Anaesth 1995;75:125-131.
55. Southall MD, Vasko MR. Prostaglandin receptor subtypes, EP3C and EP4, mediate the prostaglandin E2-induced cAMP production and sensitization of sensory neurons. J Biol Chem 2001;276:16083-16091.
56. Dubner R, Ruda MA. Activity-dependent neuronal plasticity following tissue injury and inflammation. Trends Neurosci 1992;15:96-103.
57. Hargreaves KM, Keiser K. Development of new pain management strategies. J Dent Educ (in press).
58. LaMotte RH, Lundberg LE, Torebjork HE. Pain, hyperalgesia and activity in nociceptive C units in humans after intradermal injection of capsaicin. J Physiol 1992; 448:749-764.
59. Hargreaves KM, Swift JQ, Roszkowski MT, Bowles WR, Garry MG, Jackson DL. Pharmacology of peripheral neuropeptide and inflammatory mediator release. Oral Surg Oral Med Oral Pathol 1994;78:503-510.
60. Kumazawa T, Mizumura K. Thin-fiber receptors responding to mechanical, chemical and thermal stimulation in the skeletal muscle of the dog. J Physiol 1977;273:179-194.
61. Madison S, Whitsel E, Suarez-Roca H, Maixner W. Sensitizing effects of leukotriene B4 on intradental primary afferents. Pain 1992;49:99-104.
62. Schaible H, Schmidt R. Discharge characteristics of receptors with fine afferents from normal and inflamed joints: Influence of analgesics and prostaglandins. Agents Actions 1986;19:99-117.
63. Byers M, Taylor P, Khayat B, Kimberly C. Effects of injury and inflammation on pulpal and periapical nerves. J Endod 1990;16:78-84.
64. Byers MR. Dynamic plasticity of dental sensory nerve structure and cytochemistry. Arch Oral Biol 1994;39 (suppl):13S-21S.
65. Buck S, Reese K, Hargreaves KM. Pulpal exposure alters neuropeptide levels in inflamed dental pulp: Evaluation of axonal transport. J Endod 1999;25: 718-721.
66. Närhi M, Yamamoto H, Ngassapa D. Function of intradental nociceptors in normal and inflamed teeth. In: Shimono M, Maeda T, Suda H, Takahashi K (eds). Dentin/Pulp Complex. Tokyo: Quintessence, 1996: 136-140.
67. Meyer R, Campbell J. Myelinated nociceptive afferents account for the hyperalgesia that follows a burn to the hand. Science 1981;213:1527-1529.
68. Janig W, Kollmann W. The involvement of the sympathetic nervous system in pain. Arzneimittelforschung 1984;34:1066-1073.
69. Levine J, Moskowitz M, Basbaum A. The contribution of neurogenic inflammation in experimental arthritis. J Immunol 1985;35:843S-847S.
70. Perl E. Causalgia, pathological pain and adrenergic receptors. Proc Natl Acad Sci USA 1999;96:7664-7667.
71. Neumann S, Doubell T, Leslie T, Woolf C. Inflammatory pain hypersensitivity mediated by phenotype switch in myelinated primary sensory neurons. Nature 1996;384:360-364.
72. Hargreaves KM, Roszkowski M, Jackson D, Bowles W, Richardson JD, Swift J. Neuroendocrine and immune responses to injury, degeneration and repair. In Sessle B, Dionne R, Bryant P (eds). Temporomandibular Disorders and Related Pain Conditions. Seattle: IASP Press, 1995:273-292.
73. Nakanishi T, Matsuo T, Ebisu S. Quantitative analysis of immunoglobulins and inflammatory mediators in human pulpal blood from exposed pulps. J Endod 1995;21:131-136.
74. Ahlborg K. Dose-dependent inhibition of sensory nerve activity in the feline dental pulp by anti-inflammatory drugs. Acta Physiol Scand 1978;102:434-440.
75. Eglen R, Hunter J, Dray A. Ions in the fire: Recent ion-channel research and approaches to pain therapy. Trends Pharmacol Sci 1999;20:337-342.
76. Rang H, Bevan S, Dray A. Nociceptive peripheral neurons: Cellular properties. In: Wall PD, Melzack R (eds). Textbook of Pain. Edinburgh: Churchill-Livingston, 1996:57-77.
77. Boissonade FM. Substance P expression in human tooth pulp in relation to caries and pain experience. Eur J Oral Sci 2000;108:467-474.
78. Akopian A, Soulsova V, England S, Okuse K, Ogata N, Ure J, et al. The tetrodotoxin-resistant sodium channel SNS has a specialized function in pain pathways. Nat Neurosci 1999;2:541-548.
79. Waxman S, Dib-Haji S, Cummnis T, Black J. Sodium channels and pain. Proc Natl Acad Sci USA 1999;96: 7635-7639.
80. Arbuckle JB, Docherty RJ. Expression of tetrodotoxin-resistant sodium channels in capsaicin-sensitive dorsal root ganglion neurons of adult rats. Neurosci Lett 1995;85:70-73.

81. Gold M, Reichling D, Shuster M, Levine JD. Hyperalgesic agents increase a tetrodotoxin-resistant Na+ current in nociceptors. Proc Nat Acad Sci USA 1996;93: 1108–1112.
82. Gold M. Tetrodotoxin-resistant Na currents and inflammatory hyperalgesia. Proc Natl Acad Sci USA 1999;96: 7645–7649.
83. Roy M, Narahashi T. Differential properties of tetrodotoxin-sensitive and tetrodotoxin-resistant sodium channels in rat dorsal root ganglion neurons. J Neurosci 1992;12:2104–2111.
84. Porreca F, Lai J, Bian D, Wegert S, Ossipov MH, Eglen RM, et al. A comparison of the potential role of the tetrodotoxin-insensitive sodium channels, PN3/SNS and NaN/SNS2, in rat models of chronic pain. Proc Natl Acad Sci USA 1999;96:7640–7644.
85. Coggeshall RE, Lekan HA, White FA, Woolf CJ. A-fiber sensory input induces neuronal cell death in the dorsal horn of the adult rat spinal cord. J Comp Neurol 2001; 435:276–282.
86. Woolf C, Bennett G, Doherty M, Dubner R, Kidd B, Koltzenburg M, et al. Towards a mechanism-based classification of pain? Pain 1998;77:227–229.
87. Garry MG, Hargreaves KM. Enhanced release of immunoreactive CGRP and substance P from spinal dorsal horn slices occurs during carrageenan inflammation. Brain Res 1992;582:139–142.
88. Galeazza M, Stucky C, Seybold V. Changes in [125I]h-CGRP binding in rat spinal cord in an experimental model of acute, peripheral inflammation. Brain Res 1992;591:198–208.
89. Garry MG, Durnett-Richardson J, Hargreaves KM. Carrageenan-induced inflammation alters levels of i-cGMP and i-cAMP in the dorsal horn of the spinal cord. Brain Res 1994;646:135–139.
90. Meller S, Gebhart G. Nitric oxide (NO) and nociceptive processing in the spinal cord. Pain 1993;52:127–136.
91. Draisci G, Iadarola M. Temporal analysis of increases in c-fos, preprodynorphin and preproenkephalin mRNAs in rat spinal cord. Brain Res Mol Brain Res 1989;6: 31–37.
92. Zhou Q, Imbe H, Dubner R, Ren K. Persistent Fos protein expression after orofacial deep or cutaneous tissue inflammation in rats: Implications for persistent orofacial pain. J Comp Neurol 1999;412:276–291.
93. Hylden J, Nahin R, Traub R, Dubner R. Expansion of receptor fields of spinal lamina. I. Projection neurons in rats with unilateral adjuvant-induced inflammation. Pain 1989;37:229.
94. Wall P, Woolf C. Muscle but not cutaneous C-afferent input produces prolonged increases in the excitability of the flexion reflex in the rat. J Physiol 1984;356: 443–458.
95. Sugimoto T, Bennett G, Kajander K. Transsynaptic degeneration in the superficial dorsal horn after sciatic nerve injury: Effects of a chronic constriction injury, transection and strychnine. Pain 1990;42:205–213.
96. Kwan C, Hu J, Sessle BJ. Effects of tooth pulp deafferentation on brainstem neurons of the rat trigeminal subnucleus oralis. Somatosens Motor Res 1993;10: 115–131.
97. Torneck C, Kwan C, Hu J. Inflammatory lesions of the tooth pulp induces changes in brainstem neurons of the rat trigeminal subnucleus oralis. J Dent Res 1996; 75:553–561.
98. Marshall J, Walton R. The effect of intramuscular injection of steroid on posttreatment endodontic pain. J Endod 1984;10:584–588.
99. Marshall J, Liesinger A. Factors associated with endodontic posttreatment pain. J Endod 1993;19: 573–575.
100. Torabinejad M, Cymerman J, Frankson M, Lemon R, Maggio J, Schilder H. Effectiveness of various medications on postoperative pain following complete instrumentation. J Endod 1994;20:345–354.
101. Suda H, Sunakawa M, Yamamoto H. Orofacial referred pain; Its physiological basis and case report. In: Shimono M, Maeda T, Suda H, Takahashi K (eds). Dentin/Pulp Complex. Tokyo: Quintessence, 1996: 79–84.
102. Sessle BJ, Hu JW, Amano N, Zhong G. Convergence of cutaneous, tooth pulp, visceral, neck and muscle afferents onto nociceptive and non-nociceptive neurons in trigeminal subnucleus caudalis (medullary dorsal horn) and its implications for referred pain. Pain 1986;27: 219–235.
103. Travell G, Simons D. Myofascial Pain and Dysfunction. Baltimore: Williams and Wilkins, 1983.
104. Okeson J. Orofacial Pain. Guidelines for Assessment, Diagnosis and Managment. Chicago: Quintessence,1996.
105. Ahlquist M, Franzen O. Encoding the subjective intensity of sharp dental pain. Endod Dent Traumatol 1994; 10:153–166.
106. Brännström M, Astrom A. A study on the mechanism of pain elicited from the dentin. J Dent Res 1964;43: 619–625.
107. Brännström M, Johnson G, Nordenvall KJ. Transmission and control of dentinal pain: Resin impregnation for the desensitization of dentin. J Am Dent Assoc 1979;99:612–618.
108. Trowbridge H. Review of dental pain—Histology and physiology. J Endod 1986;12:445–452.
109. Orchardson R, Gillam DG. The efficacy of potassium salts as agents for treating dentin hypersensitivity. J Orofac Pain 2000;14:9–19.
110. Matthews B, Vongsavan N. Interactions between neural and hydrodynamic mechanisms in dentine and pulp. Arch Oral Biol 1994;39:87S–92S.

111. Matthews B, Andrew D, Amess T, Ikeda H, Vongsavan N. The functional properties of intradental nerves. In: Shimono M, Maeda T, Suda H, Takahashi L (eds). Dentin/Pulp Complex. Tokyo: Quintessence, 1996: 146–153.

112. Lilja J, Nordenvall KJ, Brännström M. Dentin sensitivity, odontoblasts and nerves under desiccated or infected experimental cavities. A clinical, light microscopic and ultrastructural investigation. Swed Dent J 1982;6: 93–103.

113. Dowell P, Addy M, Dummer P. Dentine hypersensitivity: Aetiology, differential diagnosis and management. Br Dent J 1985;158:92–96.

114. Närhi M, Kontturi-Narhi V, Hirvonen T, Ngassapa D. Neurophysiological mechanisms of dentin hypersensitivity. Proc Finn Dent Soc 1992;88(suppl 1):15–22.

115. Orchardson R, Collins WJ. Clinical features of hypersensitive teeth. Br Dent J 1987;162:253–256.

116. Narhi M, Yamamoto H, Ingassapa D, Hirvonen T. The neurophysiological basis and the role of inflammatory reactions in dentine hypersensitivity. Arch Oral Biol 1994;39:23S–30S.

117. Rowe A, Pitt Ford T. The assessment of pulp vitality. Int Endod J 1990;23:77–83.

118. Cohen S, Liewehr F. Diagnostic procedures. In: Cohen S, Burns R (eds). Pathways of the Pulp, ed 8. St Louis: Mosby, 2002:3–30.

119. Daskalov I, Indjov B, Mudrov N. Electrical dental pulp testing. IEEE Eng Med Biol 1997;16:46–50.

120. Virtanen A, Huopaniemi T, Narhi M. Excitation of tooth pulp afferents with electrical current. Acupunct Electrother Res Int J 1984;9:127–134.

121. Virtanen ASJ. Electrical stimulation of pulp nerves comparison of monopolar and bipolar electrode coupling. Pain 1985;23:279–288.

122. Mumford JM, Bowsher D. Pain and protopathic sensibility. A review with particular reference to the teeth. Pain 1976;2:223–243.

123. Mumford JM, Newton AV. Zone of excitation when electrically stimulating human teeth. Arch Oral Biol 1969;14:1383–1388.

124. Jacobson JJ, Arbor A. Probe placement during electric pulp-testing procedures. Oral Surg Oral Med Oral Pathol 1984;58:242–247.

125. Bender IB, Landau MA, Fonsecca S, Trowbridge HO. The optimum placement-site of the electrode in electric pulp testing of the 12 anterior teeth. J Am Dent Assoc 1989;118:305–310.

126. Hoch S, Tismentetskiy V, Bender IB. Optimal placement of the electrode in electrical pulp testing of posterior teeth. J Dent Res (submitted) 2002.

127. Ghione S, Rosa C, Panattoni E, Nuti M, Mezzasalma L, Giuliano G. Comparison of sensory and pain threshold in tooth pulp stimulation in normotensive man and essential hypertension. J Hypertens 1985;3(suppl 3): S113–S115.

128. Ikeda H, Sunakawa M, Suda H. Three groups of afferent pulpal feline nerve fibres show different electrophysiological response properties. Arch Oral Biol 1995;40:895–904.

129. Ikeda H, Suda H. Subjective sensation and objective neural discharges recorded from clinically nonvital and intact teeth. J Endod 1998;24:552–556.

130. Ahlquist ML, Edwall LGA, Franzen OG, Haegerstam GAT. Perception of pulpal pain as a function of intradental nerve activity. Pain 1984;19:353–366.

131. Ahlquist M, Franzen O. Pulpal ischemia in man: Effects on detection threshold, A-Delta neural response and sharp dental pain. Endod Dent Traumatol 1999;15: 6–16.

132. Hyman J, Cohen M. The predictive value of endodontic diagnostic tests. Oral Surg Oral Med Oral Pathol 1984;58:343–346.

133. Petersson K, Soderstrom C, Kiani-Araaraki M, Levy G. Evaluation of the ability of thermal and electrical tests to register pulp vitality. Endod Dent Traumatol 1999; 19:127–131.

134. Moody A, Browne R, Robinson P. A comparison of monopolar and bipolar electrical stimuli and thermal stimuli in determining the vitality of human teeth. Arch Oral Biol 1989;34:701–704.

135. Peters D, Baumgartner J, Lorton L. Adult pulpal diagnosis. I. Evaluation of the positive and negative responses to cold and electrical pulp tests. J Endod 1990;20: 606–611.

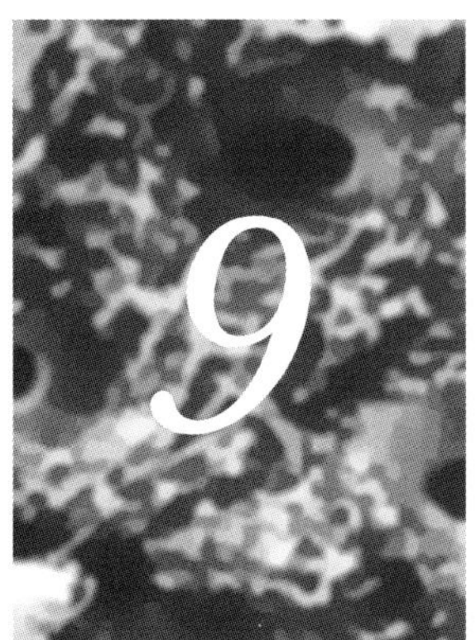

Pharmacologic Control of Dental Pain

Kenneth M. Hargreaves, DDS, PhD
Samuel Seltzer, DDS

A major theme of this book is the relationship between dental pulp and other tissues in health and disease. Perhaps the best example of this theme is dental pain. As detailed in chapters 7 and 8, pain is the predominant sensation following activation of those sensory neurons that innervate dental pulp and dentinal tubules. Although patients may report their pain as a "toothache," the skilled clinician understands that this single response may be an integration of pain originating from pulpal and periradicular nociceptors (eg, acute apical periodontitis) in addition to central mechanisms of hyperalgesia. Moreover, in some cases, the noxious input may not even occur from the tooth in question; it may actually represent pain referred to the site from a distant tissue and integrated in the central nervous system (CNS) (see chapter 20).

Given this complexity, it is perhaps not surprising that many patients view dentistry and pain as synonymous. Indeed, studies surveying more than 45,000 households in the United States indicate that odontalgia, or toothache, is the most common form of pain in the orofacial region, afflicting 12% of the study population.[1] This percentage corresponds to about 20 million people in the US alone.

In this chapter, studies on treating the two major forms of dental pain—dentinal sensitivity and inflammatory pulpal pain—will be reviewed. For each pain condition, we will review evidence supporting pharmacologic and nonpharmacologic treatment regimens for managing dental pain in the context of clinical interventions.

Management of Dentinal Hypersensitivity

Overview

As reviewed in chapter 8, the predominant hypothesis for dentinal hypersensitivity is Brännström's fluid flow hypothesis. Indeed, scanning electron microscope (SEM) analyses[2] of teeth with dentinal hypersensitivity demonstrate significantly greater numbers of patent dentinal tubules/mm^2 and significantly greater mean diameter per tubule than in control teeth (Fig 9-1). Identified risk factors for dentinal hypersensitivity include erosion, abrasion, attrition, gingival recession, periodontal treatment, and anatomic defects.[3-5] Accordingly, inter-

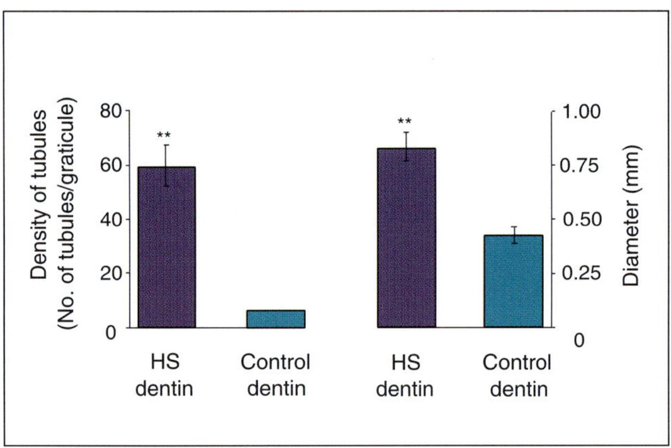

Fig 9-1 Comparison of the density of dentinal tubules and the mean diameter of dentinal tubules in teeth taken from 34 patients with hypersensitive (HS) dentin and 37 patients with normal dentin. Teeth were extracted and then examined under a scanning electron microscope $^{**}P < .01$ vs control dentin. (Data from Absi et al.[2])

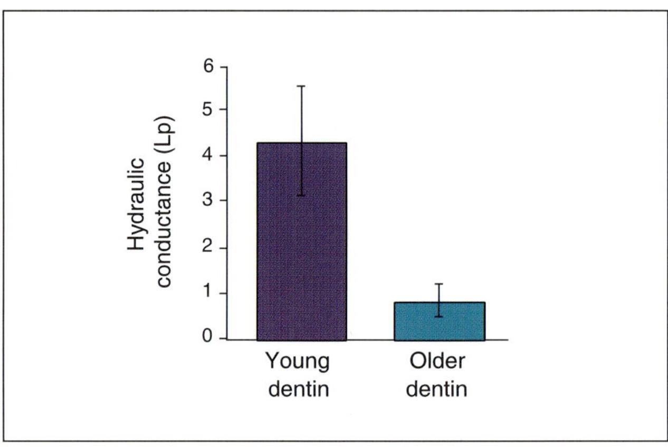

Fig 9-2 Hydraulic conductance of dentin disks taken from young (22 to 27 years old) and older (45 to 62 years old) patients. Lp, liquid permeability. (Data from Tagami et al.[12])

ventions that reduce either fluid flow or the activity of the neurons that innervate dentinal tubules would be predicted to be effective in reducing dentinal hypersensitivity.

Several cross-sectional studies have reported on the clinical characteristics of dentinal hypersensitivity. The reported prevalence of dentinal hypersensitivity ranges from 3.8% (N = 3,593, United Kingdom) to 17% (N = 635, Brazil) to about 55% (N = 250, Ireland; N = 277, United Kingdom).[6–9] The wide variation in the reported prevalence may relate to cultural or genetic factors or to experimental variations in methods of assessment or sampling. Indeed, several investigators have proposed standardized methods for assessing dentinal hypersensitivity and conducting randomized controlled clinical trials.[10,11] Dentinal hypersensitivity has been reported in some studies to be greater in female patients.[5,7,8] The location and teeth most often affected tend to be the cervical region of incisors and premolars, often on the side opposite the dominant hand. This latter finding is consistent with toothbrush abrasion as an etiologic factor. The peak reported period for dentinal hypersensitivity is the third to fourth decades of life. Most studies report a decline in the prevalence of dentinal hypersensitivity in older patients, which may be related to reductions in dentinal tubule permeability (Fig 9-2). Dentinal pain is elicited by cold stimuli in up to 90% of patients, although mechanical (eg, toothbrushing) and chemical (eg, candy) stimuli are also effective.[6,8,9] Several treatments have been evaluated for management of dentinal hypersensitivity.

Interventions that reduce dentinal tubule permeability

Because fluid flow is a major stimulus for activating nociceptors that innervate dentinal tubules, it is not surprising that interventions that reduce the permeability of dentinal tubules have been evaluated for reducing dentinal hypersensitivity. The application of resins to exposed dentinal tubules has been reported to reduce dentinal hypersensitivity of multiple etiologies at up to 12 months follow-up.[11,13–16] One study[14] developed an experimental model of dentinal sensitivity by

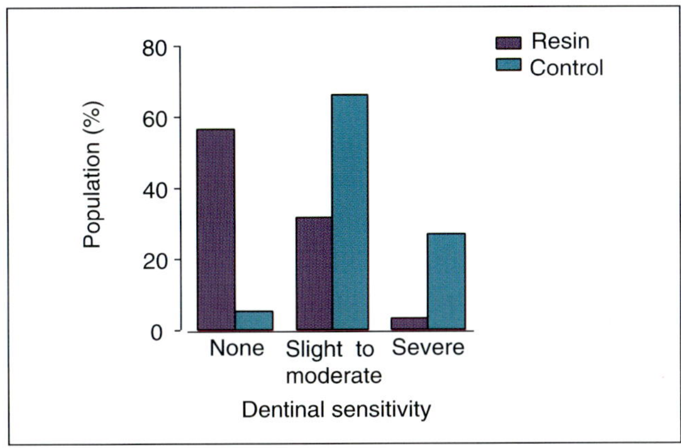

Fig 9-3 Effect of applying an unfilled resin (Concise Enamel Bond) to exposed dentin in 51 pairs of contralateral premolars in an experimental clinical model of dentinal hypersensitivity. A consistent amount of dentin exposure was made on the premolars, which then were either covered with resin or served as a no-treatment control. Dentinal sensitivity was assessed by a short pulse of compressed air onto the exposed dentin. (Data from Nordenvall et al.[14])

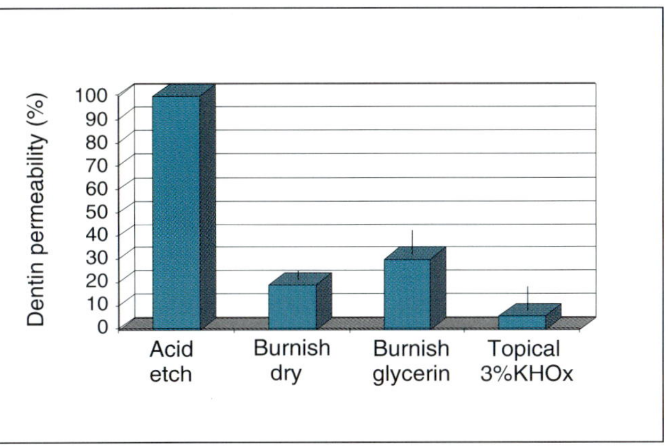

Fig 9-4 Effect of burnishing on in vitro dentin permeability. Dentin permeability after original acid etching is assigned a value of 100%. (Redrawn from Pashley et al[23] with permission.)

producing uniform dentin exposures in premolars (prior to tooth extraction for an orthodontic indication). These investigators demonstrated that the application of Concise Enamel Bond (3M, St. Paul, MN) to the exposed tubules produced about a twofold reduction in dentinal sensitivity as compared with control teeth (Fig 9-3). Similar results were reported by the same group for actual clinical cases of dentinal hypersensitivity.[13]

Other interventions that block fluid flow have also been reported to be effective in treating dentinal hypersensitivity. Examples include the application of materials such as Gluma Dentin Bond (Heraeus Kulzer, South Bend, IN), oxalate salts, isobutyl cyanoacrylate, and fluoride-releasing resins or varnishes; CO_2 lasers; and the use of devices that burnish exposed dentin and even coronally positioned mucogingival flaps[16-22] (Fig 9-4). The dominant factors contributing to the efficacy of these interventions are the longevity of effective blockage of tubules and the limited potential for cytotoxicity. For example, patients who report continued efficacy of resins at 6 months after application have evidence of resin tags still blocking their dentinal tubules; patients who have recurrence of dentinal sensitivity have few to no resin tags remaining in their tubules at that point.[24] Figure 9-5 presents SEM photomicrographs of hypersensitive dentin and dentinal tubules occluded with resin 6 months after treatment.[24]

However, it should be recognized that many studies are simply before-and-after comparisons and few studies directly compare efficacy and adverse effects among several active treatments. The lack of direct comparisons and systematic evaluations makes it difficult to determine which of the proposed treatment regimens offers the greatest efficacy and duration with the least potential for adverse effects. Thus, further research is required in this important therapeutic area.

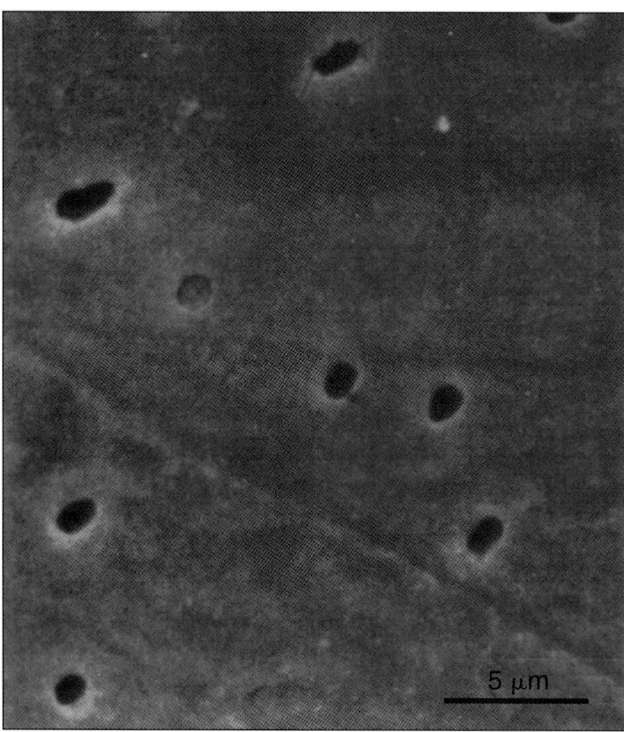

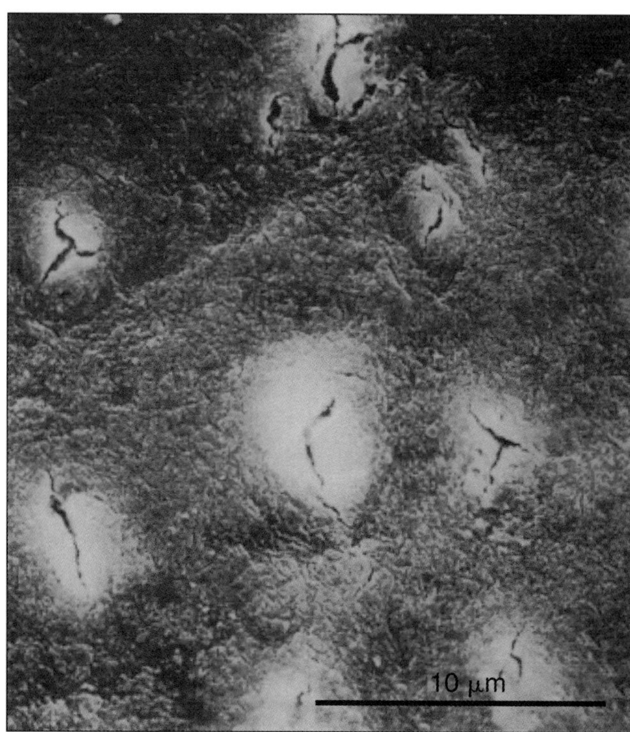

Fig 9-5 Scanning electron photomicrographs of the surface of human radicular dentin. *(left)* Hypersensitive dentin. *(right)* A tooth 6 months after application of resin liner. Note occluded tubules. Patient reported a lack of dentinal sensitivity after application of resin. (Reprinted from Yoshiyama et al[24] with permission.)

Interventions that reduce sensitivity of dentinal neurons

The second general method to reduce dentinal sensitivity employs interventions that reduce neuronal responsiveness to dentinal stimuli. Both preclinical studies and clinical trials have been used to evaluate these agents.

The preclinical studies often employ multiunit intradental electrophysiologic recordings of fibers that innervate dentinal tubules. For example, some researchers have used an anesthetized feline model with multiunit recordings of dentinal neurons using a pretreatment design.[25,26] In this design, desensitizing agents were applied to exposed dentinal tubules prior to stimulation by application of excitatory agents (eg, hypertonic NaCl). This model has been used to evaluate the efficacy of numerous compounds for reducing activation of dentinal neurons. In general, these studies indicate that application of potassium reduces neuronal activity regardless of the paired anion, that divalent cations are effective inhibitors of dentinal neurons, and that NO_3 is not effective in altering neuronal activity (Fig 9-6). However, it should be noted that the deep-cavity preparations of this model (ie, 20 to 50 µm of remaining dentin) might lead to an overestimate of drug efficacy because diffusion through dentinal fluid has been minimized. Moreover, no clinical studies to date have demonstrated that the concentrations of the test agents achieved in these experimental models are similar to actual concentrations achieved during therapeutic use in human dentinal fluid.

Several major reviews have recently summarized the outcomes of clinical trials evaluating desensitizing agents.[15,27-29] As discussed above, variations in clinical trial methodology or design (ie, techniques for assessing hypersensitivity, study duration, data analysis, comparison to active controls) may often lead to differences in study outcome. Accordingly, the following review will focus on those interventions that are successful in multiple double-blind randomized studies in an attempt to identify treatments with high efficacy.

Potassium-containing dentifrices are found to be effective in a majority of double-blind randomized clinical trials. The placebo controls in these studies consist of the dentifrice without the potassium nitrate (KNO_3) component. In a recent review of the literature,[29] 73% of formulations of potassium nitrate–containing dentifrices were significantly better than placebo for reducing dentinal hypersensitivity to application of cold air pulses (see Table 9-1). When analyzed on a sample-weighted basis, the overall results indicate that placebo dentifrices reduce sensitivity to cold by about 35%; 3.75% KNO_3 dentifrices reduce sensitivity to cold by about 60.8%; and 5% KNO_3 dentifrices reduce sensitivity to cold by about 61.2% (see Table 9-1). This finding is clinically relevant because cold is reported to be the most common stimulus of dentinal hypersensitivity.[6,8,9] Moreover, 64% of formulations of potassium nitrate–containing dentifrices were significantly better than placebo for overall global reduction in dentinal hypersensitivity symptoms (Table 9-2). Thus, the majority of randomized controlled clinical trials indicate that potassium-containing dentifrices are effective in reducing dentinal hypersensitivity.[30–40]

The efficacy of other agents for reducing dentinal hypersensitivity has also been evaluated in clinical trials. For example, 10% strontium chloride ($SrCl_2$) has been evaluated in numerous studies. In two-cell studies (ie, $SrCl_2$ versus placebo dentifrice), the weighted mean efficacy of $SrCl_2$ was a 72.5% reduction in hypersensitivity while the mean efficacy of the placebo dentifrice was a 34.3% reduction in hypersensitivity.[28] However, in studies consisting of three or more cells (ie, at least two active groups and a placebo dentifrice), the weighted mean efficacy of $SrCl_2$ was only 51.8% reduction in hypersensitivity while the mean efficacy of the placebo dentifrice was a 41% reduction in hypersensitivity.[28] Combining both types of studies, $SrCl_2$ produced about a 50% reduction in dentinal hypersensitivity. Clearly, experimental design issues contribute to the variations in efficacy estimates for desensitizing dentifrices.

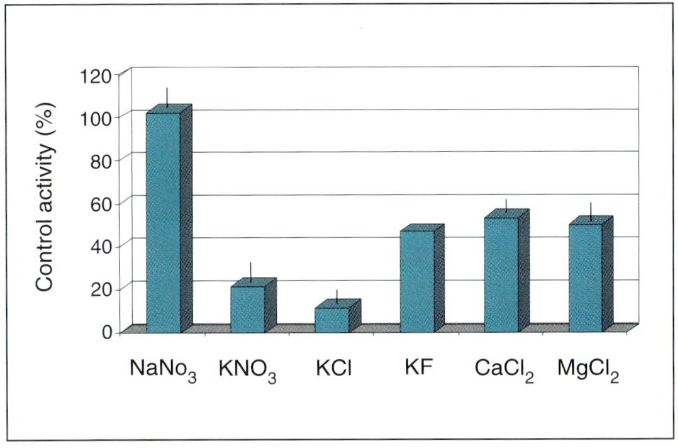

Fig 9-6 Effect on dentinal neuron activity of test desensitizing agents on exposed dentin. Data are presented as percentage of neuron activity compared with that of control (ie, application of hypertonic [3 M] sodium chloride is defined as 100%). The test agents include sodium nitrate ($NaNO_3$) (1.10 M), potassium nitrate (KNO_3) (1.0 M), potassium chloride (KCl) (0.76 M), potassium fluoride (KF) (0.05 M), calcium chloride ($CaCl_2$) (0.76 M), and magnesium chloride ($MgCl_2$) (0.76 M). (Adapted from Markowitz and Kim[26] with permission.)

The efficacy of fluoride-containing medicaments on dentinal hypersensitivity has been evaluated in several clinical trials. One meta-analysis of seven clinical trials reported that the application of 0.717% tin(II) fluoride (SnF_2) gel to exposed dentin for 3 to 5 minutes produced a significant and prolonged reduction in dentinal hypersensitivity.[41] Application of 0.4% SnF_2 gel produced a delayed effect, requiring repeated applications for several weeks. Fluoride-containing dentifrices also have been reported to reduce dentinal hypersensitivity in some but not all studies.[42–44]

Guanethidine has also been evaluated for management of dentinal hypersensitivity. In a double-blind randomized study,[45] the application of a 1% solution of guanethidine to exposed dentinal

Table 9-1 Efficacy of various potassium dentifrice formulations on cold air–induced dentinal hypersensitivity*

Study†	% Active agent (KNO_3)	N	Duration (weeks)	Active (%)	Placebo (%)	Significance
Tarbet et al (1980)[30]	5	27	4	65‡	20‡	< .05
Manochehr-Pour et al (1984)[31]	5	75	12	63	37	NS
Manochehr-Pour et al (1984)[31]	5	75	12	52	37	NS
Silverman (1985)[32]	5	68	12	75	40	< .001
Silverman (1985)[32]	5	68	12	78	40	< .001
Salvato et al (1992)[33]	3.75	41	12	66	32	.001
Nagata et al (1994)[34]	5	36	12	80	27	< .01
Schiff et al (1994)[35]	5	60	12	61	0	< .001
Silverman et al (1994)[36]	3.75	62	8	66	28	< .05
Silverman et al (1994)[36]	3.75	62	8	61	28	< .05
Silverman et al (1996)[37]	5	220	8	54	30	< .001
Gillam et al (1996)[38]	3.75	56	6	51	48	NS
West et al (1997)[39]	5	112	6	48	53	NS
Schiff et al (1998)[40]	5	39	8	82	40	< .0001

*Data from Orchardson and Gillam.[29]
†Note: Those studies in which different formulations were compared have separate listings.
‡Percent reduction in sensitivity to cold-air stimulus from baseline values.

Table 9-2 Efficacy of various potassium dentifrice formulations on patients' global subjective ratings of dentinal hypersensitivity*

Study†	% Active agent (KNO_3)	N	Duration (weeks)	Active (%)	Placebo (%)	Significance
Tarbet et al (1980)[30]	5	27	4	92‡	21‡	.001
Manochehr-Pour et al (1984)[31]	5	75	12	54	60	NS
Manochehr-Pour et al (1984)[31]	5	75	12	36	60	NS
Silverman (1985)[32]	5	68	12	71	36	< .001
Silverman (1985)[32]	5	68	12	75	36	< .001
Salvato et al (1992)[33]	3.75	41	12	75	23	.001
Nagata et al (1994)[34]	5	36	12	82	28	< .01
Schiff et al (1994)[35]	5	60	12	52	30	< .01
Silverman et al (1994)[36]	3.75	62	8	61	32	< .1
Silverman et al (1994)[36]	3.75	62	8	52	32	< .05
Silverman et al (1996)[37]	5	220	8	55	29	< .001
Gillam et al (1996)[38]	3.75	56	6	54	29	.001
West et al (1997)[39]	5	112	6	54	43	NS
Schiff et al (1998)[40]	5	39	8	30	19	NS

*Data from Orchardson and Gillam.[29]
†Note: Those studies in which different formulations were compared have separate listings.
‡Percent reduction in patients' subjective ratings to overall dentinal sensitivity as compared with baseline values.

tubules produced about a 50% reduction in sensitivity as compared with baseline values (Fig 9-7). This effect was similar to a preliminary study by the same investigators.[46] Guanethidine is known to act by inhibiting exocytosis from peripheral terminals of sympathetic fibers and has been shown previously to block sympathetically regulated blood flow in dental pulp.[47] However, guanethidine may also alter the activity of nociceptors. The application of guanethidine to human skin increases pricking pain thresholds, an effect not observed with other vasodilators.[48] Mashimo et al[48] concluded that guanethidine directly alters human nociceptors, a process that may involve A-delta nociceptors, for these neurons are thought to encode for pricking pain sensation. However, other studies have suggested that guanethidine also acts on the capsaicin-sensitive class of unmyelinated nociceptors.[49] Collectively, these studies suggest that further research is warranted on the potential application of guanethidine for treating dentinal hypersensitivity.

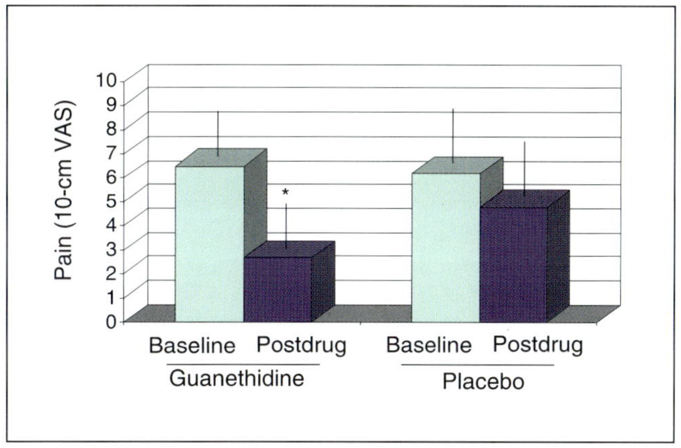

Fig 9-7 Effect of topical application of a 1% solution of guanethidine or vehicle on dentinal hypersensitivity to cold-air stimulation. N = 39 patients; $^*P < .05$ vs vehicle posttreatment. (Data from Dunne and Hannington-Kiff.[45])

Conclusions

Dentinal hypersensitivity represents a common, widespread form of odontogenic pain that is believed to be mediated primarily by activation of neurons that innervate dentinal tubules. The diagnosis of dentinal hypersensitivity is based on the eliciting stimuli, the duration of the pain, the location, and the absence of pulpal (ie, symptoms) or radiographic (ie, changes seen) pathoses. The management of dentinal hypersensitivity involves the application of therapies that either reduce flow of dentinal fluid (see also chapter 4) or reduce the activity of dentinal neurons.[15] In addition, patients should be advised to avoid habits or agents that increase dentinal permeability. For example, studies have reported that tartar-control dentifrices and toothbrushing in the presence of dietary acids or certain mouthwashes (eg, those containing hexetidine or fluoride/antiseptic) may present risk factors for dentinal sensitivity by removing the smear layer of exposed dentinal tubules.[50-52]

Management of Pulpitis and Related Pain Conditions

Overview

Another common form of odontalgia is due to pulpitis or periradicular pain pathoses. For the purposes of this chapter, we will consider this form to include pain resulting from activation of pulpal as well as periradicular nociceptors. It is appropriate to include periradicular nociceptors in this examination because the elaboration of bacteria and bacterial by-products from necrotic root canal systems constitutes the predominant etiologic factor for periradicular inflammation and pain (see chapter 17), another good example of the relationship between dental pulp and other tissues during disease. Thus, relevant clinical diagnoses will include odontogenic pain of inflammatory etiologies, such as irreversible pulpitis, pulpal necrosis with acute apical periodontitis, etc.

This section will review both pharmacologic and nonpharmacologic methods for pain control. Importantly, the clinician uses an integrated approach in combining these methods to control

Box 9-1 **"3D" strategy for managing acute odontogenic pain**

1. Diagnosis
2. Definitive dental treatment
   a. Pulpotomy, pulpectomy
   b. Extraction
   c. Incision for drainage
3. Drugs
   a. Pretreat with NSAIDs or acetaminophen when appropriate
   b. Prescribe by the clock rather than as necessary
   c. Use long-acting local anesthetics when indicated
   d. Use a flexible prescription plan

*Based on Hargreaves and Hutter.[53]

dental pain, which has been called the "3D" method for pain control: diagnosis, definitive dental treatment, and drugs.[53] This approach is summarized in Box 9-1.

Diagnosis of odontalgia

The first "D" is for *diagnosis*. Diagnosis is of obvious importance in managing acute pain because effective treatment is directed at removing the etiology of pain. For example, nitroglycerin is effective for reducing anginal pain, yet it has comparatively little analgesic activity in most other pain conditions. Similarly, if a patient has pain associated with an abscess, then an incision for drainage may prove effective in reducing pain. In both examples, the treatments are effective because they reduce the etiologic factors that elicit the pain. In treating the acute pain patient, an accurate diagnosis generally leads to predictable treatment strategies, but in the management of the chronic pain patient, the etiologies of pain are less well understood and probably multifactorial in nature.[54] Therefore, the first step in treating the acute pain patient is establishing the diagnosis. This information is reviewed extensively in several excellent endodontic texts and need not be covered here.[55-57] The clinician should be aware of differential diagnoses for patients who present with a chief complaint of tooth pain since etiologies, treatment strategies, and prognoses vary considerably (see also chapter 20).[54,58-60]

Nonpharmacologic methods that reduce pain due to pulpitis and related pain conditions

The second "D" is for *definitive dental treatment*. Numerous studies indicate that definitive dental treatment alone provides predictable and substantial relief from odontogenic pain. In patients with irreversible pulpitis, pulpotomy treatment, regardless of the coronal medicament, has been reported to abolish pain symptoms in 88% of patients evaluated 1 day after treatment.[61] The efficacy of definitive dental treatment for reducing acute pain symptoms has been confirmed by many other studies. Figure 9-8 summarizes the results of more than 1,000 patients in clinical trials to evaluate the efficacy of pulpotomy or pulpectomy for relieving odontogenic pain.[62] The horizontal bars for each group of studies indicate the sample size weighted mean reduction in pain. Since pulpotomies are only performed in vital endodontic cases (eg, pain of pulpal origin) while pulpectomies are performed in more complex pain conditions (ie, pain of pulpal and/or periradicular origin), it is not surprising that pulpotomies appear more effective than pulpectomies for relieving pain.[61-70]

Other forms of definitive dental treatment include occlusal adjustment, trephination, and incision for drainage procedures. In one study of 117 patients,[70] occlusal adjustment resulted in about twice as many patients reporting no posttreatment pain as compared with the no-treatment controls (Fig 9-9). The authors concluded that occlusal adjustment was particularly effective for reducing postoperative pain in patients with preoperative pain who had vital pulps and percussion sensitivity.

Another nonpharmacologic approach is to reduce intraosseous pressure. Although trephination has been advocated to reduce postendodontic pain, several randomized clinical trials have failed to demonstrate a significant effect of trephination with pulpectomy compared with pulpectomy alone.[67,71,72] In one study, patients were randomly placed in either of two groups:

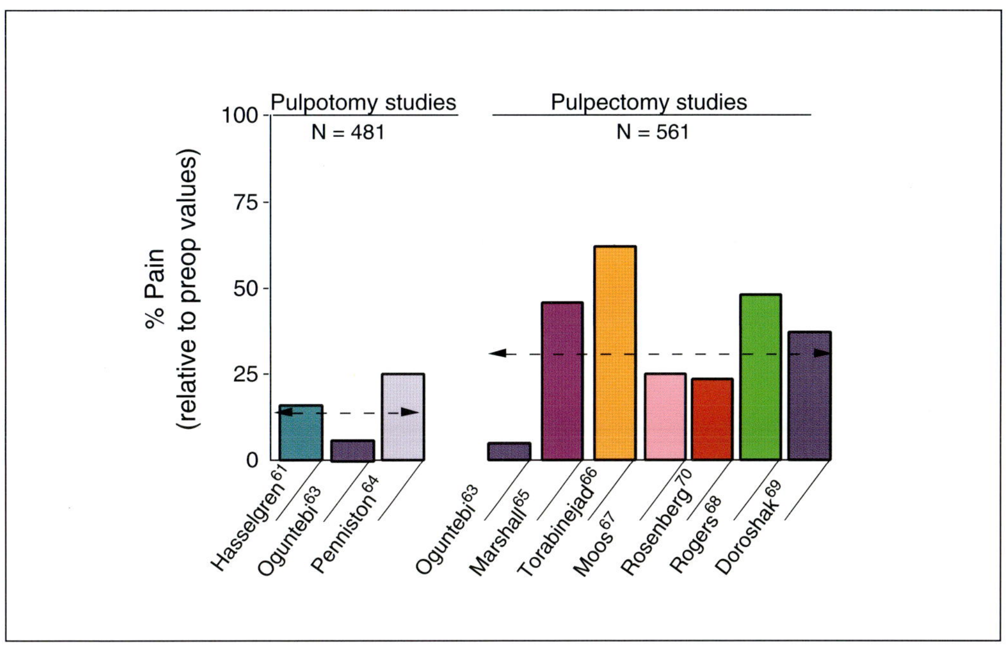

Fig 9-8 Effects of pulpotomy or pulpectomy on endodontic-related pain. Preoperative pain values are normalized to 100%. The two horizontal bars for pulpotomy and pulpectomy groups represent the sample size–weighted mean reduction in pain. Only the first author of each study is named. (Reprinted from Hargreaves and Baumgartner[62] with permission.)

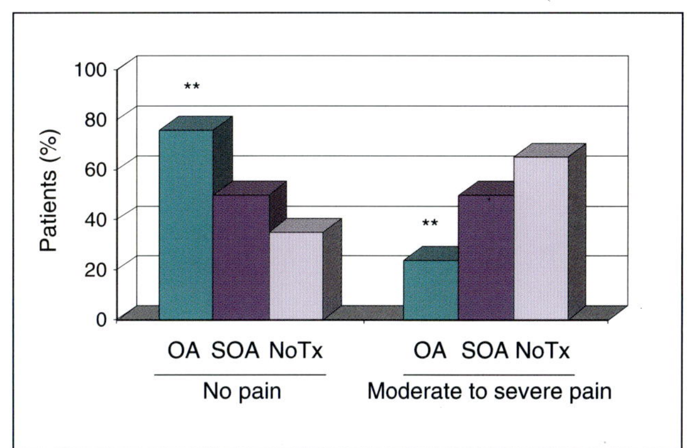

Fig 9-9 Effect of occlusal adjustment (OA), simulated occlusal adjustment (SOA, by reduction of nonfunctional cusp), or no treatment (NoTx) on the incidence of posttreatment pain in 117 endodontic patients. $^{**}P < .01$. (Redrawn from Rosenberg et al[70] with permission.)

pulpotomy or pulpotomy with periapical trephination. There was no difference between groups for postoperative pain, swelling, percussion pain, or use of analgesic tablets.[72] Thus, this technique does not appear to result in a clinically reproducible reduction in inflammatory mediators or interstitial pressure.

The rationale for the pain-relieving benefits of these definitive dental treatments is based on reducing tissue levels of factors that stimulate peripheral terminals of nociceptors (see chapters 7, 8, and 11) or reducing mechanical stimulation of sensitized nociceptors (eg, occlusal adjustment). Effective chemomechanical debridement

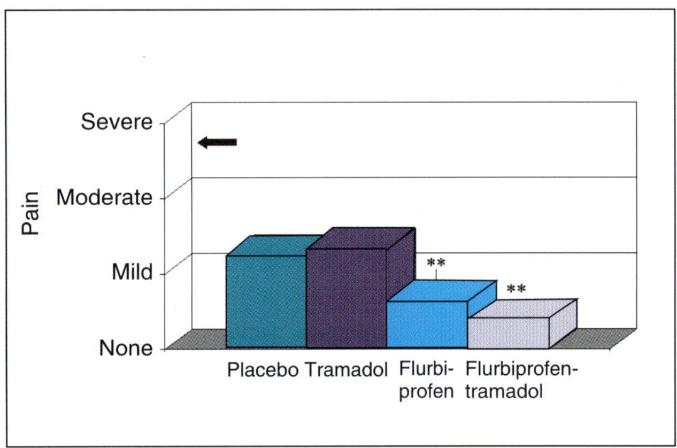

Fig 9-10 Comparison of flurbiprofen (100-mg loading dose, then 50 mg every 6 h), tramadol (100-mg initial dose, then 100 mg every 6 h), and combination flurbiprofen and tramadol (same dosages) to placebo in endodontic patients. Patients received local anesthesia, pulpectomies, and drugs. Pain levels were reported 24 hours after treatment. *Arrow* represents mean preoperative pain levels. N = 11 to 12 per group; $^{**}P < .01$ vs placebo. (Redrawn from Doroshak et al[69] with permission.)

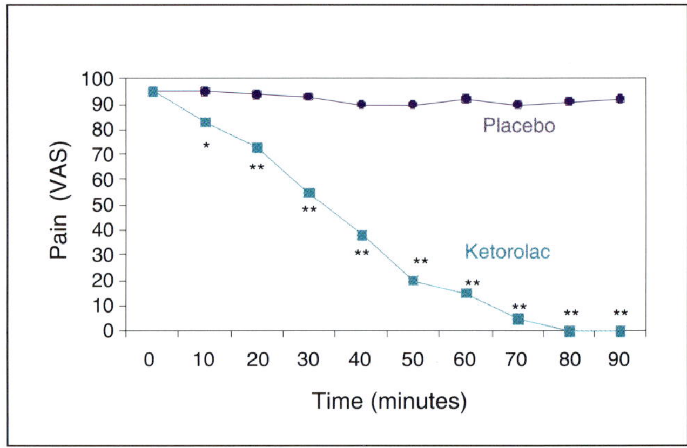

Fig 9-11 Comparison of ketorolac (60-mg intramuscular injection) to placebo for relief of endondontic pain. Patients (N = 40) completed a baseline pain scale, received drug injection, and then completed postdrug pain scales (ie, no endodontic treatment or local anesthetics were provided). $^{*}P < .05$ vs placebo; $^{**}P < .01$ vs placebo. (Redrawn from Curtis et al[82] with permission.)

of the infected root canal system, combined, when indicated, with incision for drainage procedures provides predictable pain-reduction strategies in endodontic emergency patients. Of course, if the tooth has a hopeless prognosis, then extraction will also reduce pain by reducing tissue levels of these factors. From this perspective, it can be concluded that treating the unscheduled emergency patient by the "prescription pad" (ie, drugs alone) is not a definitive intervention. Instead, the pharmacologic management of pain should be considered together with definitive dental treatment as a combined therapeutic approach for managing odontogenic pain.

Although space limitations preclude a thorough review, it should be noted that additional nonpharmacologic approaches have been evaluated for reduction of dental pain. These approaches include cognitive, motivational, and affective interventions and range from simple approaches such as establishing a confident doctor-patient relationship to more complex procedures.[73] For example, hypnosis has been reported to be an effective adjunct for management of dental pain in endodontic patients.[73-75] Other studies have demonstrated that instructing patients to focus on sensory stimuli significantly reduces intraoperative endodontic pain.[76,77] This effect was most evident in patients who were characterized as having a high desire for control and low perceived control over their clinical care. Thus, a number of nonpharmacologic approaches may be considered as a component of the overall strategy of managing dental inflammatory pain.

Drugs that block inflammatory mediators that sensitize or activate pulpal nociceptors

The third "D" in the 3D strategy of pain control is for *drugs*. Three primary pharmacologic approaches will be reviewed in this section: *(1)* drugs that block inflammatory mediators that sensitize or activate pulpal nociceptors, *(2)* drugs that block the propagation of impulses along peripheral nerves, and *(3)* drugs that block central mechanisms of pain perception and hyperalgesia.

Although numerous clinical pharmacology studies have evaluated analgesics for treating dental pain, it should be recognized that the majority of these studies employ a clinical model of acute inflammatory pain elicited by surgical trauma. Acute surgery-induced inflammation is mediated largely by release of eicosanoids such as prostacyclin and prostaglandin E_2, as well as other inflammatory mediators such as bradykinin.[78] In contrast, pulpal and periradicular pain is often associated with chronic inflammation, characterized by the presence of bacterial by-products, an influx of immune cells with activation of the cytokine network, and other inflammatory mediators (see chapters 10, 11, and 17). These considerations suggest that the composition and concentrations of inflammatory mediators that activate and sensitize nociceptors likely differ between these two models of orofacial pain. Moreover, the chronicity of pulpal inflammation permits sprouting of nociceptor terminals, and thus the peripheral anatomy of the pain system changes during pulpal inflammation (see chapter 7). Therefore, it is likely that the relative efficacy of analgesics differs between surgery-induced pain and pulp-related pain. Accordingly, this review will focus on clinical trials of endodontic pain, incorporating clinical trials on surgery-induced pain only to illustrate additional concepts.

One major class of drugs for managing endodontic pain is the non-narcotic analgesics, which include both the nonsteroidal anti-inflammatory drugs (NSAIDs) and acetaminophen. Recent studies have indicated that these drugs produce analgesia by actions in both the peripherally inflamed tissue as well as in certain regions in the brain and spinal cord.[79-81] The NSAIDs have been shown to be very effective for managing pain of inflammatory origin due to either surgery-induced trauma or pulpal and periradicular pain.[53,62,64,66,69,79,82] Indeed, the results of several double-blind randomized placebo-controlled clinical trials in endodontic pain patients[64,66,69,82] indicate that ibuprofen (400 mg), ketoprofen (50 mg), flurbiprofen (100 mg), and ketorolac (30 to 60 mg) all produce significant analgesia compared to a placebo medication (Figs 9-10 and 9-11). In interpreting these studies, it is important to realize that endodontic treatment alone (eg, pulpectomy) has a major effect on reducing pain regardless of pharmacologic treatment (see Fig 9-8). This reduction in posttreatment pain, combined with variable levels of preoperative pain, reduces the statistical power of endodontic clinical trials for detecting active analgesics over time or in all patient groups (the so-called floor effect). This limitation is a problem in interpreting clinical pain studies[83] in general and may explain why some endodontic clinical trials fail to detect analgesic treatment or only detect it in those patients with moderate to severe preoperative pain.[66,68]

Although many NSAIDs are available in the marketplace, comparatively few endodontic studies directly compare one NSAID with another for analgesia and side-effect liability. In one postendodontic study, ibuprofen (400 mg) was similar to ketoprofen (50 mg) for the time course in superiority to placebo treatment.[66] The lack of comprehensive comparative studies of endodontic pain means that only general recommendations can be made, and thus the clinician is encouraged to be familiar with several of these drugs. Ibuprofen is generally considered the prototype of NSAIDs and has a well-documented efficacy and safety profile.[84] The advantages of NSAIDs include their well-established analgesic efficacy for inflammatory pain. Indeed, many NSAIDs have been shown to be more effective than traditional acetaminophen-opioid combination drugs such as acetaminophen 650 mg with codeine 60 mg (for review, see Hargreaves and Hutter[53]).

It should be recognized that NSAIDs have a relatively high affinity to plasma proteins and that they are preferentially distributed to inflamed tissue by local vasodilation and plasma extravasation.[85] Thus NSAIDs are preferentially distributed into inflamed dental pulp compared with control

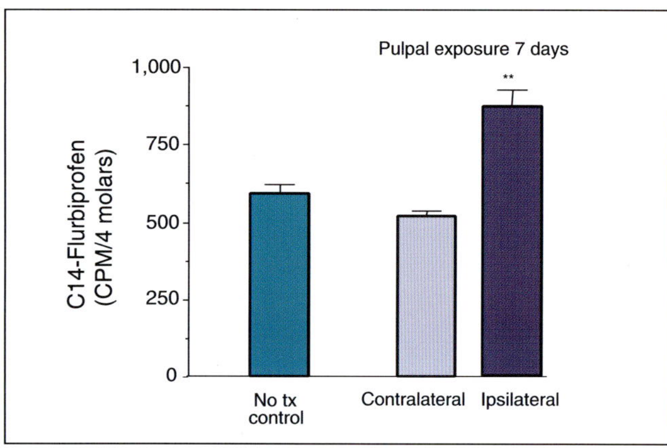

Fig 9-12 Preferential distribution of NSAIDs into inflamed pulp. Rats were anesthetized and underwent either no treatment or pulpal exposure of the first mandibular molar. Seven days later, rats were anesthetized and received an intravenous injection of C14-flurbiprofen. No-treatment control (a separate group of animals), ipsilateral (pulp exposure), and contralateral (no pulp exposure) teeth were extracted, homogenized, and analyzed for C14-flurbiprofen. N = 7 rats per group; $^{**}P < .01$ vs both the contralateral and no-treatment control groups. (Redrawn from Bunczak-Reeh and Hargreaves[85] with permission.)

dental pulp (Fig 9-12). This may improve the relative efficacy of NSAIDs compared with other analgesic drug classes.

Recent studies indicate that the two isoforms of cyclo-oxygenase (COX) differ in tissue distribution and potential for side-effect mediation.[86] One selective COX-2 inhibitor, rofecoxib, produced significant analgesia in a surgery-induced pain model. However, rofecoxib was not superior to ibuprofen 400 mg in this study.[87] Moreover, other COX-2 inhibitors (eg, celecoxib) have not received approval by the US Food and Drug Administration for treatment of acute inflammatory pain. COX-2 inhibitors may have analgesic efficacy in pulpal pain conditions because the COX-2 enzyme is elevated in inflamed human dental pulp as compared with control pulpal tissue.[88] However, concern has been raised that the COX-2 inhibitors may also display at least some gastrointestinal irritation in patients with pre-existing disease, suggesting these drugs should be used with some caution in certain patients.[89] More research is warranted on the potential efficacy and side-effect liability of COX-2 inhibitors in endodontic pain.

Although space limitations preclude an extensive review of contraindications for the NSAIDs, the clinician should be aware of these issues and understand that acetaminophen, either alone or as an acetaminophen-opioid combination, may represent an alternative for those patients unable to take NSAIDs.[90,91] Extensive reviews are available on the pharmacology and adverse effects of this important class of analgesics.[90-94] Other venues (eg, web-based drug search engines) are also available for evaluating newly released analgesics as well as potential adverse effects, contraindications, and drug interactions, including www.rxlist.com; www.pharminfo.com; www.epocrates.com; and www.endodontics.UTHSCSA.edu among others.

Steroids, or more properly glucocorticoids, form an additional class of drugs that interfere with the production or release of mediators that activate or sensitize nociceptors. Glucocorticoids are known to reduce the inflammatory response by suppressing vasodilation, neutrophil migration, and phagocytosis and by inhibiting the formation of arachidonic acid from neutrophil and macrophage-cell membrane phospholipids, thereby blocking the cyclo-oxygenase and lipoxygenase pathways and respective synthesis of prostaglandins and leukotrienes. Thus, it is not surprising that a number of investigations have evaluated the efficacy of corticosteroids on the prevention or control of postoperative endodontic pain.

Several clinical trials have evaluated the efficacy of glucocorticoids on reducing postendodontic pain after intracanal, oral, or intramuscular administration. In general, intracanal steroids appear to have the most consistent effects for reducing postoperative pain or flare-ups when used in vital cases.[68,95-97] The reduced efficacy in necrotic cases may be due to poor absorption due to this route of administration, to diffusion of inadequate amounts of the drug into the peri-

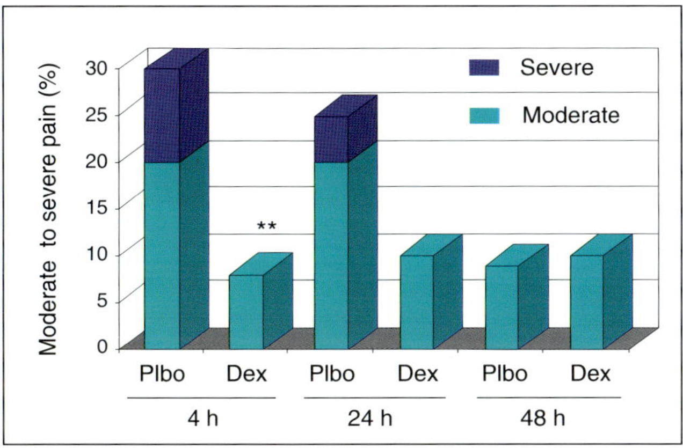

Fig 9-13 Comparison of dexamethasone (Dex) (4-mg intramuscular injection) to placebo (Plbo) for pain after endodontic instrumentation. N = 50; $^{**}P < .01$ vs placebo. (Redrawn from Marshall and Walton[98] with permission.)

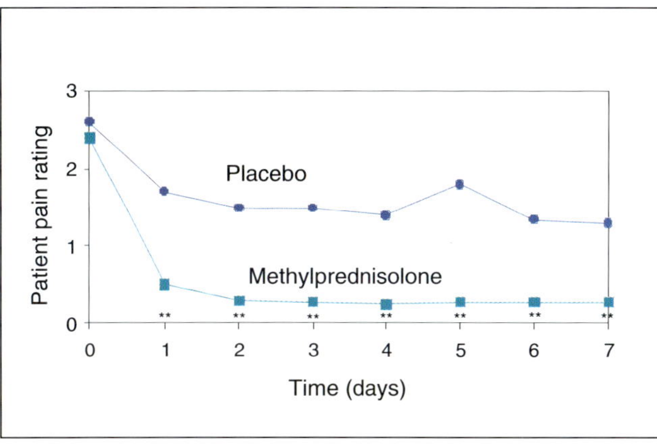

Fig 9-14 Comparison of the effects of methylprednisolone (40 mg intraosseous) to placebo for relief of pain due to irreversible pulpitis. After diagnosis and drug injection, patients reported pain levels for 7 days before any endodontic treatment was started. N = 40; $^{**}P < .01$ vs placebo. (Redrawn from Gallatin et al[103] with permission.)

radicular tissue, or to other factors such as experimental design or statistical power.

Other studies have evaluated the systemic administration of corticosteroids on postoperative pain or flare-ups. In general, these studies indicate that systemically administered corticosteroids reduce the severity of posttreatment endodontic pain as compared to placebo treatment, but with a time course of approximately 8 to 24 hours.[98-102] This point is illustrated in Fig 9-13, where dexamethasone (4 mg intramuscular injection) produced a significant effect at 4 hours and tended to separate from placebo at 24 hours. As described above, the lack of a drug effect at later time points may be due in part to the pain-relieving effects of endodontic instrumentation. In support of this point, a recent study evaluated the effects of intramuscular steroid injection on untreated pulpitis pain[101] and demonstrated that steroids produced a significant reduction in pulpitis pain over a 7-day observation period (Fig 9-14). Thus, steroids can elicit long-term reduction of pulpal pain when observed in patients with no endodontic treatment. Interestingly, 95% of steroid-treated dental pulps and 81% of the placebo-treated dental pulps were still vital at the 7-day observation period.

Taken together, these studies indicate that drugs that suppress the release or actions of inflammatory mediators on nociceptors have analgesic effect in treating pain due to inflammation of pulpal and periradicular tissue. The design of a pain-management plan is considered later in this chapter.

Drugs that block propagation of impulses along peripheral nerves

Local anesthetics represent an important component in the third "D" of pain control (drugs). Local anesthetics offer the benefit of prolonged pain control following completion of the endodontic appointment. Long-acting local anesthetics, etidocaine or bupivacaine, offer prolonged pain control 6 to 8 or more hours after injection.[104-107] However, research on pain mechanisms has revealed the existence of a central component to hyperalgesia, which can be established by an intense barrage of activity from peripheral noci-

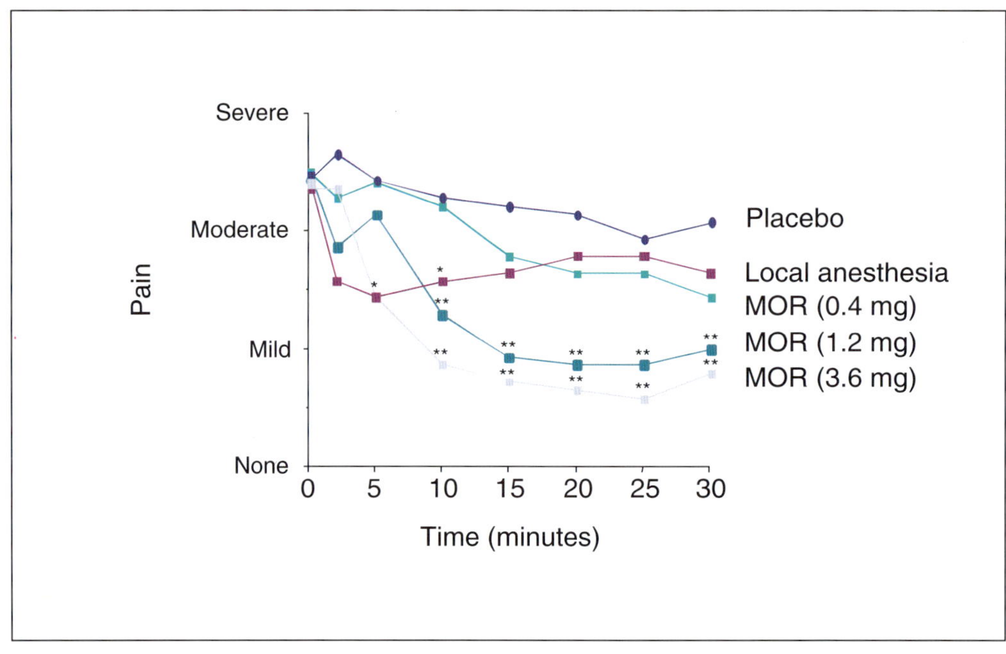

Fig 9-15 Effects of intraligamentary injection of morphine on patient levels of pain. Patients with irreversible pulpitis reported baseline pain levels and were then injected, on a double-blind randomized basis, with either placebo, local anesthetic (2% mepivacaine with 1:20,000 levonordefrin), or morphine (MOR; 0.4, 1.2, or 3.6 mg) using a standard intraligamentary route of injection. N = 8 to 10 per group; *$P < .05$ vs placebo; **$P < .01$ vs placebo. (Redrawn from Dionne et al[124] with permission.)

ceptors, particularly the unmyelinated C nociceptors (see chapter 8). The preemptive analgesia hypothesis states that clinical pain is reduced when the peripheral barrage of nociceptors is reduced.[108] Subsequent studies on orofacial pain have provided support for this concept. For example, patients given an inferior alveolar nerve block injection with bupivacaine prior to an oral surgical procedure reported less pain at 24 and 48 hours after the procedure as compared with placebo-injected patients.[109] This result is not restricted to extraction procedures, for infiltration with bupivacaine prior to tonsillectomy reduced postoperative pain for 7 days as compared with patients given placebo injections.[110] Collectively, these studies indicate that long-acting local anesthetics should be considered for treating endodontic pain and that they may reduce post-treatment pain even days after a single injection. Of course, the clinician should be aware of the potential adverse side-effect profile of the long-acting local anesthetics, including contraindications for cardiovascular patients.[111,112]

Another important application of local anesthetics is by the intraosseous route of injection. Several important pharmacokinetic and pharmacodynamic characteristics of intraosseous local anesthetic injection have been determined using normal volunteers with pulpal anesthesia defined using an electrical pulp tester. First, intraosseous injection of 1.8 mL of 2% lidocaine with 1:100,000 epinephrine provides significant anesthesia for 74% of first molars.[113] The dosage of 2% lidocaine with epinephrine produces a transient (4-minute) period of tachycardia with an average increase in rate of 28 beats/minute.[114] For intraosseous injection of 3% mepivacaine, the administration of a 1.8-mL volume produced a 45%

anesthesia rate in mandibular first molars, and anesthetic success increased with a second injection of 3% mepivacaine.[113,115] The intraosseous injection of 3% mepivacaine had no significant cardiovascular effects.[114] About 5% of patients had delayed healing at the site of injection.[113]

Additional studies have evaluated the efficacy of a supplemental intraosseous injection of local anesthetics in clinical patients with pain due to irreversible pulpitis.[115-117] In one study of 48 patients with irreversible pulpitis in mandibular teeth, an inferior alveolar block of 2% lidocaine with 1:100,000 epinephrine was only 25% successful for pulpal anesthesia; a supplementary intraosseous injection of 3% mepivacaine increased anesthetic success to 80%.[115] In a parallel study of 51 patients with irreversible pulpitis of mandibular teeth, an inferior alveolar block of 2% lidocaine with 1:100,000 epinephrine was only 19% successful for pulpal anesthesia; a supplementary injection of 2% lidocaine with 1:100,000 epinephrine increased anesthetic success to 91%.[116] Similar results have been observed in another clinical trial of irreversible pulpitis in the maxillary and mandibular teeth.[115] Collectively, these studies indicate that the intraosseous injection of either 3% mepivacaine or 2% lidocaine with 1:100,000 epinephrine can lead to a three- to fourfold improvement in anesthetic success in patients with irreversible pulpitis.

Space restrictions preclude a detailed review of the technique for intraosseous injection or other routes of injection and the relative indications and contraindications of various local anesthetics. The clinician is encouraged to seek this information in several excellent clinical texts.[118,119]

Several recent studies have suggested that the local application of peripheral opioids may have utility in treating pain due to irreversible pulpitis. Opioid receptors are present on afferent neurons and undergo a peripherally directed transport.[120,121] These observations may have clinical utility because pulpal neurons express opioid receptors, and local administration of opioids is analgesic in animal models of inflammatory pain.[122,123] Therefore, clinical trials have evaluated whether intraligamentary injection of opioids is analgesic in patients with irreversible pulpitis.[124-126] The results indicate that opioids produce significant analgesia in this model (Fig 9-15) and act locally in inflamed tissue.[124]

Drugs that block central mechanisms of pain perception and hyperalgesia

Opioids are potent analgesics, often used in dentistry in combination with acetaminophen, aspirin, or ibuprofen. Most clinically available opioids activate the mu opioid receptor. Although opioids are effective as analgesics for moderate to severe pain, their usage is generally limited by their adverse side-effect profile. Opioids induce numerous side effects, including nausea, emesis, dizziness, drowsiness, and the potential for respiratory depression and constipation. Chronic usage is associated with tolerance and dependence. Because the dose of opioids is limited by their side-effect profile, opioids are almost always used in combination drugs for management of dental pain. A combination formulation is preferred because it permits a lower dose of the opioid to reduce patient side effects.

Codeine is often considered the prototype opioid for orally available combination drugs. Most studies using surgery-induced inflammatory pain have found that a 60-mg dose of codeine produces significantly more analgesia than placebo, although it often produces less analgesia than either aspirin 650 mg or acetaminophen 600 mg.[90,91,127]

Summary of Pain Management Strategies

When managing pain in an individual patient, the skilled clinician must customize the treatment plan to the patient, balancing knowledge of pulp biology with general principles of endodontics and restorative dentistry, mecha-

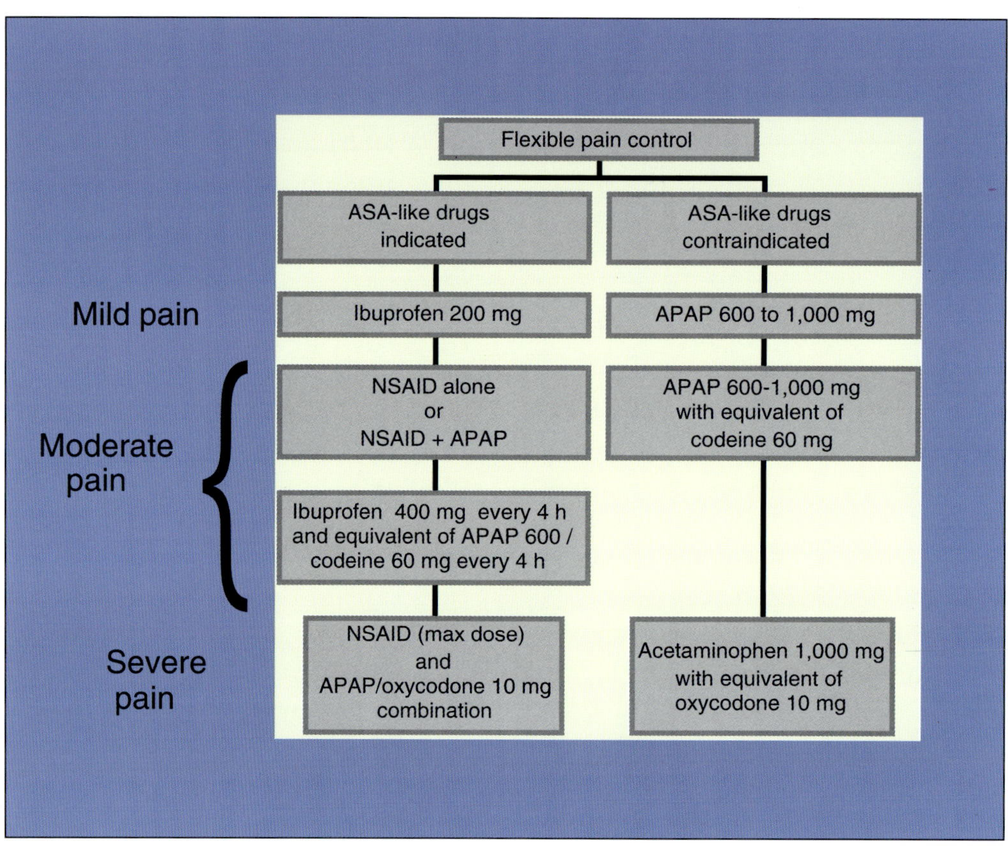

Fig 9-16 A flexible prescription plan for managing postendodontic pain based on the patient's ability to tolerate NSAIDs and designed to minimize pain and side-effect exposure. APAP, acetaminophen; ASA, acetylsalicylic acid.

nisms of hyperalgesia, pain-management strategies, and the individual's particular factors (eg, medical history, concurrent medications, etc). The following discussion reviews general considerations for pain-management strategies.

Effective management of endodontic pain starts with the three "Ds": diagnosis, definitive dental treatment, and drugs (see Box 9-1). As described earlier in this chapter, the management of endodontic pain should focus on removal of peripheral mechanisms of hyperalgesia, which generally requires treatment that removes or reduces etiologic factors (eg, bacterial-immunologic factors) and nerve terminals. As described, pulpotomy and pulpectomy represent rational and effective treatments for initial removal of these factors (see Fig 9-8). However, pharmacotherapy is often required to interrupt continued nociceptor input (eg, NSAIDs, local anesthetics) and to suppress central hyperalgesia (eg, opioids).

Administration of NSAIDs alone is usually sufficient for most patients who can tolerate this drug class because of its effectiveness in managing inflammatory pulpal pain and the relatively low incidence of postendodontic pain. (Up to 80% of patients report postendodontic pain as none to slight[128,129]). Thus, an NSAID prescription, such as ibuprofen 600 mg taken every 6 hours, is optimal for the majority of patients who can tolerate this drug class. For patients who cannot tolerate an NSAID, a 1,000-mg dosage of acetaminophen is often suitable for managing posttreatment pain.

About 20% of patients may have moderate to severe postendodontic pain,[129] and thus some patients may not be adequately relieved by a single-drug approach.

In general, a flexible analgesic prescription strategy offers the best combination of pain relief and minimal side effects while offering the clinician a rational approach for customizing an analgesic plan to a particular patient's needs (Fig 9-16). A flexible prescription plan serves to minimize both postoperative pain and side effects. With this goal in mind, the strategy is first to achieve a maximally effective dose of the nonnarcotic analgesic (either an NSAID or acetaminophen for patients who cannot take NSAIDs). Second, in those rare cases when the patient still experiences moderate to severe pain, the clinician should consider adding drugs that increase NSAID analgesia. Given its predictive value, the presence of preoperative hyperalgesia may serve as an indication for considering these NSAID combinations.[53] There are two general analgesic approaches for such patients. One approach is to co-prescribe an NSAID with acetaminophen. This strategy provides predictable control for severe pain and can be used to modify a standard NSAID-only regimen if pain control is inadequate.[130,131] The concurrent and short-term administration of acetaminophen and NSAIDs appears to be well tolerated in most patients with no apparent increase in side effects or alterations in pharmacokinetics.[130-135] A second general approach is to co-prescribe an NSAID with an acetaminophen-opioid combination. Importantly, all three drugs (the NSAID, the acetaminophen, and the opioid) are active analgesics that can have additive effects when combined.[130-132]

Of course, not all patients require concurrent use of NSAIDs with acetaminophen-opioid combinations or combinations of NSAIDs and opioids. Indeed, the basic premise of a flexible prescription plan is that the analgesic prescribed should be matched to the patient's need. The major advantage of a flexible plan is that the clinician is prepared for those rare cases when additional pharmacotherapy is indicated, increasing both the overall efficiency and efficacy of pain control. As described in chapter 8, the presence of preoperative hyperalgesia may serve as an indication for more comprehensive pharmacotherapy.

The information and recommendations provided in this chapter were selected to aid the clinician in the management of pulpal pain due to dentinal hypersensitivity or pulpitis and related periradicular pain. However, clinical judgment must also take into account other sources of information, including patient history, concurrent medications, nature of the pain, and the comprehensive treatment plan to design the best pain-management program for an individual patient. Integrating these general principles of pain mechanisms and management with the clinician's assessment of each patient's needs provides an effective approach for the successful management of pulpal pain.

References

1. Lipton J, Ship JA, Larach-Robinson D. Estimated prevalence and distribution of reported orofacial pain in the United States. J Am Dent Assoc 1993;124(10):115–121.
2. Absi E, Addy M, Adams D. Dentine hypersensitivity: A study of the patency of dentinal tubules in sensitive and non-sensitive cervical dentine. J Clin Periodontol 1987;14:280–284.
3. Cox C. Etiology and treatment of root hypersensitivity. Am J Dent 1994;7:266–270.
4. Bissada N. Symptomatology and clinical features of hypersensitive teeth. Arch Oral Biol 1994;39(suppl): 31S–32S.
5. Addy M. Etiology and clinical implications of dentine hypersensitivity. Dent Clin North Am 1990;34: 503–514.
6. Rees J. The prevalence of dentinal hypersensitivity in general dental practice in the UK. J Clin Peridontol 2000;27:860–865.
7. Fischer C, Fischer R, Wennberg A. Prevalence and distribution of cervical dentine hypersensitivity in a population in Rio de Janeiro, Brazil. J Dent 1992;20:272–276.
8. Irwin C, McCusker P. Prevalence of dentine hypersensitivity in a general dental population. J Irish Dent Assoc 1997;43:7–9.
9. Gillam D, Seo H, Bulman J, Newman H. Perceptions of dentine hypersensitivity in a general practice population. J Oral Rehabil 1999;26:710–714.

10. Holland G, Narhi M, Addy M, Gangarosa L, Orchardson R. Guidelines for the design and conduct of clinical trials on dentine hypersensitivity. J Clin Periodontol 1997;24:808–813.
11. Gillam D, Newman H. Assessment of pain in cervical detinal sensitivity studies: A review. J Clin Periodontol 1993;20:383–394.
12. Tagami J, Hosoda H, Burrow MF, Nakajima M. Effect of aging and caries on dentin permeability. Proc Finn Dent Soc 1992;88(1, suppl):149–154.
13. Brannstrom M, Johnson G, Nordenvall K. Transmission and control of dentinal pain: resin impregnation for the desensitization of dentin. J Am Dent Assoc 1979;99: 612–618.
14. Nordenvall K, Malmgren B, Brannstrom M. Desensitization of dentin by resin impregnation: A clinical and light-microscopic investigation. ASDC J Dent Child 1984;51:274–276.
15. Sommerman M. Desensitizing agents. In: ADA Guide to Dental Therapeutics. Chicago: American Dental Association, 1998:226–234.
16. Felton DA, Bergenholtz G, Kanoy BE. Evaluation of the desensitizing effect of Gluma Dentin Bond on teeth prepared for complete-coverage restorations. Int J Prosthodont 1991;4:292–298.
17. Narhi M, Kontturi-Narhi V, Hirvonen T, Ngassapa D. Neurophysiologic mechanisms of dentin hypersensitivity. Proc Finn Dent Soc 1992;88(1, suppl):15–22.
18. Javid B, Barkhordar R, Bhinda S. Cyanoacrylate: A new treatment for hypersensitive dentin and cementum. J Am Dent Assoc 1987;114:486–488.
19. Tavares M, DePaula P, Soparkar P. Using a fluoride-releasing resin to reduce cervical sensitivity. J Am Dent Assoc 1994:125:1337–1342.
20. Zhang C, Matsumoto K, Kimura Y, Harashima T, Takeda F, Zhou H. Effects of CO_2 laser in treatment of dentinal hypersensitivity. J Endod 1998;24:595–597.
21. Thompson B, Meyer R, Singh G, Mitchell W. Desensitization of exposed root surfaces using a semilunar coronally positioned flap. Gen Dent 2000;48:68–71.
22. Burke F, Combe E, Douglas W. Dentin bonding systems 2: Clinical uses. Dent Update 2000;27:124–126.
23. Pashley DH, Leibach JG, Horner JA. The effects of burnishing NaF/kaolin/lycerin paste on dentin permeability. J Periodontol 1987;58:19–23.
24. Yoshiyama M, Ozaki K, Ebisu S. Morphological characteristics of hypersensitive human radicular dentin and the effect of a light curing resin liner on tubular occlusion. Proc Finn Dent Soc 1992;88(1, suppl):337–344.
25. Bilotto G, Markowitz K, Kim S. Experimental procedures to test the efficacy of chemical agents in altering intradental nerve activity. J Endod 1987;13:458–465.
26. Markowitz K, Kim S. Hypersensitive teeth: Experimental studies of dentinal desensitizing agents. Den Clin North Am 1990;34:491–501.
27. Kanapka J. Over-the-counter dentifrices in the treatment of dentinal hypersensitivity. Review of clinical studies Dent Clin North Am 1990;34:545–560.
28. Orchardson R. Strategies for the management of hypersensitive teeth. In: Shimono M, Maeda T, Suda H, Takahashi K (eds). Dentin/Pulp Complex. Tokyo: Quintessence, 1996:85–89.
29. Orchardson R, Gillam D. The efficacy of potassium salts as agents for treating dentin hypersensitivity. J Orofacial Pain 2000;14:9–19.
30. Tarbet W, Silverman G, Stolman J, Fratarcangelo P. Clinical evaluation of a new treatment for dentinal hypersensitivity. J Periodontol 1980;51:535–540.
31. Manochehr-Pour M, Bhat M, Bissada N. Clinical evaluation of two potassium nitrate toothpastes for the treatment of dentinal hypersensitivity. Periodontol Case Rep 1984;6:25–30.
32. Silverman G. The sensitivity reducing effect of brushing with a potassium nitrate–sodium monofluorophosphate dentifrice. Compend Contin Educ Dent 1985;6: 131–133.
33. Salvato A, Clark G, Gingold J, Curro F. Clinical effectiveness of a dentifrice containing potassium chloride as a desensitizing agent. Am J Dent 1992;5:303–306.
34. Nagata T, Ishida H, Shinohara H, Nishikawa S, Kasahara S, Wakano Y, et al. Clinical evaluation of a potassium nitrate dentifrice for the treatment of dentinal hypersensitivity. J Clin Periodontol 1994;21:217–221.
35. Schiff T, Dotson M, Cohen S, de Vizio W, McCool J, Volpe A. Efficacy of a dentifrice containing 5% potassium nitrate, 1.3% soluble pyrophosphate, 1.5% PVM/MA copolymer, and 0.243% sodium fluoride in a silica base on dentinal hypersensitivity. J Clin Dent 1994;5(special issue):87–92.
36. Silverman G, Gingold J, Curro F. Desensitizing effects of a potassium chloride dentifrice. Am J Dent 1994;7: 9–12.
37. Silverman G, Berman E, Hanna C, Slavato A, Fratarcangelo P, Bartizek R. Assessing the efficacy of three dentifrices in the treatment of dentinal hypersensitivity. J Am Dent Assoc 1996;127:191–201.
38. Gillam DG, Bulman JS, Jackson RJ, Newman HN. Comparison of 2 desensitising dentifrices with a commercially available fluoride dentifrice in alleviating cervical dentine sensitivity. J Periodontol 1996;67:737–742.
39. West NX, Addy M, Jackson RJ, Ridge DB. Dentine hypersensitivity and the placebo response. A comparison of the effect of strontium acetate, potassium nitrate and fluoride toothpastes. J Clin Periodontol 1997;24: 209–215.
40. Schiff T, Dos Santos M, Laffi S, Yoshioka M, Baines E, McCool J, de Vizio W. Efficacy of a dentifrice containing 5% potassium nitrate and 1500 ppm sodium monofluorophosphate in a precipitated calcium carbonate base on dentinal hypersensitivity. J Clin Dent 1998;9:22–25.

41. Thrash W, Dodds M, Jones D. The effect of stannous fluoride on dentinal hypersensitivity. Int Dent J 1994; 44(1, suppl):107–118.
42. Plagmann H, Konig J, Bernimoulin J, Rudhart A, Deschner J. A clinical study comparing two high-fluoride dentifrices for the treatment of dentinal hypersensitivity. Quintessence Int 1997;28:403–408.
43. Bolden T, Volpe A, King W. The desensitizing effect of a sodium monofluorophosphate dentifrice. Periodontics 1968;6:112–115.
44. Haven S, Volpe A, King W. Comparative desensitizing effect of dentrifices containing sodium monofluorophosphate, stannous fluoride and formalin. Periodontics 1968;6:230–236.
45. Dunne S, Hannington-Kiff J. The use of topical guanethidine in the relief of dentine hypersensitivity: A controlled study. Pain 1993;54:165–168.
46. Hannington-Kiff J, Dunne S. Topical guanethidine relieves dentinal hypersensitivity and pain. J Royal Soc Med 1993;86:514–515.
47. Raab W, Magerl W, Muller H. Changes in dental blood flow following electrical tooth pulp stimulation: Influences of capsaicin and guanethidine. Agents Actions 1988;25:237–239.
48. Mashimo T, Pak M, Choe H, Inagaki Y, Yamamoto M, Yoshiya I. Effects of vasodilators guanethidine, nicardipine, nitroglycerin and prostaglandin E1 on primary afferent nociceptors in humans. J Clin Pharmacol 1997;37:330–335.
49. Zheng Z, Shimamura K, Anthony T, Kreulen D. Guanethidine evokes vasodilation in guinea pig mesenteric artery by acting on sensory neurons. Neurosci Lett 2000;288:231–235.
50. Lavigne S, Gutenkunst L, Williams K. Effects of tartar-control dentifrice on tooth sensitivity: A pilot study. J Dent Hyg 1997;71:105–111.
51. Absi E, Addy M, Adams D. Dentine hypersensitivity: The effect of toothbrushing and dietary compounds on dentin in vitro: An SEM study. J Oral Rehabil 1992;19: 101–110.
52. Addy M, Loyn T, Adams D. Dentine hypersensitivity: Effects of some proprietary mouthwashes on the dentine smear layer: A SEM study. J Dent 1991;19:148–152.
53. Hargreaves K, Hutter J. Endodontic pharmacology. In: Cohen S, Burns R (eds). Pathways of the Pulp, ed 8. St. Louis: Mosby, 2002:665–682.
54. Okeson J. Bell's Orofacial Pains, ed 5. Chicago: Quintessence, 1995.
55. Cohen S, Liewehr F. Diagnostic procedures. In: Cohen S, Burns R (eds). Pathways of the Pulp, ed 8. St. Louis: Mosby, 2002:1–30.
56. Walton R, Torabinejad M. Diagnosis and treatment planning. In: Walton R, Torabinejad M (eds). Principles and Practice of Endodontics, ed 3. Philadelphia: Saunders, 2002:49–70.
57. Bellizzi R, Hartwell G, Ingle J, Goerig A, Neaverth E, Marshall FJ, et al. Diagnostic procedures. In: Ingle J, Bakland L (eds). Endodontics, ed 4. Baltimore: Williams & Wilkins, 1994:465–519.
58. Eversole L, Chase P. Nonodontogenic facial pain and endodontics: Pain syndromes of the jaws that simulate odontalgia. In: Cohen S, Burns R (eds). Pathways of the Pulp, ed 8. St. Louis: Mosby, 2002:77–90.
59. Schwartz S, Cohen S. The difficult differential diagnosis. Dent Clin North Am 1992;36:279–292.
60. Lavigne F, Lund J, Sessle B, Dubner R. Orofacial Pain: Basic Sciences to Clinical Management. Chicago: Quintessence, 2001.
61. Hasselgren G, Reit C. Emergency pulpotomy: Pain relieving effect with and without the use of sedative dressings. J Endod 1989;15:254–256.
62. Hargreaves KM, Baumgartner JC. Endodontic therapeutics. In: Walton R, Torabinejad M (eds). Principles and Practice of Endodontics, ed 3. Philadelphia: Saunders, 2002:533–544.
63. Oguntebi BR, DeSchepper EJ, Taylor TS, White CL, Pink FE. Postoperative pain incidence related to the type of emergency treatment of symptomatic pulpitis. Oral Surg Oral Med Oral Pathol 1992;73:479–483.
64. Penniston SG, Hargreaves KM. Evaluation of periapical injection of Ketorolac for management of endodontic pain. J Endod 1996;22:55–59.
65. Marshall JG, Liesinger AW. Factors associated with endodontic posttreatment pain. J Endod 1993;19: 573–575.
66. Torabinejad M, Cymerman J, Frankson M, Lemon R, Maggio J, Schilder H. Effectiveness of various medications on postoperative pain following complete instrumentation. J Endod 1994;20:345–354.
67. Moos HL, Bramwell JD, Roahen JO. A comparison of pulpectomy alone versus pulpectomy with trephination for the relief of pain. J Endod 1996;22:422–425.
68. Rogers M, Johnson B, Remeikis N, BeGole E. Comparison of effect of intracanal use of ketorolac tromethamine and dexamethasone with oral ibuprofen on post treatment endodontic pain. J Endod 1999;25: 381–384.
69. Doroshak A, Bowles W, Hargreaves K. Evaluation of the combination of flurbiprofen and tramadol for management of endodontic pain. J Endod 1999;25:660–663.
70. Rosenberg PA, Babick PJ, Schertzer L, Leung A. The effect of occlusal reduction on pain after endodontic instrumentation. J Endod 1998;24:492–496.
71. Nist E, Reader A, Beck M. Effect of apical trephination on postoperative pain and swelling in symptomatic necrotic teeth. J Endod 2001;27:415–420.
72. Houck V, Reader A, Beck M, Nist R, Weaver J. Effect of trephination on postoperative pain and swelling in symptomatic necrotic teeth. Oral Surg Oral Med Oral Pathol Oral Radiol Endod 2000;90:507–513.

73. Cunningham C, Mullaney T. Pain control in endodontics. Dent Clin North Am 1992;36:393–408.
74. Morse D. Use of meditative state for hypnotic induction in the practice of endodontics. Oral Surg Oral Med Oral Pathol Oral Radiol Endod 1976;41:664–672.
75. Morse D, Wilcko J. Nonsurgical endodontic therapy for a vital tooth with meditation-hypnosis as the sole anesthetic: Case report. Am J Clin Hypn 1979;21:258–262.
76. Baron R, Logan H, Hoppe S. Emotional and sensory focus as mediators of dental pain among patients differing in desired and felt dental control. Heath Psych 1993;12:381–389.
77. Logan H, Baron R, Kohout F. Sensory focus as therapeutic treatments for acute pain. Psychosom Med 1995;57: 475–484.
78. Hargreaves KM, Roszkowski M, Jackson DL, Swift JQ. Orofacial pain: Peripheral mechanisms. In: Fricton J, Dubner R (eds). Advances in Pain Research and Therapy. Vol 21: Orofacial pain and temporomandibular disorders. New York: Raven Press, 1995:33–42.
79. Roszkowski, MT, Swift JQ, and Hargreaves KM. Effect of NSAID administration on tissue levels of immunoreactive prostaglandin E2, leukotriene B4, and (S)-flurbiprofen following extraction of impacted third molars. Pain 1997;73:339–346.
80. Malmberg A, Yaksh T. Antinociceptive actions of spinal nonsteroidal anti-inflammatory agents on the formalin test in rats. J Pharmacol Exp Ther 1992;263:136–146.
81. Samad TA, Moore KA, Sapirstein A, Billet S, Allchorne A, Poole S, et al. Interleukin-1beta-mediated induction of COX-2 in the CNS contributes to inflammatory pain hypersensitivity. Nature 2001;410:471–475.
82. Curtis P, Gartman L, Green D. Utilization of ketorolac tromethamine for control of severe odontogenic pain. J Endod 1994;20:457–460.
83. Max M, Portenoy R, Laska E (eds). The Design of Analgesic Clinical Trials. New York: Raven Press, 1990.
84. Dionne R, Campbell R, Cooper SA, Hall D, Buckinham B. Suppression of postoperative pain by preoperative administration of ibuprofen in comparison to placebo, acetaminophen and acetaminophen plus codeine. J Clin Pharmacol 1983;23:37–43.
85. Bunczak-Reeh M, Hargreaves KM. Effect of inflammation on delivery of drugs to dental pulp. J Endod 1998; 24:822–825.
86. Dionne RA. COX-2 inhibitors: Better than ibuprofen for dental pain? Compend Contin Educ Dent 1999;20: 518–522.
87. Ehrich E, Dallob A, DeLepeleire I, Van Hecken A, Riendeau D, Yuan W, et al. Characterization of rofecoxib as a cyclooxygenase inhibitor and demonstration of analgesia in the dental pain model. Clin Pharmacol Ther 1999;65:336–347.
88. Nakanishi T, Shimuzu H, Matsuo T. An immunohistological study on cyclooxygenase-2 in human dental pulp. J Endod 2001;27:385–388.
89. Wallace J. Selective COX-2 inhibitors: Is the water becoming muddy? Trends Pharmacol Sci 1999;20:4–5.
90. Cooper SA. New peripherally acting oral analgesics. Ann Rev Pharmacol Toxicol 1983;23:617–647.
91. Dionne RA, Berthold CW. Therapeutic uses of nonsteroidal anti-inflammatory drugs in dentistry. Crit Rev Oral Biol Med 2001;12:315–330.
92. Drug Facts and Comparisons, ed 54. St. Louis: Facts and Comparisons, 2000:848–919.
93. Gage T, Pickett F. Mosby's Dental Drug Reference, ed 4. St. Louis: Mosby, 2000:786.
94. Wynn R, Meiller T, Crossley H. Drug Information Handbook for Dentistry. Hudson: Lexi-Comp, 1999-2000:1399.
95. Moskow A, Morse D, Krasner P, Furst M. Intracanal use of a corticosteroid solution as an endodontic anodyne. Oral Surg Oral Med Oral Pathol 1984;58:600–604.
96. Chance K, Lin L, Shovlin FE, Skribner J. Clinical trial of intracanal corticosteroid in root canal therapy. J Endod 1987;13:466–468.
97. Trope M. Relationship of intracanal medicaments to endodontic flare-ups. Endod Dent Traumatol 1990;6: 226–229.
98. Marshall J, Walton R. The effect of intramuscular injection of steroid on posttreatment endodontic pain. J Endod 1984;10:584–588.
99. Liesinger A, Marshall F, Marshall J. Effect of variable doses of dexamethasone on posttreatment endodontic pain. J Endod 1993;19:35–39.
100. Kaufman E, Heling I, Rotstein I, Friedman S, Sion A, Moz C, Staboltz A. Intraligamentary injection of slow-release methylprednisolone for the prevention of pain after endodontic treatment. Oral Surg Oral Med Oral Pathol 1994;77:651–654.
101. Krasner P, Jackson E. Management of posttreatment endodontic pain with oral dexamethasone: A double-blind study. Oral Surg Oral Med Oral Pathol 1986;62: 187–190.
102. Glassman G, Krasner P, Morse DR, Rankow H, Lang J, Furst ML. A prospective randomized double-blind trial on efficacy of dexamethasone for endodontic interappointment pain in teeth with asymptomatic inflamed pulps. Oral Surg Oral Med Oral Pathol 1989;67:96–100.
103. Gallatin E, Reader A, Nist R, Beck M. Pain reduction in untreated irreversible pulpitis using an intraosseous injection of Depo-Medrol. J Endod 2000;26:633–638.
104. Dionne R. Suppression of dental pain by the preoperative administration of flurbiprofen. Am J Med 1986;80: 41–49.
105. Dunsky JL, Moore PA. Long-acting local anesthetics: A comparison of bupivacaine and etidocaine in endodontics. J Endod 1984;10:457–460.

106. Moore P, Dunsky J. Bupivacaine anesthesia: A clinical trial for endodontic therapy. Oral Surg Oral Med Oral Pathol Oral Radiol Endod 1983;55:176–179.
107. Moore P. Long acting anesthetics: A review of clinical efficacy in dentistry. Compend Contin Educ Dent 1990;11:22–30.
108. Woolf C. Transcriptional and posttranslational plasticity and the generation of inflammatory pain. Proc Natl Acad Sci USA 1999;96:7723.
109. Gordon S, Dionne R, Brahim J, Jabir F, Dubner R. Blockade of peripheral neuronal barrage reduces postoperative pain. Pain 1997;70:209–215.
110. Jebeles J, Reilly J, Gutierrez J, Bradley E, Kissin I. Tonsillectomy and adenoidectomy pain reduction by local bupivacaine infiltration in children. Int J Pediatr Otorhinolaryngol 1993;25:149–154.
111. Bacsik C, Swift J, Hargreaves KM. Toxic systemic reactions of bupivacaine and etidocaine: Review of the literature. Oral Surg Oral Med Oral Pathol 1995;79:18–23.
112. Saxen M, Newton C. Anesthesia for endodontic practice. Dent Clin North Am 1999;43:247–261.
113. Replogle K, Reader A, Nist R, Beck M, Weaver J, Meyers W. Anesthetic efficacy of the intraosseous injection of 2% lidocaine (1:100,000 epinephrine) and 3% mepivacaine in mandibular first molars. Oral Surg Oral Med Oral Pathol Oral Radiol Endod 1997;83:30–37.
114. Replogle K, Reader A, Nist R, Beck M, Weaver J, Meyers W. Cardiovascular effects of intraosseous injections of 2 percent lidocaine with 1:100,000 epinephrine and 3 percent mepivacaine. J Am Dent Assoc 1999;130: 649–657.
115. Reisman D, Reader A, Nist R, Beck M, Weaver J. Anesthetic efficacy of the supplemental intraosseous injection of 3% mepivacaine in irreversible pulpitis. Oral Surg Oral Med Oral Pathol Oral Radiol Endod 1997;84: 676–682.
116. Nusstein J, Reader A, Nist R, Beck M, Meyers W. Anesthetic efficacy of the supplemental intraosseous injection of 2% lidocaine with 1:100,000 epinephrine in irreversible pulpitis. J Endod 1998;24:487–491.
117. Parente SA, Anderson R, Herman W, Kimbrough W, Weller RN. Anesthetic efficacy of the supplemental intraosseous injection for teeth with irreversible pulpitis. J Endod 1998;24:826–828.
118. Jastak JT, Yagiela J, Donaldson D. Local Anesthesia of the Oral Cavity. Philadelphia: Saunders, 1995.
119. Malemed S. Handbook of Local Anesthesia, ed 3. St. Louis: Mosby, 1990.
120. Ji R, Zhang Q, Law P, Low H, Elde R, Hokfelt T. Expression of mu-, delta- and kappa-opioid receptor-like immunoreactivities in rat dorsal root ganglia after carrageenan induced inflammation. J Neurosci 1995;15: 8156–8166.
121. Laduron P. Axonal transport of opiate receptors in the capsaicin sensitive neurons. Brain Res 1984;294: 157–160.
122. Taddese A, Nah A, McCleskey E. Selective opioid inhibition of small nociceptive neurons. Science 1995;270: 1366–1369.
123. Joris J, Dubner R, Hargreaves KM. Opioid analgesia at peripheral sites: A target for opioids released during stress and inflammation? Anesth Analg 1987;66: 1277–1281.
124. Dionne RA, Lepinski AM, Jaber L, Gordon SM, Brahim JS, Hargreaves KM. Analgesic effects of peripherally administered opioids in clinical models of acute and chronic inflammation. Clin Pharmacol Ther 2001;70:66–73.
125. Uhle R, Reader A, Nist R, Beck M, Meyers W. Peripheral opioid analgesia in teeth with symptomatic inflamed pulps. Anesth Prog 1997;44:90–95.
126. Likar R, Koppaert W, Blatnig H, Chiari F, Stiil R, Stein C. Efficacy of peripheral morphine analgesia in inflamed, non-inflamed and perineural tissue of dental surgery patients. J Pain Sympt Manage 2001;21:330–337.
127. Cooper SA. Treating acute dental pain. Postgrad Dent 1995;2:7–10.
128. Harrison JW, Baumgartner CJ, Zielke DR. Analysis of interappointment pain associated with the combined use of endodontic irrigants and medicaments. J Endod 1981;7:272–276.
129. Georgopoulou M, Anastassiadis P, Sykaras S. Pain after chemomechanical preparation. Int Endod J 1996;19: 309–314.
130. Cooper S. The relative efficacy of ibuprofen in dental pain. Compend Contin Educ Dent 1986;7:578–588.
131. Breivik E, Barkvoll P, Skovlund E. Combining diclofenac with acetaminophen or acetaminophen-codeine after oral surgery: A randomized, double-blind, single oral dose study. Clin Pharmacol Ther 2000;66:625–635.
132. Wideman G, Keffer M, Morris E, Doyle R, Jiang J, Beaver W. Analgesic efficacy of a combination of hydrocodone with ibuprofen in postoperative pain. Clin Pharmacol Ther 1999;65:66–76.
133. Lanza F, Royer G, Nelson R, Rack M, Seckman C, Schwartz J. Effect of acetaminophen on human gastric mucosal injury caused by ibuprofen. Gut 1986;27: 440–443.
134. Stambaugh J, Drew J. The combination of ibuprofen and oxycodone/acetaminophen in the management of chronic cancer pain. Clin Pharmacol Ther 1988;44: 665–669.
135. Wright C, Antal E, Gillespie W, Albert KS. Ibuprofen and acetaminophen kinetics when taken concurrently. Clin Pharmacol Ther 1983;34:707–710.

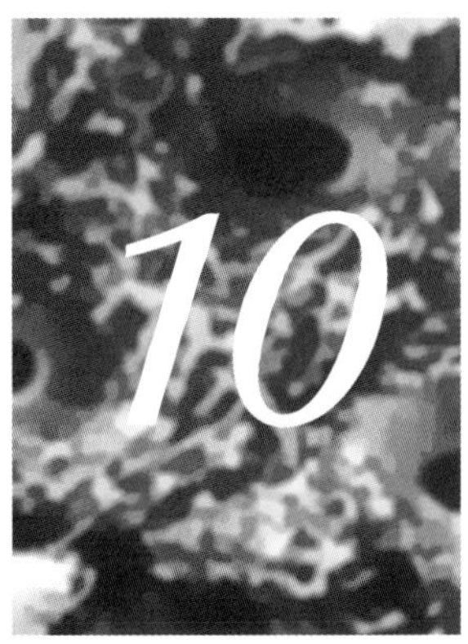

Histology of Pulpal Inflammation

Henry O. Trowbridge, DDS, PhD

The inflammatory response to pulpal injury or infection has major clinical significance. Injury may be caused by dental procedures (iatrogenic), by trauma, or by attrition. Infection may be caused by bacteria originating from caries, microleakage from restorations, or other routes of entry into the pulp. To provide a comprehensive review of this clinically important topic, this chapter describes pulpal inflammation at a histologic level; chapter 11 reviews pulpal inflammation at an inflammatory mediator level; and chapters 12 and 17 review the consequences of pulpal necrosis, namely the development of apical periodontitis.

Inflammation: General Considerations

Today it is recognized that there is no clear-cut difference between inflammation and immunity. Acute inflammation, innate immunity, humoral immunity, and cell-mediated immunity together provide the host with a wide array of weapons with which to combat pathogens and bring about healing. The major role of these systems is to protect the individual from invasion by infectious organisms that can cause disease. Neutrophils and macrophages are motile phagocytes that constitute the body's first line of defense against invading microorganisms.

For convenience, inflammation is usually divided into three stages: acute inflammation, chronic inflammation, and healing. Here we will consider only acute and chronic inflammation. Acute inflammation is abrupt in onset and of short duration, whereas chronic inflammation is persistent in nature. Usually acute inflammation precedes the chronic form, but chronic inflammation can be primary in some cases, as in immunologic reactions such as hypersensitivity and cell-mediated immune reactions.

The acute inflammatory response is primarily a vascular reaction. In the acute response, arterioles dilate and venules become more permeable so that fluid and plasma proteins can leave the bloodstream and enter the tissue, a process termed *exudation*. Important chemical mediators of the acute vascular response (and their origin) include histamine (mast cells); 5-hydroxytryptamine (serotonin, platelets); bradykinin (bloodstream); complement components C4, C3, and C5 (bloodstream); prostaglandins E_1 and E_2 (pulpal cells); leukotrienes C_4, D_4, and E_4 (primarily immune cells); platelet- activating factor (multiple sources); nitrous oxide (pulpal and immune cells); calcitonin gene-related peptide (sensory neurons); and substance P (sensory neurons)

In addition, phagocytes (neutrophils and macrophages) often emigrate from the bloodstream to the site of acute inflammation. This response can occur relatively rapidly, prior to activation of T cells and B cells, and is referred to as *innate immunity*. Innate immunity differs from *adaptive immunity* in that it lacks immunologic memory. Whereas the adaptive immune system can recognize every possible antigen, the innate system focuses on a few highly conserved antigens present in a large number of microorganisms.[1] These antigens are known as *pathogen-associated molecular patterns*. Receptors of the innate immune system are called *pattern-recognition receptors*, the best known of which bind to bacterial lipopolysaccharide (endotoxin). Other pattern-recognition receptors bind to ligands such as peptidoglycan, lipoteichoic acids, and mannans.

Another component of innate immunity is activation of the alternative pathway of the complement system.[2] Substances such as endotoxin and plasmin can activate this pathway prior to the appearance of specific antibodies. The complement system greatly enhances the ability of phagocytes to engulf infectious agents by providing chemotactic factors and the opsonin C3b. Following activation of the adaptive immune system, the complement system can be activated via the classical pathway.

A chronic inflammatory reaction differs from an acute response in that it is typically persistent and lasts for more than a week or so. For example, an abscess is an acute inflammatory response involving neutrophils. However, when the causative organisms are not eliminated, the abscess becomes persistent and is described as a chronic abscess. But, there is no clear dividing line between acute and chronic inflammation. It takes 3 to 5 days for clones of lymphocytes to be produced and to differentiate into effector cells,[2] sufficient time for pathogens to injure the host. During the time it takes for the adaptive immune system to get into high gear, host defense depends upon innate immunity. Once the adaptive immune system is activated, T helper cells, cytotoxic lymphocytes, macrophages, and specific antibody-producing plasma cells supplement the innate immune system.

The two arms of the immune system are humoral and cell-mediated immunity. With the assistance of T_H2 helper T cells, clones of activated B cells undergo maturation and become antibody-producing plasma cells. Macrophages, T_H1 helper T cells, and cytotoxic T cells are involved in cell-mediated immunity.

Just as there is no clear dividing line between acute and chronic inflammation, the overall process of inflammation overlaps with the process of healing. Tissue healing begins when the macrophages first begin to debride damaged tissue. If regeneration of new cells is unable to replace lost tissue, healing then takes place in the form of connective tissue repair.

It is important to understand that chronic inflammation can develop in the absence of an antecedent acute response. Thus, under certain conditions, chronic inflammation occurs as a distinct process from the outset, with minimal acute inflammation, as in the release of antigenic bacterial products that activate an immune response. Dental caries exemplifies this process, wherein bacterial products diffuse through the dentinal tubules and reach the pulp long before bacteria themselves invade it. Such chronic inflammatory reactions are often associated with dental restorative procedures in which microleakage develops.

Another example of "immediate" chronic inflammation is infection by certain intracellular parasites such as *Mycobacterium tuberculosis* and *M leprae*. Since these organisms have a low toxicity, tissue damage is due almost entirely to activation of a cell-mediated immune response in which macrophages play a prominent role. A third example is the introduction of inert foreign bodies such as splinters, asbestos, or silica into tissues. Indeed, the presence of almost any inanimate, particulate, persistent foreign material will provoke a chronic response, termed a *foreign-body reaction*. Additional examples of this type of immediate chronic inflammation include deposition of products of metabolism (eg, urate crystals in gout, cholesterol crystals) and autoimmune reactions (eg, rheumatoid arthritis, lupus erythematosus).

With the possible exception of the foreign-body reaction, chronic inflammation is an immune response orchestrated by macrophages and T helper cells. Macrophages play several key roles in chronic inflammatory reactions (see also chapters 5 and 11). Macrophages are the primary defense against certain intracellular pathogens. Activated macrophages can function as class II antigen-presenting cells, similar to pulpal dendritic and B cells. In addition, activated macrophages secrete many inflammatory mediators, such as complement components, plasminogen activator, IL-1, IL-12, prostaglandins, and leukotrienes.

Macrophages become activated after receiving two signals. The first is a priming stimulus and the second is an activating signal.[3] The priming stimulus is interferon-γ secreted by activated T helper cells. Activating stimuli include bacterial lipopolysaccharide (endotoxin), muramyl dipeptide, and other chemical mediators. Activated macrophages can then secrete cytotoxic mediators such as IL-1, tumor necrosis factor-α (TNF-α), cytolytic proteases, lysozyme, platelet-activating factor, and oxygen-derived radicals.

Dendritic cells are required to process and present antigen to immunocompetent T cells. Thus, they are known as *antigen-presenting cells* (APCs). Subgroups of monocytes are thought to travel to tissues and differentiate into immature dendritic cells.[4] These cells have long processes and large amounts of cell-surface major histocompatibility complex (MHC) Class II molecules. Other APCs include macrophages, activated B cells, and Langerhans cells (dendritic cells of the epidermis). Antigens entering the tissues are captured and engulfed by APCs. Once they have engulfed antigen, these cells travel to local lymph nodes through afferent lymph vessels. When they are exposed to inflammatory stimuli, they undergo further maturation, during which they lose their receptors for inflammatory chemokines and increase the number of receptors for lymphoid chemokines.[4] In this way, they are guided to the T-cell area of lymph nodes, where they present the processed antigen to naïve T helper cells. Presentation requires that the antigen be processed (degraded) intracellularly by proteolytic enzymes into antigenic determinates (epitopes) that are then presented by MHC molecules on the surface of the APC. Epitopes are recognized by antigen-specific T-cell receptors, which leads to activation of signaling pathways that induce the expression of cytokines, chemokines, and costimulatory molecules by the T helper cell. These in turn regulate and recruit other cells of the immune system.

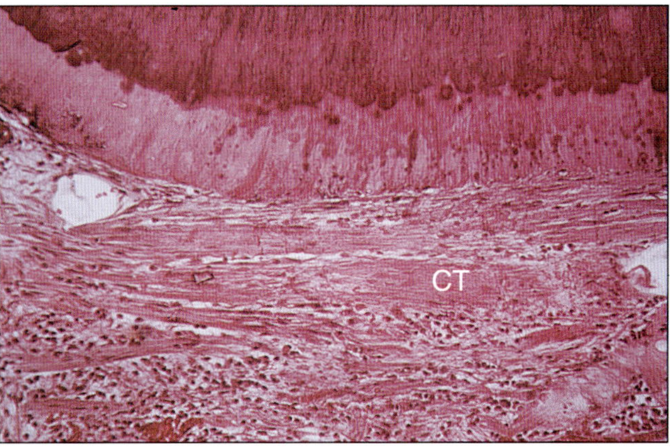

Fig 10-1 Bands of fibrous connective tissue (CT) in a chronically inflamed pulp (H&E stain, original magnification ×56).

This process ultimately results in an infiltration of the tissue by immunocompetent T and B lymphocytes as well as macrophages, neutrophils, and often, but not always, plasma cells. Whereas neutrophils are the predominant inflammatory cells in an acute inflammatory response, lymphocytes and macrophages outnumber them in chronic inflammatory reactions.

Fibroblasts frequently play an important role in chronic inflammatory reactions. In many chronic diseases, the production of collagen is responsible for loss of function. Examples are cirrhosis of the liver, scleroderma, silicosis, and pulmonary fibrosis. Growth factors that are mito-

Box 10-1	**Factors that influence the rate of caries**

- Age of the host (eating habits, maturation of hydroxyapatite crystals)
- Composition of the tooth, particularly fluoride content
- Nature of the bacterial flora in the lesion
- Rate of salivary flow (patients with xerostomia generally develop rampant caries)
- Antibacterial substances in the saliva (eg, IgA antibodies, lysozyme)
- Oral hygiene
- Cariogenicity of the diet (refined fermentable carbohydrates) and the frequency with which acidogenic foods are ingested
- Caries-inhibiting factors in the diet (eg, phosphates, calcium-containing foods, chocolate)

genic for fibroblasts include platelet-derived growth factor (PDGF), transforming growth factor-α, epidermal growth factor, and IL-1. Chemoattractants for fibroblasts include fibronectin, PDGF, transforming growth factor-β, and IL-1. An example of pulpal fibrosis is shown in Fig 10-1.

Under certain stimuli, fibroblasts are able to express genes for the production of metalloproteinases.[5] Secretion of these enzymes can be induced by several growth factors, such as PDGF, fibroblast growth factor, and IL-1. In inflammatory reactions, these enzymes can degrade fibrillar and soluble collagen, proteoglycans, laminin, and fibronectin. Thus, fibroblasts are able to participate in tissue breakdown during an inflammatory reaction.

Etiology of Pulpal Inflammation

A major etiologic factor for pulpal inflammation is the invasion of bacteria or bacteria-derived factors into the dental pulp (see also chapter 12). Bacteria can invade dental pulp tissue after caries or tooth fracture, via anomalous dentinal tracts, or following dental restorative procedures. The following section reviews each of these causes of pulpal inflammation.

Dental caries

Dental caries is a microbial disease affecting the calcified tissues of the teeth as well as the pulp. For caries to develop, specific bacteria must become established on the tooth surface. Without doubt, bacterial invasion from a caries lesion is the most common cause of pulpal inflammation.

Diagnostic tools to determine the extent of pulpal inflammation beneath a caries lesion are imprecise. Many factors play a role in determining the nature of the process, so the individuality of each caries lesion must be recognized. The response of the pulp may vary depending on whether the caries process progresses rapidly (acute caries) or slowly (chronic caries), or is completely inactive (arrested caries). In addition, caries tends to be an intermittent process, with periods of rapid activity alternating with periods of quiescence.[6] Box 10-1 lists factors that influence the rate of caries attack.

Conditions for growth and availability of nutrients are quite different in enamel caries than in dentinal caries. Lactobacilli thrive in sites of cavitation,[7] and the low pH in dentinal lesions allows only aciduric organisms to flourish there, where the microbial flora is also rather nonspecific and the environmental conditions for growth vary at different times and in different locations within the lesion.

Products of bacterial metabolism, notably organic acids and proteolytic enzymes, destroy enamel and dentin. It has been shown that exposure of the pulp to bacterial products on the dentin can elicit an inflammatory response in the pulp.[8,9] It has further been demonstrated that a relatively large bacterial product, bacterial endotoxin, is able to diffuse through dentinal tubules to the pulp chamber in vitro.[10] Bacterial antigens diffusing from the lesion to the pulp through the dentinal tubules are captured and processed by APCs as described above, which leads to the activation of the immune system. Deep penetration of dentin by bacteria results in acute inflammation and eventually infection and necrosis of the pulp.

As bacteria invade enamel and enter the dentin, changes commence in the pulp. The first reaction of odontoblasts to superficial caries lesions in enamel is a marked reduction in the cytoplasm: nucleus ratio, suggesting an altered metabolism.[11] In active lesions, primary odontoblasts are involved in the formation of reactionary dentin (see also chapter 3). Initially, there is an increase in metabolic activity in odontoblasts, which are stimulated to produce more collagen.[12] Soon, however, even before the appearance of inflammatory changes, the size and number of odontoblasts decrease, at which time their metabolic activity is reduced while cellular proliferative activity in the cell-free zone of the pulp increases.

Although normally tall columnar cells, odontoblasts adversely affected by caries become flat to cuboidal in shape (Fig 10-2). This figure also demonstrates a so-called hyperchromatic (calciotraumatic) line indicating where the odontoblasts were first subjected to injury. Reactionary dentin can be seen between the hyperchromatic line and the odontoblast layer. This form of dentin differs from reparative dentin in that it is formed by primary rather than replacement odontoblasts. It can be recognized because there is no disruption in the lumens of the dentinal tubules (ie, they are continuous with the pulp). On the other hand, the boundary zone between primary and reparative dentin is atubular and lacks continuity of tubules.[13]

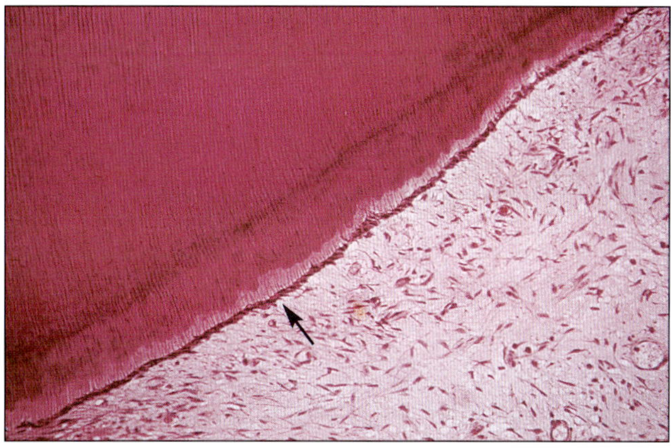

Fig 10-2 Atrophic odontoblasts beneath a superficial caries lesion in dentin. A hyperchromatic line can be seen in the dentin *(arrow)*. Note the absence of inflammation (H&E stain, original magnification ×56).

Electron microscopic examination of the odontoblasts beneath a superficial caries lesion revealed cellular injury in the form of ballooning degeneration of mitochondria and a reduction in the number and size of other cytoplasmic organelles.[14] Eventually, the primary odontoblasts die, usually followed by proliferation of replacement odontoblasts and reparative dentin formation.

It is important to point out that bacteria infect some tubules long before others are infected, as shown in Fig 10-3. The distribution of infected tubules is not uniform, as neighboring uninfected tubules are frequently found interspersed among infected tubules. Figure 10-4 shows an infected tubule deep in the dentin. At the completion of cavity or crown preparation, some infected tubules may not have been eliminated. However, if the restorative procedure adequately protects the dentin from microleakage, bacteria in the tubules will eventually die for a lack of substrate.

The reason some dentinal tubules are invaded by bacteria sooner than others remains obscure. It would appear that tubules exhibit a certain re-

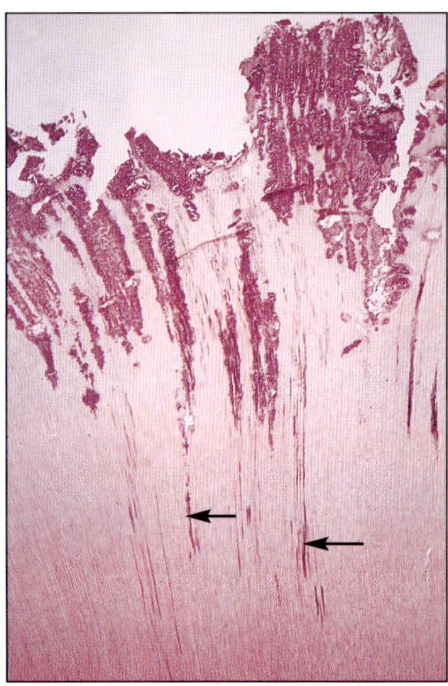

Fig 10-3 Infected tubules in dentin. Note how infected tubules *(arrows)* are interspersed with uninfected tubules (H&E stain, original magnification ×16).

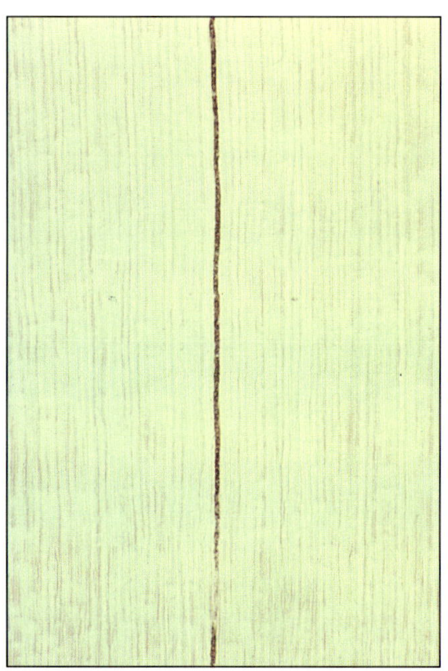

Fig 10-4 A single infected tubule deep in the dentin surrounded by uninfected tubules (Glynn modified Gram stain, original magnification ×88).

sistance to infection. For example, the resistance to bacterial invasion is greater in dentinal tubules of vital teeth than those in nonvital teeth.[15] One reason might be that dentinal fluid in the tubules may contain antibodies (see also chapter 4). This interesting phenomenon is deserving of further study.

Basic reactions that tend to protect the pulp against caries include a decrease in the permeability of the dentin due to dentinal sclerosis, the formation of new dentin (tertiary dentin), and the effectiveness of inflammatory and immunologic reactions. The following three sections describe these forms of protective reactions to caries.

Dentinal sclerosis

Dentinal sclerosis is the most common response to caries[16] (see also chapters 3, 4, and 16). Dentinal sclerosis develops at the periphery of almost all caries lesions. Antigenic and other irritating substances reach the pulp by diffusing through the dentinal tubules. Therefore, the permeability of the tubules is of critical importance in determining the extent of pulpal injury (chapters 3 and 4). In dentinal sclerosis, the dentinal tubules become partly or completely filled with mineral deposits consisting of both hydroxyapatite and whitlockite crystals (see Fig 3-11). A study[17] using dyes and radioactive ions showed that dentinal sclerosis reduces the permeability of dentin, thus shielding the pulp from irritation. In order for sclerosis to occur, vital odontoblast processes must be present within the tubules.[18]

In highly active caries lesions, odontoblast may die before sclerosis has occurred. Disintegration of odontoblast processes within the tubules results in a dead tract. A dead tract appears black in dried ground sections because the empty tubules are filled with air and are therefore refractive, as seen in Fig 10-5. Providing the pulp is relatively healthy, reparative dentin is deposited over the pulpal end of the dead tract.

Tertiary dentin

Chapter 3 provides a detailed description of tertiary dentin formation from a biochemical perspective; this chapter reviews the histology of that response to pulpal inflammation. Developmental (primary) dentin is formed during tooth development. Dentin that forms following the completion of tooth development is termed *physiologic secondary dentin.* Tertiary dentin differs from developmental and physiologic secondary dentin in that it is produced in response to some form of irritation. It is deposited at the base of the dentinal tubules corresponding to the area of the tooth that is subjected to irritation. Irritants include extensive wear of the tooth surface, erosion, cracks in the enamel and dentin, dental caries, loss of cementum from the root surface, and dental operative procedures. Thus, tertiary dentin represents a defense mechanism against loss of enamel, dentin, or cementum.

There are two types of tertiary dentin based upon the cell type responsible for dentin production (chapter 3). *Reactionary dentin* is defined as a tertiary dentin formed by surviving odontoblast cells, typically to milder stimuli. In contrast, *reparative dentin* is defined as a tertiary dentin formed by a new generation of odontoblast-like cells. Such a response will normally be seen after stronger stimuli.[19]

In primate studies, pulp exposure initiates increased mitotic activity among fibroblasts in the cell-rich zone.[19] These cells migrate to the dentin surface, mature into pre-odontoblasts, and finally become replacement odontoblasts. Characteristically, the cell bodies of these new cells are flat to cuboidal in shape, and the odontoblast layer they form has a lower density of cells than the original odontoblast layer. Reparative dentinogenesis in rat molars involves odontoblast-like cells that synthesize type I but not type III collagen and are immunopositive for dentin sialoprotein, a dentin-specific protein that marks the odontoblast phenotype.[20] Following the loss of primary odontoblasts in human teeth, there is a time lag of about 20 to 40 days before reparative dentin formation commences.[21]

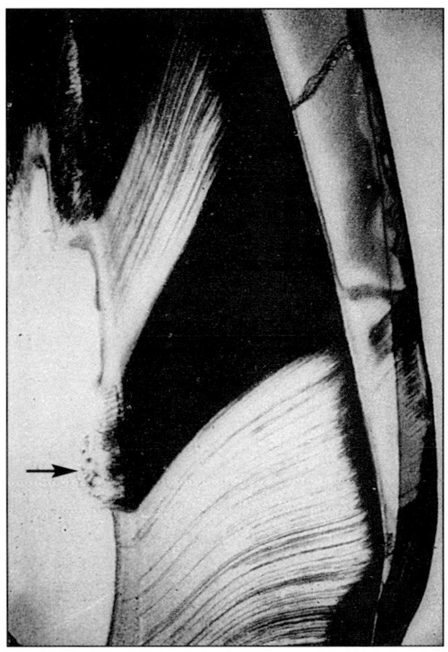

Fig 10-5 A dead tract in dentin beneath caries lesions. Note the presence of reparative dentin *(arrow)* covering the tract (ground section, original magnification ×4).

Compared with primary dentin, reparative dentin is less tubular and less well calcified. At times no tubules are formed; this type of tertiary dentin has been characterized as a form of fibrodentin.[22] The quality of reparative dentin (ie, the degree to which it resembles primary dentin) is highly variable. Factors influencing its formation include the nature and magnitude of the irritant and the status of the pulp. If the pulp is relatively healthy, the tertiary dentin is generally of good quality since the matrix is secreted by surviving odontoblasts (ie, reactionary dentinogenesis, see chapter 3). If the pulp is inflamed or has undergone degenerative changes, the quality of the dentin is more variable. An example of poor-quality dentin is shown in Fig 10-6. Note the "Swiss cheese" appearance of the dentin. The holes represent soft tissue that was trapped in the matrix and subsequently underwent necrosis.

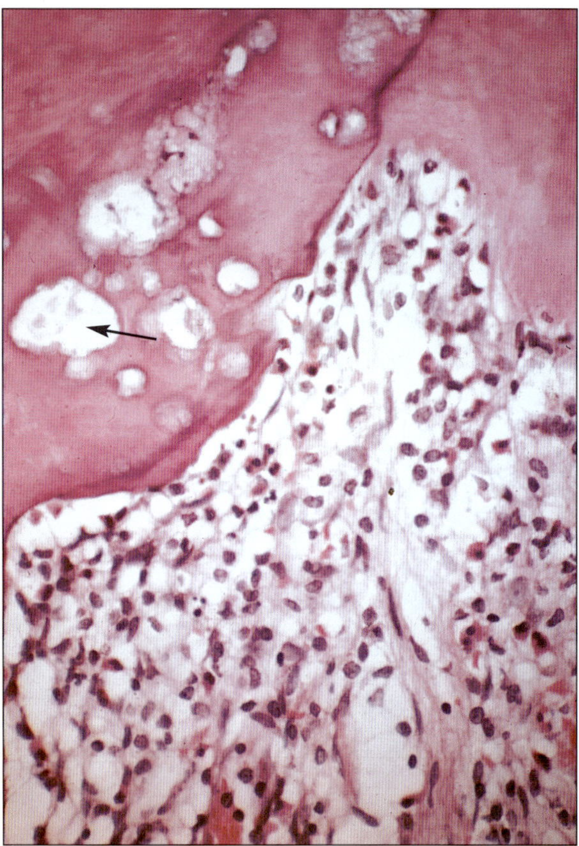

Fig 10-6 Poor-quality reparative dentin with soft tissue *(arrow)* entrapped within dentin matrix (H&E stain, original magnification ×88).

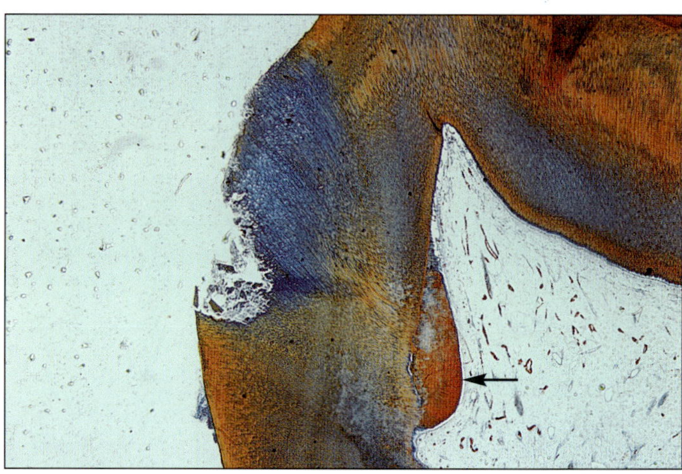

Fig 10-7 Reparative dentin *(arrow)* beneath a deep caries lesion. No inflammation is apparent (H&E stain, original magnification ×6).

Does tertiary dentin protect the pulp, or is it simply a form of scar tissue? In most cases, it seems to have a protective effect, providing it is of good quality. For example, in severe cases of attrition, the pulp can retreat into the root canal, laying down a barrier of dentin as it goes. At times, because the boundary between the primary and tertiary dentin is usually atubular, destruction of much of the coronal portion of the tooth by caries induces sufficient tertiary dentin formation that the pulp retains its vitality. Research has shown that the walls of dentinal tubules along the junction between primary and reparative dentin are thickened and many are occluded.[23,24] Presumably, this junction represents an area of very low permeability that blocks the diffusion of irritants that might otherwise elicit pulpal inflammation.

Figure 10-7 shows tertiary dentin that has formed in response to an extensive caries lesion. A thick layer of tertiary dentin has formed between the infected primary dentin and the pulp. Note that there is no discernible inflammation in the pulp underlying the tertiary dentin. This absence of inflammation clearly demonstrates the protective nature of this type of dentin. In general, the amount of tertiary dentin formed is proportional to the amount of primary dentin that was destroyed. The rate of caries attack also seems to be an influencing factor, as more dentin is formed in response to slowly progressing caries than to caries that is rapidly advancing.

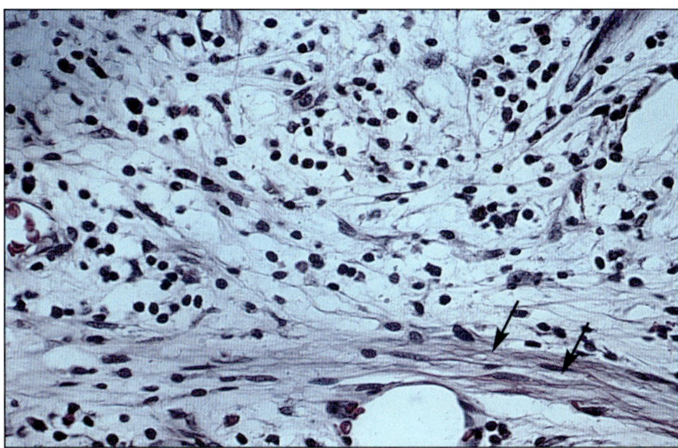

Fig 10-8 Chronic inflammatory reaction beneath a moderately deep caries lesion in dentin. Note the presence of chronic inflammatory cells, proliferating blood vessels, and numerous collagen fibers *(arrows)* (H&E stain, original magnification ×88).

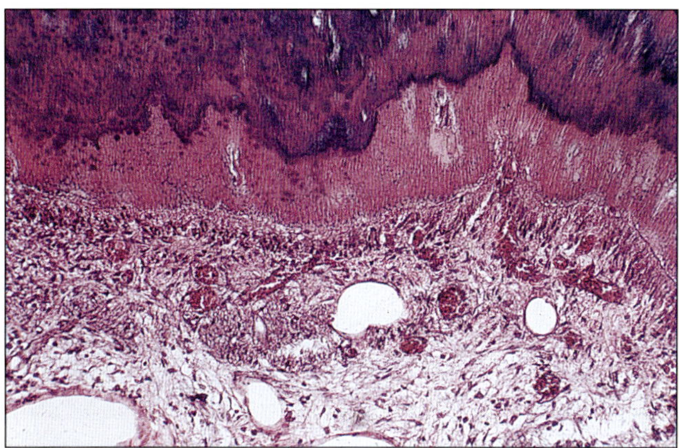

Fig 10-9 Acute inflammatory reaction beneath reparative dentin. Note numerous dilated vessels and presence of inflammatory cells (H&E stain, original magnification ×56).

Inflammatory and immunologic reactions

The tooth is rather unique in that bacteria that have invaded enamel and dentin can grow and multiply without being assaulted by host defenses. It is only after bacteria invade the pulp that they are vulnerable to inflammatory and immune mechanisms.

Caries is a prolonged process, and lesions progress slowly over a period of years. Consequently, pulpal inflammation evoked by caries lesions begins as a low-grade immunologic response to bacterial antigens rather than an acute inflammatory reaction. The initial inflammatory cell infiltrate consists almost entirely of lymphocytes, macrophages, and plasma cells[25] (see also chapters 5 and 12). This infiltrate is typical of a chronic inflammatory reaction. Additionally, there is a proliferation of small blood vessels and fibroblasts with deposition of collagen fibers, as seen in Fig 10-8.

Not all pulpal inflammatory reactions result in permanent damage to the pulp. Chronic inflammation is generally regarded as an inflammatory-reparative reaction, as all of the elements needed for healing are present. In fact, chronic inflammation is sometimes regarded as "frustrated repair." When the caries lesion is eliminated or becomes arrested before bacteria reach the pulp, inflammation undergoes resolution and healing will occur. Consequently, a major goal of restorative dentistry should be to rid the dentin of bacteria so that the inflamed pulp may heal. This is the rationale for the use of indirect pulp-capping techniques.

The severity of pulpal inflammation beneath a caries lesion depends to a great degree on the depth of bacterial penetration as well as the extent to which dentin permeability has been reduced by dentinal sclerosis and/or reparative dentin formation. According to one study,[26] when the distance between the invading bacteria and the pulp (including the thickness of reparative dentin) was 1.1 mm or more, the inflammatory response to bacterial infection of dentinal tubules was negligible.[26] However, when the lesions reached to within 0.5 mm of the pulp, there was a significant increase in the extent of inflammation. The pulp became acutely inflamed only when bacteria had invaded the reparative dentin that had formed beneath the lesion. Figure 10-9 shows an acute inflammatory response beneath infected reparative dentin. During this response, neutrophils begin to marginate in venules and migrate toward the reparative dentin (Fig 10-10).

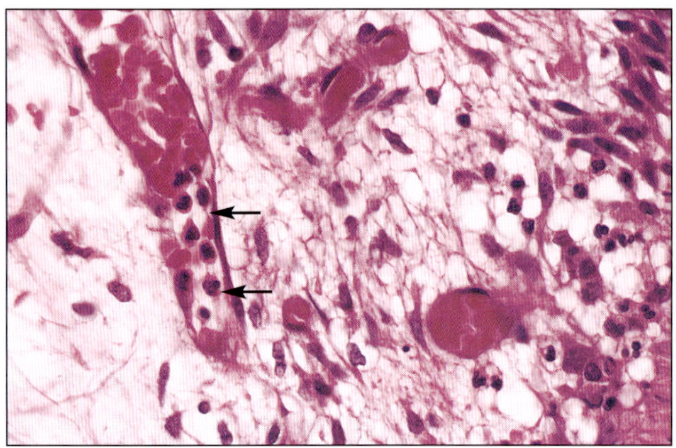

Fig 10-10 Marginating neutrophils *(arrows)* in a venule close to infected dentin (H&E stain, original magnification ×220).

Several lymphocyte subtypes are found in inflamed pulp, including T4 (helper), T8 (cytotoxic, suppressor), and B cells.[27] In reversibly inflamed pulps, 90% of the lymphocytes were T cells, with a T4:T8 ratio of 0.56. In irreversibly inflamed pulps, a ratio 1.14 was observed, indicating a twofold increase in the relative proportion of T4 helper cells. It was not determined what percentage of T8 lymphocytes were cytotoxic cells versus suppressor cells. The presence of B cells indicated that local antibody was being produced, but the exact role of these antibodies was unclear.

Helper T cells can be divided into two populations. Type 1 (T_H1) helper T cells secrete interferon-γ and IL-2.[28] These mediators activate macrophages and cytotoxic T cells. Type 2 (T_H2) helper T cells secrete cytokines IL-4, 5, and 6, which help B cells to mature into plasma cells and to secrete antibodies. B cells recognize antigen directly or in the form of immune complexes on the surface of follicular dendritic cells in the germinal centers of lymph nodes.

It has been shown that dendritic cells are located in the odontoblast layer and throughout the pulps of normal teeth[29-31] (see also chapter 5). Macrophages are also Class II antigen-presenting cells, but they are located more centrally in the pulp.[29,30] In experimentally induced superficial caries in rats, the initial pulpal response was a local accumulation of dendritic cells beneath the corresponding dentinal tubules (Fig 10-11).[32] Dendritic cells patrol the tissues and endocytose any antigens they encounter. Because most antigens arrive in the pulp through the dentinal tubules, it is fortuitous that dendritic cells are nearby to initiate an immune response.

Suppuration

Exposure of the pulp to caries often results in suppurative inflammation, depending upon the nature of the invasive bacteria. The generation of chemotaxins by pyogenic (ie, pus-producing) bacteria produces a massive accumulation of neutrophils (Fig 10-12). Pyogenic bacteria include a wide variety of organisms such as streptococci, staphylococci, pneumococci, meningococci, and gonococci (see chapter 12 for further discussion). Neutrophils are the most numerous of the circulating leukocytes, accounting for 50% to 70% of the normal white cell count. Once they leave the bone marrow, they have a relatively short life span, only about 1 or 2 days. The number of neutrophils in the blood can increase quite rapidly in response to infection.

Exogenous as well as endogenous substances can act as chemoattractants for neutrophils.[33] For example, bacterial peptides that possess an *N*-formyl-methionine terminal amino acid are exogenous chemoattractants. Important endogenous chemoattractants include complement component C5a, leukotriene B_4, and cytokines of the IL-8 family.

During the process of phagocytosis, neutrophils consume molecular oxygen in order to produce reactive oxygen metabolites such as superoxide anion, hydrogen peroxide (H_2O_2), hydroxyl radical, and hypochlorous acid (HOCl). This reaction is catalyzed by an enzyme that oxidizes reduced nicotinamide-adenine dinucleotide phosphate (NADPH) and in the process reduces oxygen to superoxide. Superoxide is then converted

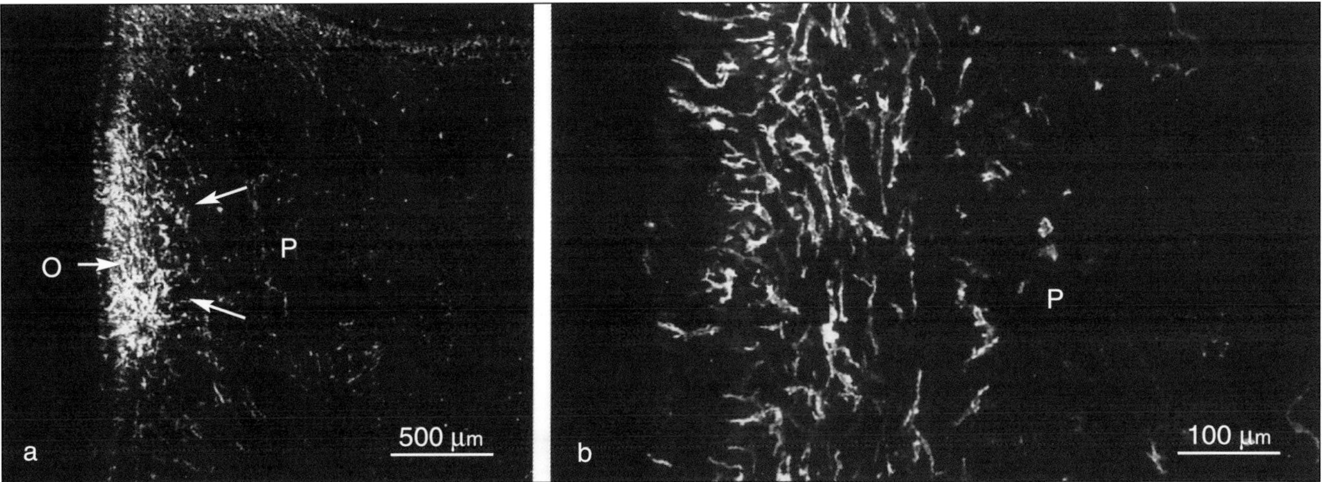

Fig 10-11 Confocal laser scanning micrograph indicating dendritic cells (HLA DR-positive cells) in a human pulp affected by early caries. O, odontoblastic layer; P, pulp. *(a)* An aggregation of dendritic cells *(arrows)* in the subodontoblastic areas corresponding to the caries lesion. *(b)* Higher magnification reveals that the cells consist of slender dendritic cells with long processes. (Reprinted from Yoshiba et al[32] with permission.)

to H_2O_2, mostly by spontaneous dismutation. The amount of H_2O_2 produced in the neutrophil's phagolysosomes is generally insufficient to effectively kill bacteria. However, H_2O_2 can be converted to HOCl by the H_2O_2-halide-myeloperoxidase system. Myeloperoxidase is contained within the neutrophil's azurophilic granules and released when the neutrophil degranulates. HOCl destroys bacteria by halogenation or by oxidation of proteins and lipids (lipid peroxidation). This system constitutes the neutrophil's major weapon against bacteria. A similar process is employed in endodontics with the use of sodium hypochlorite (NaOCl) for irrigation, for the active form of this compound (HOCl) is the same as that released from neutrophils.

Contact between neutrophils and chemoattractants results in stimulation of glucose metabolism via the hexose monophosphate (HMP) shunt. The adenosine triphosphate (ATP) that is generated by this metabolic pathway provides most of the energy necessary for chemotaxis. It has been estimated that approximately 85% of the glucose consumed by neutrophils is converted to lactic acid.[34] Glucose is derived from the breakdown of glycogen that is stored in the neutrophil's cytoplasmic granules. The pH in the neutrophil's phagolysosomes drops to a level of 4 to 4.5. By diffusing out of the neutrophil, lactic acid contributes to the acid environment of an abscess. Many bacteria are unable to tolerate such a low pH.

The ability to avoid phagocytosis is of key importance in the virulence of pyogenic bacteria. Because of certain antiphagocytic virulence factors such as lipopolysaccharide, the M protein of group A β-hemolytic streptococci, and protein A of *Staphylococcus aureus*, it is difficult for neutrophils to kill pyogenic bacteria, and as a result more and more neutrophils are mobilized in an attempt to overwhelm the invading organisms. As bacteria invade deep into the dentin, neutrophils begin to accumulate adjacent to the dentinal tubules. Figure 10-13 shows neutrophils entering the tubules, an indication of the potency of chemotactic factors derived from bacteria within the caries lesion. By this time, the odontoblasts have undergone necrosis. Because bacteria in the tubules are virtually unassailable by host defenses, there is a constant supply of chemotaxins to mobilize neutrophils.

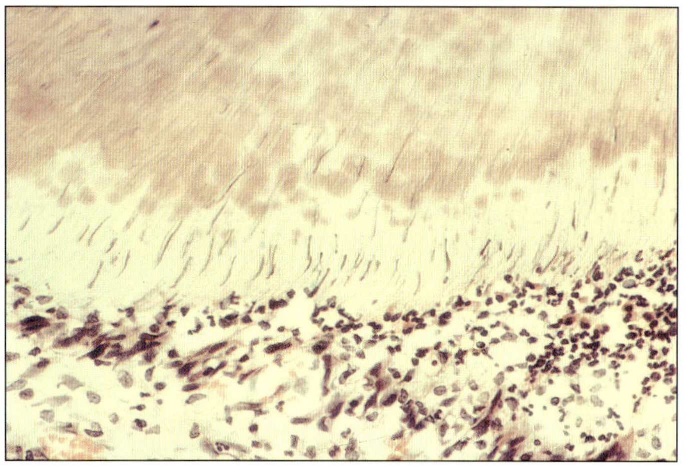

Fig 10-12 *(above)* Neutrophils accumulating beneath a deep caries lesion. Some neutrophils have entered dentinal tubules (H&E stain, original magnification ×88).

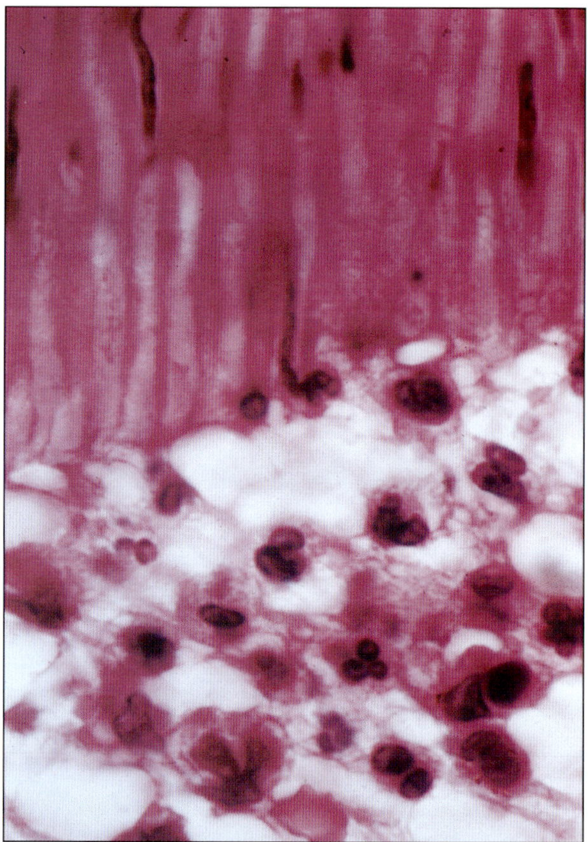

Fig 10-13 *(right)* High-power view of neutrophils entering dentinal tubules (H&E stain, original magnification ×220).

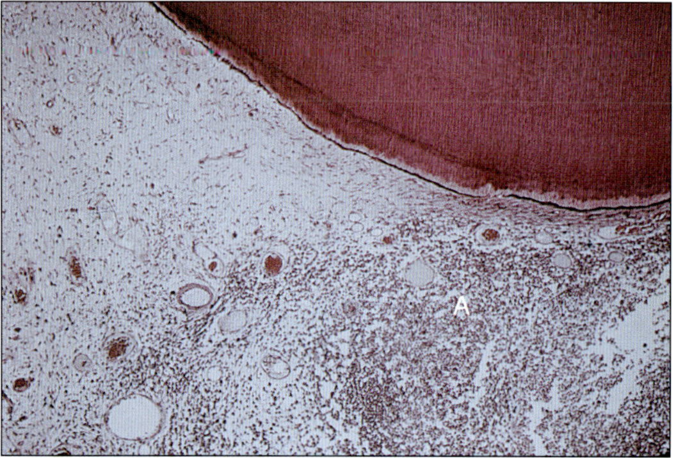

Fig 10-14 *(above)* Recently developed abscess. Note the abscess cavity (A) and surrounding connective tissue containing dilated blood vessels (H&E stain, original magnification ×56).

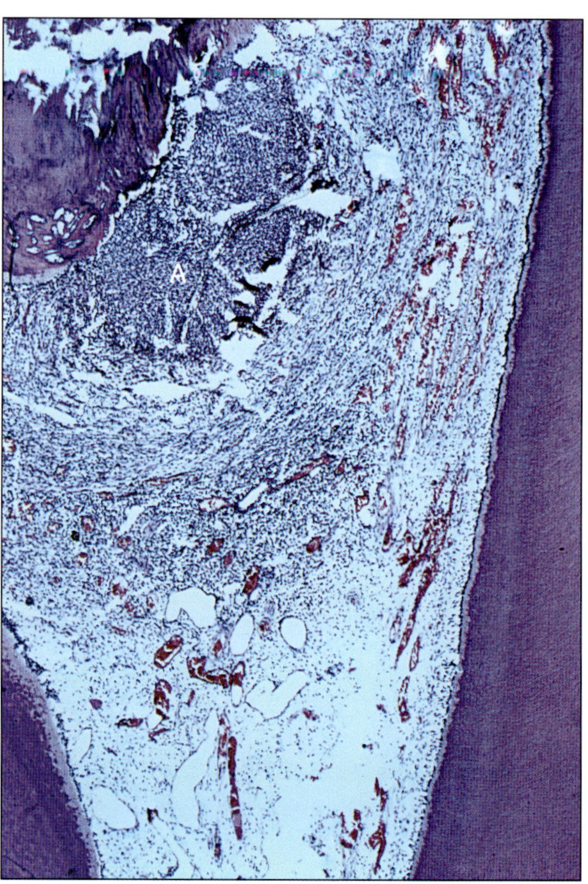

Fig 10-15 *(right)* Pulpal abscess (A). Note the way in which blood vessels encircle the abscess cavity. Relatively uninflamed pulp tissue is seen below (H&E stain, original magnification ×16).

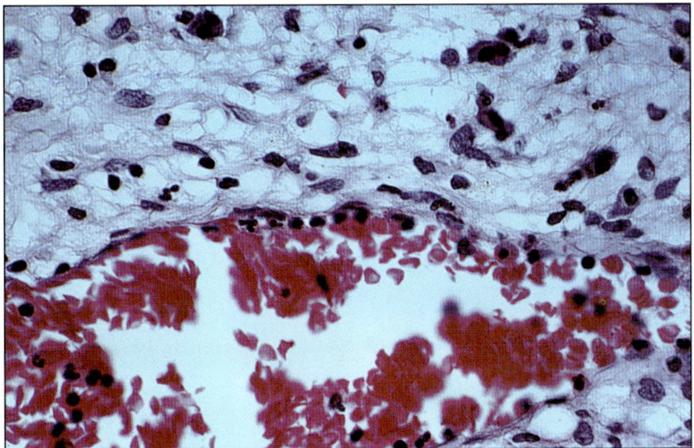

Fig 10-16 High-power view of a venule within tissue shown in Fig 10-14. Note marginating neutrophils and neutrophils that have migrated into the surrounding tissue (H&E stain, original magnification ×220).

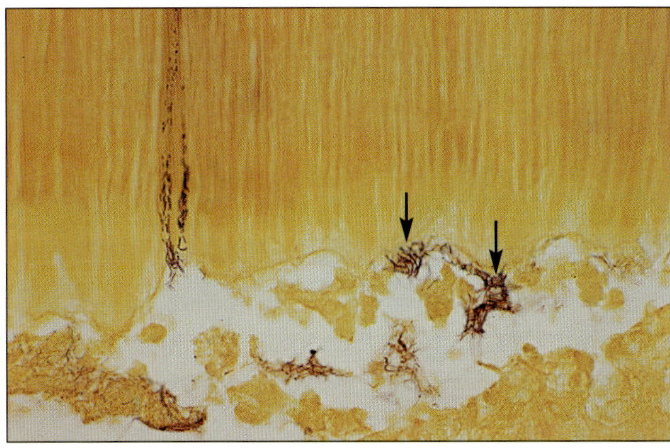

Fig 10-17 Bacterial stain showing bacteria entering the pulp from infected tubules. Bacteria can also be seen in the pulp chamber *(arrows)* (Glynn modified Gram stain, original magnification ×220).

In the case of suppuration caused by exposure of the pulp to caries, mobilization of neutrophils is due to the massive number of bacteria entering the pulp. If the number of neutrophils reaches a critical mass, an abscess, a walled-off area of suppuration, will develop (Fig 10-14). The death of neutrophils in situ gives rise to purulence, formed chiefly by autolysis of neutrophils by their own lysosomal enzymes. As this process continues, an abscess cavity is formed. The causative bacteria vary, but infection with multiple anaerobes is common. Figure 10-15 shows the highly vascularized connective tissue that surrounds an abscess. This tissue is sometime referred to as a *pyogenic membrane*. The vessels provide a delivery system for the replenishment of neutrophils that have died and must be replaced in order to sustain the abscess (Fig 10-16). Failure to do so will result in colonization of bacteria in the pulp chamber and tissue degeneration.

Tissue necrosis develops when neutrophils release activated oxygen metabolites and proteases. The neutrophil contains more than 20 proteases, of which the most important are elastase, gelatinase, and collagenase. This combined assault results in liquefaction necrosis. The area where tissue digestion is occurring has a greater osmotic pressure than the surrounding tissue, and this pressure differential together with direct actions of the mediators on nerve terminals increases the sensitivity of sensory nerve endings, explaining why abscesses are often painful and why drainage frequently provides relief (see also chapters 7 to 9).

Neutrophils are responsible for the color of a purulent discharge, particularly the free nucleic acids released from the neutrophil when it undergoes autolysis. A purulent discharge consists of neutrophils—living, dying, and dead—as well as tissue debris and inflammatory exudate from the surrounding inflamed connective tissue. Staphylococci produce a creamy purulent discharge; streptococci produce a thin discharge.

As the caries exposure enlarges and an ever-increasing number of bacteria enter the pulp, the defending forces are eventually overwhelmed. It must be remembered that the pulp has a relatively limited blood supply in relation to the volume of tissue present in the pulp chamber and root canal space. Therefore, when blood flow can no longer meet the demand for inflammatory elements, the inflammatory response can no longer be sustained and bacteria may grow unopposed within the pulp chamber (Fig 10-17). This ultimately leads to total pulp necrosis.

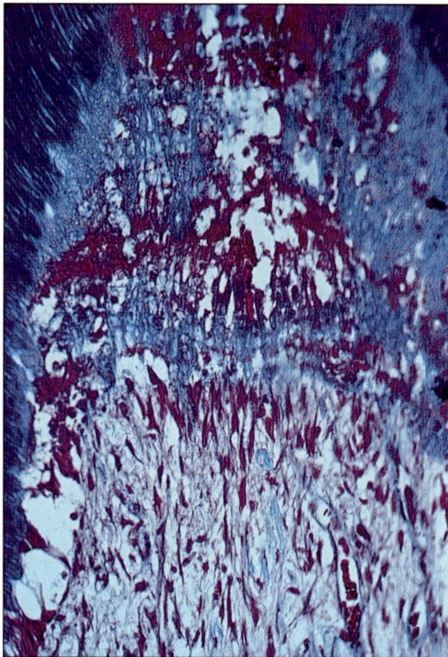

Fig 10-18 Connective tissue stain showing fibroblasts producing a collagenous matrix beneath an area of necrotic pulp tissue. This matrix may calcify to become reparative dentin (Masson stain, original magnification ×88).

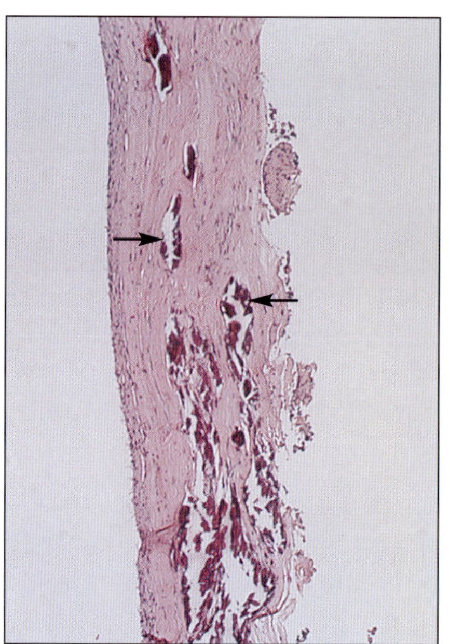

Fig 10-19 Fibrotic radicular pulp. The tooth had been referred for endodontic treatment because of carious pulp exposure. The tooth tested vital. *Arrows* indicate areas of calcification (H&E stain, original magnification ×6).

Exposure of the pulp to caries does not invariably result in suppuration. In the absence of a sufficient number of pyogenic bacteria, a localized area of necrosis may develop. The body responds to this necrotic debris by attempting to produce reparative dentin (Fig 10-18). Exposure of the pulp may also trigger extensive fibrosis of the pulp (Fig 10-19),[35] presumably due to immunologic mechanisms that lead to the proliferation and activation of fibroblasts. Other pulpal lesions that are chronic in nature include ulcerative pulpitis and hyperplastic pulpitis.

Chronic ulcerative pulpitis

The histologic term *ulcerative* is actually a misnomer in these cases because no surface epithelium is involved. This condition is the result of local excavation of the surface of the pulp resulting from liquefaction necrosis of pulp tissue (Fig 10-20).[36] Excavation is likely to occur when drainage of inflammatory exudate is established through a pathway of decomposed dentin. The inflammation tends to remain localized and asymptomatic because drainage prevents a buildup of pressure. Eventually a space is created between the area of tissue destruction and the wall of the pulp chamber. The base of the lesion consists of necrotic debris and a dense accumulation of neutrophils. A zone of chronic inflammatory tissue forms subjacent to the neutrophils in an attempt to keep the lesion localized.

Chronic hyperplastic pulpitis (pulp polyp)

This uncommon condition occurs most often in primary and immature permanent teeth with incompletely formed roots. At this stage of develop-

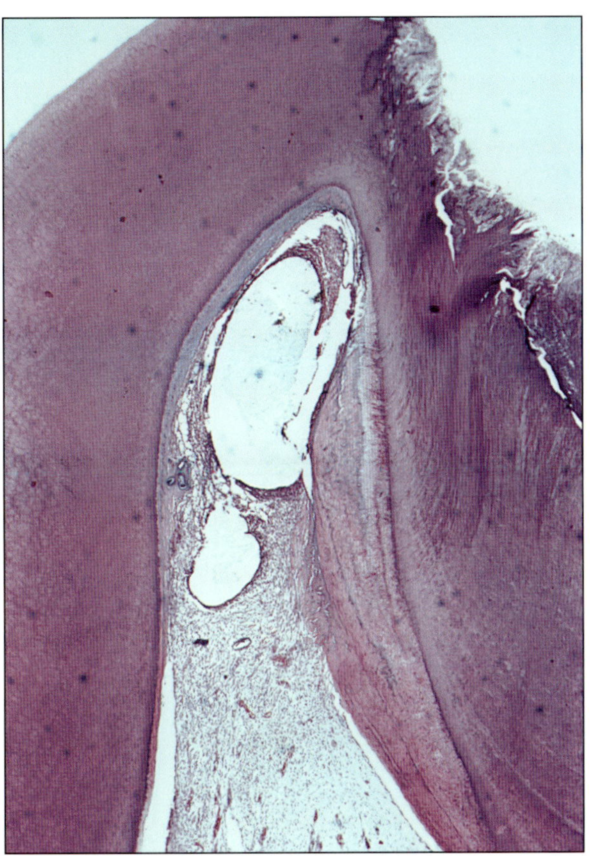

Fig 10-20 Chronic ulcerative pulpitis. Note the large space between pulp and dentinal walls (H&E stain, original magnification ×6). (Reprinted from Kim and Trowbridge[36] with permission.)

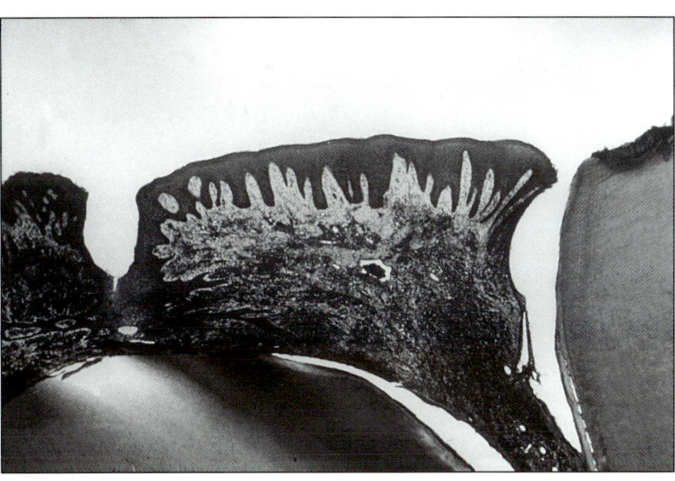

Fig 10-21 Chronic hyperplastic pulpitis. Note epithelialization of the chronically inflamed connective tissue. Space between lesion and dentin is due to fixation artifact (H&E stain, original magnification ×6).

ment, numerous blood vessels enter the pulp through the wide apical foramen. Because of its rich blood supply, the young pulp seems better able to resist bacterial infection than older pulps.[37] Its histologic characteristics are identical to those of other types of inflammatory hyperplasia, ie, a proliferation of small vessels and fibroblasts and a chronic inflammatory cell infiltrate. Eventually the lesion acquires a stratified squamous covering, presumably because of grafting of vital desquamated epithelial cells from the oral mucosa.

Chronic hyperplastic pulpitis develops when carious pulp exposure creates a large open cavity. This opening establishes a pathway for drainage of the inflammatory exudate. When drainage is established, acute inflammation subsides and chronic inflammatory tissue proliferates through the opening created by the exposure to form a polyp (Fig 10-21). The polyp may cover most of what remains of the crown of the tooth, giving the lesion the appearance of a fleshy mass. The management of this lesion consists either of conservation of the tooth through endodontic treatment or extraction of the tooth. The lesion produces little or no pain; however, masticatory forces may produce irritation and bleeding.

Tooth fracture

Pulpal death following complete coronal fractures is incidental to the invasion of bacteria, which fol-

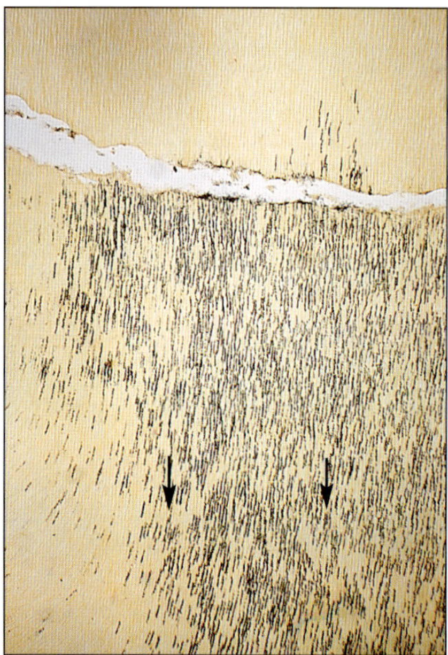

Fig 10-22 Bacteria within dentinal tubules in a cracked tooth. *Arrows* indicate the direction of the pulp. (Glynn modified Gram stain, original magnification ×88).

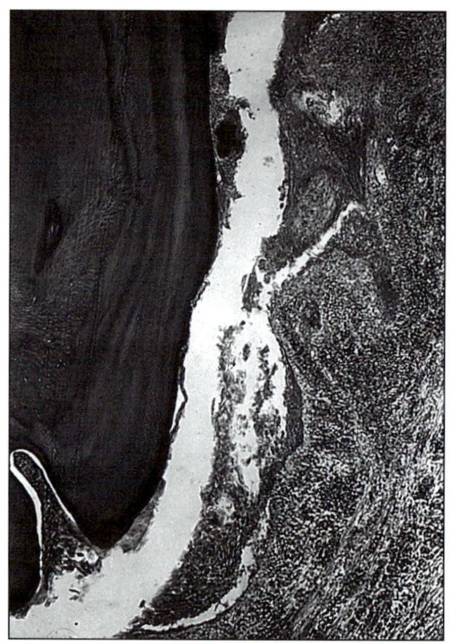

Fig 10-23 Periodontally involved tooth. The pocket has involved the apical foramen. The space between the tooth and the lining of the pocket is due to shrinkage of the tissue during fixation (H&E stain, original magnification ×22).

lows the injury. Most accidental fractures occur in children between the ages of 9 and 13. Male children suffer nearly twice the number of fractures as females. Maxillary anterior teeth are particularly susceptible, especially when there is maxillary protrusion.

Incomplete fractures most often occur in the molar teeth of middle-aged and elderly individuals, particularly teeth in which deep restorations have been placed. Cracks, or minute defects in the dentin, may produce an incomplete tooth fracture through a typically slow process. Figure 10-22 shows bacteria within the dentin of a cracked tooth. As the crack gradually enlarges, bacteria may reach the pulp through the dentinal tubules, or the crack may extend to the pulp chamber, thus exposing the pulp. Eventually the fracture either becomes clinically detectable or a portion of the tooth breaks off along the fracture line, usually producing no pain. Pulpal infection will depend upon the extent of fracture, ie, whether the fracture involves the pulp chamber or is only through the enamel.

Anomalous tracts

Infection may occur through developmental tracts such as accessory canals and channels produced by invagination of tooth structure, as in the case of dens in dente. If, during tooth development, the continuity of the epithelial root sheath is broken before dentin forms, odontoblasts do not differentiate and dentin fails to form opposite the defect. This results in a small acces-

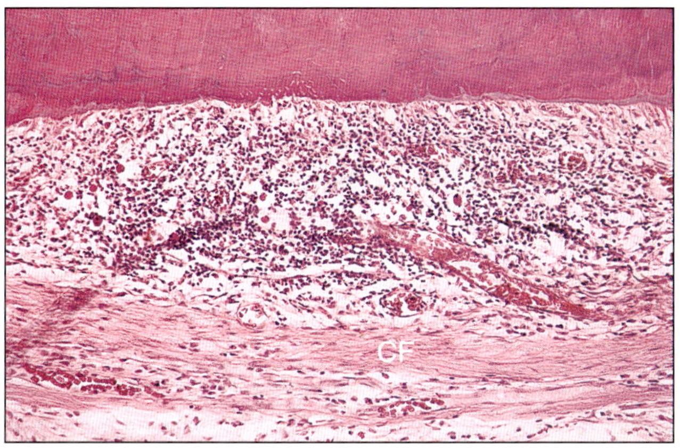

Fig 10-24 Chronic inflammatory reaction beneath an experimental cavity filled with zinc phosphate cement. Note the presence of blood vessels and collagen fibers (CF) at the periphery of the lesion (H&E stain, original magnification ×88).

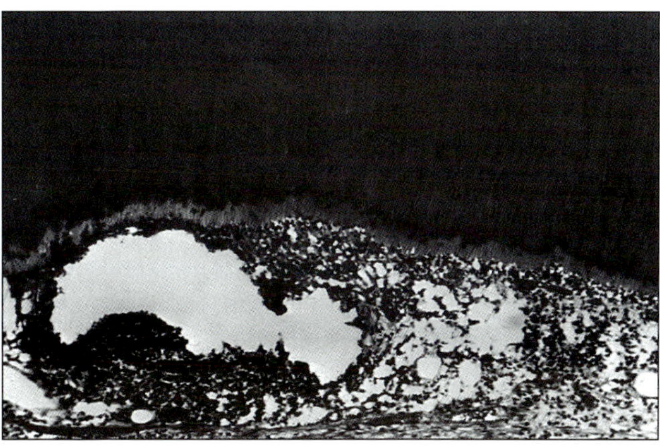

Fig 10-25 Microabscess that developed beneath an experimental restoration. Space is due to fixation artifact (H&E stain, original magnification ×88).

sory canal connecting the periodontal ligament with the root canal. Accessory canals are usually extremely narrow, permitting only small-diameter arterioles to pass. Although accessory canals may occur anywhere along the root, they most often occur in the apical third.

It has often been stated that accessory canals can transmit toxic substances into the pulp. Theoretically, when a deep periodontal pocket exposes the opening of an accessory canal, a pathway is created that could lead to infection of the pulp. However, there is no consensus as to the effect of periodontal disease on the pulp (see also chapter 18). On the other hand, when periodontal disease involves the root apex, pulpal inflammation and necrosis will develop (Fig 10-23).

Dens in dente is a condition that may range from a slight lingual pit to an enamel-lined anomalous tract that may extend most of the way to the pulp. The tooth most often involved is the maxillary lateral incisor. This tract provides cariogenic bacteria with a haven in which to multiply and produce caries. In such cases, the caries lesion often goes undetected until pulp exposure produces symptoms of pulpitis.

Dental Restorative Procedures

Restorative procedures may injure the pulp in several ways (see also chapters 4, 14, and 15). The most common cause of injury is microleakage. If a restoration fails to provide a good hermetic seal, bacteria can enter the gap between the restorative material and the walls of the cavity. Bacterial products are then able to diffuse to the pulp through the dentinal tubules and produce inflammation. Depending on the severity of the leakage and the permeability of the underlying dentin, leakage may evoke inflammatory reactions ranging from a chronic inflammatory reaction (Fig 10-24) to abscess formation (Fig 10-25).

Germ-free animal studies[38] have shown that in the absence of bacteria, restorative materials placed directly on the pulp produce little or no inflammation. Moreover, primate studies have demonstrated that restorative materials are well tolerated by the pulp if the cavity margins are sealed with zinc oxide–eugenol to prevent bacteria from infecting the cavity (see also chapters 13, 14, and 15).

With the possible exception of the latest generation of dentin-bonding agents, no permanent restorative material adapts to tooth structure well enough to reliably prevent marginal leakage. Even if there is good marginal adaptation at the time of insertion, shrinkage resulting from physical or chemical changes may cause gaps to form between the restoration and tooth structure. Other causes of microleakage include elastic deformation of tooth structure produced by masticatory forces[39] and contraction due to thermal changes. A rational approach to the problem of leakage is to seal the dentin with a liner, base, or dentin-bonding agent prior to restoring the tooth.

References

1. Janeway CA Jr. Approaching the asymptote? Evolution and revolution in immunology. Cold Spring Harbor Symp Quant Biol 1989;54:1-13.
2. Medztov R, Janeway C Jr. Innate immunity. New Eng J Med 2000;343:338-344.
3. Verret CR. Specific and nonspecific cell-mediated cytotoxicity. In: Sigal LH, Yacov R (eds). Immunology and Inflammation. New York, McGraw-Hill;1994:165.
4. Von Andrian UH, Mackay CR. T-cell function and migration. N Engl J Med 2000;343:1020-1034.
5. Birkedal-Hansen H. Proteolytic remodeling of extracellular matrix. Curr Opin Cell Biol 1995;7:728-735.
6. Massler M. Pulpal reactions to dentinal caries. J Dent Res 1967;17:441-460.
7. McKay GS. The histology and microbiology of acute occlusal dentin lesions in human permanent premolar teeth. Arch Oral Biol 1976;21:51.
8. Bergenholtz G. Effect of bacterial products on the inflammatory reactions in the dental pulp. Scand J Dent Res 1977;85:122-129.
9. Warfvinge J, Dahlen G, Bergenholtz G. Dental pulp response to bacterial cell wall material. J Dent Res 1985; 64:1046-1050.
10. Nissan R, Segal H, Pashley D, Stevens R, Trowbridge H. The ability of bacterial endotoxin to diffuse through human dentin. J Endodon 1995;21:62-64.
11. Bjorndal L, Darvann T, Thylstrup A. A quantitative microscopic study of the odontoblast and subodontoblast reactions to active and arrested enamel caries without cavitation. Caries Res 1998;32:59-69.
12. Larmas M. Response of the pulpo-dentinal complex to caries attack. Proc Finn Dent Soc 1986;82:298-304.
13. Wang YN, Ashrafi SH, Weber DF. Scanning electron microscope observations of casts of human dentinal tubules along the interface between primary and secondary dentin. Anat Rec 1985;211:149-155.
14. Magloire H, Bouvier M, Joffre A. Odontoblast response under carious lesions. Proc Finn Dent Soc 1992;88 (Suppl 1):257-274.
15. Nagaoka S, Miyazaki Y, Liu H-J, Iwamoto Y, Kitano M, Kawagoe M. Bacterial invasion into dentinal tubules of human vital and nonvital teeth. J Endodon 1995;21: 70-73.
16. Stanley HR, Pereira JC, Spiegel E, Broom C, Schultz M. The detection and prevalence of reactive and physiologic sclerotic dentin, reparative dentin and dead tracts beneath various types of dental lesions according to tooth surface and age. J Oral Pathol 1983;12:257-289.
17. Barber D, Massler M. Permeability of active and arrested caries to dyes and radioactive isotopes. J Dent Child 1964;31:26-33.
18. Johnson NW, Taylor BR, Berman DS. The response of deciduous dentine to caries studied by correlated light and electron microscopy. Caries Res 1969;3:348-368.
19. Fitzgerald M, Chiego DJ, Heys DR. Autoradiographic analysis of odontoblast replacement following pulp exposure in primate teeth. Arch Oral Biol 1990;35:707-715.
20. D'Souza RN, Bachman T, Baumgardner KR, Butler WT, Litz M. Characterization of cellular responses involved in reparative dentinogenesis in rat molars. J Dent Res 1995;74:702-709.
21. Stanley HR, White CL, McCray L. The rate of tertiary (reparative) dentin formation in the human tooth. Oral Surg 1966;21:180-189.
22. Baume LJ. The biology of pulp and dentine. In: Myers HM (ed). Monographs in Oral Science. Basel: S Karger, 1980:170.
23. Scott JN, Weber DF. Microscopy of the junctional region between human coronal primary and secondary dentin. J Morphol 1977;154:133-145.
24. Fish EW. Experimental investigation of the enamel, dentin, and dental pulp. London, John Bale Sons & Danielson, 1932:35.
25. Trowbridge H. Pathogenesis of pulpitis resulting from dental caries. J Endod 1981;7:52-60.
26. Reeves R, Stanley HR. The relationship of bacterial penetration and pulpal pathosis in carious teeth. Oral Surg Oral Med Oral Pathol 1966:22:59-65.
27. Hahn C-L, Falkler WA Jr, Siegel MA. A study of T and B cells in pulpal pathosis. J Endod 1989;15:20-26.
28. Delves PJ, Roit IM. The immune system: Second of two parts. N Engl J Med 2000;343:108-117.
29. Jontell M, Bergenholtz G. Accessory cells in the immune response of the dental pulp. Proc Finn Dent Soc 1992;88:345.
30. Bergenholtz G, Nagaoka S, Jontell M. Class II antigen expressing cells in experimentally induced pulpitis. Int Endodon J 1991;24:8-14.

31. Okiji T, Kawashima N, Kosaka T, Matsumoto A, Kobayashi C, Suda H. An immunohistochemical study of the distribution of immunocompetent cells, especially macrophages and Ia antigen-expressing cells of the heterogeneous populations in normal rat molar pulp. J Dent Res 1992;71:1196–1202.
32. Yoshiba N, Yoshiba K, Nakamura H, Iwaku M, Ozawa H. Immunohistochemical localization of HLA-DR positive cells in unerupted and erupted normal and carious human teeth. J Dent Res 1996;75:1585–1589.
33. Luster AD. Chemokines—Chemotactic cytokines that mediate inflammation. N Engl J Med1998;338:436–445.
34. Munroe JF, Shipp JC. Glucose metabolism in leukocytes from patients with diabetes mellitus, with and without hypercholesterolemia. Diabetes 1965;14:584–590.
35. Trowbridge HO, Stewart JCB, Shapiro IM. Assessment of indurated, diffusely calcified human dental pulps. In: Shimono M, Maeda T, Suda H, Takahashi K (eds). Dentin/Pulp Complex. Tokyo: Quintessence, 1996: 297–300.
36. Kim S, Trowbridge HO. Pulp responses to caries and restorative procedures. In: Cohen S, Burns R (eds). Pathways of the Pulp, ed 7. St. Louis: Mosby, 1998:532–551.
37. Avery J. Repair potential of the pulp. J Endod 1981;7: 205–212.
38. Watts A. Bacterial contamination and toxicity of silicate and zinc phosphate cements. Br Dent J 1979;146:7–13.
39. Qvist V. The effect of mastication on marginal adaptation of composite restorations in vivo. J Dent Res 1983; 62:904–906.

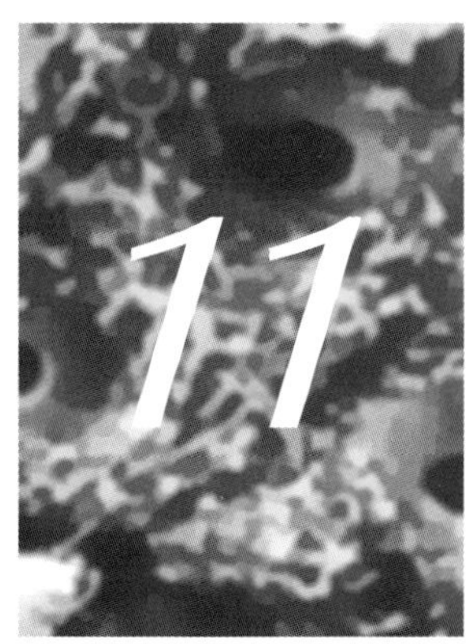

Molecular Mediators of Pulpal Inflammation

Ashraf F. Fouad, DDS, MS

Inflammation of the dental pulp is similar to that in other connective tissue in that it is mediated by cellular and molecular factors. The pulp is capable of expressing a large number of known host mediators of inflammation, as evidenced by their identification in pulp at the protein and/or gene-expression levels. The principal objective of these mediators is to combat the irritating factors and minimize their harmful effects. However, in the process of mounting the innate and adaptive inflammatory mechanisms, host factors may further injure the pulp, contributing to its ultimate demise. Unlike inflammatory events in other connective tissues, the pulp is enclosed in a noncompliant environment and has reduced collateral circulation. These anatomic restrictions, which become more exaggerated with advancing age, tend to intensify the injury that results from external irritation and the harmful side effects of host inflammatory mediators. In this chapter, the data available on the contribution of molecular mediators to the inflammatory process will be reviewed and related to clinical factors important for diagnosing and managing pulpal inflammation. The inflammatory response will be described as it progresses from vascular changes to the attraction and migration of inflammatory cells to the site of inflammation and finally to the actual processes that take place in dental pulp.

A large amount of information has been generated in the past three decades about the structural composition of dental pulp and its functional responses to external irritation. It is important as we review this information to recognize that there is a significant overlap in the functions of cellular elements and in the effects of inflammatory mediators produced by these cells (see chapters 5, 10, and 17). It is also important to note that the experimental conditions set for conducting a particular research study play an important role in determining the findings of the study. The gold standard for data generation on the inflammatory response in dental pulp would be to study these responses in humans following clinically relevant external stimulation (eg, caries, trauma, microleakage), conditions that are frequently difficult if not impossible to achieve.

Modulation of Vascular Flow

Vasodilation and increased blood flow are seen in the initial phases of pulpal inflammation. These phenomena serve to increase perfusion of the pulp, bringing needed host inflammatory factors into the area of irritation. Despite its small size, the dental pulp responds to advancing irritation in a compartmentalized manner rather than as an entire organ. Areas of the pulp closest to irritation seem to be affected the most and undergo more severe inflammatory manifestations, with resultant vascular responses (see chapter 6). In contrast, surrounding and distant pulpal regions may have milder inflammation or may even appear normal using histologic, biochemical, or molecular techniques. As the inflammatory reaction in the pulp progresses, stasis in pulp vessels eventually ensues. This result is related to the extravasation of fluid, proteins, and cells into the interstitial tissue, as well as the nonyielding dentin environment that restricts tissue edema. The vascular responses of the pulp are mediated by the following vasoactive amines.

Histamine

Histamine is found in connective tissue mast cells, basophils, and platelets that are often located near blood vessels. Histamine is present in cell granules and is released by cell degranulation in response to a variety of stimuli, including *(1)* physical stimuli such as trauma, cold, or heat; *(2)* immune reactions involving binding of antibodies (IgE) to mast cells; *(3)* complement components called *anaphylactotoxins* (C3a and C5a); *(4)* histamine-releasing proteins derived from leukocytes; *(5)* neuropeptides (eg, substance P); and *(6)* cytokines such as interleukin-1 and interleukin-8 (IL-1 and IL-8).[1]

Histamine is a potent vasodilator and mediator of vascular permeability. It acts on the microcirculation primarily by activating the H_1 receptor, although H_2 and H_3 receptors have also been implicated. Histamine is detected in small amounts in uninflamed dental pulp.[2] Thermal injury of the pulp produces a fourfold increase in histamine levels, whereas stimulation with an electric pulp tester resulted in 35% reduction in the levels of histamine.[3] Mast cells are occasionally found in inflamed pulp, although degranulation cannot be observed histologically because the cells lose their characteristic features after degranulation.[4]

The in vivo application of histamine evokes vasodilation[5] and a gradual decrease in pulpal blood flow (PBF).[6] This reduction in PBF is probably due to vascular leakage and the resultant increase in the tissue pressure in a low-compliance environment. In humans, histamine application to cavity preparations in dentin (in teeth otherwise scheduled for extraction) usually produces a dull throbbing pain, but occasionally a sharp shooting pain is reported.[7] Given the results of earlier work that histamine on its own seems to offer little stimulation to A or C fibers in the dental pulp, it is thought that the pulp tissue must first be sensitized by other inflammatory mediators, such as prostaglandins, for histamine to evoke a painful response in both types of pulp nociceptive fibers.[7] This illustrates the synergistic interactions that can occur among inflammatory mediators in dental pulp.

Serotonin

Serotonin (5-hydroxytryptamine or 5-HT) is another vasoactive mediator that generally causes vasoconstriction. It is present in endothelial cells and platelets as well as in serotinergic nerve terminals. Serotonin (and histamine) is released from stimulated platelets, often following platelet aggregation due to contact with collagen, thrombin, adenosine diphosphate (ADP), or antigen-antibody complexes. Platelet aggregation and release were also stimulated by platelet-activating factor derived from IgE-mediated degranulation of mast cells. Serotonin and its metabolite, 5-hydroxyindoleacetic acid (5-HIAA), as well as the catecholamine dopamine, are present in rat incisor pulp.[8] Unilateral surgical sympathectomy or resection of the inferior alveolar nerve did not significantly affect pulpal 5-HT levels, suggesting that serotonin in the pulp may originate primarily from extraneuronal cells and not neurons.[8] More recently, serotonin and the enzyme monoamine oxidase (MAO), which catalyze the oxidative deamination of 5-HT, have been localized in normal human dental pulp endothelium.[9] In rat dental pulp extracts, application of serotonin stimulates the synthesis of prostaglandin E_2 (PGE_2)[10] and prostacyclin (PGI_2), but not thromboxane A_2.[11] The administration of serotonin to dogs, either by intravenous injection or application to Class V cavity preparations, caused a significant increase in PBF.[12] In addition, serotonin was shown to sensitize intradental nerve fibers to various hydrodynamic stimuli,[13] indicating that it would reduce the threshold for pain in pulpal inflammation. Thus, serotonin is present in dental pulp, and its release may alter PBF and nociceptor function by both direct and indirect actions via release of other inflammatory mediators.

Neuropeptides

Several neuropeptides have been detected in the dental pulp of humans and other mammals using immunologic methods. These neuropeptides include substance P (SP),[14] calcitonin gene-related peptide (CGRP),[15] neurokinin A (NKA),[16] neuropeptide K,[17] neuropeptide Y,[18] somatostatin,[19] and vasoactive intestinal peptide (VIP).[20] These neuropeptides reside almost exclusively within the terminals of afferent neurons, sympathetic fibers, or possibly even parasympathetic fibers, neurons that typically innervate pulpal blood vessels. Tissue levels of SP immunoreactivity in the dental pulp were the highest in the body outside the CNS and were higher in adult than immature cat pulp.[21] Denervation experiments indicate that SP-, neurokinin A-, and CGRP-containing nerve fibers in the pulp originate from the trigeminal ganglion and that neuropeptide Y-containing nerve fibers come from the superior cervical ganglion. The origin of VIP-containing fibers may be parasympathetic nerve fibers because VIP has been associated with acetylcholine in other tissues (for review, see Wakisaka and Akai[22]).

Increased production and release of neuropeptides play an important role in initiating and propagating pulpal inflammation (see also chapters 6, 7, and 8). The dental pulp is very densely innervated. In the normal rat molar pulp, SP and CGRP were shown to be present in close proximity to macrophages (identified by the ED2 marker) and class II antigen-positive cells (identified by the OX6 marker) (Figs 11-1a and 11-1b), an association that was more prevalent in the odontoblastic layer than in central pulp.[23] During inflammation, sprouting of pulpal nerve fibers was shown to be associated with increased expression of neuropeptides such as SP or CGRP closely surrounding the areas of inflammation or abscess.[24,25] However, severe irritation by pulp exposures with or without acid etching was shown to cause a reduction in pulpal levels of SP and CGRP, possibly due to depletion of neuropeptide stores in the nerve endings or the development of tissue necrosis.[26] Denervation of the inferior alveolar nerve has been shown to deplete the pulp of its content of SP and CGRP but not of neuropeptide Y,[27] and was also shown to significantly increase the magnitude of pulpal necrosis following experimental pulp exposures.[28] Moreover, the addition of SP to rat pulpal cell cultures increased the proliferation of concanavalin-A-stimulated T lymphocytes while CGRP decreased it.[23] CGRP addition to human pulp cells in vitro also resulted in a twofold increase in the level of expression of bone morphogenetic protein 2 (BMP-2), a member of the transforming growth factor β (TGF-β) superfamily. Importantly, BMP-2 has the capacity to induce dentin regeneration[29] (see also chapter 3). Taken together, these findings suggest that neurogenic inflammation plays an active and dynamic role in modulating pulpal inflammation.

There are a number of mechanisms by which neuropeptides are thought to contribute to the inflammatory process: SP, CGRP,[30] and VIP are potent vasodilators, whereas neuropeptide Y is a vasoconstrictor.[22] Vasodilation following infusion of SP or VIP in the pulp was associated with a transient increase in PBF that was followed by a substantial and prolonged reduction in PBF.[6] The

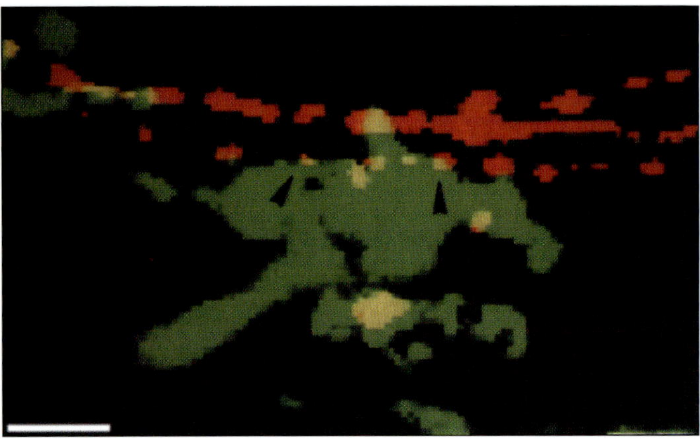

Fig 11-1a *(above)* Confocal laser-scanning micrograph of the inner portion of the pulp horn of a rat mandibular first molar after double immunofluorescence staining for ED2$^+$ cells (macrophages) *(green)* and SP-immunoreactive nerve fibers *(red)*. An ED2$^+$ cell shows some points of contact (yellow spots indicated by arrowheads). Bar = 10 μm. (Reprinted from Okiji et al[23] with permission.)

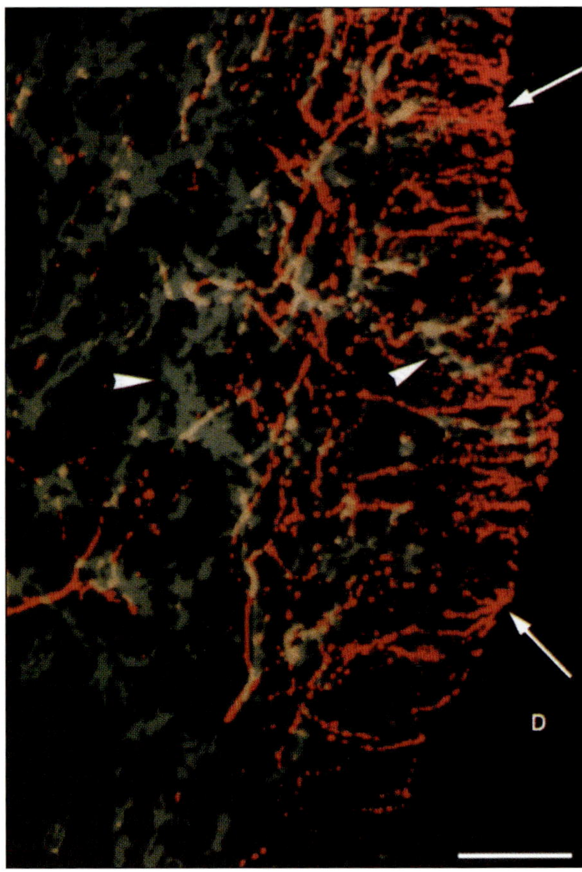

Fig 11-1b *(right)* Confocal laser-scanning micrograph of the coronal pulp of a rat mandibular first molar after double immunofluorescence staining for OX6$^+$ (rat MHC class 2 antigen) cells *(green, arrowheads)* and CGRP-immunoreactive nerve fibers *(red, arrows)*. Close association is more frequently observed at the periphery of the pulp than in the inner portion. D, dentin. Bar = 50 μm. (Reprinted from Okiji et al[23] with permission.)

intra-arterial infusion of an antagonist to the NK1 receptor for SP (SR140,333) or an antagonist to the CGRP$_1$ receptor for CGRP (h-CGRP$_{(8\text{-}37)}$) decreased basal PBF and interstitial fluid pressure in the ferret canine pulp, suggesting that these neuropeptides modulate both basal and inflammation-induced changes in these vascular indices. Moreover, administration of h-CGRP$_{(8\text{-}37)}$ eliminated the ability of tooth electrical stimulation to increase PBF and interstitial fluid pressure.[31] Administration of SP also increased vascular permeability and plasma extravasation.[32] The association between increased vascular permeability and SP content of the rat incisor pulp has been demonstrated. Vascular permeability was increased significantly after antidromic electrical stimulation of the inferior alveolar nerve in the incisor pulp and the skin of the lower lip; the content of immunoreactive SP in both tissues was increased simultaneously.[33] Furthermore, application of two antagonists to the NK1 receptor for SP ([D-Arg^1, D-Pro^2, D-Trp^{7,9}, Leu^{11}]-SP[33] and CP-96,345[34]) inhibited the neurogenic plasma extravasation induced by this antidromic stimulation. The CGRP antagonist, CGRP$_{8\text{-}37}$, significantly reduced the overall extravasation of plasma proteins in unstimulated tissues but did not affect the neurogenically induced extravasation in the stimulated pulp tissue.[34] Thus, the release of neuropeptides during pulpal inflammation evokes a complex set of vascular responses that are dependent, in part, upon the relative concentrations of these and other inflammatory mediators (see also chapter 6).

Neuropeptides may reduce the threshold of pain in the pulp, accounting for symptoms associated with certain cases of pulpitis. For example, pulpal levels of SP in permanent molars of children are positively correlated with the magnitude of caries lesions (none, moderate, or gross) and

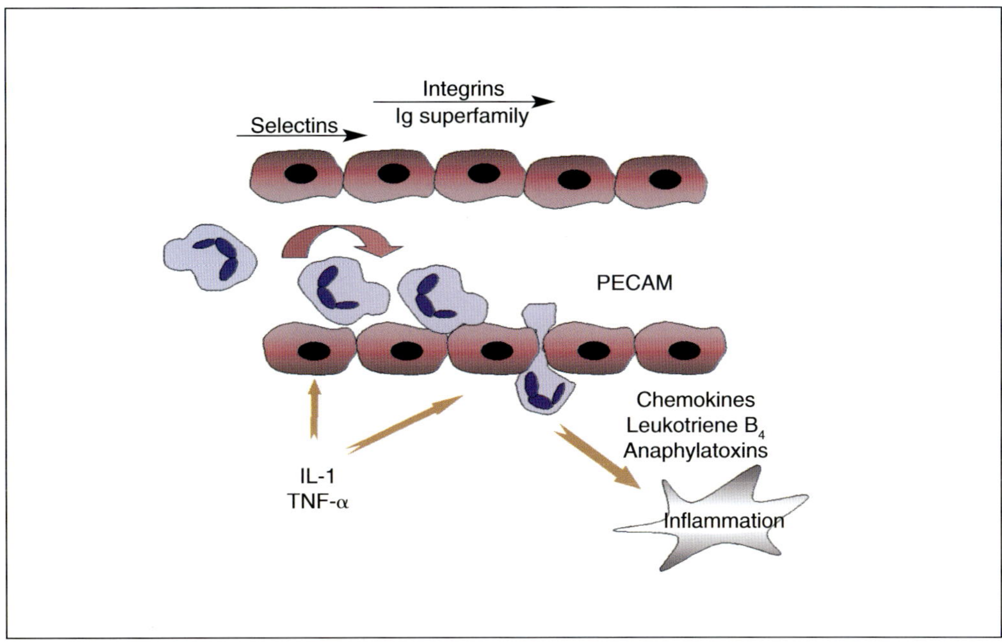

Fig 11-2 Major groups of adhesion molecules responsible for rolling, adhesion, transmigration, and chemotaxis. (Redrawn from Collins[1] with permission.)

whether or not the tooth is symptomatic.[35] The percentage of neuronal areas that positively stained for SP was found to be significantly greater in areas of gross caries lesions than in areas of moderate or no lesions and in painful versus nonpainful lesions. These findings were true at all levels of coronal pulp studied, including the pulp horn, subodontoblastic nerve plexus, and midcoronal pulp. The fact that not all cases of irreversible pulpitis are associated with pain may be explained by the actions of inhibitory neurotransmitters like γ-aminobutyric acid (GABA) or gastrin-releasing peptide (GRP). GABA-like and GRP-like immunoreactivity have been identified in the dental pulp[36] (see also chapter 8).

Neuropeptides may contribute to the inflammatory process via additional mechanisms. These include the release of inflammatory mediators such as histamine, PGE_2, collagenase, IL-1, IL-6, and tumor necrosis factor (TNF); the potentiation of chemotaxis, phagocytosis, and the expression of adhesion molecules; and lymphocyte proliferation and IL-2 production.[32,37,38] It is interesting to note that animal studies have shown a reduction of the neuropeptides SP and CGRP with age.[39]

Leukocyte Adhesion and Transmigration

The recruitment and activation of leukocytes constitute critical early steps in mounting an immune response to bacterial infection. Indeed, certain stimuli such as the dentinal transport of bacteria or bacterial by-products can directly stimulate a chronic form of inflammation, characterized by leukocyte migration into the inflamed area, without a preceding acute inflammatory response (see chapter 10).

One of the critical processes in inflammation is the delivery of leukocytes to the site of irritation. As PBF slows down at the site of inflammation (due to vasodilation and increased vascular permeability, as discussed above), leukocytes assume a more peripheral position in the vessels, a condition called *margination*. Eventually, the leukocytes roll along the endothelial wall and finally adhere to the endothelial lining (pavementing). They then insert pseudopods into gaps between the endothelial cells and transmigrate along the chemotactic gradient through the basement membrane toward the site of inflammation (Fig 11-2).

Table 11-1 Principal molecules involved in leukocyte adhesion and transmigration during inflammation*

Molecular family	Site	Ligand	Primary functions
Selectins			
L selectin (CD62L; LAM-1)	Leukocytes; high expression on naïve T cells	Glycan-bearing cell-adhesion molecule-1 (GlyCAM-I); mucosal addressin cell-adhesion molecule-1 (MAdCAM-I); and CD34, a proteoglycan	Lymphocyte homing to lymph nodes. It has low affinity and mediates the initial attachment and rolling of leukocytes. On neutrophils, binds cells to endothelial cells that are activated by IL-1, TNF-α and IFN-γ found at sites of inflammation.
E selectin (CD62E; ELAM-1)	Cytokine-activated endothelial cells, hence the designation E	Complex sialylated carbohydrate groups related to the Lewis X or Lewis A family found on surface proteins of granulocytes, monocytes, and memory T cells	Endothelial cell expression of E selectin is a hallmark of acute cytokine-mediated inflammation, and antibodies to E selectin can block neutrophil accumulation in vivo.
P selectin (CD62P; GMP-140)	Secretory granules of platelets (hence the designation P) and of endothelial cells (Weibel-Palade) bodies	Complex carbohydrate ligands similar to those recognized by E selectin	After cell stimulation, P selectin is translocated to the cell surface as part of the exocytic secretory process. It mediates binding of neutrophils, T lymphocytes, and monocytes. P-selectin expression is regulated by cytokines, similar to the regulation of E selectin.
Immunoglobulin superfamily			
Intercellular adhesion molecule 1, 2, 3 (ICAM-1, -2, -3) (CD54, CD102, CD50)	Endothelial cells	LFA-1	ICAM-1 is upregulated with inflammation, but ICAM-2 is constitutively expressed; functions in secondary adhesion and transmigration.
Vascular cell adhesion molecule (VCAM-1) (CD106)	Endothelial cells	$\alpha 4\beta 1$ integrins	Inflammation induced. Expression is heterogeneous, suggesting the possibility of tissue- or microenvironment-selective function.

*Data from Paul[40] and Abbas et al.[43]

Adhesion molecules

Several important molecules are essential in the adhesion and transmigration of leukocytes: selectins, integrins, endothelial adhesion molecules, and CD44 (Table 11-1). Selectins are the molecules that initially bind to circulating leukocytes and cause them to roll along the endothelial lining (see Fig 11-2). L-selectins are found on leukocytes, whereas endothelial cells express P and E selectins. Selectins are classified by lectins that bind to carbohydrate ligands on the corresponding cell type.[40] Mouse knock-out studies have shown that the absence of either P selectin or E selectin individually does not cause significant disruption in cell adhesion. However, the absence of both molecules causes a condition called *leukocyte adhesion deficiency-II* (LAD-II). In normal dental pulp, only a few blood vessels located in the pulp core react weakly with an immunohistochemical stain for E or P selectin. However, in the pulp of teeth with pericoronitis

Table 11-1 (cont) Principal molecules involved in leukocyte adhesion and transmigration during inflammation*

Molecular family	Site	Ligand	Primary functions
Mucosal addressin (MAdCAM-1)	Endothelial adhesion molecule on high endothelial venules (HEVs)	$\alpha 4\beta 7$ integrins	Binds mucosa-homing lymphoid subsets.
Platelet endothelial cell-adhesion molecule (PECAM-1) (CD31)	Intercellular junction of endothelium and leukocytes	PECAM-1 (self)	Antibodies to soluble forms of this molecule inhibit transmigration.
Integrins: β_2-class (CD18)			
$\alpha_L\beta_2$ (LFA-1)		ICAM-1, -2, and -3 on endothelial cells and leukocytes	Leukocyte adhesion to endothelium; T-cell antigen-presenting cell adhesion; T-cell co-stimulation.
$\alpha_M\beta_2$ (MAC-1, CR3)		Inactivated C3b, fibrinogen, factor X, ICAM-1	Leukocyte adhesion and phagocytosis; cell-matrix adhesion.
$\alpha_X\beta_2$ (p150,95, CR4)		Inactivated C3b, fibrinogen	Leukocyte adhesion and phagocytosis; cell-matrix adhesion.
Integrins: α_4-class (CD49D)			
$\alpha_4\beta_1$ (VLA-4)		VCAM-1	Memory lymphocyte homing to sites of chronic inflammation, potentially functioning in primary adhesion, rolling velocity reduction, and secondary adhesion. Also cell-matrix adhesion.
$\alpha_4\beta_7$		MAdCAM-1 is the predominant endothelial ligand.	Mucosal homing receptor for naïve lymphocyte functions in primary adhesion, rolling velocity reduction, and secondary adhesion.
Proteoglycan-cartilage-link protein: CD44 (HCAM, Pgp-1)		Hyaluronate	Mediates primary adhesion of activated (by not resting) lymphocytes; participates in the homing of memory-effector blasts to sites of inflammation.
Other: vascular adhesion protein-1 (VAP-1)			Constitutively expressed by peripheral lymph node HEV and widely upregulated on inflamed venules.

*Data from Paul[40] and Abbas et al.[43]

but no caries, a large number of vessels located in the subodontoblastic layer react strongly with the antibody for these molecules.[41] Thus, selectins can be upregulated in human dental pulp and are vital in the adhesion of leukocytes to endothelial cells.

Intercellular adhesion molecules (ICAMs) are members of the immunoglobulin superfamily and include ICAM-1, ICAM-2, ICAM-3, VCAM-1, and PECAM-1. ICAM-1 is strongly induced on leukocytes and endothelial cells. Endothelial cells constitutively express ICAM-2, VCAM-1, and PECAM-1, whereas resting leukocytes bear ICAM-3 and PECAM-1 on their surfaces. ICAM-1 interacts with the integrins LFA-1 and Mac-1; ICAM-2 and ICAM-3 with LFA-1; and VCAM-1 with VLA-4. PECAM-1 is engaged in homophilic interactions. In one study,[41] subodontoblastic and pulp-core blood vessels had increased expression of immunoreactive PECAM-1, ICAM-1 and -3, and VCAM-1 in teeth with pericoronitis compared with normal teeth. Immunohistochemical studies have also localized the presence of the following adhesion molecules in normal human pulp: PECAM-1, endoglin, (CD105) ICAM-1, ICAM-2, and MUC-18 (CD146) on endothelium of capillaries, arterioles, and venules; ICAM-3 (CD50) on peripheral blood cells; and VCAM-1 weakly on venule endothelium. P selectin (CD62-P) was mostly found on venule endothelium and platelets.[42] Thus, several ICAMs found on pulpal cells appear to be upregulated under certain conditions.

Integrins mediate cell-cell or cell-matrix binding (see Fig 11-2). The integrins are transmembrane glycoproteins expressed on many cell types, including leukocytes and endothelial cells. Their cytoplasmic domains bind to the cytoskeleton. The integrin superfamily consists of about 30 structurally homologous proteins that promote cell-cell or cell-matrix binding. All integrins are heterodimeric cell–surface proteins consisting of noncovalently linked α and β chains. The most notable integrins are LFA-1, Mac-1, and VLA-4 (see Table 11-1). Integrins mediate stable adhesion of leukocytes to endothelial cells, T cells to antigen-presenting cells, cytolytic T cells to target cells, and connective tissue cells to extracellular matrix proteins such as fibronectin, vitronectin, osteopontin, and collagen.[43] The affinity of leukocytes to bind integrins is increased by chemokine secretion from either the endothelial cells or the inflamed tissue. Patients who have a defect in the biosynthesis of the β_2 chain, shared by LFA-1 and Mac-1 integrins, develop leukocyte adhesion deficiency-I (LAD-I). Patients with LAD-I or LAD-II develop immunodeficiency and recurrent bacterial infections.[1] A recent case report of a patient with LAD-I described multiple dental pulp infections and severe periodontitis.[44] The authors recommended treating such patients with prophylactic antibiotics. Human dental pulp cells express multiple integrins, including the $\alpha_{1,}\alpha_{3,}\alpha_{5,}\alpha_{6,}\alpha_{V}$ and β_1, but not α_4 integrin subunits; the α_2 subunit is found in some but not all studies.[45,46] In these studies, blockage of the β_1 integrin with an anti-β_1 monoclonal antibody completely inhibited pulp cell adhesion to laminin but not to fibronectin. Leukocyte transmigration is mediated by interactions between ICAM-1 and integrins as well as PECAM-1 on leukocytes and endothelial cells.[1]

Thus, several classes of adhesion molecules, including the selectins, ICAMs, and integrins, are found in normal dental pulp, where they coordinate the cellular organization of the tissue via cell-cell and cell-matrix binding. During pulpal inflammation, many of these adhesion molecules are selectively upregulated and play major roles in organizing the immune-cell response to pulpal inflammation. A genetic deficiency in these molecules, as in the case of LAD-I, leads to functional immunodeficiency because leukocytes do not undergo the critical step in binding to endothelium. The multiple dental abscesses and severe periodontitis found in these patients emphasize the importance of adhesion molecules in mounting an effective immune-cell response to pulpal infection.

Chemotactic factors

After transmigration across the vasculature, leukocytes undergo chemotaxis to the site of inflammation along a chemical gradient. Bacterial products may act as chemoattractants. All of the following induce the chemotaxis of neutrophils to the subjacent pulp region when applied to the base of a Class V cavity preparation in monkeys: plaque extract,[47] crude homogenates from gram-positive and gram-negative bacteria,[48] and purified gram-positive or gram-negative cell-wall complexes.[49] Different endodontically relevant bacteria were found to have comparable chemotactic abilities when tested at the bacterial cell[50]

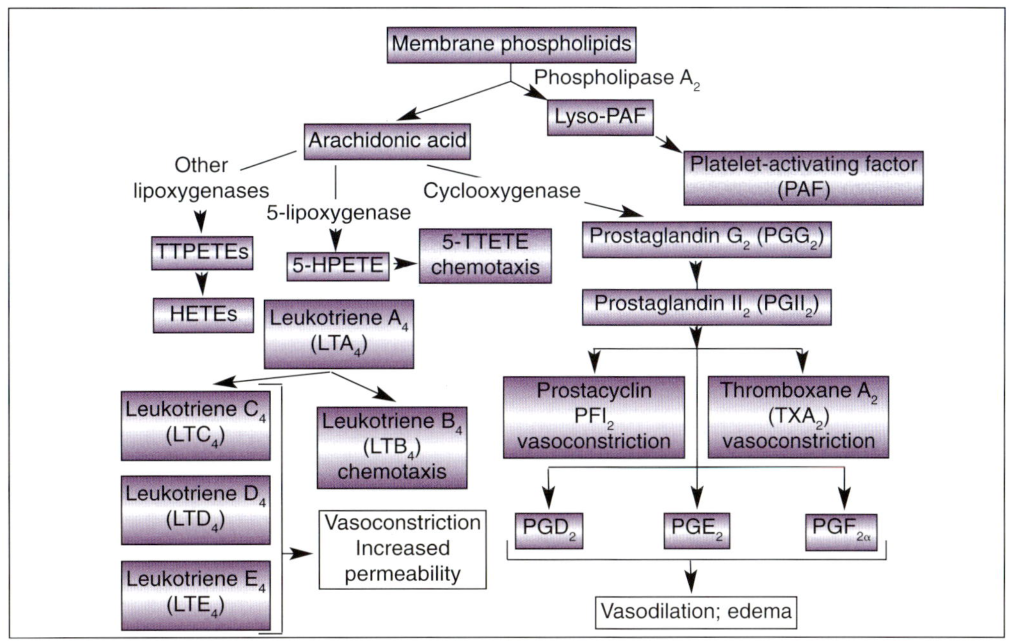

Fig 11-3 Phospholipid metabolism and arachidonic acid pathways.

or bacterial cell wall-extract[49] levels. However, in an in vitro pulp-chamber model, *Fusobacterium nucleatum* was found to be more chemoattractant than *Treponema denticola*.[51] Agents that are chemotactic for neutrophils should be associated with the formation of abscesses; thus it is not surprising that the presence of *F nucleatum* along with black-pigmented bacteria is significantly associated with the development of pus and abscesses (see chapter 12).

Endogenous molecules may also serve as chemotactic factors. For example, complement components C3a and C5a, leukotrienes (especially leukotriene B_4 or LTB_4), and chemokines (such as IL-8) all serve as chemotactic agents. (A more detailed discussion of these factors will follow). Vascular endothelial growth factor (VEGF), an angiogenic growth factor that induces proliferation and migration of vascular endothelial cells, was recently shown to promote chemotaxis and proliferation of human pulp cells.[52] These effects were in part mediated by the activation of the DNA-binding protein AP-1 and to a lesser degree nuclear factor-kappa B (NF-κB).

Other Mediators of the Inflammatory Response

Arachidonic acid metabolites

When cells are activated, their membrane phospholipids are rapidly remodeled to generate biologically active lipid inflammatory mediators. Products derived from the metabolism of arachidonic acid (AA), a 20-carbon polyunsaturated fatty acid, affect a variety of biologic processes, including inflammation and hemostasis. AA metabolites, also called *eicosanoids*, are synthesized by two major classes of enzymes: cyclo-oxygenases (prostaglandins and thromboxanes) and lipoxygenases (leukotrienes and lipoxins) (Fig 11-3).

Prostaglandins and thromboxanes

The cyclo-oxygenase (COX) pathway leads to the generation of prostaglandins. This process takes place in the normal pulp. It may be blocked by the addition of indomethacin, a prostaglandin synthetase inhibitor, or augmented by application of exogenous arachidonic acid or serotonin.[10,53] The most important prostaglandins in inflammation are PGE_2, PGD_2, $PGF_{2\alpha}$, PGI_2 (prostacyclin), and TXA_2 (thromboxane). It has been known for decades that prostaglandins play a critical role in the pathogenesis of pulpal disease[54,55] (see also chapter 8). In the rat incisor, application of bacterial lipopolysaccharide (LPS) induces pulpal inflammation and evokes a ninefold increase in PGE_2 and about a fourfold increase in 6-keto-$PGF_{1\alpha}$, a stable metabolite of PGI_2.[56] The increase in pulpal levels of PGE_2, $PGF_{2\alpha}$, and 6-keto-$PGF_{1\alpha}$ after induced inflammation was also shown immunohistochemically.[57] Prostaglandins generally cause vasodilation while thromboxane causes vasoconstriction. Elevated PGE_2 and 6-keto-$PGF_{1\alpha}$ levels are associated with a significant increase in vascular permeability of LPS-inflamed rat pulp, which may be inhibited in a dose-dependent manner by administration of indomethacin prior to the application of the LPS.[58] The increased level of hydroxyeicosatetraenoic acids (HETEs), a lipoxygenase metabolite, was not affected by indomethacin administration. It is of clinical interest that systemic administration of LPS also caused an increase in baseline pulpal PGI_2 and TXA_2 biosynthesis (measured indirectly by its stable metabolite TXB_2).[59] This phenomenon may be important in cases of endotoxemia during dentinogenesis.

Prostaglandins may also induce the production of other inflammatory mediators or regenerative molecules. In the dental pulp, PGE_2 significantly increased the bradykinin-evoked release of immunoreactive CGRP[60] and was found to increase significantly the production of hepatocyte growth factor, which stimulates DNA synthesis, and which was shown to increase in pulpal inflammation.

Prostaglandins are also involved in the pathogenesis of pain (see chapters 8 and 9). The direct involvement of prostanoids in pulpal pain was proposed when the intravenous administration of nonsteroidal anti-inflammatory drugs (NSAIDs), which are known to block the COX pathway, resulted in significant inhibition of stimulated nerve activity in cat pulp.[62] Furthermore, patients with acute forms of pulpal pain had significantly increased pulpal levels of both PGE_2 and PGF_{2a} compared with patients presenting nonpainful pulpitis or normal pulp.[63] In the rat incisor model, cavity preparation without coolant caused a significant rise in pulpal levels of PGE_2, 6-keto-$PGF_{1\alpha}$, and TXB_2, but sealing the cavities with zinc oxide and eugenol (ZnOE) halted any increase in prostaglandin.[64] This result was not found with zinc oxide and water, however, suggesting that eugenol released from ZnOE fillings may reduce the amount of pulp prostaglandins, and this may be one of the mechanisms by which it reduces pulpal pain. Because prostaglandins are so abundant in pulpal inflammation, it has been suggested that their level could be used as a biochemically based diagnostic test to determine the degree of pulpal inflammation in patients undergoing pulpotomy procedures.[65]

Glucocorticoids block the breakdown of membrane phospholipids to arachidonic acid by phospholipases, whereas NSAIDs block the COX pathway (see Fig 11-3). Numerous investigations have shown the effectiveness of corticosteroids[66-68] or NSAIDs[69-71] on pulpal pain, particularly in the apical inflammation that occurs following pulpectomy.

Recently, research into the pathophysiology of inflammatory pain led to the recognition that the COX pathway is mediated by at least two different enzymes, COX-1 and COX-2. COX-1 is thought to be constitutively expressed and to perform beneficial homeostatic functions on the gastric mucosa and the kidneys; however, COX-2 is an induced pro-inflammatory enzyme.[72] Therefore, the recent introduction of the selective COX-2 inhibitor class of NSAIDs purports to allow the anti-inflammatory properties while suppressing the harmful side effects on the gastric mucosa and the kidneys. The inhibition of PGE_2 production in induced rat molar pulpal inflammation by the primarily COX-2 inhibitor nabumetone was similar to that of ibuprofen.[71] While the effectiveness of commericially available COX-2 inhibitors in controlling pulpal pain has not been reported, it appears that their efficacy in other models of oral pain is not different from that of traditional NSAIDs.[73]

Leukotrienes and lipoxins

Products of the lipoxygenase pathway are synthesized only by inflammatory cells such as neutrophils, eosinophils, mast cells, basophils, macrophages, and monocytes. This exclusivity is distinctly different than COX products, which are present in all mammalian cells except erythrocytes (ie, all nucleated cells). The predominant enzyme in neutrophils is 5-lipoxygenase. The main product, 5-HETE, which is chemotactic for neutrophils, is converted into a family of compounds collectively called *leukotrienes*. LTB_4 is a potent chemotactic agent and activator of neutrophil functional responses, such as aggregation and adhesion of leukocytes to venule endothelium, generation of oxygen free radicals, and release of lysosomal enzymes.[1] Inflammation induced in the rat incisor,[74] rat molar,[74] or dog canine[75] stimulates the increased production of LTB_4[71,74] or LTC_4.[75] Administration of a dual inhibitor of the COX and lipoxygenase pathways blocks the stimulatory effects of LPS on both neutrophil chemotaxis and LTB_4 levels in dental pulp.[74] Interestingly, this effect was not seen with a traditional inhibitor of the COX pathway (indomethacin).[74] The clinical implications of these results are that dual-inhibitor NSAID-like drugs may have clinical applications for reducing the development of pulpal inflammation and abscesses.

The results of studies on whether leukotrienes reduce the pain threshold in dental pulp have not been conclusive. LTB_4 and LTC_4 were found to significantly reduce spontaneous and evoked nerve excitability of cat dental pulp in one study,[76] but LTB_4 was found to increase pulpal nerve excitability under similar conditions in another study.[77] The concentrations of sodium chloride used to evoke pulpal responses in these two studies were different and a ceiling effect of sodium chloride was detected in the latter study. The changes from baseline observed in both studies indicate that leukotrienes may modulate the excitability of nerves brought about by neurogenic inflammation.

Lipoxins are the most recent addition to the family of bioactive products generated from arachidonic acid. Lipoxins A_4 and B_4 (LXA_4 and LXB_4) are generated by the action of platelet 12-lipoxygenase on neutrophil LTA_4.[1] Lipoxins may be negative regulators of leukotrienes, inhibiting neutrophil chemotaxis and adhesion in acute inflammation[78] and causing vasodilation to attenuate leukotriene LTC_4-mediated vasoconstriction.[79] The actions of lipoxins in the pulp have not been reported.

Platelet-activating factor

Platelet-activating factor (PAF) is another bioactive mediator derived from phospholipids (see Fig 11-3). It is secreted by platelets, basophils (and mast cells), monocytes/macrophages, neutrophils, and endothelial cells. Its actions include platelet stimulation, leukocyte adhesion to endothelial cells by integrins, chemotaxis, and the stimulation of an oxidative burst. At low doses, PAF is a potent vasodilator, 100 to 1,000 times more potent than histamine.[1,80] At higher doses, PAF is a vasoconstrictor.[1,80] PAF stimulates the production of PGI_2 and TXA_2 from homogenates of rat incisor pulp.[81] Furthermore, antagonists of the PAF receptor block the stimulatory effects of LPS on TXA_2 synthesis in tooth pulp.[59] Thus, PAF appears to be released from dental pulp after exposure to stimuli such as LPS, and this phospholipid mediator may initiate early inflammatory processes such as vasodilation, leukocyte transmigration, chemotaxis and activation, and the release of other inflammatory mediators.

Plasma proteins and proteases

The development of plasma extravasation during inflammation results in the outflow of fluid, plasma proteins, and blood-borne cells into dental pulp. These plasma proteins include constituents of the kinin system, the complement system, the clotting and fibrinolytic systems, lysosomal enzymes, and protease inhibitors. Collectively, these factors play important roles in mediating and modulating pulpal inflammation.

The kinin system and bradykinin

The precursors to the kinin system circulate in the vascular compartment and can be activated at any location where vascular integrity is lost. During the inflammatory process, prekallikrein is activated by the Hageman factor (coagulation factor XII) to become the active enzyme kallikrein. Kallikreins, which are specific proteases, generate vasoactive peptides from plasma proteins called *kininogens*. The most important peptide released from the kininogens is bradykinin (BK). BK has four main proinflammatorypro-inflammatory actions: vasodilation, increased vascular permeability, activation of nociceptors, and the attraction of leukocytes.[82] Bradykinin performs its actions through binding with two receptors: B_1 and B_2. The B_1 receptor is involved in certain forms of persistent hyperalgesia or chronic pain, whereas the B_2 receptor is the main BK receptor that is constitutively present in normal tissues and plays a role in acute inflammatory pain.[83] B_2 is also the principal BK receptor in dental pulp.[60,84,85]

Numerous studies have shown that BK is one of the major molecular mediators of inflammation in the dental pulp. In the dog canine model, it was shown that BK, like PGE_2, increases PBF and vascular permeability (probably at the postcapillary venule site). Bradykinin caused a smaller flow increase but produced more leakage than PGE_2.[86] During pulpal inflammation, a complex interaction takes place between BK and a number of other molecular mediators, frequently eliciting synergy among the actions of the different mediators and an exaggeration of the inflammatory response. Bradykinin was shown to increase the release of arachidonic acid and its metabolites from rat-pulp cell lines[84] by stimulating the intracellular signaling mediators cAMP, Ca^{++}, and inositol phosphate.[87] In both these studies, the use of indomethacin abrogated this effect, and BK had no effect on the proliferation of the cells as did thrombin[84] and epidermal growth factor.[87] BK also enhanced the formation of PGE_2 by IL-1α, IL-1β, TNF-α, and TNF-β.[85] PGE_2 on the other hand was recently shown using the bovine pulp superfusion model to increase the release of BK-evoked immunoreactive CGRP by more than 50%.[60] Thus, the process of plasma extravasation leads directly to several key inflammatory events mediated in part by the kinin system.

Once released, BK is rapidly metabolized by specific kininases.[88] Therefore, it has been difficult to measure BK levels in vivo. However, in a recent study, BK levels in the pulp interstitial fluid were measured directly in humans using the elegant technique of microdialysis.[89] This technique utilizes a narrow probe with a semipermeable membrane that allows dialysis of smaller molecules, thus eliminating contamination by the much larger kininogens and proteases. In that study, a comparison between BK levels in individuals with normal pulp and those with irreversible pulpitis revealed a 13-fold increase in BK levels in irreversible pulpitis. Interestingly, when patients who had pain at the time of sampling were compared with those who had a history of pain, significantly more BK was reported in the latter group (a 17-fold increase vs a 3-fold increase above normal levels). This apparent lack of correlation between pain intensity at the time of sampling and BK levels was attributed to either the presence of other algesiogenic mediators in the pulp or the desensitization of BK receptors after chronic exposure to BK.[89]

Anti-inflammatory drugs such as the corticosteroid methylprednisolone[90] or NSAIDs such as flurbiprofen[91] reduce the level of BK in inflamed tissue. Also, the addition of BK to homogenized rat pulp led to the release of the endogenous opiate metenkephalin in a dose-dependent manner, an effect that was inhibited by a BK receptor antagonist.[92] Thus homeostatic mechanisms may contribute to the control of BK release in vivo.

The complement system

The complement system consists of 20 different plasma proteins and their cleavage products that

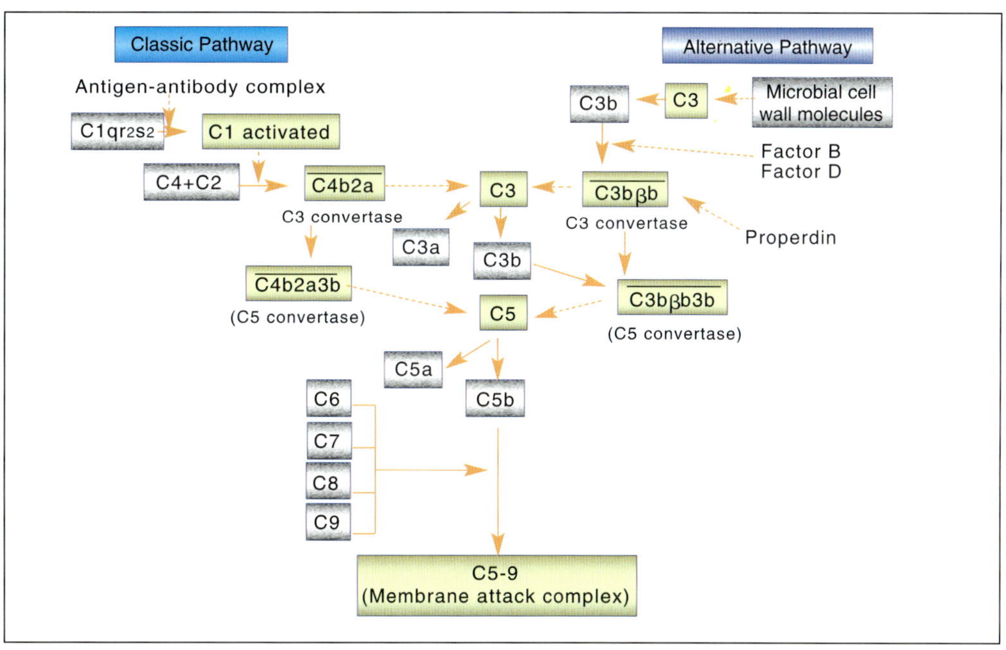

Fig 11-4 The complement cascade.

function in both adaptive and innate immune responses and aid in the lysis of microbial cells. Two complement activation pathways have been described: the classical and the alternative (Fig 11-4). The pathways differ in how C3b is produced but are otherwise similar. Complement activation promotes phagocytosis because phagocytes express receptors for C3b. The terminal components of the complement system, whose activation is dependent on C3b, generate a lipid-soluble macromolecular protein complex called the *membrane attack complex* (MAC), which causes osmotic lysis of target cells. Peptides produced by proteolysis of C3 and other complement proteins stimulate inflammation.[43] C3a and C5a, also known as anaphylactotoxins, stimulate histamine release from mast cells, thereby causing vasodilation and increased vascular permeability. C5a activates the lipoxygenase pathway of arachidonic acid in neutrophils and monocytes and is itself a potent chemotactic agent for these cells.[1]

Early studies revealed weak complement activity in the dental pulp.[93-95] One report indicates positive staining for C3 and C4 complement proteins in dentin in normal and carious teeth.[96] More recently it was shown that complement staining in caries lesions is more on the external surface and is probably of plaque origin.[97] The relative paucity of direct observational evidence for the presence of complement components in the pulp may be because most complement proteins are present only transiently in the inflammatory process and are easily denatured during processing of specimens. The effects of bacterial irritants placed in Class V cavities on the dental pulp were studied in primates, a group of which was injected with purified cobra venom factor, which has known anticomplement activity. The results did not reveal histologic differences between the two animal groups.[48] Therefore, the role of complement activity in pulpal inflammation is not clear at this time.

The clotting and fibrinolytic systems

The clotting system is closely related to the inflammatory process. As discussed previously, Hageman factor (coagulation factor XII) is a protease that initiates the kinin system by releasing

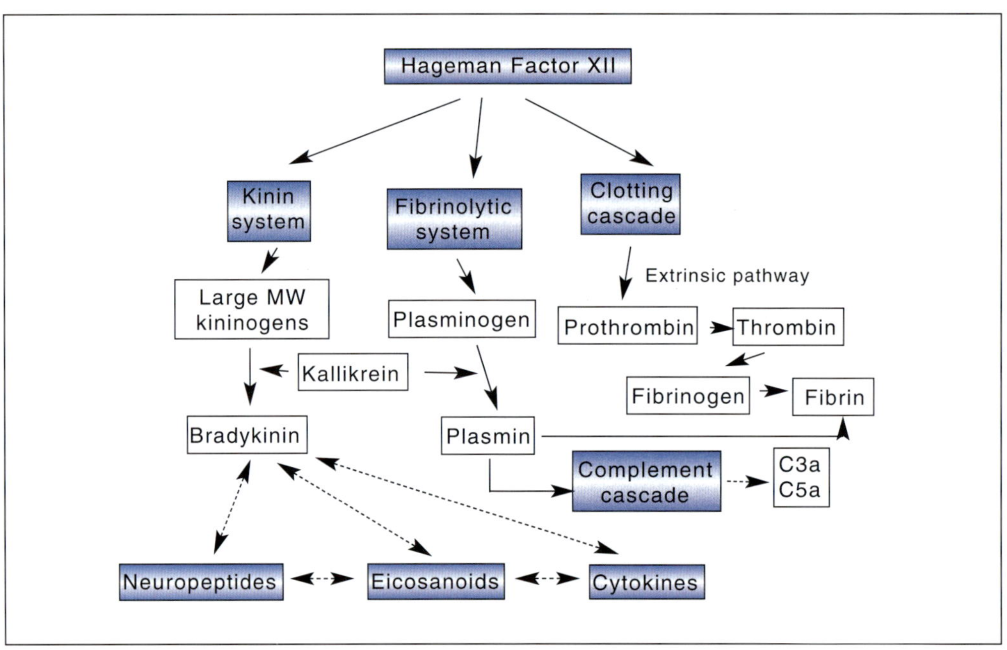

Fig 11-5 Interaction between selected groups of inflammatory systems. The dotted arrows indicate synergy and/or potentiation. MW, molecular weight.

kallikrein from prekallikrein; it also initiates the extrinsic pathway of the coagulation cascade[98] (Fig 11-5). A number of intermediary steps result in the formation of thrombin (factor II, a serine protease) from prothrombin. Thrombin has many pro-inflammatory effects: it cleaves fibrinogen to form fibrin, activates factor XIII to cross-link the fibrin polymer and aggregate platelets, acts as a chemotactic factor, stimulates leukocyte adhesion to endothelial cells, and induces fibroblast proliferation.[99] The addition of thrombin to pulpal fibroblasts caused a burst in the production of PGE_2 and 6-keto-$PGF_{1\alpha}$, an effect that was very similar to the addition of BK.[84] It was also shown that thrombin increases DNA synthesis, protein synthesis, and the proliferation of pulp fibroblasts and that these effects may be modulated by PGE_2.[100-102] Factor XIIIa expressed by dendritic pulpal cells was recently shown immunohistochemically to co-accumulate with increased neural elements in close relation to areas of carious dentin.[103] Thus, both thrombin and Hageman factor are key enzymatic steps in the development of inflammation.

In addition to activating the extrinsic clotting system, Hageman factor also initiates the fibrinolytic system that destabilizes the fibrin clot by breaking the cross-linked polymer (see Fig 11-5). A plasminogen activator is secreted from leukocytes and endothelial cells to cleave plasminogen into plasmin, a protease. Plasmin's main action is to lyse fibrin clots. However, it also cleaves C3 into its fragments, participating in the initiation of the complement cascade (see Fig 11-5). Fibrinolytic activity was demonstrated in the dental pulp several decades ago.[104] A fibrin clot is formed under cavity preparations, particularly when the pulp is exposed.[105,106] Fibrinogen has been localized in the pulp and inside dentinal tubules under cavity preparations when the pulp was not exposed.[107,108] It may reduce dentinal permeability to advancing microbial irritants[109] (see also chapter 4). It is also conceivable that the fibrinolytic system plays an important role in the early organization of healing pulp under acute injury such as a cavity preparation. The administration of IL-6 to human pulp cells increases plasminogen activity.[110] It is noteworthy that a number of pathogenic endodontic microorganisms have been found to specifically degrade fibrin or fibrinogen or both.[107] This property may play an important role in determining virulence of microorganisms infecting the dental pulp and surrounding tissue.

Lysosomal enzymes and metalloproteases

Neutrophils and monocytes/macrophages have lysosomal granules containing a number of enzymes that contribute to the inflammatory process. Neutrophils contain two types of granules: the smaller or specific granules contain lysozyme, collagenase, lactoferrin, plasminogen activator, histaminase, and alkaline phosphatase; the larger or azurophil granules contain myeloperoxidase, lysozyme, defensins, acid hydrolases, and neutral hydrolases such as collagenase, elastase, cathepsin G, and other proteinases.[1] Most of these enzymes have potent antimicrobial properties, thus eliminating microbial irritants, yet they may also lead to excessive tissue destruction during an inflammatory episode.

Lysosomes and phagosomes have been observed in the ultrastucture of the inflamed pulp.[111] Excessive neutrophil accumulation in the pulp may increase the likelihood of tissue necrosis.[49] Cathepsin D was observed in the odontoblastic layer of normal pulp,[112] and cathepsin G (along with elastase and lactoferrin) was shown to increase during pulp inflammation.[113-115] In these latter studies the protease inhibitor α_2-macroglobulin was also observed to increase with inflammation, indicating an attempt to control the tissue destruction aspect of these enzymes.

A tissue inhibitor of metalloproteinases (TIMP) from cultured bovine dental pulp was identified and found to be destroyed by the serine proteinases, human neutrophil elastase, trypsin, and alpha-chymotrypsin, but not by cathepsin G or plasmin.[116] The intensity of pulpal inflammation may determine the neutrophil/monocyte infiltration, their release of lysosomal enzymes, and the final outcome of the balance between inflammation and regeneration.

Metalloproteinases (MMPs) are an important family of 11 or more zinc-dependent endopeptidases responsible for the degradation of extracellular matrix components, which takes place during normal and pathologic remodeling of tissues, such as during embryonic development, inflammation, tumor invasion, etc. They include collagenases (MMP-1, -8, and -13), stromelysins (MMP-3, -10, -11, and -12), gelatinases (MMP-2 and -9), and membrane MMP.[117] These enzymes are upregulated by cytokines such as IL-1β and TNF-α and by growth factors such as platelet-derived growth factor (PDGF), epidermal growth factor (EGF), and nerve growth factor (NGF) and are abrogated by interferon gamma (IFN-γ) and TGF-β. They are also inhibited by TIMP and α_2-macroglobulin as mentioned before.

Interstitial collagenase (MMP-1) was detected in ameloblasts and odontoblasts of the developing enamel organ,[118] and its expression was upregulated in dental pulp cells stimulated in vitro with IL-1 or TNF-α[119,120] and with bacterial sonicates or LPS[121,122] but was reduced by TGF-β.[119] Host MMP-8 (collagenolytic) and MMP-2 and 9 (gelatinolytic) (probably of salivary rather than pulpal origin) were recently shown to participate in the degradation of demineralized dentin under a caries lesion.[123] It was also shown using reverse transcriptase-polymerase chain reaction (RT-PCR) that MMP-8 was expressed by native and cultured odontoblasts and pulp tissue and cultured pulp fibroblasts.[124] Clearly, MMPs may contribute to the remodeling of dentin and pulp that takes place in physiologic as well as pathologic situations. Collectively, these studies indicate that the release of proteases into dental pulp orchestrates a complex series of responses leading to tissue inflammation and possibly tissue destruction. Regulation of this enzymatic activity is clearly an important factor in the transition from tissue inflammation to healing.

Protease inhibitors

Protease inhibitors serve the important function of limiting the normal protease, including metalloproteinase, that may damage the host tissue if left unchecked. A number of protease inhibitors have been identified in the dental pulp. Examples of these include collagenase inhibitor[125]; dipep-

Table 11-2 Modulation of inflammation by nitric oxide*

Pro-inflammatory properties	Anti-inflammatory properties
Promotes vasodilation and vascular leakiness	Inhibits leukocyte adhesion to endothelium
Promotes hypotension or vascular collapse in sepsis	Inhibits P-selectin expression by platelets, endothelium
Cytotoxic	Inhibits microvascular thrombosis
Activates cyclo-oxygenase†	Inhibits lymphocyte proliferation
Reacts with O_2 to form toxic peroxynitrite	Inhibits mast cell degranulation
Inhibitors of NO synthesis ameliorate experimental models of arthritis	Inhibits oxidant production by phagocytes
Simulates tumor necrosis factor alpha production by synoviocytes	Inhibits cyclo-oxygenase†

*Based on data from Clancy et al.[131]
†Depends on the dose.

tidyl peptidase II, a lysosomal peptidase active on collagen-related peptides[126]; alpha-1-antitrypsin and alpha-2-macroglobulin, which inhibit polymorphonuclear neutrophil (PMN) elastase and other proteases[115,127]; and alpha-1-antichymotrypsin, a protease inhibitor secreted by activated macrophages.[128]

Nitric oxide and oxygen-derived free radicals

Free radicals are highly reactive, short-lived molecules that can damage nearby cells of either host or bacterial origin. Due to their reactivity, these compounds in general have extremely short half-lives and are therefore synthesized in proximity to their targets. Free radicals are chemically similar in the addition of an unpaired electron but vary in structure from gases such as nitric oxide to oxygen-derived factors such as superoxide anions.

Nitric oxide

Nitric oxide (NO) has received a lot of attention since its discovery in the late 1980s. Despite its high reactivity and short life, NO modulates a large array of biologic functions. It is a soluble gas that was first identified by its action of relaxing smooth muscle, causing vasodilation. This effect was also shown to be true in the dental pulp.[129,130] Nitric oxide is synthesized via L-arginine oxidation by a family of NO synthases (NOSs) and several cofactors, including nicotinamide adenine dinucleotide phosphate (NADPH). Three different isoforms of the NOS enzyme exist: neuronal NOS (ncNOS, NOS-I), inducible NOS (iNOS, NOS-II), and endothelial NOS (ecNOS, NOS-III).[1] The calcium-dependent neuronal and endothelial NOS is constitutively expressed in the respective tissues, whereas the calcium-independent inducible NOS is induced in macrophages and a number of other cells, primarily by cytokines such as IL-1, and TNF-α or microbial products such as LPS. The cytokines IL-4, IL-10, and TGF-β regulate the expression of iNOS in macrophages.[131]

Depending on the site of production, the amount of NO produced, and the targets within the local environment, NO can exert very different effects. A small quantity of NO released by the vascular endothelium regulates the relaxation of adjacent smooth muscle and protects against the adhesion of leukocytes and platelets to the blood-vessel wall. These properties may be considered protective and anti-inflammatory (Table 11-2). In contrast, the much larger amounts of NO released by cells in response to cytokines can destroy host tissues and impair discrete cellular responses. Finally, by affecting functions of lymphocytes and macrophages, induced NO can exert an immunomodulatory influence that modifies the course of disease[131] (see Table 11-2).

In a recent study, NO activity was investigated in the inflamed pulp of rat molars.[132] The ncNOS isoform could not be seen in either normal or in-

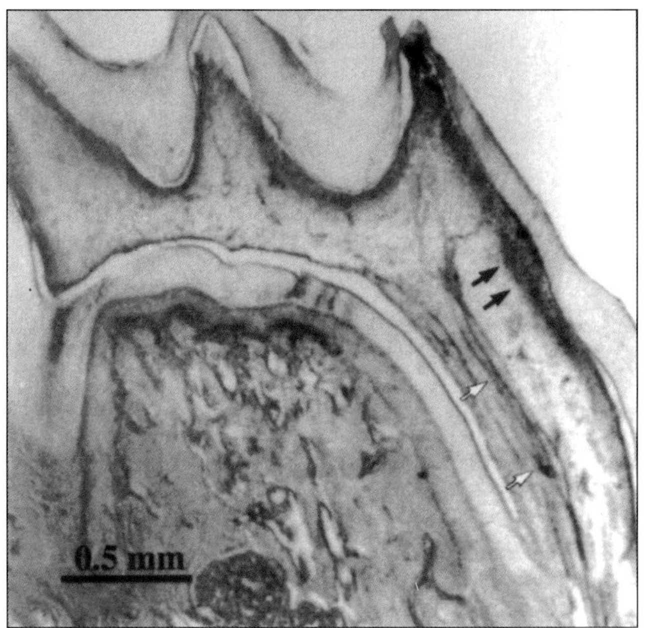

Fig 11-6a Maxillary first molar stained for NADPH-d activity 1 day following cavity preparation. Note increased NADPH-d intensity in the pulp tissue adjacent to the prepared dentin *(black arrows)* and in blood vessels of mesial root *(white arrows)*; however, only the blood vessels showed a statistically significant increase in intensity as compared with controls. (Reprinted from Law et al[132] with permission.)

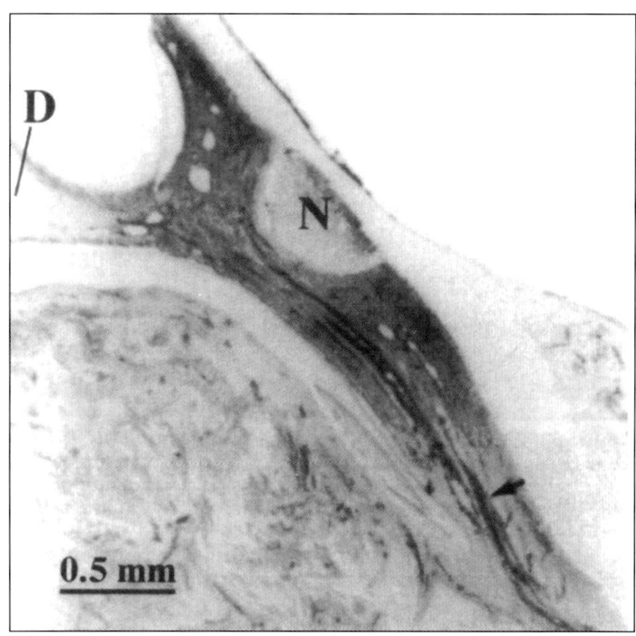

Fig 11-6b Maxillary first molar stained for NADPH-d activity 4 days following cavity preparation. Note that an area of leukocytic infiltration and necrosis (N) has developed in the mesial pulp under the prepared dentin. This area is surrounded by pulp tissue with significantly increased NADPH-d intensity in the mesial pulp horn as well as in the mesial root, whereas the NADPH-d intensity of the distal pulp (D) has remained at control values. Blood vessels *(arrow)* of the mesial root also had significantly increased NADPH-d intensity. (Reprinted from Law et al[132] with permission.)

flamed rat pulp tissue as it had been previously shown in feline teeth,[133] possibly due to species differences. However, there was evidence of a dramatic increase in NO activity as evidenced by an increase in the iNOS isoform and the NADPH cofactor at the site of pulp irritation (Fig 11-6). There was also an increase in NADPH staining in pulpal blood vessels, indicating that under inflammatory conditions there may be induction of NOS activity in the endothelium and vascular smooth muscle.

Oxygen-derived free radicals

Oxygen-derived free radicals (ODFR) are potent inflammatory mediators released from neutrophils that are challenged with antigen-antibody complexes or chemotactic agents. The superoxide anion ($O_2^{\bullet-}$), hydrogen peroxide (H_2O_2), and hydroxyl radical ($OH^{\bullet}$) are the most important species. These combine with NO to form peroxynitrite and other toxic nitrogen intermediates. Oxygen-derived free radicals, also known as reactive oxygen intermediates, induce the synthesis of IL-8; antioxidants are known to reduce this cytokine.[134] The enzyme superoxide dismutase (SOD) is the main intracellular scavenger of ODFRs, particularly $O_2^{\bullet-}$. The $OH^{\bullet}$ radical has been shown to reduce PBF,[135] possibly due to its effect on the endothelium, following the rise in tissue pressure in the low-compliance pulp environment that accompanies pulpal inflammation. Copper-and-zinc-containing SOD (CuZnSOD) is found in the cytoplasm, whereas manganese-containing SOD (MnSOD) is located in the nucleus or the mitochondria. In humans, CuZnSOD activity was identified in low quantities in normal pulp[136] but increased significantly in

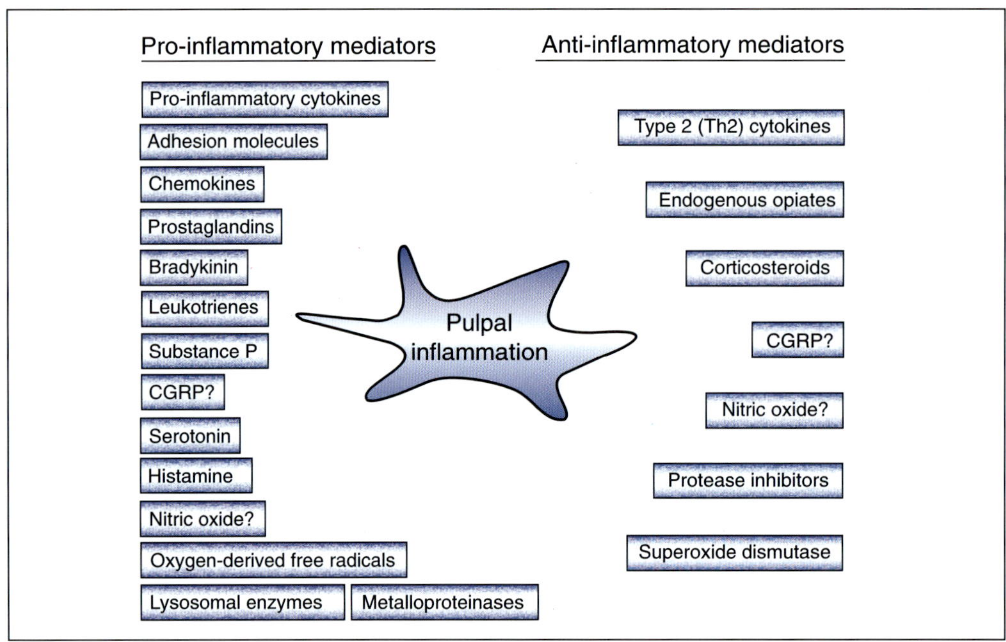

Fig 11-7 Important pro-inflammatory and anti-inflammatory mediators of pulpal inflammation.

inflamed pulp.[137] The latter study noted that the enzyme activity decreased with the advancing age of the patient in both the normal and inflamed pulp groups. More recently, the rat molar model was used to show a dramatic increase in levels of both CuZnSOD and MnSOD activity that was closely associated with areas of intense inflammation and with leukocytic infiltrates.[138]

Collectively, these studies suggest that pulpal inflammation may be modulated to a large extent by the activation of free radicals. Based on their chemistry, these substances are made locally in pulp tissue and act locally to damage bacterial or host cells and modulate the inflammatory process. The clinical significance of these substances may lie, in part, in the use of antioxidants to control their level of activity following injury due to caries or traumatic injuries.

Cytokines

The inflammatory response represents a closely regulated balance between pro-inflammatory and anti-inflammatory mediators that are titrated to neutralize the harmful effects of an advancing irritant while minimizing damage to host tissues (Fig 11-7). This concept is very well illustrated by a discussion of cytokines in pulp inflammation. Cytokines are proteins released from cells in an inflammatory process that activate, mediate, or potentiate actions of other cells or tissues. Their actions may be effected in an autocrine (self-activating), paracrine (local-acting), or endocrine (systemically acting) manner.

Although most of the cytokines present in an inflammatory process are produced by inflammatory cells like monocytes/macrophages, lymphocytes, and neutrophils, they may also be produced by a number of noninflammatory cells, which in the dental pulp would include fibroblasts and endothelial cells. Cytokine secretion is a brief, self-limited event initiated by new gene transcription with messenger RNA encoding that is transient in the activated cell.[43] Cytokines have numerous overlapping, and sometimes seemingly redundant, functions that mediate either pro-inflammatory or anti-inflammatory activities to effect a closely regulated, well-orchestrated inflammatory process.

There are two main classifications of cytokines. A structural classification addresses the

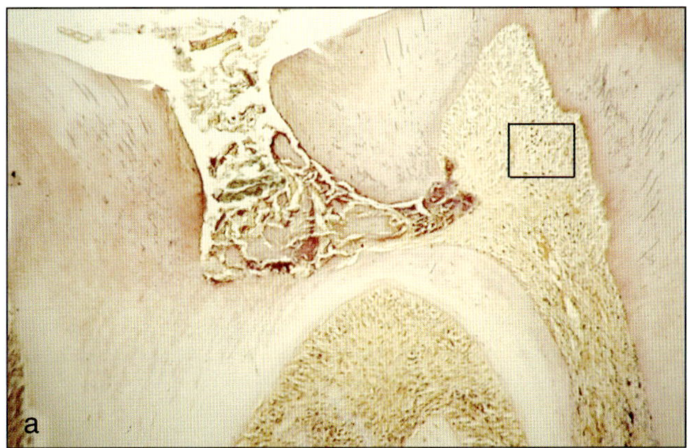

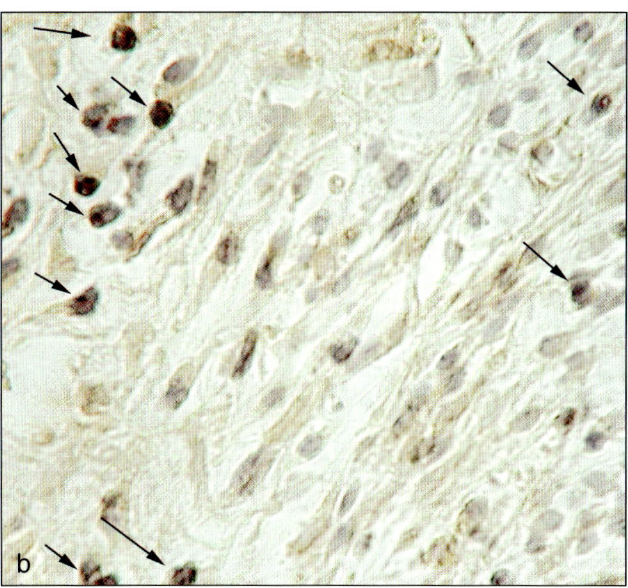

Fig 11-8 Mouse molar with pulp exposure of 1-week duration in the mesial pulp horn (stained for IL-1α). Distal portion of the chamber and the pulp in the distal canal showed an inflammatory infiltrate. *(a)* Low magnification showing pulp exposure (original magnification ×100). *(b)* High magnification of boxed area in *(a)* showing IL-1α–positive cells *(arrows)* (original magnification ×1,000).

molecular structure and the types of cells that produce the cytokine; for example, type I cytokines are produced by T-helper 1 (Th1) cells and share a four-α helical structure and receptor structure. In contrast, type II cytokines are produced by Th2 lymphocytes.[40] A functional classification describes their role in inflammation: either pro-inflammatory, anti-inflammatory, or as effectors of chemotaxis or chemokines. A modification of the latter classification will be used here.

Pro-inflammatory cytokines produced by innate immune cells

Among the most important pro-inflammatory cytokines are IL-1 and TNF. The actions of these two cytokines are very similar despite the fact that they interact with structurally different receptors. IL-1 is expressed in two isoforms: IL-1α and IL-1β. IL-1 is produced mainly by monocytes/macrophages but may also be produced by PMNs, fibroblasts, and endothelial cells. IL-1 has several systemic effects such as fever and the synthesis of acute-phase proteins, prostaglandins, PAF, or NO. Locally, IL-1 activates T cells and stimulates them to produce IL-2 and prostaglandins. IL-1 and TNF also activate endothelial cells and induce the expression of adhesion molecules on their membranes, thereby aiding in the recruitment of inflammatory cells to the site of inflammation.[139]

In the pulp, IL-1 inhibits proliferation of fibroblasts[140] and induces the expression of collagenase from pulpal fibroblasts.[119] The effects of these cytokines on matrix production from pulpal cells have been studied in vitro. In one study, IL-1β was shown to have a mild stimulatory effect on the synthesis of type I collagen in the dental pulp.[140] However, others showed that in the pulp fibroblast cultures, IL-1β suppressed the production of type I collagen as well as laminin, osteonectin, DNA, and protein synthesis overall. TNF-α had similar effects in pulp fibroblast cultures except that this cytokine stimulated DNA and protein.[141]

IL-1 is heavily expressed in pulpal inflammation (Fig 11-8). Furthermore, IL-1 activity was shown to be significantly higher in human dental pulps with symptomatic caries lesions than asymptomatic carious teeth or teeth with periodontal disease.[142] In that study, impacted third molars with pain but no caries also had elevated pulpal IL-1 activity.[142] IL-1 was shown to evoke hyperalgesia after peripheral injection, primarily by increasing PGE_2 synthesis.[143] In dental pulp, IL-1α, IL-1β, TNF-α, or TNF-β all evoke the release of PGE_2; interestingly, this effect is potentiated by

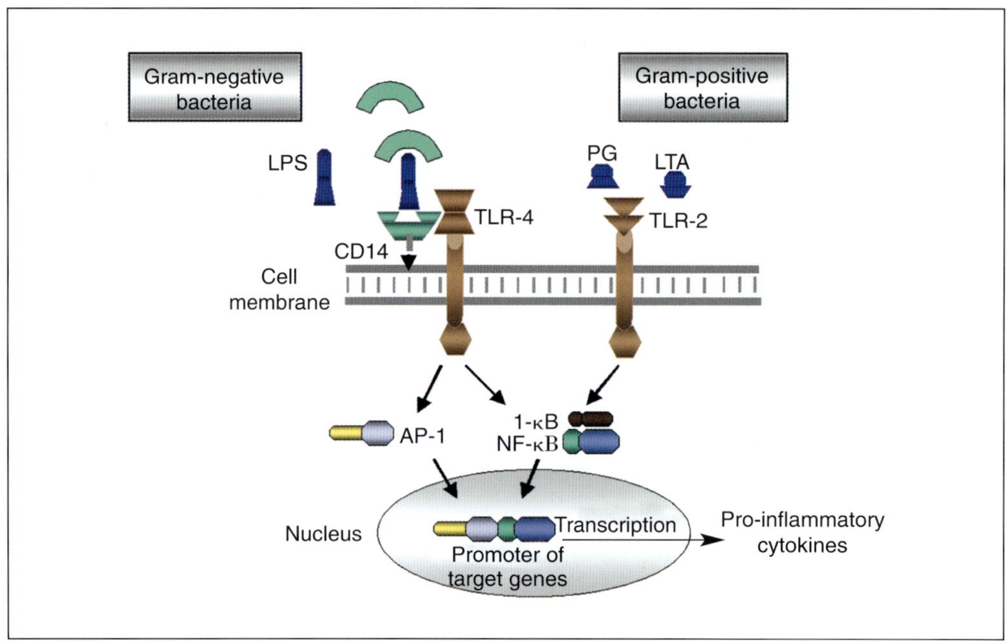

Fig 11-9 Pathway for pro-inflammatory cytokine production after stimulation by bacteria cell-wall products. LPS, lipopolysaccharide; LBP, LPS-binding protein; PG, peptidoglycan; LTA, lipoteichoic acid; TLR, *toll*-like receptor; NF-κB, nuclear factor-kappa B.

bradykinin and thrombin in dental pulp and periodontal ligament cells.[85,144]

The production of IL-1 and TNF in the pulp is probably a result of direct stimulation by bacterial virulence factors such as cell-wall products. The progression of pulpal inflammation and the tissue expression of IL-1α and TNF-α were shown to be similar in normal mice and mice that lacked any functional T or B cells, indicating that the production of these cytokines could occur without the presence of adaptive immunity.[145] LPSs from *Porphyromonas endodontalis* applied to human pulp cells in vitro evoked IL-1β synthesis in a dose-dependent manner.[146] Peptidoglycans (PGs) and lipoteichoic acid (LTA) from gram-positive bacteria were shown to have similar effects on the production of IL-1 and TNF[147] (Fig 11-9). LPS (aka endotoxin) achieves its effect by binding initially to an LPS-binding protein (LBP) in the blood. LBP attaches to cell-surface receptors on macrophages called CD14. The heterotrimer complex of LBP:LPS:CD14 then binds to cell receptors called *toll*-like receptors (TLRs). The ligands for two of these receptors are LPS (TLR-4)[148] and PG and LTA (TLR-2).[149] TLRs, which have cytoplasmic domains nearly identical to that of the IL-1 receptor, cause the translocation of two nuclear factors: NFκB and AP-1 to the nucleus, followed by the transcription of the gene signal to produce the pro-inflammatory cytokines.[150] Recently, LPS was found to be present in large amounts in carious dentin, superficial caries had more LPS than deep caries, and LPS content correlated with the incidence of pain.[151] Thus, the introduction of bacteria or bacterial by-products into the pulp plays a direct role in stimulating the production of these pro-inflammatory cytokines.

The relative importance of IL-1 and TNF in mediating pulpal responses to mixed bacterial infection was recently investigated in the mouse model.[152] Pulp exposures were created in mice deficient in IL-1 receptor, TNF p55 and p75 receptors, or both IL-1R and TNFp55 receptors (dual deficiency). The receptor-deficient mice had a significantly faster rate of pulpal degeneration and necrosis (Fig 11-10a) and microbial penetration (Fig 11-10b) than the wild-type mice. The animals with the combined deficiency had worse results than those with either deficiency alone. These findings indicate that the pro-inflammatory properties of these cytokines play an important role in protecting dental pulp against the spread of infection. It is clinically important to recognize that the production of IL-1 and TNF from pulpal macrophages in response to bacterial irritants may be suppressed by the toxic effects of dental filling materials that may come in contact with the pulp.[153,154]

Pro-inflammatory cytokines produced by Th1 cells (type 1 cytokines)

The type 1 cytokines are pro-inflammatory. This class includes IFNγ, IL-2, IL-12, and TNF-β (also known as lymphotoxin or LT-α) and are synthesized by the Th1 lymphocytes.[155] These cytokines are mostly involved in cell-mediated hypersensitivity, self-activation of T cells (IL-2), and activation of B cells and macrophages (IFNγ). IFNγ is the key cytokine produced by Th1 cells. It augments TNF activity and induces NO release.[150] IL-12 is a cytokine produced by macrophages and dendritic cells, but it will be included here because it is thought to be essential for Th1 cell differentiation. It is noteworthy that IFNγ is produced by NK cells[156] in addition to being a Th1 cytokine. This finding may explain the production of pro-inflammatory cytokines in T-cell–deficient mouse models and illustrate the multitude of cellular sources for key inflammatory cytokines.

Interleukin-2 is present in normal vital pulp and is significantly elevated in histologically verified cases of symptomatic irreversible pulpitis.[157] Shallow caries lesions, mostly colonized by *Streptococcus mutans*, were recently shown to elicit a strong type 1 cytokine response.[158] In human dental pulp, the mRNA for IFNγ is significantly greater than that of either IL-10 or IL-4. Furthermore, peripheral blood mononuclear cells (PBMCs) challenged with *S mutans* produced significantly more IFNγ and IL-12 than those challenged with *Lactobacillus casei*, an organism commonly associated with deep caries.

Immunoregulatory or anti-inflammatory cytokines (Th2, type 2 cytokines)

The type 2 cytokines are anti-inflammatory and act in many ways to regulate the actions of the type 1 pro-inflammatory cytokines. The Th2 lymphocytes produce IL-4, IL-5, IL-6, IL-9, IL-10 (also secreted by Th1 and macrophages), and IL-13. Both Th1 and Th2 produce IL-3 and granulocyte monocyte colony-stimulating factor (GM-CSF).[40] The Th2 cytokines are mostly involved in humoral immunity (production of neutralizing antibodies), mast cell degranulation (IgE production), and eosinophil activation. They also serve the very important function of inhibiting most pro-inflammatory functions caused by other cytokines, thus serving the homeostatic function of regulating the immune response.[155] This latter function is primarily effected by IL-4, IL-10, and IL-13. Peripheral blood mononuclear cells challenged with *S mutans* produced a dose-dependent increase in IL-10 production, but no change in IL-4 production.[158] The levels of mRNA expression of IL-10 and IL-4 were significantly lower than IFNγ in shallow caries lesions, but this difference disappeared in deep caries lesions.[158] An increased need for these two immunoregulatory cytokines in deep caries lesions is likely as more pro-inflammatory cytokines are produced.

IL-6 was initially thought to be pro-inflammatory but is now recognized to be an immunoregulatory and anti-inflammatory cytokine. The anti-inflammatory functions of IL-6 are caused by suppression of IL-1 and TNF, the induction of glucocorticoid release, and the induction of natural antagonists of IL-1 (IL-1 receptor antagonist) and TNF (soluble TNFR p55).[159] Peptidoglycan from the cell wall of *L casei* was shown to increase the IL-6 production by human pulp cells in a dose-dependent manner.[160] Likewise, LPS from *P endodontalis* produced IL-6 in human pulp cells that preceded and was independent of IL-1β production.[161] In human dental pulp, the mean level of IL-6 in carious, symptomatic teeth was more than

Fig 11-10 Quantitative analysis of tissue necrosis in mice lacking response to IL-1 and/or TNF. Surgical pulp exposure followed by inoculation with six oral pathogens was carried out. H&E–stained cryostat sections were examined for the presence of tissue necrosis in the dental pulp. This tissue was divided into three equal parts: coronal third, middle third, and apical third, which follows the path of necrosis from the coronal third to the apical third of the dental root. (Reprinted from Chen et al[152] with permission.)

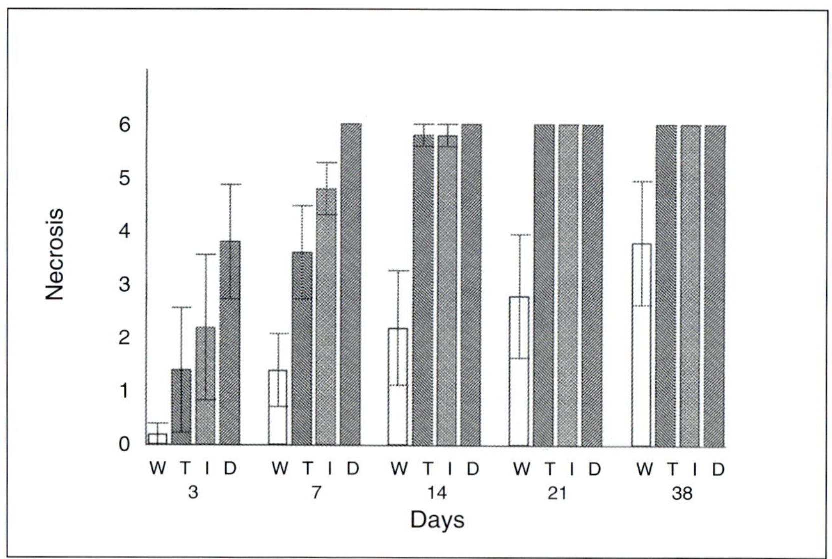

Fig 11-10a Under microscopic examination (magnification ×400), the following scale was used: 0, no necrosis; 1, partial necrosis of coronal third; 2, total necrosis of coronal third; 3, partial necrosis of middle third; 4, total necrosis of middle third; 5, partial necrosis of apical third; and 6, total necrosis of apical third. The highest score for the specimen represented the necrosis status of that tooth and was used in statistical analysis. Each value represents the mean ± SEM; n = 5 for each time point. Significant differences ($P < .01$) were noted between all receptor-deficient and wild-type mice at 7, 14, 21, and 38 days after bacterial challenge. There were no statistical differences between any of the groups at 3 days after pulpal insult. W, wild-type; T, TNFRp55$^{-/-}$-p75$^{-/-}$; I, IL-1 RI$^{-/-}$; D, TNFRp55$^{-/-}$-IL-1RI$^{-/-}$.

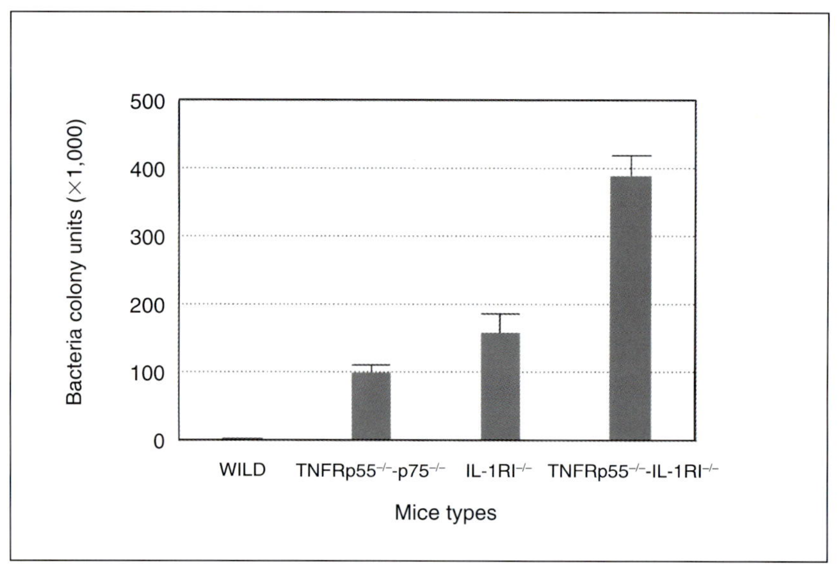

Fig 11-10b Bacterial penetration in pulpal tissue is greater in mice lacking IL-1 and/or TNF activity. The number of bacterial colonies that could be cultured from the apical portion of the distal root 8 days after exposure and inoculation with six oral pathogens was determined. Values represent the mean ± SEM; n = 10 for each group. All receptor-mutant mice showed significant differences ($P < .01$) when compared with wild-type mice. *IL-1RI$^{-/-}$ and TNFRp55$^{-/-}$-p75$^{-/-}$ mice had values that were not significantly different from each other ($P < .05$) but were significantly higher than those of wild-type mice ($P < .01$). **Significantly ($P < .01$) larger values were observed in TNFRp55$^{-/-}$-IL-1RI$^{-/-}$ mice compared with IL-1RI$^{-/-}$ and TNFRp55$^{-/-}$-p75$^{-/-}$ mice.

3,000-fold greater than that found in normal pulp.[162]

IL-6 causes the formation of acute-phase proteins such as fibrinogen and C-reactive protein (CRP) in the liver. The latter functions as an opsonin by binding to C1q or Fcγ receptors or by activating the complement classical pathway. Dental pulp with irreversible pulpitis displays significantly elevated CRP compared with uninflamed pulp, a finding that was independent of serum CRP.[163]

TGF-β1 is another cytokine considered an immunosuppressant as well as an inducer of extracellular matrix production. This cytokine is a member of the TGF-β superfamily, which includes TGF-βs, activins, and BMPs (see chapters 2 and 3). However, TGF-β1 was recently shown to play a fundamental role not only in the formation of enamel and dentin matrix but also in the prevention of spontaneous pulpal inflammation.[164] In that study, mice deficient in TGF-β1 (but treated with corticosteroids to keep them alive) developed very thin enamel and dentin with significant attrition and spontaneous pulpitis and pulp necrosis. Crossing this species with the knockout mouse deficient in the recombinase-activating gene 2 (RAG-2 mouse) that was also deficient in T- and B-cell immunity resulted in a breed that showed the same hard tissue defects but had normal pulp structure, indicating that TGF-β1 stops spontaneous inflammation mediated by the adaptive immune response.

Chemokines

Chemokines are potent pro-inflammatory cytokines that share structural similarities and act by mediating leukocyte movement and chemotaxis of inflammatory cells to the inflammatory site. A large number of chemokines have been described: IL-8 (neutrophils); regulated-on-activation normal T cell, expressed and secreted (RANTES; monocytes, T cells); monocyte chemoattractant-1, -2, -3, and -4 (MCP-1 through -4) (monocytes, basophils, T cells); and Eotaxin (eosinophils).[43]

Dental pulp cells exposed to endodontically relevant species of gram-positive or gram-negative bacteria or to *Prevotella intermedia* LPS expressed IL-8 and MCP-1 at both the protein and the mRNA levels.[165,166] Patients with symptomatic or asymptomatic irreversible pulpitis had an almost 23-fold increase in IL-8 levels in the pulp.[167] Recently, human odontoblasts cultured in vitro were shown to be capable of expressing IL-8 at both the protein and mRNA levels.[168]

Collectively, these studies indicate that cytokines interact in a coordination network and that the ultimate effect on pulpal inflammation and healing is dependent upon the integrated actions of this diverse family of inflammatory mediators.

Other classes of innate and adaptive immunity

The last class of molecular mediators of pulpal inflammation are proteins that act to recognize (ie, bind) foreign antigens. The recognition of self from nonself is an essential step in the integrated actions of the innate and adaptive immune processes.

Class I and Class II major histocompatability complex (MHC) molecules

The innate and adaptive immune responses work in synchrony to recognize and destroy foreign antigenic material. One of the fundamental mechanisms underlying this process is mediated by the MHC Class I and Class II molecules. MHC Class I proteins are expressed on all nucleated cells, whereas MHC Class II proteins are expressed on a small group of cells collectively called *antigen-presenting cells* (APCs) (see also chapter 10). These cells include macrophages, dendritic cells, Langerhans cells, B cells, endothelial cells, and a few other cell types, although only dendritic cells and macrophages have been demonstrated in the dental pulp.[169] MHC Class I proteins are recog-

Fig 11-11 Specimen with a deep caries lesion. *(a)* H&E–stained section showing formation of reparative dentin with well-mineralized *(arrows)* and poorly mineralized *(*)* portions. Boxes show the approximate positions of *(b), (c), (d),* and *(g)*. *(b)* Section stained with anti-HLA-DR showing an accumulation of positively stained cells under the reparative dentin. In addition to cells with dendritic morphology, some Schwann cells show an immunoreactivity to HLA-DR. *(c)* A semiserial section of *(b)* stained with antifactor XIIIa showing an increased density of positively stained cells not only in the paraodontoblastic region but also in the inner portion of the coronal pulp. See *(e)* for comparison. *(d)* A semiserial section of *(b)* and *(c)* stained with anti-NGFR showing an increased density of immunoreactive neural elements in the region where the accumulation of HLA-DR and factor XIIIa–immunoreactive cells is observed. *Arrows* indicate the border of the poorly mineralized portion of reparative dentin, which corresponds to *(*)* in *(a)*. Numerous fibers penetrate the poorly mineralized portion of reparative dentin. *(e,f)* Factor XIIIa–immunoreactive cells *(e)* and NGFR-immunoreactive neural elements *(f)* in the noncarious region of the same sections as *(c)* and *(d)*, respectively. The density of immunoreactive structures is lower in the noncarious region than in the carious region. *(g)* Accumulation of CD3-positive lymphocytes in the area corresponding to the smaller boxed area in *(a)*. (Reprinted from Sakurai et al[103] with permission.)

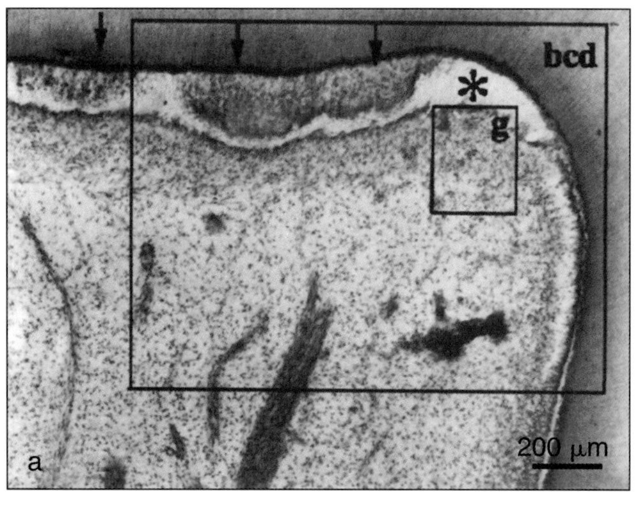

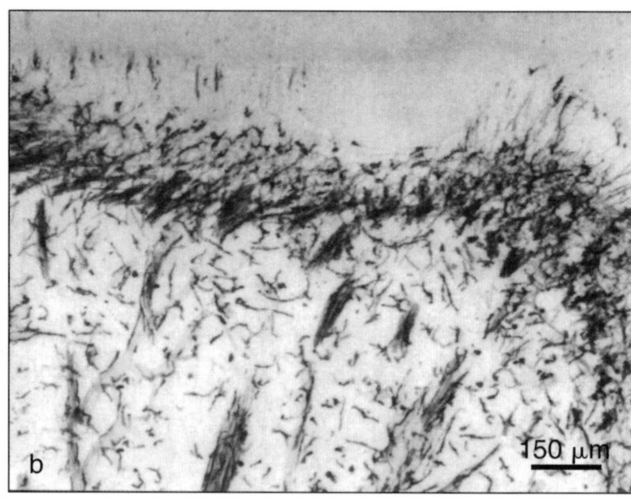

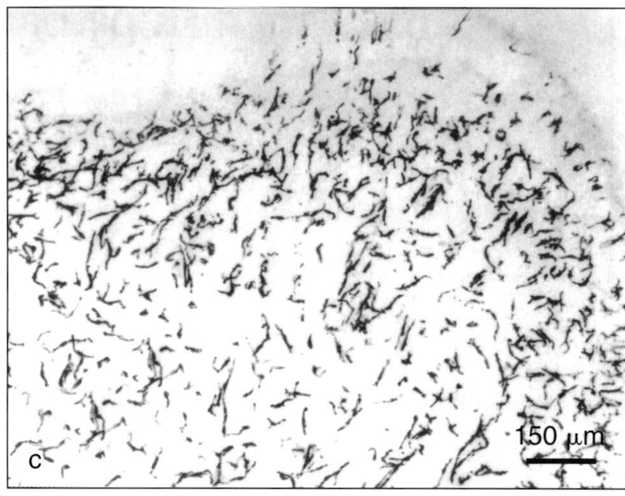

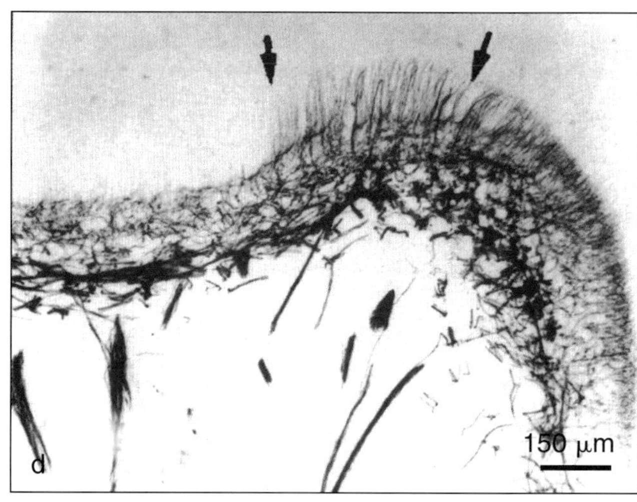

nized by CD8+ or cytolytic T cells; these cells' classification is called *Class I-restricted*. This process is best known for viral infection of any nucleated cell, in which the viral antigens are recognized by the MHC Class I-restricted CD8+ cells. However, APCs process many other antigens, including bacterial antigens, and present them to MHC Class II-restricted CD4+ T-helper cells. The processed antigens are recognized in the context of the MHC Class II molecule on the APC and the T-cell

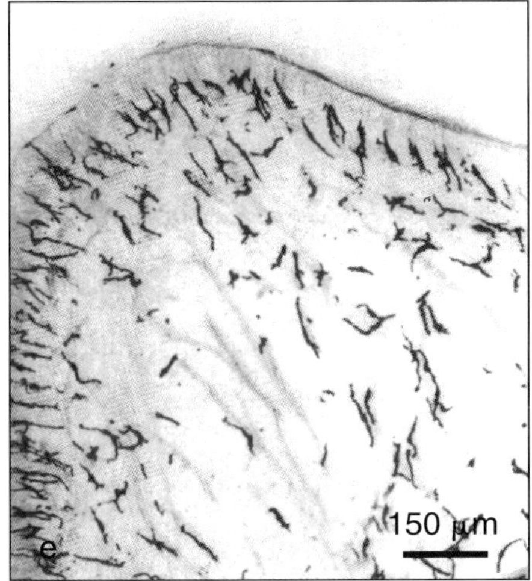

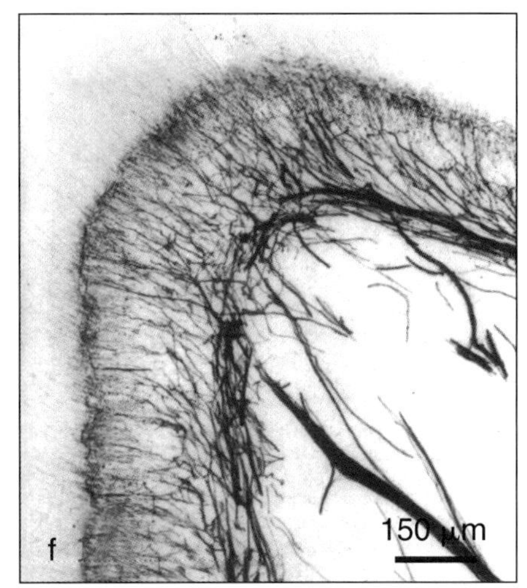

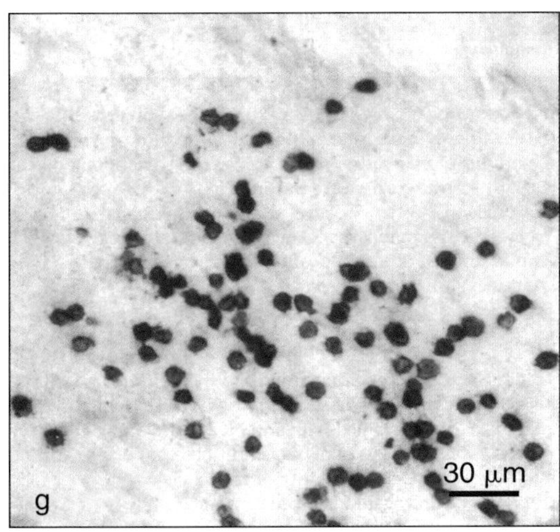

receptor (TCR) on the T cell. This mechanism is fundamental for the development of specific immunity to the presented antigen and the activation of T cells, macrophages, and B cells that follows. The expression of MHC molecules is mediated by cytokines, most notably IFN-γ.

Class II APCs are observed in normal human dental pulp, including the odontoblastic layer and the central pulp.[170] Using cell surface markers, APCs were characterized in rat pulp to be either dendritic in shape or to be tissue macrophages, with dendritic cells more concentrated in the odontoblastic layer.[171,172] Dendritic cells were also found to be much more important than macrophages in providing the antigen-presentation signals to costimulate T cells.[173] In rat molar pulp, a dramatic increase in the number of Class II APCs was seen following the induction of caries[174] and following cavity preparation alone or with the application of *P gingivalis* LPS.[175,176] There was also a significant reduction in the number of these cells when the cavity preparations were immediately restored with a self-curing dental adhesive resin.[176] This finding emphasizes the importance of appropriate restorative procedures in minimizing inflammatory pulpal changes.

A possible functional relationship was recently demonstrated between pulpal APCs, and sensory nerve fibers and their products. Sensory nerves were found in close proximity to the APCs, and subsequent experiments revealed that substance P potentiated while CGRP suppressed the proliferation of stimulated T lymphocytes in the presence of APCs.[23] This neuroimmune interaction was further studied in carious human molars in which dendritic cells and NGF (marker for nerve fibers) were both shown to increase close to carious dentin, particularly in cases with superficial caries lesions (Fig 11-11; see also chapter 7).[103]

In the rat model, pulpal macrophages and dendritic cell numbers seem to stay constant with age, whereas MHC Class II^{+} cells decline with age.[177] Taken together, these studies suggest that these immunocompetent cells play an important role in pulpal inflammation, interact with neuropeptides, and decline in number with age.

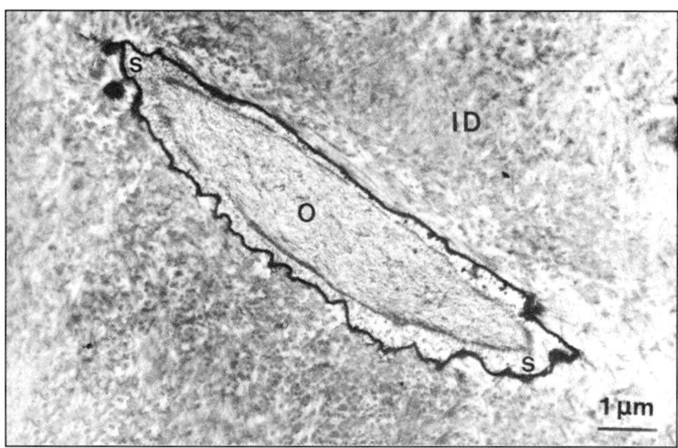

Fig 11-12a Transverse section of a dentinal tubule located in the inner face of the carious cone. A thin, dense, positive reaction for IgG is visible on the wall of the dentinal tubule. ID, intertubular dentin; O, odontoblast process; S, organic periodontoblast space. (Reprinted from Ackermans et al[178] with permission.)

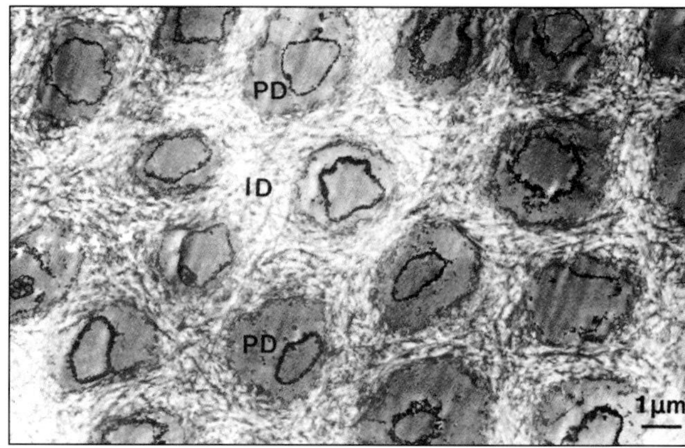

Fig 11-12b An area of carious dentin further away from the pulp. The peritubular dentin (PD) has been dissolved with ethylenediaminetetraacetic acid (EDTA), and there is a strong, ring-shaped, positive reaction for IgM along the walls of the cross-sectioned dentinal tubules. ID, intertubular dentin. (Reprinted from Ackermans et al[178] with permission.)

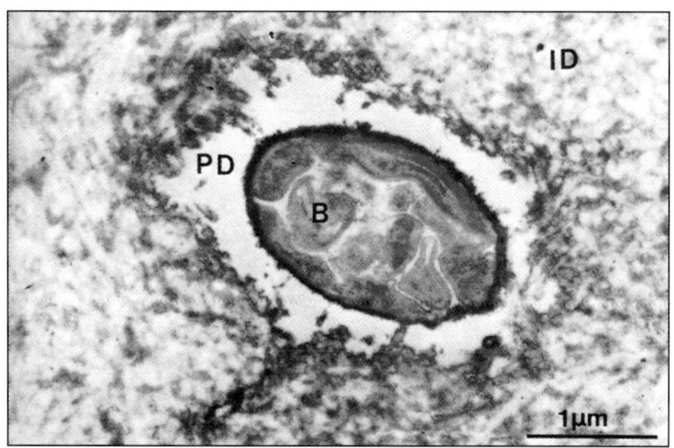

Fig 11-12c Cross section of carious dentin invaded by several microorganisms (B). A positive reaction for IgG is present on the wall of the dentinal tubule with a less marked precipitate at the border between the peritubular dentin (PD) and the intertubular dentin (ID) (Reprinted from Ackermans et al[178] with permission.)

Immunoglobulins

In addition to the specific cellular immunity factors discussed above, dental pulp has long been known to express markers for humoral immunity under inflammatory conditions, whereby B cells differentiate to plasma cells that then undergo clonal selection and produce the immunoglobulins IgG, IgA, IgE, and IgM.[93,94] Immunoglobulins participate in both recognition and effector functions. When antibodies are first expressed in a membrane-bound form on B cells, they recognize antigens in their environment. After their release, they mediate cytotoxic reactions by innate immune cells such as NK cells; opsonize bacterial and other antigens to enhance phagocytosis; form antigen-antibody complexes that activate the classical pathway of the complement cascade, leading to the secretion of anaphylatoxins and lysis of membranes of target cells as described previously; and, in the case of IgE, cause the degranulation of mast cells. The processes of opsonization and complement fixation take place via the Fc portion (nonantigen-binding portion) of the antibody molecule, which is unique for each antibody isotype and which either binds to Fc receptors on the surface of phagocytic cells for opsonization or to the C1q complement protein for complement fixation.

Immunoglobulins of pulpal origin were found in dentin beneath caries lesions.[96] Although the secretory IgA was identified in carious dentin in a subsequent study,[178] further functional experiments in rats using bovine serum albumin placed on induced caries lesions or injected into blood indicated that this protein was found in the dentin only when it was injected,[179] indicating a more likely systemic route. Immunoglobulins were also observed in large vacuoles within odontoblasts under shallow caries lesions and along the walls of dentinal tubules[178] (Figs 11-12a to 11-12c).

Plasma cells in infected dental pulp produce specific antibodies against bacteria such as *S mutans*, *Actinomyces viscosus*, *A naeslundii*, *Porphyromonas gingivalis*, and *Prevotella intermedia*, commonly found in deep caries, and the resultant antigen-antibody complexes fixed complement.[95,97] Moreover, fluid specimens from pulp explant cultures of normal and inflamed symptomatic human pulp were also shown to contain specific antibodies to bacteria commonly found in carious dentin[180] and to the bacteria cultured from the teeth from which the explants were obtained.[181] In the latter study the only differences between normal and inflamed pulps were in levels of antibodies against *Lactobacillus acidophilus*, one of the most common organisms in deep caries, but the differences were not statistically significant. The pulp did not contain antibodies to bacteria not common to caries lesions. It is not clear why normal pulp contains elevated amounts of immunoglobulins that seem to be specific to organisms involved in caries lesions; however, in another study in which the pulp was sampled directly during pulpectomy procedures, significantly elevated levels of IgG, IgA, and IgM were reported in inflamed compared with normal pulps,[182] indicating that the experimental technique may have influenced the findings in these studies. Recently, an additional protective function of immunoglobulins in the pulpodentin complex was proposed with the finding that IgG, IgA, or IgM reduced fluid filtration through dentin in vitro.[183]

Conclusions

The development of pulpal inflammation employs many of the inflammatory mediators seen in other injured connective tissues. The special features of the dental pulp, including restricted vascularity, enclosure in dentin, and susceptability to bacterial infection or trauma, play an important role in defining the inflammatory and healing potential of this tissue. It is critical to realize that the clinical outcome of an injury such as bacterial invasion secondary to caries is due to the actions of an integrated network of inflammatory mediators, immune cells, and other factors elaborated in the inflamed dental pulp. The identification of these mediators in inflamed pulp and the comprehension of their actions will likely lead to biochemically based diagnoses, prognoses, and treatment.

References

1. Collins T. Acute and chronic inflammation. In: Cotran RS, Kumar V, Collins T (eds). Robbins' Pathologic Basis of Disease. Philadelphia: Saunders, 1999:50–88.
2. Pohto P, Antila R. Assay of histamine in dental pulps. Acta Odontol Scand 1970;28:691–699.
3. DelBalso AM, Nishimura RS, Setterstrom JA. The effects of thermal and electrical injury on pulpal histamine levels. Oral Surg Oral Med Oral Pathol 1976;41:110–113.
4. Miller GS, Sternberg RN, Piliero SJ, Rosenberg PA. Histologic identification of mast cells in human dental pulp. Oral Surg Oral Med Oral Pathol 1978;46:559–566.
5. Edwall L, Olgart L, Haegerstam G. Influence of vasodilator substances on pulpal blood flow in the cat. Acta Odontol Scand 1973;31:289–296.
6. Kim S, Dorscher-Kim J. Hemodynamic regulation of the dental pulp in a low compliance environment. J Endod 1989;15:404–408.
7. Ahlquist ML, Franzen OG. Inflammation and dental pain in man. Endod Dent Traumatol 1994;10:201–209.
8. Kerezoudis NP, Nomikos GG, Olgart LM, Svensson TH. Serotonin in rat oral tissues: role of 5-HT1 receptors in sympathetic vascular control. Eur J Pharmacol 1995; 275:191–198.
9. Inoue K, Mogi M, Mori R, Naito J, Fukuda S, Creveling CR. Immunocytochemical localization of serotonin, monoamine oxidase and assessment of monoamine oxidase activity in human dental pulp. Brain Res 2000; 853:374–376.

10. Hirafuji M, Terashima K, Satoh S, Ogura Y. Stimulation of prostaglandin E2 biosynthesis in rat dental pulp explants in vitro by 5-hydroxytryptamine. Arch Oral Biol 1982;27:961–964.
11. Hirafuji M, Ogura Y. 5-Hydroxytryptamine stimulates the release of prostacyclin but not thromboxane A2 from isolated rat dental pulp. Eur J Pharmacol 1987; 136:433–436.
12. Liu M, Kim S, Park DS, Markowitz K, Bilotto G, Dorscher-Kim J. Comparison of the effects of intra-arterial and locally applied vasoactive agents on pulpal blood flow in dog canine teeth determined by laser Doppler velocimetry. Arch Oral Biol 1990;35:405–410.
13. Ngassapa D, Narhi M, Hirvonen T. Effect of serotonin (5-HT) and calcitonin gene-related peptide (CGRP) on the function of intradental nerves in the dog. Proc Finn Dent Soc 1992;88(suppl 1):143–148.
14. Olgart L, Hokfelt T, Nilsson G, Pernow B. Localization of substance P-like immunoreactivity in nerves in the tooth pulp. Pain 1977;4:153–159.
15. Uddman R, Grunditz T, Sundler F. Calcitonin gene-related peptide: A sensory transmitter in dental pulps? Scand J Dent Res 1986;94:219–224.
16. Goodis H, Saeki K. Identification of bradykinin, substance P, and neurokinin A in human dental pulp. J Endod 1997;23:201–204.
17. Casasco A, Calligaro A, Springall DR, Casasco M, Poggi P, Valentino KL, Polak JM. Neuropeptide K-like immunoreactivity in human dental pulp. Arch Oral Biol 1990;35: 33–36.
18. Uddman R, Grunditz T, Sundler F. Neuropeptide Y: Occurrence and distribution in dental pulps. Acta Odontol Scand 1984;42:361–365.
19. Casasco A, Calligaro A, Casasco M, Springall DR, Polak JM, Marchetti C. Immunocytochemical evidence for the presence of somatostatin-like immunoreactive nerves in human dental pulp. J Dent Res 1991;70:87–89.
20. Uddman R, Bjorlin G, Moller B, Sundler F. Occurrence of VIP nerves in mammalian dental pulps. Acta Odontol Scand 1980;38:325–328.
21. Brodin E, Gazelius B, Lundberg JM, Olgart L. Substance P in trigeminal nerve endings: Occurrence and release. Acta Physiol Scand 1981;111:501–503.
22. Wakisaka S, Akai M. Immunohistochemical observation on neuropeptides around the blood vessel in feline dental pulp. J Endod 1989;15:413–416.
23. Okiji T, Jontell M, Belichenko P, Dahlgren U, Bergenholtz G, Dahlstrom A. Structural and functional association between substance P- and calcitonin gene-related peptide-immunoreactive nerves and accessory cells in the rat dental pulp. J Dent Res 1997;76:1818–1824.
24. Kimberly CL, Byers MR. Inflammation of rat molar pulp and periodontium causes increased calcitonin gene-related peptide and axonal sprouting. Anat Rec 1988; 222:289–300.
25. Byers MR. Effects of inflammation on dental sensory nerves and vice versa. Proc Finn Dent Soc 1992;88 (suppl 1):499–506.
26. Grutzner EH, Garry MG, Hargreaves KM. Effect of injury on pulpal levels of immunoreactive substance P and immunoreactive calcitonin gene-related peptide. J Endod 1992;18:553–557.
27. Fristad I, Heyeraas KJ, Jonsson R, Kvinnsland IH. Effect of inferior alveolar nerve axotomy on immune cells and nerve fibres in young rat molars. Arch Oral Biol 1995;40:1053–1062.
28. Byers MR, Taylor PE. Effect of sensory denervation on the response of rat molar pulp to exposure injury. J Dent Res 1993;72:613–618.
29. Calland JW, Harris SE, Carnes DL Jr. Human pulp cells respond to calcitonin gene-related peptide in vitro. J Endod 1997;23:485–489.
30. Gazelius B, Edwall B, Olgart L, Lundberg JM, Hokfelt T, Fischer JA. Vasodilatory effects and coexistence of calcitonin gene-related peptide (CGRP) and substance P in sensory nerves of cat dental pulp. Acta Physiol Scand 1987;130:33–40.
31. Berggreen E, Heyeraas KJ. The role of sensory neuropeptides and nitric oxide on pulpal blood flow and tissue pressure in the ferret. J Dent Res 1999;78: 1535–1543.
32. Hargreaves KM, Swift JQ, Roszkowski MT, Bowles W, Garry MG, Jackson DL. Pharmacology of peripheral neuropeptide and inflammatory mediator release. Oral Surg Oral Med Oral Pathol 1994;78:503–510.
33. Ohkubo T, Shibata M, Yamada Y, Kaya H, Takahashi H. Role of substance P in neurogenic inflammation in the rat incisor pulp and the lower lip. Arch Oral Biol 1993; 38:151–158.
34. Kerezoudis NP, Olgart L, Edwall L. Involvement of substance P but not nitric oxide or calcitonin gene-related peptide in neurogenic plasma extravasation in rat incisor pulp and lip. Arch Oral Biol 1994;39:769–774.
35. Rodd HD, Boissonade FM. Substance P expression in human tooth pulp in relation to caries and pain experience. Eur J Oral Sci 2000;108:467–474.
36. Todd WM, Kafrawy AH, Newton CW, Brown CE Jr. Immunohistochemical study of gamma-aminobutyric acid and bombesin/gastrin releasing peptide in human dental pulp. J Endod 1997;23:152–157.
37. Payan DG. Neuropeptides and inflammation: The role of substance P. Ann Rev Med 1989;40:341–352.
38. Brain SD. Sensory neuropeptides: Their role in inflammation and wound healing. Immunopharmacology 1997;37:133–152.
39. Fried K. Changes in pulpal nerves with aging. Proc Finn Dent Soc 1992;88(suppl 1):517–528.
40. Paul WE. Fundamental Immunology, ed 4. Baltimore: Lippincott Williams & Wilkins, 1998.

41. Sawa Y, Yoshida S, Shibata KI, Suzuki M, Mukaida A. Vascular endothelium of human dental pulp expresses diverse adhesion molecules for leukocyte emigration. Tissue Cell 1998;30:281-291.
42. Tasman F, Dagdeviren A, Kendir B, Ozcelik B, Atac A, Er N. Endothelial cell adhesion molecules in human dental pulp: A comparative immunohistochemical study on chronic periodontitis. J Endod 1999;25:664-667.
43. Abbas AK, Lichtman AH, Pober JS. Cellular and Molecular Immunology, ed 4. Philadelphia: Saunders, 2000.
44. Majorana A, Notarangelo LD, Savoldi E, Gastaldi G, Lozada-Nur F. Leukocyte adhesion deficiency in a child with severe oral involvement. Oral Surg Oral Med Oral Pathol Oral Radiol Endod 1999;87:691-694.
45. Zhu Q, Safavi KE, Spangberg LS. Integrin expression in human dental pulp cells and their role in cell attachment on extracellular matrix proteins. J Endod 1998; 24:641-644.
46. Zhu Q, Safavi KE, Spangberg LS. The role of integrin beta 1 in human dental pulp cell adhesion on laminin and fibronectin. Oral Surg Oral Med Oral Pathol Oral Radiol Endod 1998;85:314-318.
47. Bergenholtz G, Lindhe J. Effect of soluble plaque factors on inflammatory reactions in the dental pulp. Scand J Dent Res 1975;83:153-158.
48. Bergenholtz G, Warfvinge J. Migration of leukocytes in dental pulp in response to plaque bacteria. Scand J Dent Res 1982;90:354-632.
49. Warfvinge J, Dahlen G, Bergenholtz G. Dental pulp response to bacterial cell wall material. J Dent Res 1985;64:1046-1050.
50. Sundqvist G, Johansson E. Neutrophil chemotaxis induced by anaerobic bacteria isolated from necrotic dental pulps. Scand J Dent Res 1980;88:113-121.
51. Hanks CT, Syed SA, Craig RG, Hartrick JM, Van Dyke TE. Modeling bacterial damage to pulpal cells in vitro. J Endod 1991;17:21-25.
52. Matsushita K, Motani R, Sakuta T, Yamaguchi N, Koga T, Matsuo K, et al. The role of vascular endothelial growth factor in human dental pulp cells: Induction of chemotaxis, proliferation, and differentiation and activation of the AP-1-dependent signaling pathway. J Dent Res 2000;79:1596-1603.
53. Hirafuji M, Ogura Y. Endogenous biosynthesis of prostaglandin I2 and thromboxane A2 by isolated rat dental pulp. Biochem Pharmacol 1983;32:2983-1985.
54. Torabinejad M, Bakland LK. Prostaglandins: Their possible role in the pathogenesis of pulpal and periapical diseases, part 2. J Endod 1980;6:769-776.
55. Torabinejad M, Bakland LK. Prostaglandins: Their possible role in the pathogenesis of pulpal and periapical diseases, part 1. J Endod 1980;6:733-739.
56. Okiji T, Morita I, Kobayashi C, Sunada I, Murota S. Arachidonic-acid metabolism in normal and experimentally-inflamed rat dental pulp. Arch Oral Biol 1987; 32:723-727.
57. Miyauchi M, Takata T, Ito H, Ogawa I, Kobayashi J, Nikai H, Ijuhin N. Immunohistochemical demonstration of prostaglandins E2, F2 alpha, and 6-keto-prostaglandin F1 alpha in rat dental pulp with experimentally induced inflammation. J Endod 1996;22:600-602.
58. Okiji T, Morita I, Sunada I, Murota S. Involvement of arachidonic acid metabolites in increases in vascular permeability in experimental dental pulpal inflammation in the rat. Arch Oral Biol 1989;34:523-528.
59. Hirafuji M, Shinoda H. Increased prostaglandin I2 and thromboxane A2 production by rat dental pulp after intravenous administration of endotoxin. Arch Oral Biol 1994;39:995-1000.
60. Goodis HE, Bowles WR, Hargreaves KM. Prostaglandin E2 enhances bradykinin-evoked iCGRP release in bovine dental pulp. J Dent Res 2000;79:1604-1607.
61. Ohnishi T, Suwa M, Oyama T, Arakaki N, Torii M, Daikuhara Y. Prostaglandin E2 predominantly induces production of hepatocyte growth factor/scatter factor in human dental pulp in acute inflammation. J Dent Res 2000;79:748-755.
62. Ahlberg KF. Dose-dependent inhibition of sensory nerve activity in the feline dental pulp by anti-inflammatory drugs. Acta Physiol Scand 1978;102:434-440.
63. Cohen JS, Reader A, Fertel R, Beck M, Meyers WJ. A radioimmunoassay determination of the concentrations of prostaglandins E2 and F2 alpha in painful and asymptomatic human dental pulps. J Endod 1985;11: 330-335.
64. Hashimoto S, Uchiyama K, Maeda M, Ishitsuka K, Furumoto K, Nakamura Y. In vivo and in vitro effects of zinc oxide-eugenol (ZOE) on biosynthesis of cyclo-oxygenase products in rat dental pulp. J Dent Res 1988;67: 1092-1096 [erratum 1988;67(11):inside back cover].
65. Waterhouse PJ, Whitworth JM, Nunn JH. Development of a method to detect and quantify prostaglandin E2 in pulpal blood from cariously exposed, vital primary molar teeth. Int Endod J 1999;32:381-387.
66. Chance K, Lin L, Shovlin FE, Skribner J. Clinical trial of intracanal corticosteroid in root canal therapy. J Endod 1987;13:466-468.
67. Fachin EV, Zaki AE. Histology and lysosomal cytochemistry of the postsurgically inflamed dental pulp after topical application of steroids. I. Histological study. J Endod 1991;17:457-460.
68. Rogers MJ, Johnson BR, Remeikis NA, BeGole EA. Comparison of effect of intracanal use of ketorolac tromethamine and dexamethasone with oral ibuprofen on posttreatment endodontic pain. J Endod 1999;25: 381-484.
69. Curtis P Jr, Gartman LA, Green DB. Utilization of ketorolac tromethamine for control of severe odontogenic pain. J Endod 1994;20:457-459.

70. Doroschak AM, Bowles WR, Hargreaves KM. Evaluation of the combination of flurbiprofen and tramadol for management of endodontic pain. J Endod 1999;25(10): 660–663.
71. Hutchins M, Housholder G, Suchina J, Rittman B, Rittman G, Montgomery E. Comparison of acetaminophen, ibuprofen, and nabumetone therapy in rats with pulpal pathosis. J Endod 1999;25:804–806.
72. Colville-Nash PR, Gilroy DW. COX-2 and the cyclopentenone prostaglandins: A new chapter in the book of inflammation? Prostaglandins Other Lipid Mediat 2000; 62:33–43.
73. Dionne R. COX-2 inhibitors: Better than ibuprofen for dental pain? Compend Contin Educ Dent 1999;20: 518–520, 522–524.
74. Okiji T, Morita I, Sunada I, Murota S. The role of leukotriene B4 in neutrophil infiltration in experimentally-induced inflammation of rat tooth pulp. J Dent Res 1991;70:34–37.
75. Lessard GM, Torabinejad M, Swope D. Arachidonic acid metabolism in canine tooth pulps and the effects of nonsteroidal anti-inflammatory drugs. J Endod 1986;12: 146–149.
76. Gazelius B, Panopoulos P, Odlander B, Claesson HE. Inhibition of intradental nerve excitability by leukotriene B4 and C4. Acta Physiol Scand 1984;120 (1):141–143.
77. Madison S, Whitsel EA, Suarez-Roca H, Maixner W. Sensitizing effects of leukotriene B4 on intradental primary afferents. Pain 1992;49:99–104.
78. Diamond P, McGinty A, Sugrue D, Brady HR, Godson C. Regulation of leukocyte trafficking by lipoxins. Clin Chem Lab Med 1999;37:293–297.
79. Clarkson MR, McGinty A, Godson C, Brady HR. Leukotrienes and lipoxins: Lipoxygenase-derived modulators of leukocyte recruitment and vascular tone in glomerulonephritis. Nephrol Dial Transplant 1998;13: 3043–3051.
80. Peplow PV. Regulation of platelet-activating factor (PAF) activity in human diseases by phospholipase A2 inhibitors, PAF acetylhydrolases, PAF receptor antagonists and free radical scavengers. Prostaglandins Leukot Essent Fatty Acids 1999;61:65–82.
81. Hirafuji M, Ogura Y. Distinct stimulatory effect of platelet-activating factor on prostaglandin I2 and thromboxane A2 biosynthesis by rat dental pulp. Eur J Pharmacol 1990;185:81–90.
82. Lewis GP. Bradykinin. Nature 1961;192:596–599.
83. Hall JM. Bradykinin receptors: Pharmacological properties and biological roles. Pharmacol Ther 1992;56: 131–190.
84. Sundqvist G, Rosenquist JB, Lerner UH. Effects of bradykinin and thrombin on prostaglandin formation, cell proliferation and collagen biosynthesis in human dental-pulp fibroblasts. Arch Oral Biol 1995;40: 247–256.
85. Sundqvist G, Lerner UH. Bradykinin and thrombin synergistically potentiate interleukin 1 and tumour necrosis factor induced prostanoid biosynthesis in human dental pulp fibroblasts. Cytokine 1996;8:168–177.
86. Kim S, Liu M, Simchon S, Dorscher-Kim JE. Effects of selected inflammatory mediators on blood flow and vascular permeability in the dental pulp. Proc Finn Dent Soc 1992;88(suppl 1):387–392.
87. Kawase T, Orikasa M, Suzuki A. Effect of bradykinin on intracellular signalling systems in a rat clonal dental pulp-cell line. Arch Oral Biol 1993;38:43–48.
88. Maita E, Endo Y, Ogura Y. Properties of kininase in rat dental pulp. J Dent Res 1984;63:1067–1071.
89. Lepinski AM, Hargreaves KM, Goodis HE, Bowles WR. Bradykinin levels in dental pulp by microdialysis. J Endod 2000;26:744–747.
90. Hargreaves KM, Costello A. Glucocorticoids suppress levels of immunoreactive bradykinin in inflamed tissue as evaluated by microdialysis probes. Clin Pharmacol Ther 1990;48:168–178.
91. Swift JQ, Garry MG, Roszkowski MT, Hargreaves KM. Effect of flurbiprofen on tissue levels of immunoreactive bradykinin and acute postoperative pain. J Oral Maxillofac Surg 1993;51:112–116 [discussion 116–117].
92. Kudo T, Kuroi M, Inoki R. In vitro production and release of opioid peptides in the tooth pulp induced by bradykinin. Neuropeptides 1986;7:391–397.
93. Pulver WH, Taubman MA, Smith DJ. Immune components in normal and inflamed human dental pulp. Arch Oral Biol 1977;22:103–111.
94. Speer ML, Madonia JV, Heuer MA. Quantitative evaluation of the immunocompetence of the dental pulp. J Endod 1977;3:418–423.
95. Pekovic DD, Fillery ED. Identification of bacteria in immunopathologic mechanisms of human dental pulp. Oral Surg Oral Med Oral Pathol 1984;57:652–661.
96. Okamura K, Maeda M, Nishikawa T, Tsutsui M. Dentinal response against carious invasion: Localization of antibodies in odontoblastic body and process. J Dent Res 1980;59:1368–1373.
97. Pekovic DD, Adamkiewicz VW, Shapiro A, Gornitsky M. Identification of bacteria in association with immune components in human carious dentin. J Oral Pathol 1987;16:223–233.
98. Lerner UH. Effects of kinins, thrombin, and neuropeptides on bone. In: Gowen M (ed). Cytokines and Bone Metabolism. Ann Arbor: CRC, 1992:267–298.
99. Fenton JW II. Thrombin functions and antithrombotic intervention. Thromb Haemost 1995;74:493–498.
100. Chang MC, Lan WH, Chan CP, Lin CP, Hsieh CC, Jeng JH. Serine protease activity is essential for thrombin-induced protein synthesis in cultured human dental pulp cells: Modulation roles of prostaglandin E2. J Oral Pathol Med 1998;27:23–29.

101. Chang MC, Lin CP, Huang TF, Lan WH, Yin YL, Hsieh CC, Jeng JH. Thrombin-induced DNA synthesis of cultured human dental pulp cells is dependent on its proteolytic activity and modulated by prostaglandin E2. J Endod 1998;24:709-713.
102. Chang MC, Jeng JH, Lin CP, Lan WH, Tsai W, Hsieh CC. Thrombin activates the growth, cell-cycle kinetics, and clustering of human dental pulp cells. J Endod 1999; 25:118-122.
103. Sakurai K, Okiji T, Suda H. Co-increase of nerve fibers and HLA-DR- and/or factor-XIIIa-expressing dendritic cells in dentinal caries-affected regions of the human dental pulp: An immunohistochemical study. J Dent Res 1999;78:1596-1608.
104. Southam JC, Moody GH. The fibrinolytic activity of human and rat dental pulps. Arch Oral Biol 1975;20: 783-786.
105. Mjor IA, Dahl E, Cox CF. Healing of pulp exposures: An ultrastructural study. J Oral Pathol Med 1991;20: 496-501.
106. Sasaki T, Kawamata-Kido H. Providing an environment for reparative dentine induction in amputated rat molar pulp by high molecular-weight hyaluronic acid. Arch Oral Biol 1995;40:209-219.
107. Wikstrom MB, Dahlen G, Linde A. Fibrinogenolytic and fibrinolytic activity in oral microorganisms. J Clin Microbiol 1983;17:759-767.
108. Izumi T, Yamada K, Inoue H, Watanabe K, Nishigawa Y. Fibrinogen/fibrin and fibronectin in the dentin-pulp complex after cavity preparation in rat molars. Oral Surg Oral Med Oral Pathol Oral Radiol Endod 1998;86: 587-591.
109. Pashley DH, Galloway SE, Stewart F. Effects of fibrinogen in vivo on dentine permeability in the dog. Arch Oral Biol 1984;29:725-728.
110. Hosoya S, Ohbayashi E, Matsushima K, Takeuchi H, Yamazaki M, Shibata Y, Abiko Y. Stimulatory effect of interleukin-6 on plasminogen activator activity from human dental pulp cells. J Endod 1998;24:331-334.
111. Torneck CD. Changes in the fine structure of the human dental pulp subsequent to carious exposure. J Oral Pathol 1977;6:82-95.
112. Linde A, Persliden B, Ronnback L. Cathepsin D purification from rat liver and immunohistochemical demonstration in rat incisor. Acta Odontol Scand 1978;36: 117-126.
113. Rauschenberger CR, Turner DW, Kaminski EJ, Osetek EM. Human polymorphonuclear granule components: Relative levels detected by a modified enzyme-linked immunosorbent assay in normal and inflamed dental pulps. J Endod 1991;17:531-536.
114. Cootauco CJ, Rauschenberger CR, Nauman RK. Immunocytochemical distribution of human PMN elastase and cathepsin-G in dental pulp. J Dent Res 1993; 72:1485-490.
115. Rauschenberger CR, McClanahan SB, Pederson ED, Turner DW, Kaminski EJ. Comparison of human polymorphonuclear neutrophil elastase, polymorphonuclear neutrophil cathepsin-G, and alpha 2-macroglobulin levels in healthy and inflamed dental pulps. J Endod 1994;20:546-550.
116. Okada Y, Watanabe S, Nakanishi I, Kishi J, Hayakawa T, Watorek W, et al. Inactivation of tissue inhibitor of metalloproteinases by neutrophil elastase and other serine proteinases. FEBS Lett 1988;229:157-160.
117. Birkedal-Hansen H. Proteolytic remodeling of extracellular matrix. Curr Opin Cell Biol 1995;7:728-735.
118. Caron C, Xue J, Bartlett JD. Expression and localization of membrane type 1 matrix metalloproteinase in tooth tissues. Matrix Biol 1998;17:501-511.
119. Tamura M, Nagaoka S, Kawagoe M. Interleukin-1 alpha stimulates interstitial collagenase gene expression in human dental pulp fibroblast. J Endod 1996;22: 240-243.
120. O'Boskey FJ Jr, Panagakos FS. Cytokines stimulate matrix metalloproteinase production by human pulp cells during long-term culture. J Endod 1998;24:7-10.
121. Panagakos FS, O'Boskey JF Jr, Rodriguez E. Regulation of pulp cell matrix metalloproteinase production by cytokines and lipopolysaccharides. J Endod 1996;22: 358-361.
122. Nakata K, Yamasaki M, Iwata T, K. S,[au: please confirm authors] Nakane A, Nakamura H. Anaerobic bacterial extracts influence production of matrix metalloproteinases and their inhibitors by human dental pulp cells. J Endod 2000;26:410-413.
123. Tjaderhane L, Larjava H, Sorsa T, Uitto VJ, Larmas M, Salo T. The activation and function of host matrix metalloproteinases in dentin matrix breakdown in caries lesions. J Dent Res 1998;77:1622-1629.
124. Palosaari H, Wahlgren J, Larmas M, Ronka H, Sorsa T, Sato T, Tjaderhane L. The expression of MMP-8 in human odontoblasts and dental pulp cells is down-regulated by TGF-beta1. J Dent Res 2000;79:77-84.
125. Kishi J, Hayakawa T. Purification and characterization of bovine dental pulp collagenase inhibitor. J Biochem (Tokyo) 1984;96:395-404.
126. McDonald JK, Schwabe C. Dipeptidyl peptidase II of bovine dental pulp: Initial demonstration and characterization as a fibroblastic, lysosomal peptidase of the serine class active on collagen-related peptides. Biochim Biophys Acta 1980;61:68-81.
127. McClanahan SB, Turner DW, Kaminski EJ, Osetek EM, Heuer MA. Natural modifiers of the inflammatory process in the human dental pulp. J Endod 1991;17: 589-593.
128. Izumi T, Kobayashi I, Okamura K, Matsuo K, Kiyashima T, Ishibashi Y, et al. An immunohistochemical study of HLA-DR and alpha 1-antichymotrypsin-positive cells in the pulp of human non-carious and carious teeth. Arch Oral Biol 1996;41:627-630.

129. Lohinai Z, Balla I, Marczis J, Vass Z, Kovach AG. Evidence for the role of nitric oxide in the circulation of the dental pulp. J Dent Res 1995;74:1501-1506.
130. Billiar TR. Nitric oxide: Novel biology with clinical relevance. Ann Surg 1995;221:339-349.
131. Clancy RM, Amin AR, Abramson SB. The role of nitric oxide in inflammation and immunity. Arthritis Rheum 1998;41:1141-1151.
132. Law AS, Baumgardner KR, Meller ST, Gebhart GF. Localization and changes in NADPH-diaphorase reactivity and nitric oxide synthase immunoreactivity in rat pulp following tooth preparation. J Dent Res 1999;78: 1585-1595.
133. Lohinai Z, Szekely AD, Benedek P, Csillag A. Nitric oxide synthase containing nerves in the cat and dog dental pulp and gingiva. Neurosci Lett 1997;227:91-94.
134. Remick DG, Villarete L. Regulation of cytokine gene expression by reactive oxygen and reactive nitrogen intermediates. J Leukoc Biol 1996;59:471-475.
135. Okabe E. Endogenous vasoactive substances and oxygen-derived free radicals in pulpal haemodynamics. Arch Oral Biol 1994;39(suppl):39S-45S.
136. Grossi GB, Borrello S, Giuliani M, Galeotti T, Miani C. Copper-zinc superoxide dismutase in human and animal dental pulp. J Dent 1991;19:319-321.
137. Davis WL, Jacoby BH, Craig KR, Wagner G, Harrison JW. Copper-zinc superoxide dismutase activity in normal and inflamed human dental pulp tissue. J Endod 1991;17:316-318.
138. Baumgardner KR, Law AS, Gebhart GF. Localization and changes in superoxide dismutase immunoreactivity in rat pulp after tooth preparation. Oral Surg Oral Med Oral Pathol Oral Radiol Endod 1999;88:488-495.
139. Bevilacqua MP, Nelson RM, Mannori G, Cecconi O. Endothelial-leukocyte adhesion molecules in human disease. Ann Rev Med 1994;45:361-378.
140. Lertchirakarn V, Birner R, Messer HH. Effects of interleukin-1 beta on human pulpal fibroblast proliferation and collagen synthesis. J Endod 1998;24:409-413.
141. Shiba H, Nakamura S, Shirakawa M, Nakanishi K, Okamoto H, Satakeda H, et al. Effects of basic fibroblast growth factor on proliferation, the expression of osteonectin (SPARC) and alkaline phosphatase, and calcification in cultures of human pulp cells. Dev Biol 1995;170:457-466.
142. D'Souza R, Brown LR, Newland JR, Levy BM, Lachman LB. Detection and characterization of interleukin-1 in human dental pulps. Arch Oral Biol 1989;34:307-313.
143. Schweizer A, Feige U, Fontana A, Muller K, Dinarello CA. Interleukin-1 enhances pain reflexes: mediation through increased prostaglandin E2 levels. Agents Actions 1988;25:246-251.
144. Ransjo M, Marklund M, Persson M, Lerner UH. Synergistic interactions of bradykinin, thrombin, interleukin 1 and tumor necrosis factor on prostanoid biosynthesis in human periodontal-ligament cells. Arch Oral Biol 1998;43:253-260.
145. Fouad AF. IL-1 alpha and TNF-alpha expression in early periapical lesions of normal and immunodeficient mice. J Dent Res 1997;76:1548-1554.
146. Hosoya S, Matsushima K. Stimulation of interleukin-1 beta production of human dental pulp cells by *Porphyromonas endodontalis lipopolysaccharide*. J Endod 1997;23:39-42.
147. Mattsson E, Verhage L, Rollof J, Fleer A, Verhoef J, van Dijk H. Peptidoglycan and teichoic acid from *Staphylococcus epidermidis* stimulate human monocytes to release tumour necrosis factor-alpha, interleukin-1 beta and interleukin-6. FEMS Immunol Med Microbiol 1993; 7:281-287.
148. Hoshino K, Takeuchi O, Kawai T, Sanjo H, Ogawa T, Takeda Y, et al. Cutting edge: Toll-like receptor 4 (TLR4)-deficient mice are hyporesponsive to lipopolysaccharide: Evidence for TLR4 as the Lps gene product. J Immunol 1999;162:3749-3752.
149. Schwandner R, Dziarski R, Wesche H, Rothe M, Kirschning CJ. Peptidoglycan- and lipoteichoic acid-induced cell activation is mediated by toll-like receptor 2. J Biol Chem 1999;274:17406-17409.
150. Dinarello CA. Pro-inflammatory cytokines. Chest 2000;118:503-508.
151. Khabbaz MG, Anastasiadis PL, Sykaras SN. Determination of endotoxins in caries: Association with pulpal pain. Int Endod J 2000;33:132-137.
152. Chen CP, Hertzberg M, Jiang Y, Graves DT. Interleukin-1 and tumor necrosis factor receptor signaling is not required for bacteria-induced osteoclastogenesis and bone loss but is essential for protecting the host from a mixed anaerobic infection. Am J Pathol 1999;155: 2145-2152.
153. Rakich DR, Wataha JC, Lefebvre CA, Weller RN. Effects of dentin bonding agents on macrophage mitochondrial activity. J Endod 1998;24:528-533.
154. Rakich DR, Wataha JC, Lefebvre CA, Weller RN. Effect of dentin bonding agents on the secretion of inflammatory mediators from macrophages. J Endod 1999;25: 114-117.
155. Abbas AK, Murphy KM, Sher A. Functional diversity of helper T lymphocytes. Nature 1996;383:787-793.
156. Bancroft GJ, Schreiber RD, Unanue ER. Natural immunity: A T-cell-independent pathway of macrophage activation, defined in the scid mouse. Immunol Rev 1991;124:5-24.
157. Rauschenberger CR, Bailey JC, Cootauco CJ. Detection of human IL-2 in normal and inflamed dental pulps. J Endod 1997;23:366-370.

158. Hahn CL, Best AM, Tew JG. Cytokine induction by Streptococcus mutans and pulpal pathogenesis. Infect Immun 2000;68:6785–6789.
159. Tilg H, Dinarello CA, Mier JW. IL-6 and APPs: Anti-inflammatory and immunosuppressive mediators. Immunol Today 1997;18:428–432.
160. Matsushima K, Ohbayashi E, Takeuchi H, Hosoya S, Abiko Y, Yamazaki M. Stimulation of interleukin-6 production in human dental pulp cells by peptidoglycans from Lactobacillus casei. J Endod 1998;24:252–255.
161. Hosoya S, Matsushima K, Ohbayashi E, Yamazaki M, Shibata Y, Abiko Y. Stimulation of interleukin-1beta-independent interleukin-6 production in human dental pulp cells by lipopolysaccharide. Biochem Mol Med 1996;59:138–143.
162. Barkhordar RA, Hayashi C, Hussain MZ. Detection of interleukin-6 in human dental pulp and periapical lesions. Endod Dent Traumatol 1999;15:26–27.
163. Proctor ME, Turner DW, Kaminski EJ, Osetek EM, Heuer MA. Determination and relationship of C-reactive protein in human dental pulps and in serum. J Endod 1991;17:265–270.
164. D'Souza RN, Cavender A, Dickinson D, Roberts A, Letterio J. TGF-beta1 is essential for the homeostasis of the dentin-pulp complex. Eur J Oral Sci 1998;106(suppl 1): 185–191.
165. Nagaoka S, Tokuda M, Sakuta T, Taketoshi Y, Tamura M, Takada H, Kawagoe M. Interleukin-8 gene expression by human dental pulp fibroblast in cultures stimulated with Prevotella intermedia lipopolysaccharide. J Endod 1996;22:9–12.
166. Jiang Y, Russell TR, Schilder H, Graves DT. Endodontic pathogens stimulate monocyte chemoattractant protein-1 and interleukin-8 in mononuclear cells. J Endod 1998;24:86–90.
167. Huang GT, Potente AP, Kim JW, Chugal N, Zhang X. Increased interleukin-8 expression in inflamed human dental pulps. Oral Surg Oral Med Oral Pathol Oral Radiol Endod 1999;88:214–220.
168. Levin LG, Rudd A, Bletsa A, Reisner H. Expression of IL-8 by cells of the odontoblast layer in vitro. Eur J Oral Sci 1999;107:131–137.
169. Jontell M, Okiji T, Dahlgren U, Bergenholtz G. Immune defense mechanisms of the dental pulp. Crit Rev Oral Biol Med 1998;9:179–200.
170. Jontell M, Gunraj MN, Bergenholtz G. Immunocompetent cells in the normal dental pulp. J Dent Res 1987; 66(6):1149–1153.
171. Okiji T, Kawashima N, Kosaka T, Matsumoto A, Kobayashi C, Suda H. An immunohistochemical study of the distribution of immunocompetent cells, especially macrophages and Ia antigen-expressing cells of heterogeneous populations, in normal rat molar pulp. J Dent Res 1992;71:1196–1202 [erratum 71:1760].
172. Ohshima H, Kawahara I, Maeda T, Takano Y. The relationship between odontoblasts and immunocompetent cells during dentinogenesis in rat incisors: An immunohistochemical study using OX6-monoclonal antibody. Arch Histol Cytol 1994;57:435–447.
173. Jontell M, Eklof C, Dahlgren UI, Bergenholtz G. Difference in capacity between macrophages and dendritic cells from rat incisor pulp to provide accessory signals to concanavalin-A-stimulated T-lymphocytes. J Dent Res 1994;73:1056–1060.
174. Kamal AM, Okiji T, Kawashima N, Suda H. Defense responses of dentin/pulp complex to experimentally induced caries in rat molars: An immunohistochemical study on kinetics of pulpal Ia antigen-expressing cells and macrophages. J Endod 1997;23:115–120.
175. Bergenholtz G, Nagaoka S, Jontell M. Class II antigen expressing cells in experimentally induced pulpitis. Int Endod J 1991;24:8–14.
176. Kamal AMM, Okiji T, Suda H. Response of class II molecule-expressing cells and macrophages to cavity preparation and restoration with 4-META/MMA-TBB resin. Int Endod J 2000;33:367–373.
177. Okiji T, Kosaka T, Kamal AM, Kawashima N, Suda H. Age-related changes in the immunoreactivity of the monocyte/macrophage system in rat molar pulp. Arch Oral Biol 1996;41:453–460.
178. Ackermans F, Klein JP, Frank RM. Ultrastructural localization of immunoglobulins in carious human dentine. Arch Oral Biol 1981;26:879–886.
179. Okamura K. Histological study on the origin of dentinal immunoglobulins and the change in their localization during caries. J Oral Pathol 1985;14:680–689.
180. Falkler WA, Martin SA, Tolba M, Siegel MA, Mackler BF. Reaction of pulpal immunoglobulins to oral microorganisms by an enzyme-linked immunosorbent assay. J Endod 1987;13:260–266.
181. Hahn CL, Falkler WA, Jr. Antibodies in normal and diseased pulps reactive with microorganisms isolated from deep caries. J Endod 1992;18:28–31.
182. Nakanishi T, Matsuo T, Ebisu S. Quantitative analysis of immunoglobulins and inflammatory factors in human pulpal blood from exposed pulps. J Endod 1995;21: 131–136.
183. Hahn CL, Overton B. The effects of immunoglobulins on the convective permeability of human dentine in vitro. Arch Oral Biol 1997;42:835–843.

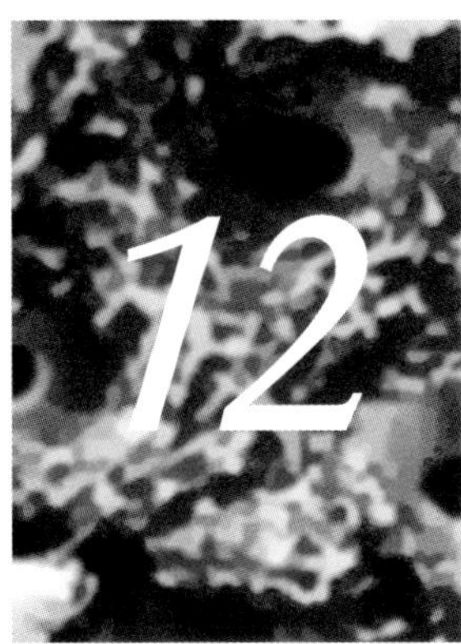

Pulpal Infections Including Caries

J. Craig Baumgartner, DDS, PhD

Dental caries remains the most prevalent infectious disease in the world. Caries is a bacterial infection that causes dissolution of the mineralized matrix of teeth. Although researchers have made significant advancements in our treatment and understanding of caries, it continues to be a worldwide epidemic. Twenty million years ago, hominids had an incidence of caries of only 1%, despite the fact that they had the same number and type of teeth as modern-day humans. During the Neolithic period, *Homo sapiens* had a caries rate of about 5%, or the same as many contemporary primitive societies.[1] A rise in caries in Europe during the Roman occupation has been correlated to an increase in the cooking of food. However, the most dramatic rise in caries took place between the Middle Ages and the 1950s, when caries affected 95% of the population in the developed world. Since the 1960s, caries in children has dropped sharply: 50% of 5- and 6-year-olds were caries free. By the late 1980s, approximately 75% of children aged 5 to 11 years were caries free, whereas approximately 70% of 12- to 17-year-olds had caries in permanent teeth. At that time, 40% of the 17-year-olds accounted for 80% of the caries.[2-4] The decline in the caries rate did not continue into the 1990s.[4] Before 1970, caries reduction was associated with fluoridation of public water supplies; since then, it seems to be related to fluoride-containing products such as toothpaste, mouth rinses, and topical gels.[5-9]

Caries has been associated with several variables, including host factors, the bacterial ecosystem, and a fermentable diet; saliva and other secondary factors are now also associated with caries. With the recent advent of new techniques in molecular biology, our understanding of the microbial agents associated with caries has grown. These findings reinforce the concept that the biofilm found on tooth surfaces, known as *dental plaque*, represents an interactive community of bacteria. Human dental plaque has more than 1×10^8 bacteria/mm^3 or about 1.7×10^{11} microbes/wet wt/g, comprising 200 to 400 different species of bacteria at each site.[10] Unlike *materia alba*, an aggregation of bacteria, leukocytes, and desquamated oral epithelium that accumulates at the surface of plaque but lacks its internal structure, dental plaque is capable of withstanding a strong water spray.

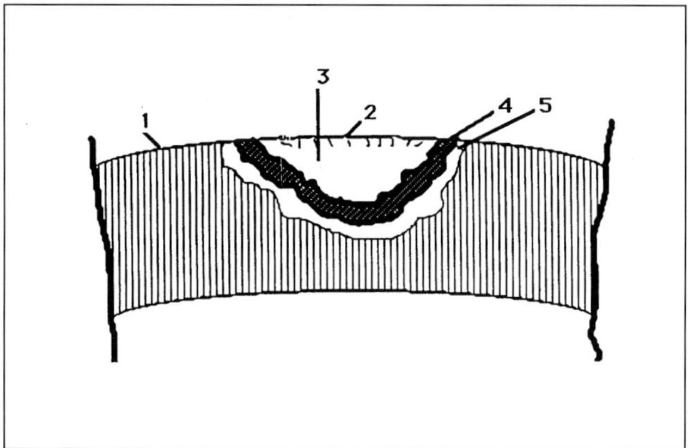

Fig 12-1 Diagrammatic representation of microscopic thin ground section showing enamel caries. Major zones are sound enamel (1), surface enamel slightly demineralized (2), body of lesion (3), dark zone (4), and translucent zone (5). (Redrawn from Newman and Nisengard[15] with permission.)

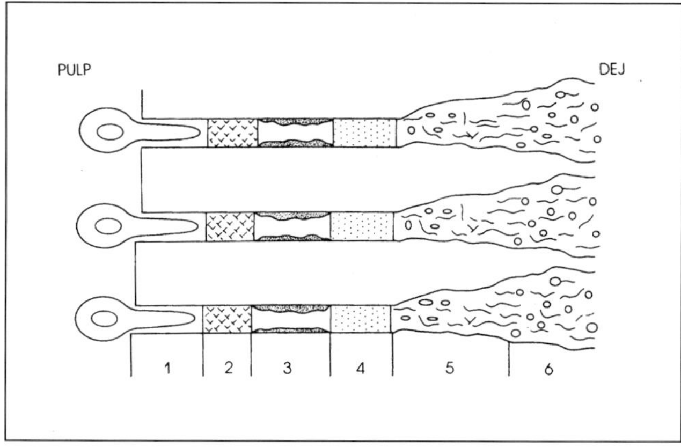

Fig 12-2 Diagrammatic illustration of Newbrun's six zones as seen in microscopic sections of dentinal caries: zone 1, retreating odontoblast process; zone 2, fatty degeneration; zone 3, dentinal sclerosis; zone 4, dentinal demineralization; zone 5, bacterial invasion; and zone 6, necrotic dentin. (Reprinted from Newman and Nisengard[15] with permission.)

Bacteria and Caries

In 1890, W. D. Miller described dental caries as the action of bacterial-produced acids on the calcium phosphate of teeth. This theory, known as the *chemoparasitic theory*, is still the most widely accepted one today; others include the proteolysis-chelation theory, the proteolytic theory, and the phosphoprotein theory. Bacteria's fundamental role in caries was demonstrated in the 1950s and 1960s, when germ-free animals failed to develop caries irrespective of their diets except in the presence of bacteria.[11] Caries is primarily the effect of lactic acid and other organic acids produced by bacteria in the dental plaque. These acids dissolve the calcium phosphate mineral of the tooth enamel or dentin in a process known as *demineralization*.[12,13]

The so-called white-spot lesion is the first clinically observed form of caries and is the result of subsurface demineralization of up to 50% of the original mineral content but with an intact surface layer beneath dental plaque.[14] Although the surface enamel appears to be intact, it in fact undergoes demineralization in the form of pitting. Enamel caries of this type has four distinct microscopic zones (Fig 12-1). It is believed that after nonionized acid diffuses through the pores and dissociates, it reacts with the hydroxyapatite crystals to produce a white spot. Eventually, through progressive dissolution of hydroxyapatite, the surface breaks down under the ingress of bacteria. Thus, early caries is aseptic and the result of the dissolution of enamel crystals by acids. Once bacteria enter the lesion, mechanical removal of the organisms is required. If left untreated, caries spreads laterally along the dentinoenamel junction (DEJ). Its rapid rate of spread is related to the fact that dentin is less mineralized than enamel and is made up of tubules that allow the movement of bacteria into deeper portions of the lesion. Six zones of dentinal caries have been described (Fig 12-2).

Fermentable carbohydrates, such as sucrose, glucose, fructose, and cooked starch, are metabolized by acidogenic bacteria to produce the acids that diffuse through the plaque into the porous enamel or dentin. The hydrogen ions chemically exchange with calcium and phosphate ions so they go into solution. The role of saliva in this process is to buffer the acid and to provide minerals that can replace those dissolved from the tooth. As described below, the process of remineralization has been replicated through similar therapeutic interventions.

Plaque is a dynamic microbial ecosystem that is influenced by host factors, other bacterial species, and the genetic potential of the individual species. The oral microbial ecosystem is the most complex in the body, comprising over 500 species. As the host surfaces change and the microbial biofilms evolve, bacterial species successively colonize the oral cavity. *Streptococcus salivarius*, the first permanent colonizer of the oral cavity, is found in infants of less than 1 week. Other early streptococci colonizers are *S mitis*, *S oralis*, and *S sanguis*. Studies based on DNA fingerprinting methods have demonstrated that close family members are the source of the bacteria that initially colonize an infant. The oral cavity is especially unique during the eruption of teeth, which are highly mineralized, nonshedding surfaces. Colonization by *S mutans* and numerous other species of bacteria does not occur until teeth erupt. At that time, children are generally colonized by one or two strains of *S mutans* that are genetically identical to bacterial strains colonizing the mother or other main caregivers. Adults often are colonized by five or more distinct strains of *S mutans*, suggesting that colonization by nonfamilial sources occurs after infancy.[16] Each genetically distinct strain is a derivative of a parent strain that has slightly different phenotypic characteristics, which maximizes its capacity to exploit changes in its environment. The composition of a climax population is remarkably stable. Adults generally retain their own community of oral flora,[17] and attempts to implant other specific strains into an established oral community usually fail.[18] The transfer and establishment of bacterial strains between adults is rare.

Research suggests that mutans streptococci are the primary etiologic agents of both coronal and root caries and that *Actinomyces* are also associated with root caries.[19,20] Table 12-1 lists the bacteria associated with different types of caries.

Table 12-1 Bacteria Associated with Caries*

Caries type	Organisms isolated
Pit and fissure	*Streptococcus mutans* *Streptococcus sanguis* *Lactobacillus* species *Actinomyces* species
Smooth surface	*Streptococcus mutans*
Dentinal caries	*Lactobacillus* species *Actinomyces viscosus* *Actinomyces naeslundii* *Streptococcus mutans*
Root caries	*Actinomyces viscosus* *Actinomyces naeslundii* *Streptococcus mutans* Filamentous rods

*Data from Newman and Nisengard,[15] Simmonds et al,[16] Marsh,[18] and van Houte et al.[21]

Mutans streptococci is a group of bacteria that includes *S mutans*, *S sobrinas*, *S creccetus*, and *S rattus*. *S mutans* and *S sobrinas* are closely associated with human caries.[21] The ability of these organisms to produce caries is directly related to their production of acid (acidogenic) and their ability to tolerate large quantities of lactic acid (aciduric). Mutans streptococci are heterofermentative in that they can produce acid other than lactic acid; that is, they can change the relative amount of enzymes in their glycolytic pathway to produce mixed acid products. This enables mutans streptococci to produce an extra 2 to 3 mol of adenosine triphosphate (ATP) per mol of glucose metabolized and thus gives them a growth advantage over other microorganisms.[16] Mutans streptococci are able to maintain their energy production even at pH levels as low as 5.0, when other plaque bacteria (with the exception of lactobacilli) are inhibited. Mutans streptococci are also able to store nonmetabolized carbohydrate in the form of intracellular polysaccharides, something else that few of the other

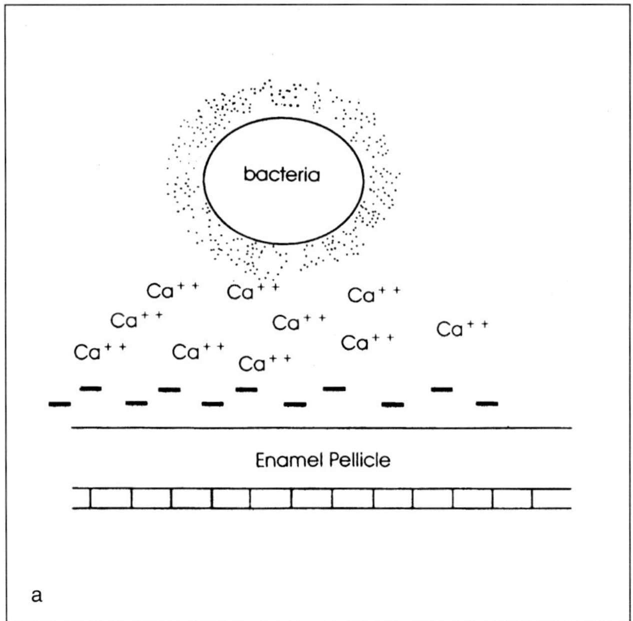

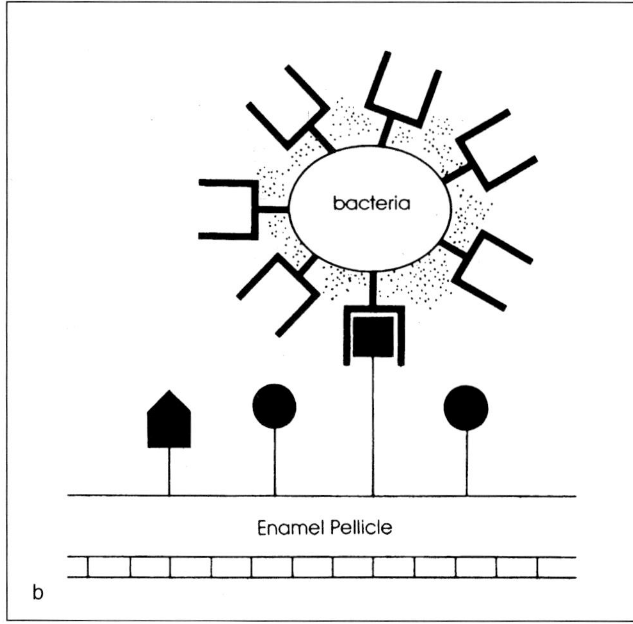

Fig 12-3 Diagrammatic representation of two proposed theories of the interaction of oral bacteria with pellicle-coated enamel surfaces: *(a)* electrostatic hypothesis; *(b)* "lectin-like"interaction. (Reprinted from Newman and Nisengard[15] with permission.)

plaque bacteria are capable of doing. When the external supply of sugar becomes limited, mutans streptococci can metabolize the stored carbohydrate and continue acid production. Other bacteria, especially lactobacilli, contribute to the cariogenic process primarily in advanced lesions.[22] The frequent intake of sucrose produces an imbalance in the plaque ecosystem by the selection of mutans streptococci.

The prevalence of root caries increases with age because most of these lesions are associated with gingival recession. Root caries is a soft progressive lesion associated with microbial plaque and must be distinguished from abrasion, erosion, and idiopathic resorption. The species *Actinomyces* has been shown to be predominant in root caries. However, no specific bacteria or group of bacteria has been associated with the initiation or progression of root caries. Patients with decreased salivary function (xerostomia), often associated with head and neck radiation, various medications, and Sjögren syndrome, may have a dramatic increase in root caries.

Bacteria-Host Interactions and Plaque Formation

Components of saliva represent the primary host factors that resist caries development. As noted earlier, saliva has excellent buffering and remineralizing properties.[23] In addition to bicarbonate and phosphate ions, which provide the major buffering capability, saliva contains immunoglobulins, glycoproteins, enzymes, and host-derived antimicrobial agents, all of which may also affect plaque formation.[22]

It is not only the presence of bacteria, but also the development of cariogenic conditions that eventually leads to the production of dental caries. A salivary pellicle will form within minutes after a tooth surface is cleaned. The salivary pellicle is an insoluble acellular layer that is less than 1 μm in thickness; it is produced by the selective adsorption of glycoproteins onto the hydroxyapatite surface.[24] Salivary components on the surface of the pellicle act as binding sites for bacteria.[25] Two theories have been advanced for the interaction of the pellicle and bacteria. The first proposes that electrostatic charges are responsible for calcium ions binding the negatively charged surface of bacteria to the negatively charged pellicle on enamel[26] (Fig 12-3). This theory fails to explain the selectivity shown by different strains of bacteria with similar surface charges. The second theory proposes that "lectin-like" interaction occurs between specific bacterial surface receptors with pellicle-bound glycoproteins (see Fig 12-3). Experimental evidence has shown that the adsorption of oral bacteria to pellicles on hydroxyapatite is inhibited by specific sugars; this suggests sugar-protein binding. The salivary pellicle selectively adsorbs bacteria with the appropriate surface fibrillar protein structures. Microbial surface adhesins are surface proteins that display distinct preferences in binding site specificity by mediating attachment to epithelial surfaces and to other bacteria.[27,28] The specificity of adhesins is further demonstrated by the finding that only strains of *S mutans* and *S gordonii* can invade dentinal tubules and attach to type I collagen.[29] It is believed that bacterial surface proteins prevent attachment of phagocytic cells or suppress complement activation.[30]

Coaggregation is the adherence of certain strains of bacteria to specific partner strains. Table 12-2 shows coaggregation reactions between oral bacteria. The strain specificity is mediated by the production of a specific protein adhesin on one species and a complementary carbohydrate ligand on a partner species. Because each bacteria cell may have numerous adhesins and ligand molecules, multiple linkages may occur. *A naeslundii*, which is usually found in plaque, adheres poorly to the salivary pellicle but adheres readily to *S sanguis*, which in turn adheres readily to the pellicle. Such adhesive mechanisms are extremely important in the development of dental plaque. Mutans streptococci are able to produce and bind glucan molecules, which result in the aggregation and accumulation of more bacteria. The insoluble glucan may mediate nonspecific entrapment of other microorganisms. *Actinomyces* can produce large amounts of plaque in the presence of carbohydrates. *A viscosus* synthesizes an extracellular heteropolysaccharide composed of N-acetylglucosamine, glucose, and galactose. The presence of *Actinomyces* or other gram-positive bacteria may be associated with the attachment and colonization of plaque with strains of black-pigmented bacteria.

Table 12-2 Coaggregation reactions between oral bacteria*

Bacterial strain	Partner strains
Streptococcus species or *Actinomyces* species (gram positive)	Gram positive: *Actinomyces viscosus* *Actinomyces naeslundii* *Actinomyces odontolticus* *Bacterionema matruchotti* *Propionibacterium acnes* Gram negative: *Bacteroides* species *Capnocytophaga* species *Fusobacterium nucleatum* *Eikenella corrodens* *Veillonella* species
Prevotella melaninogenicus (gram negative)	Gram negative: *Fusobacterium nucleatum* *Capnocytophaga* species

*Data from Whittaker et al,[25] Cisar,[31] and Newbrun.[32]

Three phases of plaque development have been described[32]: initial colonization is followed by rapid bacterial growth and then remodeling. The pellicle forms within a few minutes after tooth cleaning. Within hours, streptococci produce a thin mass covering the surface. They also produce large amounts of extracellular glucan to the height of contour and in the interproximal areas, and this incorporates other species of bacteria. Growth of plaque above the height of contour is limited by surface abrasion during mastication. After 2 to 3 days, the innermost plaque becomes more anaerobic, and a succession of anaerobic species and other bacteria appears.

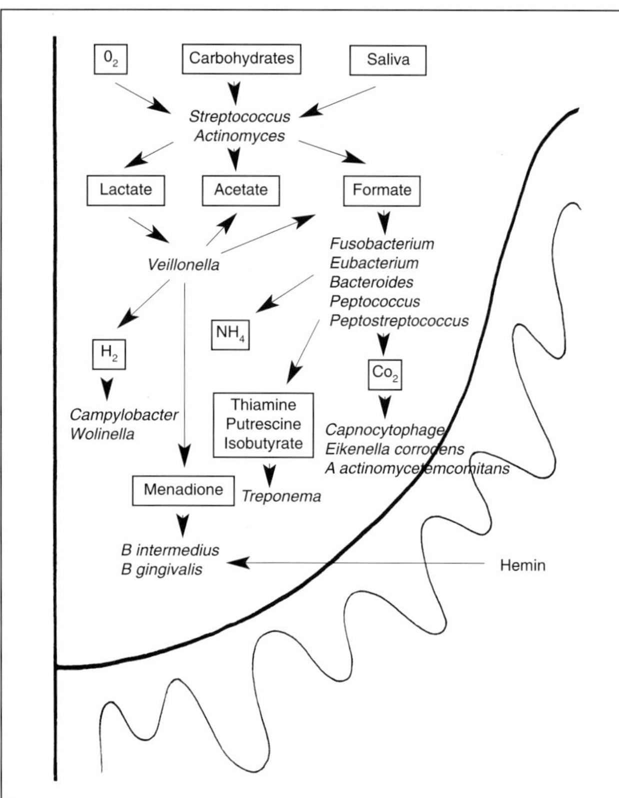

Fig 12-4 Interbacterial and host nutritional interactions influence the maturation of dental plaque. (Modified from Newman and Nisengard[15] with permission.)

Various species of bacteria produce antibacterial agents to ensure their own adaptation to the ecosystem. One strain of bacteria may produce a by-product that another strain is able to metabolize. For example, one species may produce ammonia, which is a nutrient for another species at a low concentration but lethal at a higher concentration. The production of factors, such as ammonia from urea by bacterial ureases, modifies the final pH of the plaque and affects its pathogenicity. Streptococci and lactobacilli grow under facultative conditions and produce superoxide anions, hydrogen peroxide, and hydroxyl radicals. These agents are bactericidal for some species of bacteria and hence affect the bacterial composition of the plaque. In mature plaque, the levels of these agents decreases, allowing for the growth of obligate anaerobes.

Bacteria may produce specific agents called *bacteriocins*; these are the proteins secreted by one species of bacteria that are lethal to other closely related organisms. A large number of oral bacteria are capable of producing bacteriocins.[33] Because of nutritional deficiencies, some bacteriocins may not be produced in plaque, while others may by destroyed by proteolytic enzymes. Bacteriocins experimentally administered to animals in either food or drinking water significantly reduced the level of *S mutans*.[34] Some species of bacteria have been shown to produce more than one bacteriocin that act synergistically.[35]

These agents may have clinical utility for prevention of caries. Unfortunately, the bacteriocins with the greatest potential are either difficult to produce in large quantities or their purification is not cost effective for large-scale production.[36,37] An alternative is to implant a bacteriocin-producing strain into human plaque. However, even if this method was accepted by the public, it is unlikely that such a genetically diverse population could be successfully colonized.[38] Microbial succession is a result of numerous interactions (Fig 12-4).

Saliva greatly influences the metabolism and microbial composition of dental plaque. Saliva affects plaque pH by clearance of carbohydrates, neutralization of acids, and supply of nutrients. Saliva also contains bacterial inhibitory substances such as lactoperoxidase, thiocyanate, peroxide, lactoferrin, lysozyme, and hypothiocyanate ion (OSCN−). In the presence of hydrogen peroxide and thiocyanate ion, lactoperoxidase catalyzes the formation of OSCN−, which rapidly destroys bacterial metabolic systems. Lactoferrin binds iron that bacteria find essential for growth. The major buffer system in saliva, bicarbonate-carbonate, rapidly buffers by losing carbon dioxide. It has a dissociation constant (pK) in the range of the plaque acids, and as salivary flow increases, so does the concentration of bicarbonate.

Just as chemical mediators regulate the behavior of cells in the human body, interbacterial signaling factors serve to coordinate actions among bacterial cells. More than 20 years ago, a sex pheromone was associated with bacterial conjugation in strains of *Enterococcus faecalis*. It is now believed that chemical signals regulate population-wide growth.[39] As the dental plaque approaches a critical density, cellular metabolism, DNA synthesis, and cell growth increase. This is apparently the result of chemical communication.[40] A majority of species are simultaneously triggered into a rapid growth spurt. Identification of the signaling molecule may allow the production of a chemical or antibody to inhibit the signaling and decrease the rapid maturation of dental plaque.

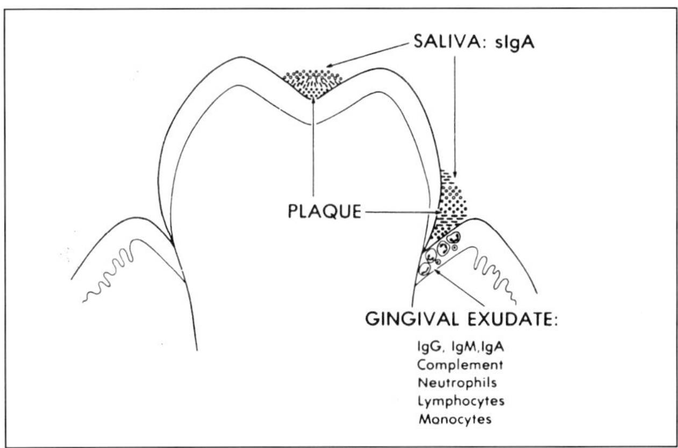

Fig 12-5 Sources of immunoglobulins in the oral cavity. (Reprinted from Newbrun[32] with permission.)

Bacterial Evolution

The genetic composition of bacteria undergoes constant change. If a strain of bacteria has a generation time of 4 to 6 hours, it undergoes in 6 weeks the equivalent of the number of generations that humans have over a period of 4,000 years.[15] Some bacteria have generation times of less than 1 hour. In addition, mechanisms exist that allow bacteria to rapidly change their genetic structure, as has been demonstrated with extracellular enzymes known as *glucosyltransferases* (GTFs). When GTF binds to sucrose, it breaks the disaccharide into units of glucosyl and fructosyl and transports the fructose unit into the cell cytoplasm. The glucosyl units are polymerized into the extracellular polysaccharide known as glucan. Only strains of *S mutans* capable of producing glucans are cariogenic in animal models.[41] Glucan is a branched structure composed of glucose units joined by alpha 1-6 and alpha 1-3 glucosidic linkages. These insoluble glucans have been described as the "universal glue" that holds plaque together.[41,42] Streptococcal GTFs are approximately 1,500 amino acids, with an additional signal peptide of about 30 amino acids, that facilitate transport across the cell membrane. The number of GTF genes in each species varies; for example, *S mutans* has three genes, while *S salivarius* has four genes. These genes can individually and independently evolve new characteristics through successive mutation and evolutionary selection. A more rapid mechanism of gene evolution is recombination between the genes. Because of homologous genes, there is a significant chance for sequence interchange (recombination), which results in novel GTFs and hybrid genes that produce different glucan products.[43] In addition, large fragments of DNA may be transferred between bacteria.[44,45] If homologous sequences are in the host bacterium, recombination with the transferred DNA may take place, yielding new functional proteins. Thus, the oral cavity may be considered a dynamic gene pool of bacteria that can rapidly evolve in response to environmental change, which clearly has clinical significance since caries, pulpitis, and periodontitis all have major bacterial etiologies.

Immunologic Control of Caries

Salivary secretions are the major source of IgA, which is the predominant immunoglobulin in the saliva. IgG and IgM are found in the saliva after their diffusion from the gingival sulcus (Fig 12-5).

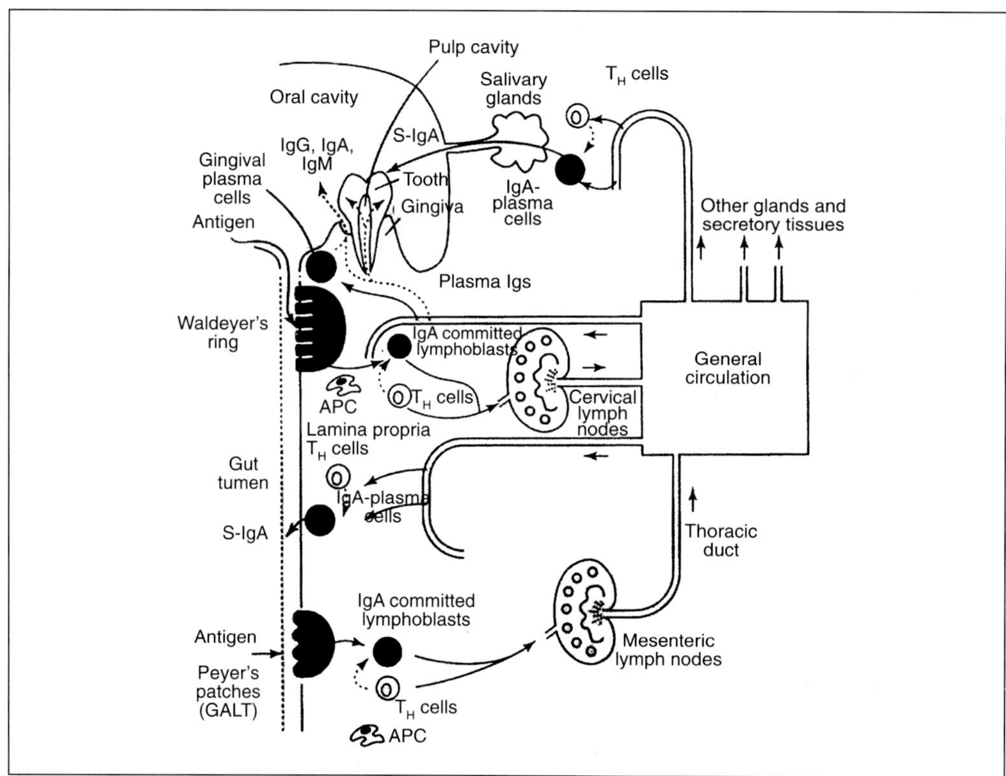

Fig 12-6 The common mucosal immune system and salivary immunity. Specialized epithelial cells covering the mucosa-associated lymphoid tissues, in the crypts of the tonsils and adenoids (Waldeyer's ring) and on intestinal Peyer's patches, take up antigenic materials and transport them to underlying antigen-processing cells (APC), which present them to T helper (T_H) cells. These in turn stimulate B cells to differentiate into precursors of IgA-secreting plasma cells. Stimulated B and T cells emigrate via the local draining lymph nodes, enter the circulation, and finally relocate in various mucosal effector sites, including the stoma of the salivary glands where terminal differentiation of the B lymphoblasts into IgA-secreting plasma cells occurs under the regulation of cytokines secreted by the T and epithelial cells. The secreted polymeric IgA is taken up by polymeric Ig receptor (secretory component) on the basolateral surface of glandular epithelial cells and transported to the apical surface, where it is released with bound secretory component to form S-IgA. Small amounts of circulating IgM, IgG, and IgA transude through the gingival crevice into the oral cavity, and may also penetrate the dentinal tubules from the pulp cavity of the teeth. In advanced periodontal disease, foci of plasma cells in the gingiva secrete IgM, IgG, and IgA, which exude into the periodontal pockets and oral cavity. (Reprinted from Russell et al[46] with permission.)

All of the cellular components of the immune system, including lymphocytes, macrophages, and neutrophils, are located in the gingival sulcus. Salivary immunoglobulins may act as specific agglutinins of bacteria and prevent colonization. They may also inactivate surface GTFs, resulting in reduced plaque formation. Antibodies that opsonize bacteria assist in phagocytosis by lymphocytes and macrophages.

The common mucosal immune system (CMIS) (Fig 12-6) produces secretory IgA (S-IgA) and consists of B and T cells, macrophages, and specialized epithelial cells that are distributed throughout the mucosa, glands, and lymph nodes.[46] Cells in the crypts of the tonsils and adenoids and on intestinal Peyer's patches in the small intestine contain B and T lymphocytes that are activated by bacteria. Lymphocytes and plasma cells are produced, and these have a homing ability to migrate to various mucosal sites, including salivary glands. Those in the salivary glands produce S-IgA specific for the bacteria that activated the lymphocytes in the CMIS. Researchers have attempted to develop vaccines that would utilize the ability of the

CMIS to produce S-IgA. Studies attempting to produce a vaccine by using a "pill" of bacteria in animal and human studies have obtained questionable results. Because IgG levels are higher than IgA levels in plaque, some investigators believe that serum IgG from the gingival sulcus may have a greater role in providing immunity to caries. While the idea of producing a caries vaccine may be a good one, several problems need to be overcome. Bacteria have the ability to rapidly change their antigenic properties, making a vaccine useless. If one strain of bacteria is eliminated, it may be replaced by an even more virulent strain. Humoral antibodies produced against specific bacteria may have cross-reactivity against body tissues such as the human heart. Finally, the question of how long the immunity might last must be asked. Although S-IgA reactive with GTF has been shown to reduce caries in rats, the possibility of developing successful vaccines against human GTF genes that can rapidly alter their structure is questionable.[47,48] To elicit protection against caries, immunization should occur before tooth eruption. Studies would need to determine whether immunization against *S mutans* is inducible in infants and whether it would be safe; what the effectiveness of the vaccines tested would be; how long it would provide protection against colonization by *S mutans*; and the cost-effectiveness of vaccines compared to other preventive measures.[46]

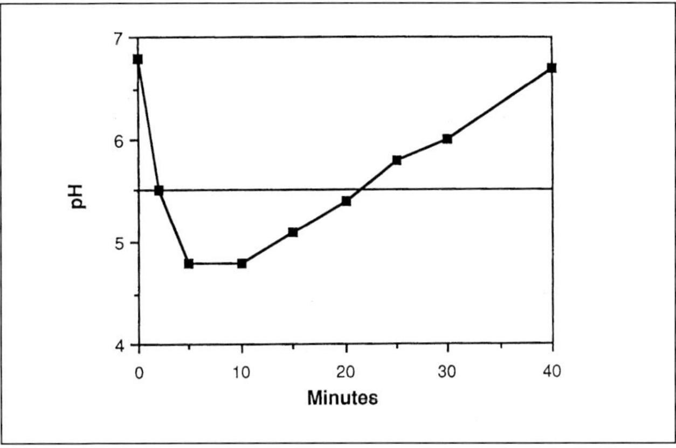

Fig 12-7 The pH of plaque was measured after rinsing the mouth with 10% glucose solution. The line at pH 5.5 is the value at which decalcification of enamel will occur, termed the *critical pH*. The curve is commonly called a *Stephan curve*. (Reprinted from Newman and Nisengard[15] with permission.)

Role of Diet and Nutrition

Diet refers to consumption of food, *nutrition* to the process whereby food is assimilated and metabolized in the production of a systemic effect. The diet's effects on the teeth are seen with the systemic incorporation of fluoride during tooth formation. Likewise, the amounts of calcium and phosphorus in the diet play an important role in tooth development.

The incidence of caries is dramatically affected by diet. Research using electrodes to measure the pH of dental plaque after rinses with glucose showed a rapid drop in pH from 6.8 to 5.0, which lasted about 20 minutes and required about 40 minutes to return to normal (Fig 12-7). The Vipeholm study in Sweden, which examined institutionalized patients,[49] found that caries increased significantly when the intake of sucrose-containing food was increased. That study also showed that sticky and adhesive forms of carbohydrates delayed clearance of the sugars and increased the risk of caries. Other epidemiologic studies of isolated populations have also found that the type and amount of carbohydrate in the diet was directly associated with the amount of caries.

Inorganic phosphates in diets also may have an effect on caries rate. An increase in phosphate ions in saliva may shift the equilibrium dissociation of hydroxyapatite toward the salt in the presence of acids. In addition, phosphate may buffer the organic acids produced by bacteria and may alter the ability of bacteria to adsorb to the pellicle. Other dietary components, including lipids, plant extracts, and trace elements, have been studied with inconclusive results.

Role of Fluoride in Caries

Fluoride has three principal mechanisms for arresting or preventing caries. First, fluoride inhibits bacterial metabolism after diffusing into the bacterial cytoplasm, not as the fluoride ion (F–) but as the unchanged form (HF).[12,50-53] Once in the bacterial cell, HF dissociates and releases the F– that interferes with enzyme activity. Second, fluoride can prevent demineralization because carbonated hydroxyapatite (CAP) is much more soluble in acid than hydroxyapatite (HAP), which in turn is much more soluble than fluorapatite (FAP). Studies have shown that when fluoride is concentrated into a new crystal surface during remineralization, it decreases enamel solubility.[54,55] If fluoride is in plaque fluid at the time of acid formation by bacteria, it will travel with the acid into the subsurface of the tooth and adsorb to the crystal surface, protecting it against demineralization. Third, fluoride enhances remineralization by adsorbing to HAP crystals and attracting calcium and phosphate ions from supersaturated saliva, leading to new mineral formation. This remineralized veneer excludes carbonate and has a composition somewhere between HAP and FAP.[55] Further acid challenges must be quite strong and prolonged to dissolve the remineralized enamel.

Antibacterial Caries Control

Because caries is a transmissible disease, it would be logical to use antibacterial therapy to control it. Traditional restorative work may remove bacteria at the site of the restoration, but caries can nonetheless continue unchecked elsewhere in the mouth. Although chlorhexidine gluconate rinses have been used for years in European countries, an antibacterial approach to the prevention of dental caries is rarely used in the US.[56-58] It is now accepted that high levels of mutans streptococci and lactobacilli constitute a "high bacterial challenge."[59] This challenge can be balanced by numerous protective factors to prevent progression of caries. If the factors are out of balance, caries either progresses or reverses. Studies have shown that the most successful antibacterial therapy for caries control is chlorhexidine gluconate.[60] Daily doses for 2 weeks reduce the cariogenic bacteria in the mouth to such a level that it takes 3 to 6 months for recolonization.[56] So-called dip slides have been used in Europe to determine whether the bacterial challenge is high, medium, or low. Two days after a saliva sample is taken on the dip slide, the levels of *S mutans* and lactobacilli bacteria in the mouth are determined.[56] More precise methods of determining the microbial challenge using molecular methods or monoclonal antibody probes should be available in the near future.

In the future, restorations for the treatment of caries will be used only as a last resort when other intervention measures have failed. Chairside bacterial probes will be used to determine the cariogenic bacterial challenge. Immunization and the production of S-IgA may be used to prevent colonization of teeth by specific bacteria. Genetically engineered plant immunoglobulins may be applied to the surfaces of teeth to inhibit recolonization by specific bacteria.[61,62] Early detection methods that may be available in the future include fluorescence, tomography, electrical impedance, and ultrasonography.[13] Early detection will allow intervention with remineralization via salivary enhancement and application of fluoride and chlorhexidine along with good oral hygiene. Lasers may be used in the future to remove caries and make the adjacent tooth structure highly resistant to acid dissolution.[63,64]

Bacteria Associated with Deep Caries

What bacteria cause pulpal death is still uncertain, partly because caries progresses so slowly, but also because the bacteria are in a dynamic ecosystem. *S mutans* is regarded as one of the main cariogenic species, but lactobacilli have also been identified as participants in deep caries lesions.[65-67] Proteolytic bacteria such as anaerobic streptococci have also been isolated from deep caries,[68,69] while anaerobic rods, such as *Bacteroides*, *Eubacterium*, and *Fusobacterium*, have been associated with symptomatic pulps or abscesses.[70-72] Thus, there is a transition from predominantly facultative gram-positive rods and cocci in shallow decay to anaerobic gram-negative rods and anaerobic gram-positive cocci in infected root canals.

In a microbiologic study of deep carious dentin in human teeth with irreversible pulpitis, gram-positive rods including lactobacilli were the most common isolate,[73] gram-positive cocci were the second most common, and *S mutans* was present in low numbers in the deep layers. Two types of deep caries lesions were detected. In the first group of 15 deep caries lesions, lactobacilli constituted 92% of the bacteria isolated, while the second most frequent isolate was gram-positive cocci; however, *S mutans* and alpha hemolytic streptococci were not cultured from these sites. The third most common organism was anaerobic, gram-positive, nonlactobacillus rods identified as *Propionibacterium*, *Bifidobacterium*, and *A viscosus*. In the second group of 14 deep caries lesions with low numbers of lactobacilli, the flora were much more diverse, consisting of gram-positive cocci, anaerobic gram-positive nonbranching rods, branching rods, and *Bacteroides*.[73] Black-pigmented bacteria were numerous in three of the low lactobacillus lesions. Invasion of the pulp by black-pigmented bacteria and other anaerobes from the periodontal sulcus or periodontal pocket is a likely source of the microorganisms.[74] Black-pigmented bacteria have been associated with symptomatic endodontic infections.[70,71,75,76] Their relationship with low lactobacillus lesions may suggest a relationship with pulpal necrosis and the presence of black-pigmented bacteria in deep caries.[73]

There has been no consistent correlation between clinical and histologic findings in pulpal disease.[77,78] Immunohistologic studies have demonstrated the presence of immune components in the pulp consistent with an immune response, including lymphocytes, plasma cells, IgG, IgA, and the third component of complement[79-82] (see also chapter 11). An investigation using electron microscopy of pulps with irreversible pulpitis found lymphocytes and macrophages as the predominant cells in the inflammatory infiltrates.[83] Another study used monoclonal antibodies to determine the types of lymphocytes in pulps extirpated from teeth clinically diagnosed as either normal, reversibly inflamed, or irreversibly inflamed (Fig 12-8).[84] Helper (T4) cells predominated in normal pulp tissue. In the group with reversible pulpitis, 90% of the lymphocyte population was T lymphocytes, with a T4/T8 ratio of 0.56. In the irreversible pulpitis group, the ratio of T4/T8 lymphocytes was 1.14.[84] In addition, the ratio of B/T lymphocytes was 1.60.[84] It appears that the T4 cells may have a regulatory effect on B cell activities. The increase in concentration of lymphokines released by T4 cells, including those inducing the production of immunoglobulin by B cells, could likely result in pathologic changes.[85,86] When IgG in the supernatant fluids from pulpal explant cultures of teeth

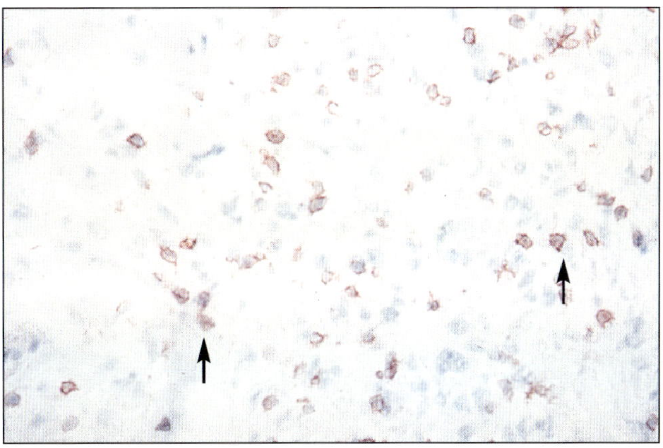

Fig 12-8 Positively stained T8 lymphocytes *(arrows)* in an irreversible pulpitis sample using anti-T8 monoclonal antibody (original magnification ×800). (Courtesy of Dr Ellen Hahn[84].)

with caries was allowed to react with a panel of bacteria implicated in endodontic infections, IgG was found to specifically react with bacteria isolated from deep caries.[86] IgG reacted with species of *Lactobacilli*, *Actinomyces*, *Eubacterium*, and *S mutans*.[85,86] The presence of immunoglobulins along the walls of dentinal tubules has been associated with the protein-adsorbing property of HAP.[86-88] Immunoglobulins have been observed near the pulpal side of the dentinal tubules under incipient caries and later seen extending toward a caries lesion as it invaded more deeply.[89] The presence of immunoglobulins in dentinal tubules has also been shown to decrease tubular permeability and perhaps protect the pulp from invasion by bacterial antigens or other toxic by-products of the bacteria[90] (see also chapter 4).

The correlation between thermal sensitivity and isolated bacteria from deep caries has been investigated.[91] Gram-positive cocci and non-black-pigmented *Bacteroides (Prevotella)* were positively associated with sensitivity to both cold and hot thermal tests. The presence of black-pigmented bacteria, *S mutans*, and high anaerobic counts were positively related to heat sensitivity.[91]

Microorganisms in Pulpal Disease

Under the proper conditions, normal oral flora may become opportunistic pathogens. Such organisms have the capability of producing disease if they gain access to normally sterile areas of the body such as the dental pulp or periradicular tissues. Virulence is the degree of pathogenicity produced by microbes. Following bacterial invasion of the dental pulp and periradicular tissues, the host responds with both nonspecific inflammatory responses and specific immunologic responses (see chapters 10 and 11). Clinicians should remember that the biologic rationale of endodontic therapy is based on disrupting and removing the microbial ecosystem that is associated with the disease process.

Pulpitis includes increased vascular permeability, vasodilation, pain, and resorption of hard tissues, and eventually leads to pulpal necrosis. Dendritic cells have been demonstrated in the pulp that activate T-lymphocytes, which in turn promote a local immune response.[92-94] If infection of the root canal system is not treated, inflammation with accompanying bone resorption spreads to the contiguous periradicular tissues.

Infection of the Root Canal System

Caries is the main source of the bacteria infecting the pulp space. When the tooth is intact, enamel and dentin provide protection against microbial invasion of the pulp space. As caries approaches the pulp, tertiary dentin is produced (see also chapter 3). Bacterial movement through the dentinal tubules is restricted by odontoblast processes, mineralized crystals, and macromolecules including immunoglobulins in the tubules[90] (chapter 4). Bacteria and their by-products may have an effect on the pulp before direct exposure[85-97] (Fig 12-9). If, as a result of trauma, a healthy vital pulp is exposed, the penetration of tissue by bacteria is relatively slow, while penetration of the dentin has been shown to be less than 2 mm after 2 weeks.[98] However, if the pulp is necrotic, "dead tracts" of empty dentinal tubules are rapidly penetrated by microorganisms (Fig 12-10). The breakdown products of a necrotic pulp—serum and tissue fluid—form the periradicular tissues, while bacterial by-products provide the nutrients for invading organisms.

Bacteria and their by-products may reach the pulp space through the apical foramen and other lateral, accessory, or furcation canals. The question of whether periodontal disease directly causes pulpal disease has been controversial.[99-102] One study found that pulpal necrosis occurs only when periodontal disease extends to the apical foramen.[101] The number of spirochetes present in exudate draining from the sulcus may be used to

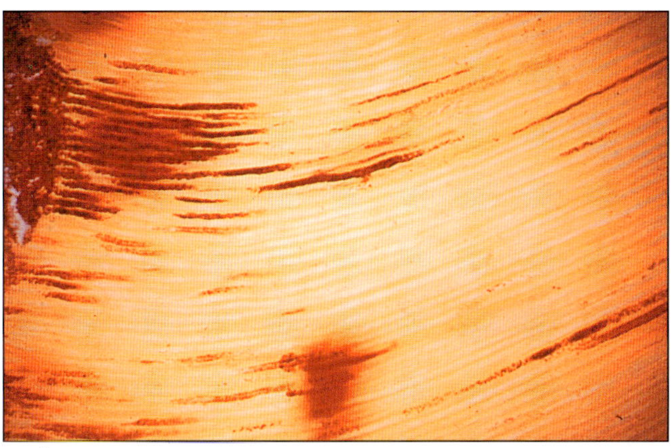

Fig 12-9 Section through tooth with caries on left side and stained bacteria penetrating into dentinal tubules (Brenn and Brown stain, original magnification ×100). (Courtesy of Dr Henry O. Trowbridge.)

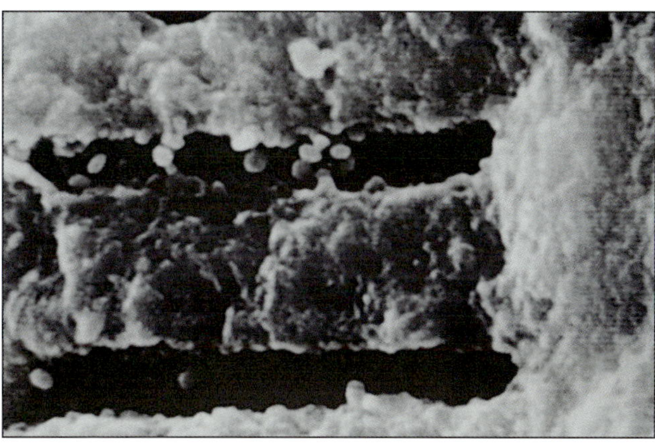

Fig 12-10 Scanning electron microscope view of cocci in dentinal tubules.

determine whether the infection is of endodontic or periodontal origin. Abscesses of periodontal origin contained 30% to 58% spirochetes, while abscesses of endodontic origin contained less than 10% spirochetes.[103]

A much less likely pathway of bacteria for endodontic infections is *anachoresis*, whereby microbes are transported through the blood or lymph to an area of inflammation such as an inflamed pulp. This phenomenon has been demonstrated in animals but is not believed to significantly produce disease in humans.[104-106] However, anachoresis may be the pathway whereby some traumatized teeth become infected.[107] Anachoresis could not be demonstrated in unfilled root canals from which the pulp had been removed.[108,109]

Microbes in Endodontic Infections

In 1894, W. D. Miller was the first to associate the presence of bacteria with pulpal disease.[110] In 1965, Kakehashi et al[111] demonstrated that bacteria cause pulpal and periradicular disease[111] (Fig 12-11). When pulps were exposed in rats with normal microbial flora, pulpal necrosis and periradicular lesions formed; however, when the pulps were exposed in germ-free rats, no pathologic changes were evident. Dentinal bridging was evident in the germ-free rats regardless of the severity of the pulpal exposure. This research conclusively demonstrated that bacteria are the cause of pulpal and periradicular disease.[111]

Modern culturing methods allow cultivation of several strains of bacteria from each endodontic infection. Polymicrobial infections of a root canal are usually associated with a periradicular inflammatory lesion. The number of colony-forming units (CFUs) cultivated from an infected root canal is usually between 10^2 and 10^8. Studies have shown a positive correlation between the number of bacteria in an infected root canal and the size of periradicular radiolucencies.[76-113]

A majority of the bacteria isolated from an endodontic infection are anaerobic (Box 12-1). Considering that there are over 500 species of cultivable bacteria in the oral cavity, only a relatively small group of bacteria has been cultured and isolated. Bacteria that are strict anaerobes only grow in an environment with low oxidation-reduction potential in an absence of oxygen. Some strains may be microaerophilic. Strict anaerobic bacteria lack the superoxide dismutase and catalase enzymes. Endodontic infections do con-

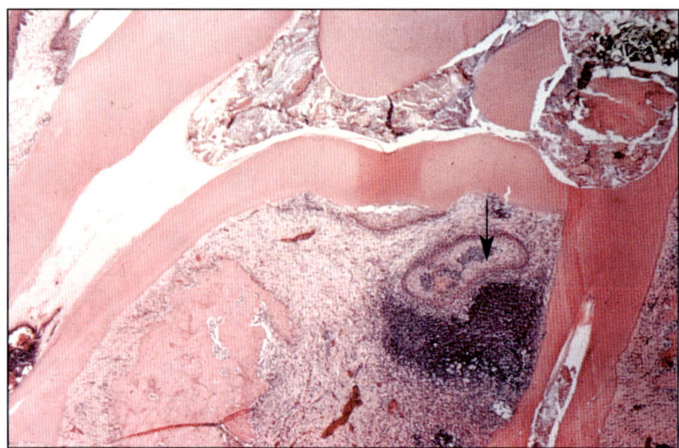

Fig 12-11a Pulp exposed in conventional rat with normal oral flora showing pulpal inflammation and necrosis *(arrow)* (H&E stain, original magnification ×40). (Courtesy of Dr Harold R. Stanley.)

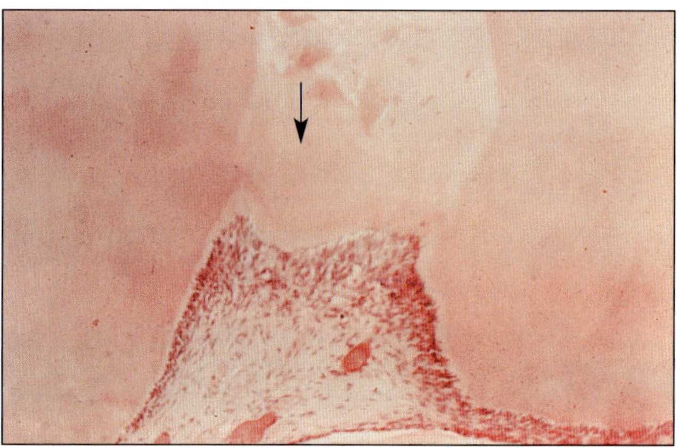

Fig 12-11b Pulp exposed in germ-free rat showing matrix production over area of pulp exposure *(arrow)*. Note completion of bridge with vital noninflamed pulp tissue under exposure site (H&E stain, original magnification ×40). (Courtesy of Dr Harold R. Stanley.)

tain some species of facultative anaerobic bacteria that can grow either in the presence or absence of oxygen. Because bacteria isolated from root canals are usually a subgroup of the bacteria found in the sulcus or periodontal pockets, it is believed that the sulcus is the source of bacteria in root canal infections.[114]

The selective process and interrelationships of bacteria have been studied in monkeys.[115-117] In the root canals of monkeys infected with indigenous oral bacteria and then sealed in the pulp space, anaerobic bacteria predominated over period of time.[115-117] After nearly 3 years of pulpal infection, 98% of the bacteria cultured from the canals were strict anaerobes. Tissue fluid, serum, necrotic pulp tissue, low oxygen tension, and bacterial by-products within an infected root canal provide a selective environment for strict anaerobes. In addition, bacterial metabolites may be antagonistic to other bacteria. As described earlier, some bacteria produce bacteriocins. When intact teeth with necrotic pulps were cultured, over 90% of the bacteria were strict anaerobes.[70] When cultures were taken from the apical 5 mm of infected root canals of carious exposed teeth, 67% of the bacteria were strict anaerobes.[118] This suggests a selective process for strict anaerobes in infected root canals.

Based on cultivation studies, several species of black-pigmented bacteria—peptostreptococci, peptococci, *Fusobacterium* sp, *Eubacterium* sp, and *Actinomyces* sp—have been implicated in causing certain clinical signs and symptoms.[70,71,75,76,119-129] However, no absolute correlation has been made between any species of bacteria and the severity of endodontic infections. This may be related to the polymicrobial nature of endodontic infections and relationships between bacteria or virulence factors that increase the overall pathogenic effect. Even current state-of-the-art culturing techniques detect and identify only a portion of the total microbial population. Conventional identification of bacteria is based on gram-staining, colonial morphology, growth characteristics, and biochemical tests. Often, the best that can be done is a presumptive identification.

Culturing and identification of bacteria has traditionally been referred to as the "gold standard." Today, the use of molecular techniques to detect and precisely identify the bacteria allows us to better understand the microbial ecosystem associated with endodontic infections; this is referred to as the "DNA standard." A recent study used the polymerase chain reaction (PCR) to detect *Porphyromonas endodontalis* in root canals associated with both symptomatic and asymptomatic infections.[130] *P endodontalis* was detected in 17 of 43 (40%) infected canals, in 4 of the 6 cases (66%) with acute periradicular abscess, and in 13 of the 37 (35%) other cases. *P endodontalis* was associated with an asymptomatic periradicular lesion in 6 cases (25%) and with tenderness to percussion in 10 of 19 teeth (53%). One investigation using PCR did not detect *P endodontalis* in closed periradicular lesions, while another study using DNA hybridization detected *P endodontalis* in 35% of the cases with pain and in 24% of the cases with swelling.[131,132] No absolute relationship between the presence of *P endodontalis* or any other species of bacteria has been identified. It is also possible that *P endodontalis* does not necessarily play an important role in the pathogenesis of acute periradicular lesions. Another study using DNA:DNA hybridization of extracts from necrotic pulps found bacterial DNA in 100% of the samples; an average of five species was identified in each necrotic pulp, of which *Bacteroides forsythus* was both the most prevalent and the most concentrated.[133] Interrelationships between species of bacteria and their virulence factors need further research. Virulence factors can vary from one strain of bacteria to another strain within the same species. These studies suggest that some species of bacteria may have the potential to progress to symptomatic pathoses.

Endodontic infections progress from an infected root canal to contiguous periradicular tissues. Periradicular abscesses of endodontic origin are mixed infections from which several strains of bacteria may be cultured.[70,71,75,76,119,129] Strains of black-pigmented bacteria in pure culture usually produce only a mild infection in animals. However, mixed with *Fusobacterium nucleatum*, multiple abscesses and even death of the animals may result[134-139] (see also chapters 11 and 17).

Box 12-1 Bacteria from the root canals of teeth with apical rarefactions*

- *Fusobacterium nucleatum*
- *Streptococcus* species
- *Bacteroides* species†
- *Prevotella intermedia*
- *Peptostreptococcus* species
- *Eubacterium* species
- *Lactobacillus* species
- *Capnocytophaga ochracea*
- *Veillonella parvula*
- *Porphyromonas endodontalis*
- *Prevotella buccae*†
- *Prevotella oralis*†
- *Proprionibacterium propionicum*
- *Prevotella denticola*
- *Prevotella loescheii*
- *Prevotella nigrescens*
- *Actinomyces* species
- *Porphyromonas endodontalis*
- *Porphyromonas gingivalis*
- *Enterococcus faecalis*

*Data from Van Winkelhoff et al,[71] Sundqvist,[76] Baumgartner and Falkler,[118] Dougherty et al,[144] Baumgartner and Watkins,[146] and Sundqvist et al.[163]

†Nonpigmenting species.

Numerous taxonomic changes have been made as improved bacterial identification methods have evolved. Based on precise identification of bacteria at a DNA level, identification of bacteria at the species level in older studies is very questionable. Black-pigmented bacteria previously placed in the genus *Bacteroides* have now been placed in the genera *Porphyromonas* (asaccharolytic) and *Prevotella* (saccharolytic) (Box 12-2). The species *Prevotella nigrescens* was recently separated from *Prevotella intermedia*.[140] It has been determined that *P nigrescens* is actually the black-pigmented bacteria most commonly cultivated from endodontic infections.[141-144]

Molecular techniques were recently used to identify five strains of black-pigmented bacte-

Box 12-2 Recent taxonomic changes for previous "*Bacteroides*" species

- *Porphyromonas* black-pigmented (asaccharolytic *Bacteroides* species):
  - *Porphyromonas asaccharolyticus* (usually nonoral)
  - *Porphyromonas gingivalis**
  - *Porphyromonas endodontalis**
- *Prevotella* black-pigmented (saccharolytic *Bacteroides* species):
  - *Prevotella melaninogenica*
  - *Prevotella denticola*
  - *Prevotella loescheii*
  - *Prevotella intermedia**
  - *Prevotella nigrescens*†
  - *Prevotella corporis*
  - *Prevotella tannerae*
- *Prevotella* nonpigmented (saccharolytic *Bacteroides* species):
  - *Prevotella buccae**
  - *Prevotella bivia*
  - *Prevotella oralis*
  - *Prevotella oris*
  - *Prevotella oulorum*
  - *Prevotella ruminicola*

*Studies have associated this species with clinical signs and symptoms.
† Most common species of black-pigmented bacteria isolated from endodontic infections.

ria.[145] Culture and biochemical tests previously identified these strains as *P intermedia*.[146] Using SDS-PAGE, they were differentiated from *P intermedia* and believed to be *P nigrescens*.[142] However, after using molecular methods and comparing gene sequences in a gene bank, they have been identified as *Prevotella tannerae*.[145] When 118 microbial samples from endodontic infections were examined using PCR with specific primers for *P tannerae*, 60% were found to be positive for the presence of the organism,[145] suggesting that *P tannerae* is commonly present in endodontic infections but not routinely cultivable. There may be many other species, including pathogenic organisms yet to be characterized, that are not cultivable.

The teleologic purpose of chronic periradicular lesions (periapical granulomas) is believed to be prevention of the spread of infection to surrounding tissues (see chapter 17). A classic statement of this belief is "a granuloma is not an area in which bacteria live, but an area in which they are destroyed."[147] However, using careful experimental methods that minimize contaminants, investigators have been able to culture bacteria from samples taken from asymptomatic chronic periradicular lesions.[148-151] More recent studies have used DNA-DNA hybridization to detect and identify bacteria in asymptomatic lesions.[152,153] Although bacterial DNA was detected in 100% of the periradicular samples collected from submarginal incisional biopsies, this finding may overestimate the incidence of bacteria in the periradicular tissue. Microbial contaminants may be present in these studies from the surgical procedure by contamination from the root end (foramen) during curettage of the sample. A microbial plaque that has been demonstrated at the root end of infected roots would be likely to contaminate any periradicular sample curetted from the root end.[154] However, evidence supports the hypothesis that under certain conditions bacteria do invade periradicular tissues since numerous strains are found in periradicular abscesses. It is possible that sometime before formation of a symptomatic abscess/cellulites, microbial invasion takes place without the inflammatory response being symptomatic. Using detection methods less sensitive than DNA:DNA hybridization (ie, light and electron microscopy), investigators[155] were able to detect bacteria in 4 symptomatic granulomas and 1 symptomatic cyst out of a total of 31 apical lesions. Taken together, current evidence indicates that bacteria exist in periradicular tissue beyond the apical foramen in necrotic teeth under at least certain conditions such as symptomatic periradicular abscesses. No consensus on their existence in the asymptomatic periradicular lesion has yet been formed.

Species of *Actinomyces* and *Propionibacterium* have been shown to persist in inflammatory tissue.[120,156,157] *Actinomyces israelii* is a species

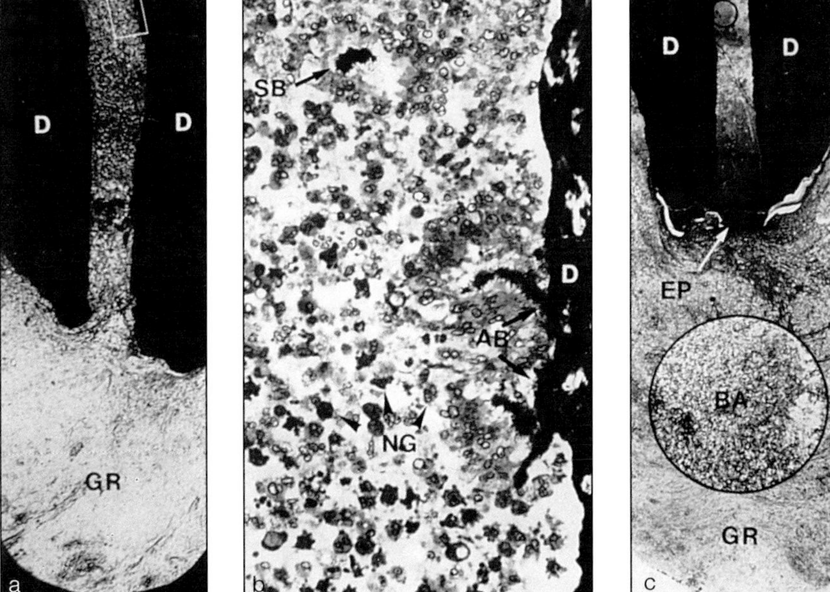

Fig 12-12 Endodontic flora in the apical third of an infected root canal with attached periradicular granuloma (GR in *a* and *c*). The foramen appears to be blocked by a wall of neutrophils (NG in *b*) or by an epithelial plug (EP in *c*) in the apical foramen. Note the dense aggregates of bacteria (AB in *b*) sticking to the dentinal wall (D) and similar ones (SB in *b*) along with loose collections of bacteria (*inset*) remaining suspended in the root canal among neutrophils (*a*, original magnification ×50; *b*, original magnification ×400; *c*, original magnification ×40). (Reprinted from Nair[155] with permission.)

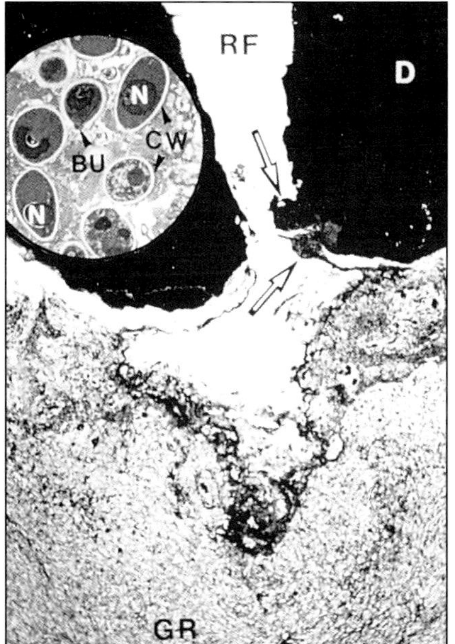

Fig 12-13 Presence of fungi in the root canal and apical foramen of a root-filled (RF) tooth with a therapy-resistant lesion (GR). Note the two clusters of microorganisms located between the dentinal wall (D) and the root filling *(arrows)*. The inset photo shows an electron microscopic view of the organisms. They are about 3 to 4 μm in diameter and reveal a distinct cell wall (CW), nuclei (N), and budding forms (BU) (original magnification ×100). (Reprinted from Nair et al[164] with permission.)

of bacteria isolated from periradicular tissues identified as unresponsive to conventional root canal therapy.[120,156,157] However, both sodium hypochlorite and calcium hydroxide have been shown to be highly effective in destroying A israelii.[158] Apparently, both nonsurgical and surgical endodontics provide a high success rate without antibiotics.[120,156,158] *Actinomyces* may be detected in histopathologic specimens as "sulfur granules," yet the apical lesion heals without antibiotic therapy. Antibiotic therapy is indicated when a periradicular infection with *A israelii* does not resolve following endodontic surgery.[158]

Enterococcus faecalis has been associated with failed endodontically treated teeth requiring retreatment.[159-163] A recent study reported that complete periradicular healing occurred in 94% of cases following a negative culture at the obturation appointment, compared with only 68% if the cultures were positive at the time of obturation.[159] These findings support previous studies suggesting that failure of healing is likely due to the presence of bacteria in the root canal at the time of obturation.[164,165]

In addition to bacteria, viruses and fungi have been the subject of recent investigations.[164,166-168] Studies have demonstrated the presence of fungi following therapy-resistant endodontic treatment[163,164-169] (Figs 12-12 and 12-13). A recent investigation showed that strains of *Candida albicans* required incubation with a saturated solution of calcium hydroxide for about 16 hours to kill 99.9% of the fungi.[170] Fungi were identified in 7% of 692 samples of therapy-resistant chronic apical periodontitis.[169] In another study, scanning electron microscopy was used to observe fungi in the dentinal tubules of 4 out of 10 extracted human molars with infected root canals.[166] In another recent study, PCR was used to detect *Candida albicans* in 5 of 24 intact teeth with infected root canals, but no fungi in 19 samples aspirated from periradicular abscesses/cellulitis.[171]

Bacterial Virulence Factors

Bacteria have numerous virulence factors, including bacterial capsules, fimbriae (pili), lipopolysaccharides (LPSs), enzymes, extracellular vesicles, fatty acids, polyamines, ammonia, and hydrogen sulfide. Both gram-positive and gram-negative bacteria have capsules that may protect the bacteria from phagocytosis (Fig 12-14).[137] Fimbriae and extracellular vesicles from the outer membrane may participate in aggregation of bacteria or attachment to tissues (Fig 12-15).[137] Sex pili are important for the exchange of DNA during conjugation. The DNA may contain a virulence factor such as a gene for resistance to an antibiotic.

When LPS is released from the outer membrane of gram-negative bacteria, it is called *endotoxin*. Endotoxin has several biologic effects, among which are the activation of complement and bone resorption.[172,173] The concentration of endotoxin has been shown to be higher in the canals of symptomatic teeth than in asymptomatic teeth.[174] LPS from black-pigmented bacteria may be involved in periradicular periodontitis by inducing cytokines or humoral immune responses.[175] Other components of the bacterial cell wall, including lipoteichoic acid, peptidoglycan, and muramyl dipeptide, have been shown to stimulate the production of cytokines.[176-179]

Bacterial enzymes may be associated with pulpal and periradicular pathogenesis. The spread of cellulitis is believed to be associated with the microbial production of collagenase.[180-182] Collagenase has been detected in strains of *Porphyromonas gingivalis*, but not in strains of *Porphyromonas endodontalis* isolated from endodontic infections.[183] Sonicated extracts of *Fusobacterium nucleatum* and strains of black-pigmented bacteria have been shown to stimulate the production of metalloproteases.[184] Bacteria produce other enzymes that neutralize immunoglobulins and the components of complement.[185-187] In addition to bacteria, the neutrophils in abscesses lyse and release their enzymes to form purulent exudates, which have an adverse effect on the surrounding tissues.

Extracellular vesicles are formed from the outer membrane of gram-negative bacteria; like the parent bacteria, they have a trilaminar structure (see Fig 12-14a). Because they have the same surface antigens as the parent bacteria, they are capable of neutralizing antibodies against the parent organism. In addition, vesicles may contain enzymes or other toxic agents. Extracellular vesicles are believed to be involved in hemagglutination, hemolysis, bacterial adhesion, and proteolytic action on host tissues.[188-189]

Propionic, butyric, and iso-butyric acids are the short-chain fatty acids most commonly produced by bacteria in endodontic infections. Short-chain fatty acids affect neutrophil chemotaxis, degranulation, chemiluminescence, and phagocytosis. Butyric acid is capable of inhibiting T-cell blastogenesis, and it stimulates the production of interleukin-1, which is associated with bone resorption.[190]

Polyamines are biologically active compounds involved in the regulation of growth, regeneration of tissues, and modulation of inflammation. They include spermine, spermidine, cadaverine, and putrescine. Polyamines, produced by both bacteria and host cells, are found in infected root canals. Teeth that are painful to percussion or have spontaneous pain have been shown to have a higher concentration of putrescine and total polyamines in necrotic pulps.[190]

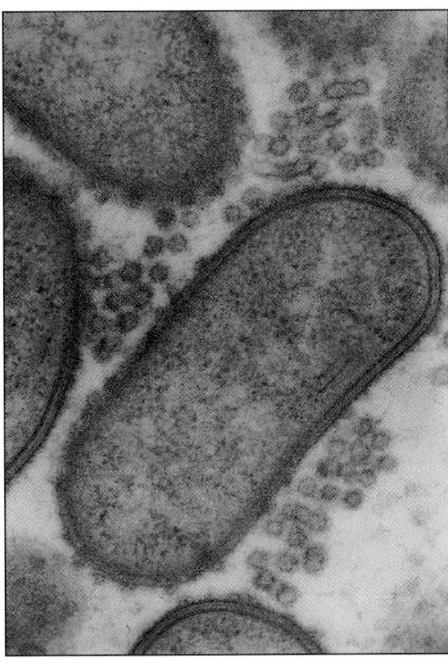

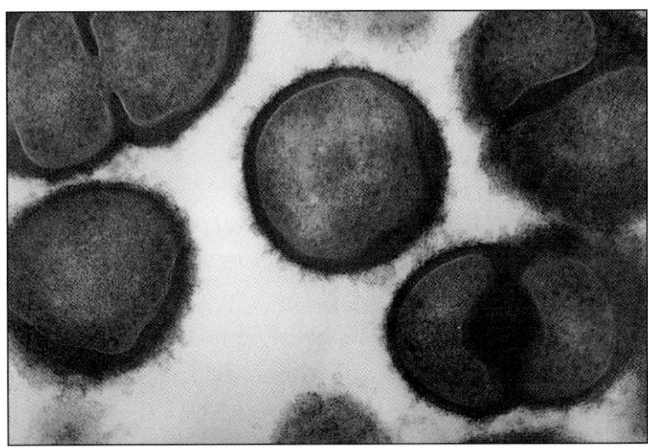

Fig 12-14b TEM view of gram-positive bacteria *(Peptostreptococcus anaerobius)*. Note cells undergoing binary fission and cell wall with thick layer of peptidoglycan and capsular material.

Fig 12-14a TEM view of gram-negative bacteria *(Prevotella intermedia)*. Note inner and outer cell wall membranes with capsular material. In addition, note vesicles extruded from the cell wall.

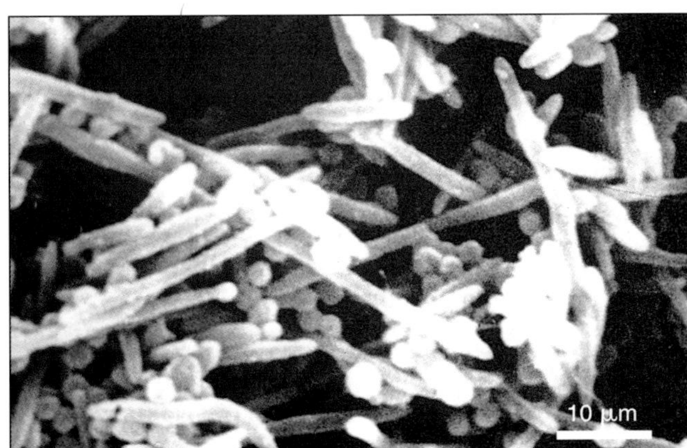

Fig 12-15a SEM view of coaggregation between *Fusobacterium nucleatum* and *Porphyromonas gingivalis*. (Reprinted from Kinder and Holt[189] with permission.)

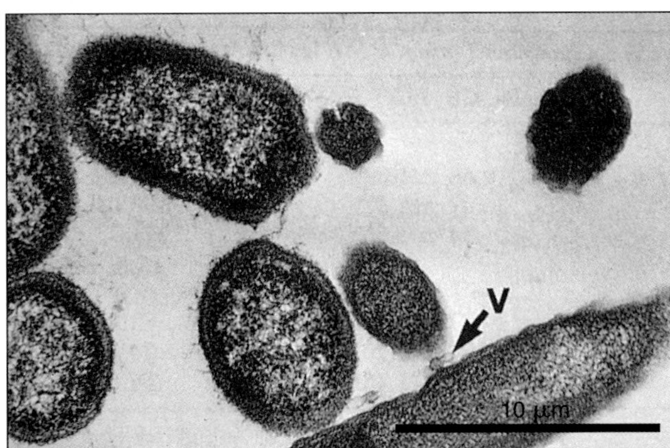

Fig 12-15b TEM view of coaggregation between *Fusobacterium nucleatum* and *Porphyromonas gingivalis* with vesicle (v) contributing to cell interaction. (Reprinted from Kinder and Holt[189] with permission.)

Management of Pulpal/Endodontic Infections

Correct diagnosis and removal of the cause of an infection from the pulp space are the keys to successful treatment. Debridement of the infected root canals and incision for drainage of a periradicular swelling in an otherwise healthy patient usually leads to rapid recovery from the original signs and symptoms. The reduction and elimination of bacteria from the root canal system following pulpal infection is necessary for successful endodontics.[111,191] Root canals obturated after a negative culture have a better prognosis than teeth filled following a positive culture.[159,165,192] Several studies have demonstrated the antimicrobial efficacy of irrigating with sodium hypochlorite and placing calcium hydroxide in infected root canals between appointments.[112,193-195] The use of modern-day obturating techniques after appropriate cleaning and shaping produces a predictably high clinical success rate.

Endodontic Abscesses/ Cellulitis Following Pulp Space Infection

If bacteria from the infected root canal space invade the periradicular tissue and the immune system is not able to suppress the invasion, an otherwise healthy patient will eventually present with the signs and symptoms of an acute periradicular abscess and/or cellulitis. An abscess is a nonspecific inflammatory response to the presence of bacteria in normally sterile tissues (Fig 12-16). The seriousness of the infection is related to the numbers and virulence of the bacteria, host resistance, and associated anatomic structures. An abscess by definition is an accumulation of purulent exudate consisting of bacteria, bacterial by-products, inflammatory cells (mainly neutrophils), lysed inflammatory cells, and the contents of those cells (enzymes, etc). A cellulitis is defined as a diffuse, erythematous mucosal or cutaneous infection that may spread to deeper facial spaces and become life threatening. A needle aspirate often reveals pockets of purulence within a diffuse cellulitis. From a clinical viewpoint, a cellulitis and an abscess may be considered a continuum of the inflammatory process.

A patient with an abscess/cellulitis usually presents with an obvious swelling and mild to severe pain. The swelling may be localized to the vestibule or extend into a fascial space. Patients may have clinical signs or symptoms indicating systemic manifestations of the infection. These include fever, chills, lymphadenopathy, malaise, headache, and nausea. The involved tooth may not show radiographic evidence of periradicular disease. In most cases, the tooth will be sensitive to biting pressure, touch, and percussion. The periradicular area will likely be tender to palpation. In general, treatment of an abscess/cellulitis includes incision and drainage and root canal debridement to remove the source of the infection. Adjunctive antibiotic therapy is indicated if there are systemic symptoms or fascial space swelling, or if the patient is medically compromised. Fascial space infections of endodontic origin are infections that have spread into the fascial spaces of the head and neck from the periradicular area of a tooth. This may be determined by the location of the root end of the involved tooth in relation to its overlying buccal or lingual cortical plate and the relationship of the apex with the attachment of a muscle. The infected root canal causing an abscess/cellulitis serves as a source of infection for the periradicular area and for possible secondary (metastatic) spread to the fascial spaces of the head and neck. The infected root canal as a source or focus of infection should be differentiated from the so-called theory of focal infection, which was advanced in the early part of the 20th century (1910–1940) and is no longer considered valid. According to this theory, pulpless and endodontically treated teeth may leak bacteria and/or toxins into the body, and this causes arthritis and diseases of the kidney; heart;

nervous, gastrointestinal, and endocrine systems; and other degenerative diseases. Most dentists and physicians accepted the theory, which resulted in the needless extraction of millions of teeth. However, it also encouraged research, which eventually led to the current scientific and biologic basis for root canal treatment. The removal of bacteria and necrotic pulpal substrate supporting the growth of bacteria is a cornerstone of endodontic treatment.

The use of antibiotics should be considered adjunctive to appropriate clinical treatment. The adjunctive prescription of antibiotics is recommended for endodontic infections that include fever (>100°F), malaise, cellulitis, unexplained trismus, and progressive/persistent swelling. The prescription of antibiotics is empirically based on knowledge of the bacteria most likely associated with endodontic infections. An antibiotic regimen should continue for 2 to 3 days following resolution of the major clinical signs and symptoms. Thus, antibiotics are usually taken for 6 to 10 days following initial diagnosis and treatment of the infection. Penicillin V, amoxicillin, and clindamycin continue to be the antibiotics of choice for treatment of an endodontic infection. Metronidazole may be used in combination with the penicillins. Clarithromycin or azithromycin may be used as alternatives to erythromycin, which does not have efficacy against strict anaerobes.[196]

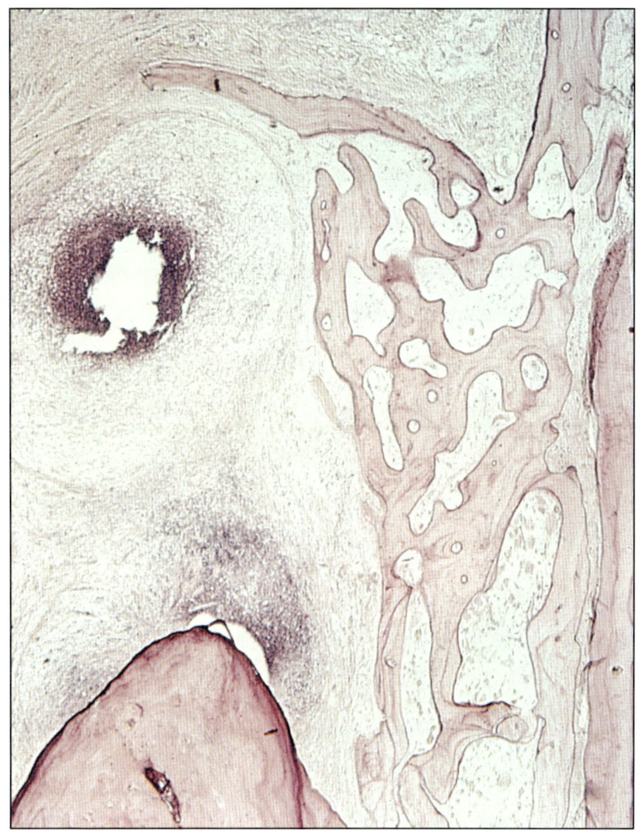

Fig 12-16 Serial section from cadaver specimen showing a periradicular abscess disassociated from the tooth believed to be the source of the infection. This supports capability of bacteria in root canal infections to invade periradicular tissue (H&E stain, original magnification ×40). (Courtesy of Dr Henry O. Trowbridge.)

References

1. Bowen W. Wither or whither caries research? Caries Res 1999;33:1-3.
2. Featherstone J. Prevention and reversal of dental caries: Role of low level fluoride. Community Dent Oral Epidemiol 1999;27:31-44.
3. Kaste L, Selwitz R, Oldakowski R, Brunella J, Winn D, Brown L. Coronal caries in the primary and permanent dentition of children and adolescents 1-17 years of age: United States, 1988-1991. J Dent Res 1996;75:61-41.
4. Speechley M, Johnston D. Some evidence from Ontario, Canada, of a reversal in the dental caries decline. Caries Res 1996;30:423-427.
5. Burt BA, Fejerskov O. Water fluoridation. In: Fejerskov O, Ekstrand J, Burt BA (eds). Fluoride in Dentistry. Copenhagen: Munksgaard, 1996.
6. Hargreaves JA, Thompson GW, Wagg BJ. Changes in caries prevalence in Isle of Lewis children between 1971 and 1981. Caries Res 1983;17:554-559.
7. Jenkins GN. Recent changes in dental caries. Br Med J 1985;291:1297-1298.
8. Murray JJ. Fluorides in Caries Prevention, ed 3. Oxford: Butterworth-Heinemann, 1991.
9. Newbrun E. Effectiveness of water fluoridation. J Public Health Dent 1989;49:279-289.
10. Sanz M, Newman MG. Dental plaque and calculus. In: Newman MG, Nisengard RJ (eds). Oral Microbiology and Immunology. Philadelphia: Saunders, 1988.
11. Keyes P. The infectious and transmissible nature of experimental dental caries. Findings and implications. Arch Oral Biol 1960;1:304-320.

12. Featherstone J, Goodman P, McLean J. Electron microscope study of defect zones in dental enamel. J Ultrastruct Res 1979;67:117–123.
13. Featherstone J. The science and practice of caries prevention. J Am Dent Assoc 2000;131:887–899.
14. Silverstone L. Structure of carious enamel, including the early lesion. Oral Sci Rev 1973;3:100–160.
15. Newman MG, Nisengard RJ (eds). Oral Microbiology and Immunology, ed 2. Philadelphia: Saunders, 1988.
16. Simmonds R, Tompkins G, George R. Dental caries and the microbial ecology of dental plaque: A review of recent advances. N Zealand Dent J 2000;96:44–49.
17. Hohwy J, Kilian M. Colonal diversity of the Streptococcus mitis biovar 1 population in the human oral cavity and pharynx. Oral Microbiol Immunol 1995;10:19–25.
18. Marsh P. Microbial ecology of dental plaque and its significance in health and disease. Adv Dent Res 1994;8: 263–271.
19. Coykendall A. Proposal to elevate the subspecies of *Streptococcus mutans* to species status, based on their molecular composition. Int J Systemat Bacteriol 1977;27:26–30.
20. Coykendall A. *Streptococcus sobrinus* nom. rev. and *Streptococcus ferus* nom. rev.: Habitat of these and other mutans streptococci. Int J Systemat Bacteriol 1983;33:883–885.
21. Van Houte J, Lopman J, Kent R. The predominant cultivable flora of sound and carious human root surfaces. J Dent Res 1994;73:1727–1734.
22. Schenkels L, Veerman E, Nieuw Amerongen A. Biochemical composition of human saliva in relation to other mucosal fluids. Crit Rev Oral Biol Med 1995;6: 161–175.
23. Mandel I, Wotman S. The salivary secretions in health and disease. Oral Sci Rev 1976;8:25–47.
24. Tabak L, Bowen W. Roles of saliva (pellicle), diet and nutrition on plaque formation. J Dent Res 1989;68: 1560–1566.
25. Whittaker C, Klier D, Kolenbrander P. Mechanisms of adhesion by oral baceria. Ann Rev Microbiol 1996;50: 513–552.
26. Rolla S, Bonesvoll P, Opermann R. Interactions between oral streptococci and salivary proteins. In: Kleinberg I, Ellison S (eds). Saliva and Dental Caries. Stony Brook, NY: State Univ of New York, 1979:227.
27. Brooks W, Demuth D, Gil S, Lamont R. Identification of a *Streptococcus gordonii* SspB domain that mediates adhesion to *Porphromonas gingivalis*. Infect Immun 1997;65:3753–3758.
28. Talay S, Valentin-Weigand P, Jerlstrom P, Timmis KN, Chhatwal GS. Fibronectin-binding protein of *Streptococcus pyogenes*: Sequence of the binding domain involved in adherence of streptococci to epithelial cells. Infect Immun 1992;60:3837–3844.
29. Love R, McMillan M, Jenkinson H. Invasion of dentinal tubules by oral streptococci is associated with collagen recognition mediated by the antigen I/II family of polypeptides. Infect Immun 1997;65:5157–5164.
30. Fischetti V. Streptococcal M protein: Molecular design and biological behavior. Clin Microbiol Rev 1989;2: 285–314.
31. Cisar JO. Coaggregation reactions between oral bacteria. In: Genco RJ, Mergenhagen SE (eds). Host-Parasite Interactions in Periodontal Diseases. Washington: ASM, 1982:121–131.
32. Newbrun E. Cariology, ed 3. Chicago: Quintessence, 1989.
33. James S, Tagg J. The prevention of dental caries by BIS-mediated inhibition of mutans streptococci. New Zealand Dent J 1991;87:80–83.
34. Kelstrup J, Gibbons R. Inactivation of bacteriocins in the intestinal canal and oral cavity. J Bacteriol 1969;99: 888–890.
35. Jack R, Tagg J, Ray B. Bacteriocins of Gram-positive bacteria. Microbiologic Rev 1995;59:171–200.
36. Hillman J, Novak J, Sagura E, Gutierrez JA, Brooks TA, Crowley PJ, et al. Genetic and biochemical analysis of mutacin 1140, an antibiotic from *Streptococcus mutans*. Infect Immun 1998;66:2743–2749.
37. Loyola-Rodriguez J, Morisaki I, Kitamura K, Hamada S. Purification and properties of extracellular mutacin, a bacteriocin from *Streptococcus sobrinus*. J Gen Microbiol 1992;138:269–274.
38. Hillman J, Dzuback A, Andrews S. Colonization of the human oral cavity by a *Streptococcus mutans* mutant producing increased bacteriocin. J Dent Res 1987;66: 1092–1094.
39. Dunny G, Craig R, Carron R, Clewell D. Plasmid transfer in *Streptococcus faecalis*: Production of multiple sex pheromones by recipients. Plasmid 1979;2:454–465.
40. Liljemark W, Bloomquist C. Human oral microbial ecology and dental caries and periodontal diseases. Crit Rev Oral Biol Med 1996;7:180–198s.
41. Yamashita Y, Bowen W, Burne R, Kuramitsu H. Role of the *Streptococcus mutans* gtf genes in caries induction in the specific-pathogen-free rat model. Infect Immun 1993;61:3811–3817.
42. Loesche W. Role of *Streptococcus mutans* in human dental decay. Microbiologic Rev 1986;50:353–380.
43. Chia J, Lin S, Hsu T, Chen JY, Kwan HW, Yang CS. Analysis of a DNA polymorphic region in the gtfB and gtfC genes of *Streptococcus mutans*. Infect Immun 1993; 61: 1563–1566.
44. Jenkinson H, Lamont R. Streptococcal adhesion and colonization. Crit Rev Oral Biol Med 1997;8:175–200.
45. Poulsen K, Reinholdt J, Jespersgaard Cea. A comprehensive genetic study of streptococcal immunoglobulin A1 proteases: Evidence for recombination within and between species. Infect Immun 1998;66:181–190.

46. Russell M, Hajishengallis G, Childers N, Michalek S. Secretory immunity in defense against cariogenic mutans streptococci. Caries Res 1999;33:4–15.
47. Bork P. Mobile modules and motifs. Curr Opin Struct Biol 1992;2:413–421.
48. Childers N, Zhang S, Harokopakis E, Harmon C, Michalek S. Properties of practical oral liposome-*Streptococcus mutans* glucosyltransferase vaccines for effective induction of caries protection. Oral Microbiol Immunol 1996;11:172–180.
49. Gustafsson B, Quensel C, Lanke L, Lundquist C, Grahnen H, Bonow B, et al. The Vipeholm dental caries study. The effect of different levels of carbohydrate intake on caries activity in 436 individuals observed for five years. Acta Odontol Scand 1954;11:232.
50. Featherstone J, Nelson D, McLean J. An electron microscope study of modifications to defect regions in dental enamel and synthetic apatites. Caries Res 1981;15:278–288.
51. Hamilton I, Bowden G. Fluoride Effects on Oral Bacteria. Copenhagen: Munksgaard, 1996.
52. Van Louveren C. The antimicrobial action of fluoride and its role in caries inhibition. J Dent Res 1990;69:676–681.
53. Whitford G, Shuster G, Pashley D, Venkateswarlu P. Fluoride uptake by *Streptococcus mutans* 6715. Infect Immunol 1977;18:680–687.
54. Fejerskov O, Thylstrup A, Larsen M. Rational use of fluorides in caries prevention. A concept based on possible cariostatic mechanisms. Acta Odontol Scand 1981;39:241–249.
55. Ten Cate J, Featherstone J. Mechanistic aspects of the interactions between fluoride and dental enamel. Crit Rev Oral Biol Med 1991;2:283–296.
56. Anderson M, Bales D, Omnell K. Modern management of dental caries: The cutting edge is not the dental bur. J Am Dent Assoc 1993;124:37–44.
57. Anusavice K. Treatment regimens in preventive and restorative dentistry. J Am Dent Assoc 1995;129:727–743.
58. Anusavice K. Efficacy of nonsurgical management of the initial caries lesion. J Dent Educ 1997;61:895–905.
59. Leverett D, Proskin H, Featherstone J. Caries risk assessment in a longitudinal discrimination study. J Dent Res 1993;72:538–543.
60. Featherstone J, Zero D. Laboratory and Human Studies to Elucidate the Mechanism of Action of Fluoride-Containing Dentifrices. Oxford: Oxford University Press, 1992.
61. Ma J, Lehner T, Stabila P, Bux C, Hiatt A. Assembly of monoclonal antibodies with IfF1 and IgA heavy chain domains in transgenic tobacco plants. Eur J Immunol 1994;24:131–138.
62. Ma J, Hikmat B, Wycoff K, Vine ND, Chargelegue D, Yu L, et al. Characterization of a recombinant plant monoclonal secretory antibody and preventive immunotherapy in humans. Nat Med 1998;4:601–606.
63. Featherstone J, Barrett-Vesone N, Fried D, Kantorowitz Z, Seka W. CO_2 laser inhibitor of artificial caries-like lesion progression in dental enamel. J Dent Res 1998;77:1397–1403.
64. Kantorowitz Z, Featherstone J, Fried D. Caries prevention by CO_2 laser treatment: Dependency on the number of pulses used. JADA 1998;129:585–591.
65. Edwardsson S. Bacteriological studies on deep areas of carious dentine. Odontol Revy 1974;25:1–143.
66. Hoshino E. Predominant obligate anaerobes in human dentin. J Dent Res 1985;64:1195–1199.
67. McKay G. The histology and microbiology of acute dentine lesions in human permanent molar teeth. Arch Oral Biol 1976;21:51–58.
68. Burnett G, Scherp H. Bacteriologic studies of the advancing lesion. J Dent Res 1951;30:766–777.
69. Parikh S, Toto P, Grisamore T. Streptococcal hyaluronidase in dentin caries. J Dent Res 1965;44:996–1001.
70. Sundqvist G, Johansson E, Sjögren U. Prevalence of black-pigmented *Bacteroides* species in root canal infections. J Endod 1989;15:13–19.
71. Van Winkelhoff AJ, Carlee AW, de Graaff J. *Bacteroides endodontalis* and other black-pigmented *Bacteroides* species in odontogenic abscesses. Infect Immun 1985;49:494–497.
72. Zavistoski J, Dzink J, Onderdonk A, Bartlett J. Quantitative bacteriology of endodontic infections. Oral Surg 1980;49:171–174.
73. Hahn C-L, Falkler WA Jr, Minah GE. Microbiological studies of carious dentine from human teeth with irreversible pulpitis. Arch Oral Biol 1991;36:147–153.
74. Adriaens PA. Ultrastructural observations on bacterial invasion in cementum and radicular dentin of periodontally diseased human teeth. J Periodontol 1988;59:493.
75. Griffee MB, Patterson SS, Miller CH, Kafrawy AH, Newton CW. The relationship of *Bacteroides melaninogenicus* to symptoms associated with pulpal necrosis. Oral Surg 1980;50:457–461.
76. Sundqvist GK. Bacteriological Studies of Necrotic Dental Pulps [odontological dissertation no. 7]. Umea, Sweden: Univ of Umea; 1976.
77. Baum BJ. Has modern biology entered the mouth? The clinical impact of biological research. J Dent Educ 1991;55:299–303.
78. Seltzer S, Bender IB, Ziontz M. The dynamics of pulp inflammation: Correlations between diagnostic data and actual histologic findings in the pulp. Oral Surg 1963;16:846–977.

79. Honjo H, Tsubakimoto K, Utsumi N, Tsutsui M. Localization of plasma proteins in the human dental pulp. J Dent Res 1970;49:888.
80. Pulver WH, Taubman MA, Smith DJ. Immune components in normal and inflamed human dental pulp. Arch Oral Biol 1977;22:103-111.
81. Pekovic DD, Fillery ED. Identification of bacteria in immunopathologic mechanisms of human dental pulp. Oral Surg 1984;57:652-661.
82. Speer ML, Madonia JV, Heuer MA. Quantitative evaluation of the immunocompetence of the dental pulp. J Endod 1977;3:418-423.
83. Mendoza MM, Reader A, Meyers WJ, Foreman DW. An ultrastructural investigation of the human apical pulp in irreversible pulpitis. I. Nerves. J Endod 1987;13: 267-276.
84. Hahn CL, Falkler WAJ, Siegel M. A study of T and B cells in pulpal pathosis. J Endod 1989;15:20-26.
85. Falkler WA, Jr, Martin SA, Tolba M, Siegel MA, Mackler BF. Reaction of pulpal immunoglobulins to oral microorganisms by an enzyme-linked immunosorbent assay. J Endod 1987;13:260-266.
86. Hahn C, Falkler WAJ. Antibodies in normal and diseased pulps reactive with microorganisms isolated from deep caries. J Endod 1992;18:28-31.
87. Ackermans F, Klein JP, Frank RM. Ultrastructural localization of immunoglobulins in carious humane dentine. Arch Oral Biol 1981;26:879.
88. Pashley D, Nelson R, Kepler E. The effects of plasma and salivary constituents on dentin permeability. J Dent Res 1982;61:978-981.
89. Okamura K. Histological study on the origin of dentinal immunoglobulins and the change in their localization during caries. J Oral Pathol 1985;14:680-689.
90. Hahn CL, Overton B. The effects of immunoglobulins on the convective permeability of human dentine *in vitro*. Arch Oral Biol 1997;42:835-843.
91. Hahn CL, Falkler WAJ, Minah GA. Correlation between thermal sensitivity and microorganisms isolated from deep carious dentin. J Endod 1993;19:26-30.
92. Jontell M, Okiji T, Dahlgren U, Bergenholtz G. Immune defense mechanisms of the dental pulp. Crit Rev Oral Biol Med 1998;9:179-200.
93. Jontell M, Bergenholtz G, Scheynius A, Ambrose W. Dendritic cells and macrophages expressing Class II antigens in the normal rat incisor pulp. J Dent Res 1988; 67:1263-1266.
94. Jontell M, Gunraj MN, Bergenholtz G. Immunocompetent cells in the normal dental pulp. J Dent Res 1987; 66:1149-1153.
95. Langeland K. Tissue changes in the dental pulp. Odontol Tidskr 1957;65:239-244.
96. Bergenholtz G, Lindhe J. Effect of soluble plaque factors on inflammatory reactions in the dental pulp. Scand J Dent Res 1975;83:153.
97. Warfvinge J, Bergenholtz G. Healing capacity of human and monkey dental pulps following experimentally induced pulpitis. Endo Dent Traumatol 1986;2: 256-262.
98. Cvek M, Cleaton-Jones PE, Austin JC, Andreason JO. Pulp reactions to exposure after experimental crown fractures or grinding in adult monkeys. J Endod 1982;8: 391-397.
99. Torabinejad M, Kiger RD. A histologic evaluation of dental pulp tissue of a patient with periodontal disease. Oral Surg 1985;59:198-200.
100. Mazur B, Massler M. Influence of periodontal disease on the dental pulp. Oral Surg 1964;17:592-603.
101. Langeland K, Rodrigues H, Dowden W. Periodontal disease, bacteria, and pulpal histopathology. Oral Surg 1974;37:257-270.
102. Czarnecki RT, Schilder H. A histological evaluation of the human pulp in teeth with varying degrees of periodontal disease. J Endod 1979;5:242-253.
103. Trope M, Rosenberg E, Tronstad L. Darkfield microscopic spirochete count in the differentiation of endodontic and periodontal abscesses. J Endod 1992;18:82-86.
104. Gier RE, Mitchell DF. Anachoretic effect of pulpitis. J Dent Res 1968;47:564.
105. Allard U, Nord CE, Sjoberg L, Stromberg T. Experimental infections with *Staphylococcus aureus*, *Streptococcus sanguis*, *Pseudomonas aeruginosa*, and *Bacteroides fragilis* in the jaws of dogs. Oral Surg 1979;48:454-463.
106. Robinson HB, Boling LR. The anachoretic effect in pulpitis. JADA 1941;28:268-270.
107. Grossman LI. Origin of microorganisms in traumatized pulpless sound teeth. J Dent Res 1967;46:551-553.
108. Delivanis PD, Snowden RB, Doyle RJ. Localization of blood-borne bacteria in instrumented unfilled root canals. Oral Surg 1981;52:430-432.
109. Delivanis PD, Fan VSC. The localization of blood-borne bacteria in instrumented unfilled and overinstrumented canals. J Endod 1984;10:521-524.
110. Miller W. An introduction in the study of the bacteriopathology of the dental pulp. Dent Cosmos 1894;36: 505.
111. Kakehashi S, Stanley HR, Fitzgerald RJ. The effects of surgical exposures of dental pulps in germ-free and conventional laboratory rats. Oral Surg 1965;20:340-348.
112. Byström A, Happonen RP, Sjögren U, Sundqvist G. Healing of periapical lesions of pulpless teeth after endodontic treatment with controlled asepsis. Endod Dent Traumatol 1987;3:58-63.
113. Sundqvist G. Taxonomy, ecology, and pathogenicity of the root canal flora. Oral Surg 1994;78:522-530.
114. Kobayashi T, Hayashi A, Yoshikawa R, Okuda K, Hara K. The microbial flora from root canals and periodontal pockets of non-vital teeth associated with advanced periodontitis. Int Endod J 1990;23:100-106.

115. Moller AJR. Influence on periapical tissues of indigenous oral bacteria and necrotic pulp tissue in monkeys. Scand J Dent Res 1981;89:475–484.
116. Fabricius L, Dahlén G, Öhman AE, Möller ÅJR. Predominant indigenous oral bacteria isolated from infected root canals after varied times of closure. Scand J Dent Res 1982;90:134–144.
117. Fabricius L, Dahlén G, Holm SE, Möller ÅJR. Influence of combinations of oral bacteria on periapical tissues of monkeys. Scand J Dent Res 1982;90:200–206.
118. Baumgartner JC, Falkler WA, Jr. Bacteria in the apical 5 mm of infected root canals. J Endod 1991;17:380–389.
119. Yoshida M, Fukushima H, Yamamoto K, Ogawa K, Toda T, Sagawa H. Correlation between clinical symptoms and microorganisms isolated from root canals of teeth with periapical pathosis. J Endod 1987;13:24–28.
120. Happonen RP. Periapical actinomycosis: A follow-up study of 16 surgically treated cases. Endo Dent Traumatol 1986;2:205–209.
121. Heimdahl A, Von Konow L, Satoh T, Nord CE. Clinical appearance of orofacial infections of odontogenic origin in relation to microbiological findings. J Clin Microbiol 1985;22:299–302.
122. Hashioka K, Yamasaki M, Nakane A, Horiba N, Nakamura H. The relationship between clinical symptoms and anaerobic bacteria from infected root canals. J Endod 1992;18:558-561.
123. Drucker D, Lilley J, Tucker D, Gibbs C. The endodontic microflora revisited. Microbios 1992;71:225–234.
124. Gomes B, Lilley J, Drucker D. Clinical significance of dental root canal microflora. J Dent 1996;24:47–55.
125. Gomes B, Drucker D, Lilley J. Positive and negative associations between bacterial species in dental root canals. Microbios 1994;80:231–243.
126. Brook I, Frazier E. Clinical features and aerobic and anaerobic microbiological characteristics of cellulitis. Arch Surg 1995;130:786–792.
127. Brook I, Frazier E, Gher MJ. Microbiology of periapical abscesses and associated maxillary sinusitis. J Periodontol 1996;67:608–610.
128. Haapasalo M, Ranta H, Rantah K, Shah H. Black-pigmented *Bacteroides* spp. in human apical periodontitis. Infect Immun 1986;53:149–153.
129. Haapasalo M. *Bacteroides* spp. in dental root canal infections. Endod Dent Traumatol 1989;5:1–10.
130. de Oliveira J, Siqueira JF Jr, Alves G, Hirata R Jr, Andrade A. Detection of *Porphyromonas endodontalis* in infected root canals by 16s rRNA gene-directed polymerase chain reaction. J Endod 2000;26:729–732.
131. Bogen G, Slots J. Black-pigmented anaerobic rods in closed periapical lesions. Int Endod J 1999;32:204–210.
132. Makkar S, Nissan R, Wilkinson D, Sela M, Stevens R. *Porphyromonas endodontalis* and symptoms from teeth with endodontic infections [abstract]. J Endod 1999; 25:283–287.
133. Siqueira JF Jr, Rocas JN, Souto R, de Uzeda M, Colombo AP. Checkerboard DNA-DNA hybridization analysis of endodontic infections. Oral Surg Oral Med Oral Pathol Oral Radiol Endod 2000;89:744–748.
134. Baumgartner JC, Falkler WA. Experimentally induced infection by oral anaerobic microorganisms in a mouse model. Oral Microbiol Immunol 1992;7:253–256.
135. Brook I, Walker RI. Infectivity of organisms recovered from polymicrobial abscesses. Infect Immunol 1983;42: 986–989.
136. Price SB, McCallum RE. Studies on bacterial synergism in mice infected with *Bacteroides intermedius* and *Fusobacterium necrophorum*. J Basic Microbiol 1987; 27:377–386.
137. Sundqvist G, Bloom GD, Enberg K, Johansson E. Phagocytosis of *Bacteroides melaninogenicus* and *Bacteroides gingivalis in vitro* by human neutrophils. J Periodontal Res 1982;17:113–121.
138. Sundqvist GK, Eckerbom MI, Larsson ÅP, Sjögren UT. Capacity of anaerobic bacteria from necrotic dental pulps to induce purulent infections. Infect Immunol 1979;25:685–693.
139. Van Steenbergen TJM, Kastelein P, Touw JJA, De Graaff J. Virulence of black-pigmented *Bacteroides* strains from periodontal pockets and other sites in experimentally induced skin lesions in mice. J Periodontal Res 1982;17: 41–49.
140. Shah HN, Gharbia SE. Biochemical and chemical studies on strains designated *Prevotella intermedia* and proposal of a new pigmented species, *Prevotella nigrescens* sp. nov. Int J Syst Bacteriol 1992;42:542–546.
141. Gharbia S, Haapasalo M, Shah H, Kotiranta A, Lounatmaa K, Pearce M, et al. Characterization of *Prevotella intermedia* and *Prevotella nigrescens* isolates from periodontic and endodontic infections. J Periodontol 1994; 65:56–61.
142. Bae K, Baumgartner J, Xia T, Whitt B, David L. SDS-PAGE and PCR for differentation of *Prevotella intermedia* and *P nigrescens*. J Endod 1997;25:324–328.
143. Bae K, Baumgartner J, Shearer T, David L. Occurence of *Prevotella nigrescens* and *Prevotella intermedia* in infections of endodontic origin. J Endod 1997;23: 620–623.
144. Dougherty W, Bae K, Watkins B, Baumgartner J. Black-pigmented bacteria in coronal and apical segements of infected root canals. J Endod 1998;24:356–358.
145. Xia T, Baumgartner JC, David LL. Isolation and identification of *Prevotella tannerae* from endodontic infections. Oral Microbiol Immunol 1999;15:273–275.
146. Baumgartner JC, Watkins BJ. Prevalence of black-pigmented bacteria associated with root canal infections. J Endod 1994;20:191.
147. Kronfeld R. Histopathology of the Teeth and Their Surrounding Structures. Philadelphia: Lea & Febiger, 1920.

148. Tronstad L, Barnett F, Riso K, Slots J. Extraradicular endodontic infections. Endod Dent Traumatol 1987;3: 86–90.

149. Iwu C, MacFarlane TW, MacKenzie D, Stenhouse D. The microbiology of periapical granulomas. Oral Surg 1990; 69:502–505.

150. Abou-Rass M, Bogen G. Microorganisms in closed periapical lesions. Int Endod J 1998;31:39–47.

151. Wayman BE, Murata SM, Almeida RJ, Fowler CB. A bacteriological and histological evaluation of 58 peripical lesions. J Endod 1992;18:152–155.

152. Gatti J, Dobrik J, Smith C, White R, Socransky S, Skobe Z. Bacteria of asymptomatic periradicular endodontic lesions identified by DNA-DNA hybridization. Endod Dent Traumatol 2000;16:197–204.

153. Sunde P, Tronstad L, Eribe E, Lind P, Olsen I. Assessment of periradicular microbiota by DNA-DNA hybridization. Endod Dent Traumatol 2000;16:191–196.

154. Tronstad L, Barnett F, Cervone F. Periapical bacterial plaque in teeth refractory to endodontic treatment. Endod Dent Traumatol 1990;6:73–77.

155. Nair PNR. Light and electron microscopic studies of root canal flora and periapical lesions. J Endod 1987;13: 29–39.

156. Sundqvist G, Reuterving CO. Isolation of *Actinomyces israelii* from periapical lesion. J Endod 1980;6:602–605.

157. O'Grady JF, Reade PC. Periapical actinomycosis involving *Actinomyces israelii*. J Endod 1988;14:147–149.

158. Barnard D, Davies J, Figdor D. Susceptibility of *Actinomyces israelii* to antibiotics, sodium hypochlorite and calcium hydroxide. Int Endod J 1996;29:320–326.

159. Sjögren U, Figdor D, Persson S, Sundqvist G. Influence of infection at the time of root filling on the outcome of endodontic treatment of teeth with apical periodontitis. Int Endod J 1997;30:297–306.

160. Ranta H, Haapasalo M, Kontiainen S, Kerosuo E, Valtonen V. Bacteriology of odontogenic apical periodontitis and effect of penicillin treatment. Scand J Infect Dis 1988; 20:187–192.

161. Molander A, Reit C, Dahlen G, Kvist T. Microbiological status of root-filled teeth with apical periodontitis. Int Endod J 1998;31:1–7.

162. Siren E, Haapasalo M, Ranta K, Salmi P, Kerosuo N. Microbiological findings and clinical treatment procedures in endodontic cases selected for microbiological investigation. Int Endod J 1997;30:91–95.

163. Sundqvist G, Figdor D, Persson S, Sjögren U. Microbiologic analysis of teeth with failed endodontic treatment and the outcome of conservative re-treatment. Oral Surg 1998;85:86–92.

164. Nair PNR, Sjögren U, Krey G, Kahnberg KE, Sundqvist G. Intraradicular bacteria and fungi in root-filled, asymptomatic human teeth with therapy-resistant periapical lesions: A long-term light and electron microscopic follow-up study. J Endod 1990;16:580–587.

165. Sjögren U. Success and Failure in Endodontics [dissertation]. Umea, Sweden: Umea Univ, 1996.

166. Sen B, Safavi K, Spangberg L. Growth patterns of *Candida albicans* in relation to radicular dentin. Oral Surg 1997;84:68–73.

167. Glick M, Trope M, Pliskin M. Detection of HIV in the dental pulp of a patient with AIDS. J Am Dent Assoc 1989;119:649–650.

168. Glick M, Trope M, Pliskin E. Human immunodeficiency virus infection of fibroblasts of dental pulp in seropositive patients. Oral Surg 1991;71:733–735.

169. Waltimo TMT, Sirén EK, Torkko HLK, Olsen I, Haapasalo MPP. Fungi in therapy-resistant apical periodontitis. Int Endod J 1997;30:96–101.

170. Waltimo T, Sirén E, Orstavik D, Haapasalo M. Susceptibility of oral *Candida* species to calcium hydroxide in vitro. Int Endod J 1999;32:94–98.

171. Baumgartner JC, Watts CM, Xia T. Occurrence of *Candida albicans* infections of endodontic origin. J Endod 1999;26:695–698.

172. Horiba N, Maekawa Y, Yamauchi Y, Ito M, Matsumoto T, Nakamura H. Complement activation by lipopolysaccharides purified from gram-negative bacteria isolated from infected root canals. Oral Surg 1992;74:648–651.

173. Dwyer TG, Torabinejad M. Radiographic and histologic evaluation of the effect of endotoxin on the periapical tissues of the cat. J Endod 1981;7:31–35.

174. Horiba N, Maekawa Y, Abe Y, Ito M, Matsumoto T, Nakamura H. Correlations between endotoxin and clinical symptoms or radiolucent areas in infected root canals. Oral Surg 1991;71:492–495.

175. Matsushita K, Tajima T, Tomita K, Takada H, Nagaoka S, Torii M. Inflammatory cytokine production and specific antibody responses to lipopolysaccharide from endodontopathic black-pigmented bacteria in patients with multilesional periapical periodontitis. J Endod 1999;25: 795–799.

176. Dewhirst FE. N-acetyl muramyl dipeptide stimulation of bone in tissue culture. Infect Immun 1982;35:133–137.

177. Hausmann E, Weinfield N, Miller W. Effects of lipopolysaccharides on bone resorption in tissue culture. Calcif Tissue Res 1972;9:272–282.

178. Hausmann E, Luderitz O, Knox K, Weinfeld N. Structural requirements for bone resorption by endotoxin and lipoteichoic acid. J Dent Res 1975;54:94–99.

179. Safavi K, Nichols F. Effects of a bacterial cell wall fragment on monocyte inflammatory function. J Endod 2000;26:153–155.

180. Topazian R, Goldberg M. Oral and Maxillofacial Infections, ed 3. Philadelphia: Saunders, 1994.
181. Tamura M, Nagaoka S, Kawagoe M. Interleukin-1 stimulates interstitial collagenase gene expression in human dental pulp fibroblast. J Endod 1996;22:240–243.
182. Barkhordar RA. Determining the presence and origin of collagenase in human periapical lesions. J Endod 1987; 13:228–232.
183. Odell L, Baumgartner J, Xia T, David L. Survey of collagenase gene *prtC* in *porphyromonas gingivalis* and *porphyromonas endodontalis* isolated from endodontic infections. J Endod 1999;25:555–558.
184. Nakata K, Yamasaki M, Iwata T, Suzuki K, Nakane A, Nakamura H. Anaerobic bacterial extracts influence production of matrix metalloproteinases and their inhibitors by human dental pulp cells. J Endod 2000; 26:410–413.
185. Sundqvist GK, Carlsson J, Herrmann BF, Höfling JF, Väätäinen A. Degradation in vivo of the C3 protein of guinea-pig complement by a pathogenic strain of *Bacteroides gingivalis*. Scand J Dent Res 1984;92:14–24.
186. Sundqvist G, Carlsson J, Herrmann B, Tärnvik A. Degradation of human immunoglobulins G and M and complement factors C3 and C5 by black-pigmented *Bacteroides*. J Med Microbiol 1985;19:85–94.
187. Sundqvist G, Carlsson J, Hänström L. Collagenolytic activity of black-pigmented *Bacteroides* species. J Periodontal Res 1987;22:300–306.
188. Shah HH. Biology of the Species *Porphyromonas gingivalis*. Ann Arbor, MI: CRC Press, 1993.
189. Kinder SA, Holt SC. Characterization of coaggregation between *Bacteroides gingivalis* T22 and *Fusobacterium nucleatum* T18. Infect Immun 1989;57:3425–3433.
190. Eftimiadi C, Stashenko P, Tonetti M, Mangiante PE, Massara R, Zupo S, et al. Divergent effect of the anaerobic bacteria by-product butyric acid on the immune response: Suppression of T-lymphocyte proliferation and stimulation of interleukin-1 beta production. Oral Microbiol Immunol 1991;6:17–23.
191. Bergenholtz G. Micro-organisms from necrotic pulp of traumatized teeth. Odontol Rev 1974;25:347–358.
192. Engstrom B, Segerstad LHA, Ramstrom G, Frostell G. Correlation of positive cultures with the prognosis of root canal treatment. Odontol Rev 1964;15:257–270.
193. Byström A, Sundqvist G. Bacteriologic evaluation of the efficacy of mechanical root canal instrumentation in endodontic therapy. Scand J Dent Res 1981;89: 321–328.
194. Byström A, Sundqvist G. The antibacterial action of sodium hypochlorite and EDTA in 60 cases of endodontic therapy. Int Endod J 1985;18:35–40.
195. Shuping GB, Orstavik D, Sigurdsson A, Trope M. Reduction of intracanal bacteria using nickel-titanium rotary instrumentation and various medications. J Endod 2000; 26:751–755.
196. Riley MR. Drug Facts and Comparisons, ed 5. St. Louis: Facts and Comparisons, 2001.

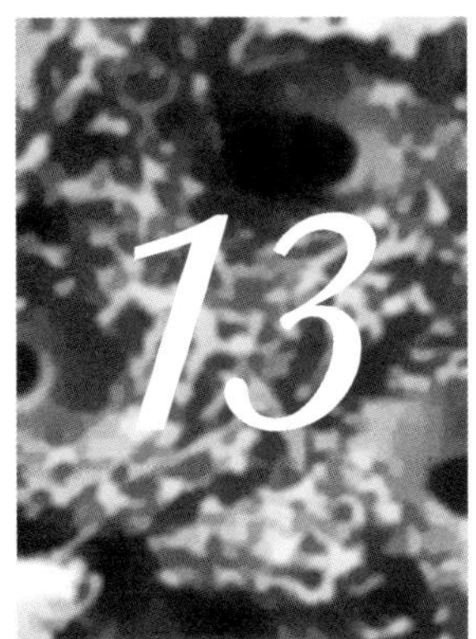

13 Calcium Hydroxide and Vital Pulp Therapy

Harold Stanley, BS, MS, DDS

Vital pulp therapy includes direct and indirect pulp-capping, pulpotomy, and any therapy that minimizes pulpal injury by protecting the pulp from the toxic effects of chemical, bacterial, mechanical, or thermal insult.[1] Vital pulp therapy therefore is aimed at treating reversible pulpal injuries by sealing the pulp and stimulating the formation of tertiary dentinal formation.[2] Pathologic stimuli that may induce reversible pulpitis include attrition, erosion, caries, and restoration placement.[3]

This chapter first explores the factors that affect the success of vital pulp therapy, and then specifically discusses calcium hydroxide treatment, comparing it with treatments using other materials that have been developed and evaluated for vital pulp therapy. Finally, indirect pulpal treatment is reviewed. Elsewhere in this text, see related discussions on mechanisms of dentinal repair (chapter 3) and on materials used in repair of pulpal injury (chapter 14) and restoration of the tooth (chapter 15).

Factors Affecting the Success of Vital Pulp Procedures

Several factors have been shown to influence the success of vital pulp procedures. Some of these are influenced by the clinician's choice of material and technique, and others relate to critical factors influencing case selection. An understanding of these factors is important since they will guide the selection of cases appropriate for vital pulp therapy.

Relative importance of bacteria versus toxicity of dental materials

The classic studies of Kakehashi et al[4] clearly emphasize the pathologic role of bacteria in pulpal exposures (Figs 13-1 to 13-4). In the presence of bacteria, exposed pulpal tissue in conventional rats is partially necrotic by 8 days (Fig 13-1) and completely necrotic with formation of periradicular abscesses by 14 days (Fig 13-2). This response is not seen in germ-free animals with pulpal exposures. Figure 13-3 presents dental pulp at 7 days after exposure in germ-free animals; although food

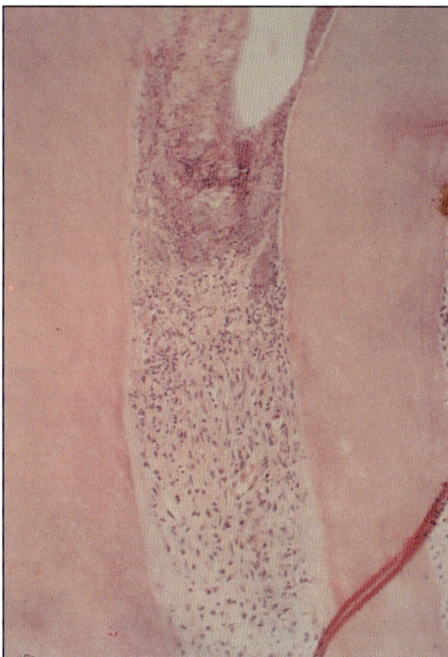

Fig 13-1 Dental pulp 8 days after pulpal exposure in conventional rats. Note the necrotic and vital pulp tissue juxtaposed in the root canal system (H&E stain, original magnification ×100). (Reprinted from Kakehashi et al[4] with permission.)

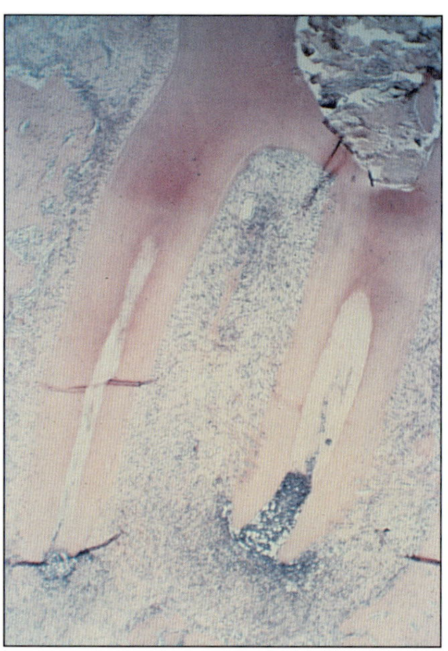

Fig 13-2 Dental pulp 14 days after pulpal exposure in conventional rats. Note the complete necrosis of dental pulp with the development of a periradicular abscess (H&E stain, original magnification ×40). (Reprinted from Kakehashi et al[4] with permission.)

debris has been impacted into the dental pulp, the tissue appears normal. By 32 days after pulpal exposure in germ-free rats, an intact dentinal bridge has developed with subjacent normal dental pulp tissue (Fig 13-4). Thus, bacterial infection of dental pulp constitutes a dominant etiologic factor for pulpal necrosis (see also chapter 12). Vital pulp therapy must, therefore, include those materials and methods that reduce or eliminate this etiologic factor.

The following section reviews those factors that modify pulpal healing for the purpose of developing clinical therapeutic guidelines for vital pulp therapy. Two related issues are considered. First, does the duration of pulpal exposure to the oral environment modify the success of pulp-capping procedures? And second, in comparing various pulp-capping materials, is the ability to form an effective seal against bacterial invasion more important than the toxicity of the material itself?

The duration of pulpal contamination is an important factor in the success of pulp-capping procedures. Many clinicians believe that only uncontaminated pulpal exposures should be treated, and that longer periods of contamination by oral microorganisms and debris lead to reduced success.[5-11] Indeed, the results from animal studies indicate that the success of calcium hydroxide ($Ca[OH]_2$) pulp-capping is reduced from 93% to 56% when microbial contamination is extended from 1 hour to 7 days.[8] However, clinical studies

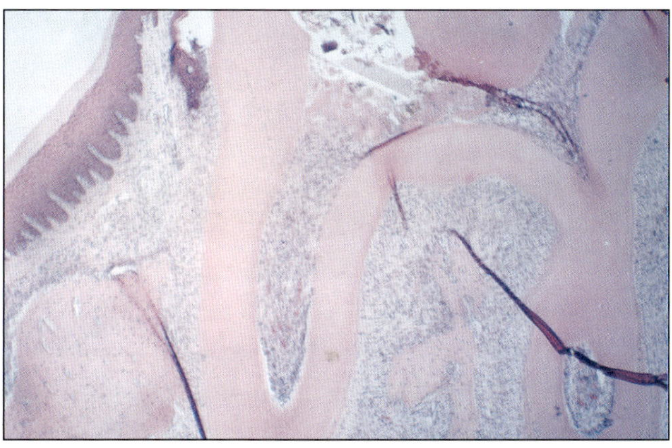

Fig 13-3 Dental pulp 7 days after pulpal exposure in germ-free rats. The dental pulp remains vital even though food debris has been impacted into the exposure site and pulpal tissue (H&E stain, original magnification ×40). (Reprinted from Kakehashi et al[4] with permission.)

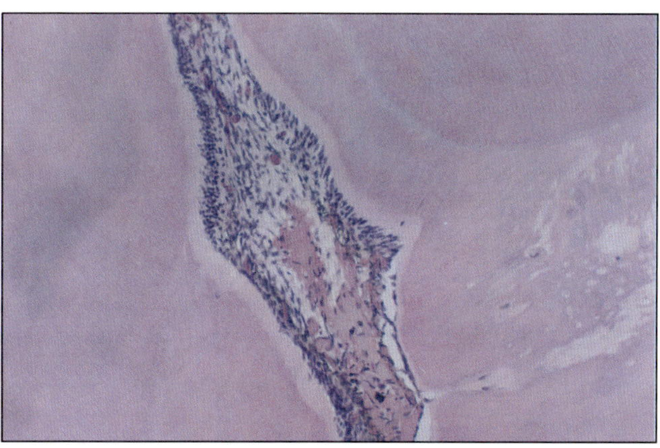

Fig 13-4 Dental pulp 32 days after pulpal exposure in germ-free rats. Note the formation of a dentinal bridge across the exposure with vital and uninflamed dental pulp beneath the bridge (H&E stain, original magnification ×100). (Reprinted from Kakehashi et al[4] with permission.)

in younger patients have shown that the superficial pulp is resistant to bacterial invasion and that partial pulpotomy with $Ca(OH)_2$ dressing results in a 93% radiographic success rate at a mean follow-up of more than 4.5 years.[12,13] In these studies, treatment of pulp that was exposed for up to 2,160 hours had success rates similar to those associated with treatment of pulp exposed for a shorter period of time.[12] Collectively, these studies illustrate that duration of contamination remains an important yet controversial factor in terms of successful pulp-capping.

The second issue concerns the relative importance of bacterial microleakage versus material toxicity. Various materials differ in these properties; some (eg, zinc oxide–eugenol) show greater ability to prevent microleakage while others (eg, zinc phosphate cement) show greater tissue toxicity. Early research focused on tissue toxicity of materials, but in 1971, Brännström and Nyborg[14] demonstrated that infection due to the microleakage of microorganisms around the restoration was the greatest threat to the pulp.[15] Other investigators[16–18] have suggested that pulpal devitalization following a restorative procedure probably results from the combined effect of bacteria, the mechanical injury induced during cutting of the tooth substance, the extent and depth of the cavity preparation, and the toxicity of the restorative materials. However, bacteria are believed to be the predominant factor.[16–18] Pulpal mechanisms proposed to reduce the threat of bacterial invasion include increased outward flow of dentinal fluid (see also chapter 4), emigration of neutrophils into dentinal tubules, and the sequestering of toxic substances (of either restorative or bacterial origin) by their binding to or reacting with dentinal tubule walls.[18]

Taken together, these studies indicate that both bacteria and material toxicity contribute to the development of pulpal pathosis. Dating back to the classic work of Kakehashi and coworkers[4,7] using germ-free animals, an obvious relationship has been established between the presence of microorganisms and the degree of pulpal response. In an excellent review, Bergenholtz[18] states that even a thin wall of primary dentin, if intact, often prevents the deleterious effects of both toxic materials and bacterial leakage. The biocompatibility of materials is directly affected by bacterial contamination (eg, leakage) and their intrinsic toxicity (eg, effects of constituents such as acids and components such as catalysts and photoinitiators). Therefore, both sealing ability and the toxicity of the material are important factors in predicting pulpal responses to vital pulp therapy.[18,19]

Histologic features to be considered when evaluating pulp-capping studies

Size of pulpal exposure

Several studies suggest that the size of the pulpal exposure may influence case selection. Many dentists believe that for pulp-capping to be successful the exposure must be less than 1.0 mm in size and the patient must be young.[20,21] Pulpal exposures that are too large may have greater risk of microleakage or may be very difficult to restore. However, partial pulpotomies after traumatic crown fractures have been shown to produce a 96% success rate with an average 31-month follow-up, even with pulpal exposures ranging from 0.5 to 4.0 mm in size.[12] Thus, the size of the exposure, within a range of 0.5 to 4.0 mm, does not appear to be a major limiting factor in the success of vital pulp therapy. Similar success rates were observed in teeth with immature and mature roots.[12,21] However, it also may be possible for an exposure to be too small for successful pulp-capping. This is based on the author's hypothesis that contact between the pulp-capping agent and dental pulp tissue is essential for stimulating formation of tertiary dentin (see chapter 3). In a minute exposure, it is possible that the dressing may not come into contact with the pulp.[22]

Presence of dentinal chips

The restorative field is usually contaminated with dentinal chips resulting from the use of rotating instruments in caries removal and tooth preparation procedures. The question of whether these dentinal chips promote or retard healing remains controversial. Some researchers believe that dentinal chips encourage the formation of a dentinal bridge, leading some clinicians to use dentinal chips as a dressing material for pulp-capping procedures.[23-25] However, if dentinal chips are forced into the deeper coronal pulp tissue by a rotating instrument, they may produce a pulpitis with abscess formation. Dentinal chips infected with oral microflora may be part of the cause. Another study found that unintentional deep impaction of the medicament and dentinal chips in primary teeth leads to an increased inflammatory response.[26]

Control of hemorrhage and plasma exudate

Pulp-capping agents should never be placed against a bleeding pulp or a clinically observed blood clot. (The use of materials to control hemorrhage and to chemically clean the wound is reviewed in chapter 14.) The need for hemorrhage control was first examined by Marzouk and Van Huysen[27] in 1966, and others have since confirmed its necessity.[28-30] Chiego[31] has suggested that operative trauma may evoke very rapid changes in the dental pulp, leading to permeation and leakage of plasma proteins out of the tubules to the cut dentinal surface (see also chapter 4). Such leakage could inhibit wound healing (ie, dentinal bridge formation).

Extruded pulpal tissue

Pulpal exposure can promote pulpal edema by evoking an acute inflammatory response and, by virtue of the mechanical opening, increasing tissue compliance via the exposure (see chapters 5 and 6). The development of pulpal edema can have several deleterious effects, including extrusion of pulpal tissue, dislodgement of the pulp-capping material, loss of an effective seal against bacterial invasion, development of a chronic inflammatory infiltrate, and inhibition of tertiary dentinal formation. Accordingly, the use of a hemostatic agent may be recommended in the future for all vital pulp procedures. Ideally, clotting of the capillaries within the subjacent pulpal tissue should occur. In contrast, the formation of a macroscopic clot subjacent to the pulp-capping material is not desired because the pulp-capping agent may become intertwined with the extruded pulpal tissue.[21]

Impaction of pulp-capping agents

Impaction of particles of pulp-capping agents into pulpal tissue causes similar effects as impaction of dentinal chips. Ideally, the agent should be placed gently onto the exposed pulpal surface and not into the deeper pulpal tissue, since deep impaction of particles of the pulp-capping material can reduce the success of dentinal bridge formation and healing. Controlling or minimizing impaction is a clinical challenge and one that is not always achieved (Fig 13-5). Several studies have shown that particles of certain $Ca(OH)_2$ formulas can be phagocytosed. Particles no longer chemically active can be retained indefinitely in macrophages and giant cells in the healed area beneath the bridge and adjacent normal areas.[21] One study used a cell culture model system to evaluate the ability of $Ca(OH)_2$ to alter macrophage function.[33] Inflammatory macrophages were obtained from rats, and substrate adherence capacity assays were then carried out. $Ca(OH_2)$ was shown to decrease substrate adherence in a time- and dose-dependent manner. The investigators concluded that $Ca(OH)_2$ could inhibit macrophage function and reduce inflammatory reactions when used in direct pulp-capping and pulpotomy procedures. This may explain, at least in part, the mineralized tissue induction property of the agent.

In another study, an adhesive system applied to exposed human pulp caused large areas of neutrophil infiltration with death of odontoblasts.[34] The inflammatory infiltrate was subsequently replaced with fibroblasts, macrophages, and giant cells in the coronal pulp tissue; this response inhibits pulpal repair or dentinal bridging. Together, these studies suggest that the sealing ability of the agent, the method of placement (eg, minimizing the impaction of pulp-capping agents into dental pulp), and the chemical nature of the pulp-capping material all comprise critical factors in pulpal healing.

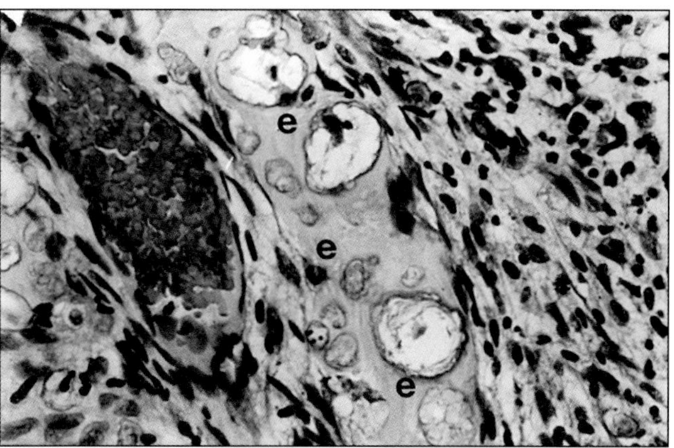

Fig 13-5 The pulpal tissue of an adult patient's premolar extracted 24 hours after the application of a $Ca(OH_2)$ mixture because of the development of an acute pulpitis. Note emboli (e) of $Ca(OH_2)$ mixture lodged within vascular channels (H&E stain, original magnification ×370). (Reprinted from Stanley[32] with permission.)

Embolization of pulp-capping agents

As stated earlier, hemorrhage must be controlled prior to placement of the pulp-capping agent. If open or cut vessels are present, venules can carry capping material particles into the deeper pulpal tissue. In a large mechanical exposure, especially one resulting from a traumatic injury or following a pulpotomy, many vessels may be dilated or transsected. Sometimes particles of the capping material may enter these vessels and travel as emboli until they are lodged in areas where a vessel is diminishing in size as it approaches the apical portion of the root canal (Fig 13-6). At these sites the chemical or caustic effects of agents such as the fresh particles of $Ca(OH)_2$ (if still chemically active and especially if from high-pH formulations) produce perivascular foci of mummification and inflammation. If the particles are from low-pH $Ca(OH)_2$ formulations, they merely block the vessels and decrease pulpal blood flow, which leads to delayed or inadequate healing.

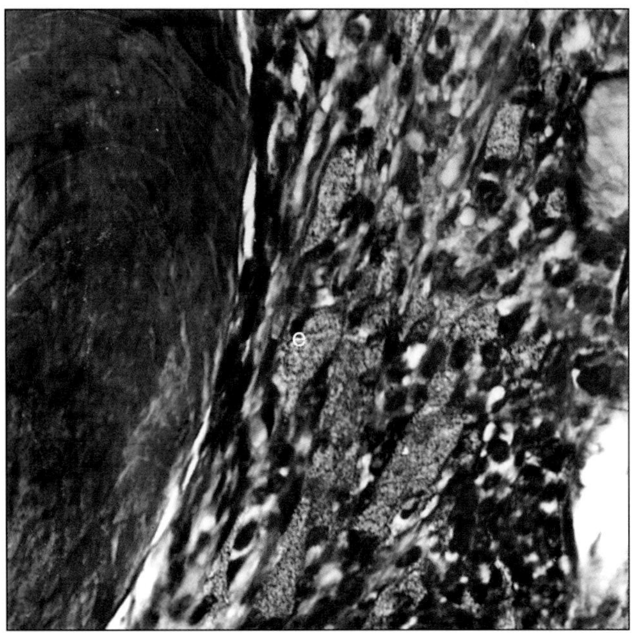

Fig 13-6 Emboli (e) of $Ca(OH_2)$ (Prisma VLC Dycal [Dentsply, York, PA]) in numerous blood vessels far removed from the exposure surface (H&E stain, original magnification ×480). (Reprinted from Stanley and Pameijer[35] with permission.)

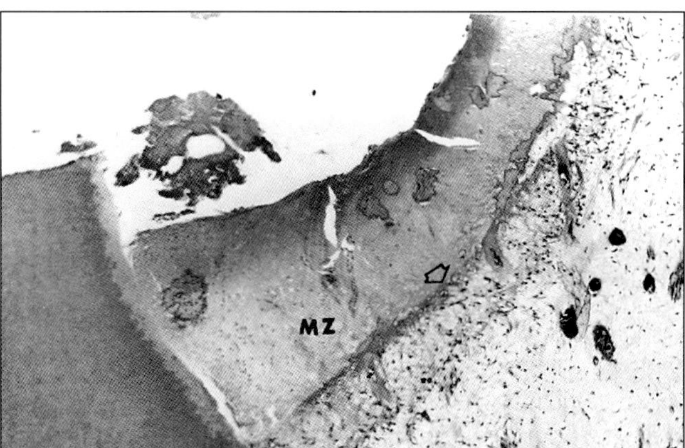

Fig 13-7 Pulpal response to a $Ca(OH_2)$ saline paste at 7 days. Note the thickness of the mummified zone (MZ). The *arrow* denotes the line of demarcation between the mummified zone and the dental pulp. Note also the new layer of odontoblast-like cells forming subjacent to the mummified zone (H&E stain, original magnification ×80). (Reprinted from Turner et al[26] with permission.)

Quality of dentinal bridge

If dentinal bridge formation is essential, then the presence and quality of the dentinal bridge are important prognostic factors for success. A dentinal bridge will form with appropriate $Ca(OH)_2$ treatment, permitting intimate contact with remaining pulpal tissue (Fig 13-7). Although the integrity of a dentinal bridge may be suspect, it nevertheless serves as a physical barrier to protect the pulp. Figures 13-8 and 13-9 show examples of dense, thick bridges that formed over a period of more than 60 days; these can be compared to Fig 13-10, which shows a thin, porous dentinal bridge that formed in 4 weeks. Thus, dentinal bridges may continue to form over time, and most pulps survive despite the presence of a porous dentinal bridge.[21]

Additional studies demonstrate that exposed pulps survive even in the absence of dentinal bridges. The theory is that acid etching and bonding techniques adequately seal the exposure sites from bacterial invasion so that no inflammatory pulpal response can occur, obviating the need for a dentinal bridge. This theory is based on the observation that the fourth-generation (and newer) dentin bonding agents can prevent recontamination of the exposed pulpal surface by forming a seal that protects against bacterial invasion. The bonding agent will penetrate the dentinal tubules approximating the exposure site and create an impenetrable permanent hybrid layer that prevents subsequent microleakage when followed by placement of a permanent restoration. Cox and coworkers[37] demonstrated that when the so-called toxic restorative materials (zinc phosphate, silicate cement, and visible light-cured composite) were placed directly on pulpal exposures, but peripherally sealed with zinc oxide–eugenol to prevent marginal leakage of microorganisms into the pulp, the bridging of the exposures that

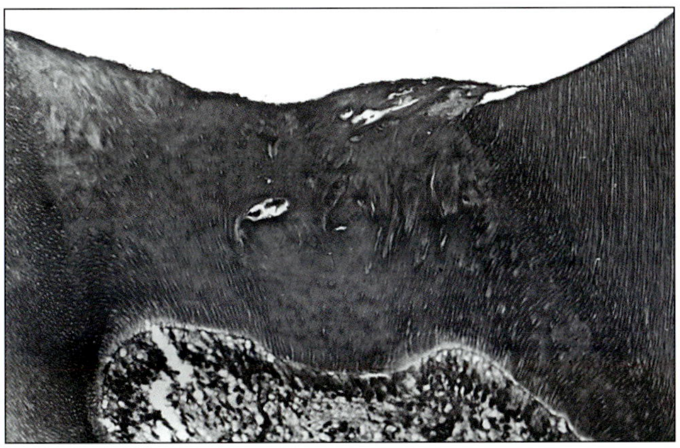

Fig 13-8 Example of a high-quality, dense dentinal bridge in which only one inclusion or tunnel has formed during the 63 days following application of an experimental $Ca(OH)_2$ agent (H&E stain, original magnification ×160). (Reprinted from Stanley[36] with permission.)

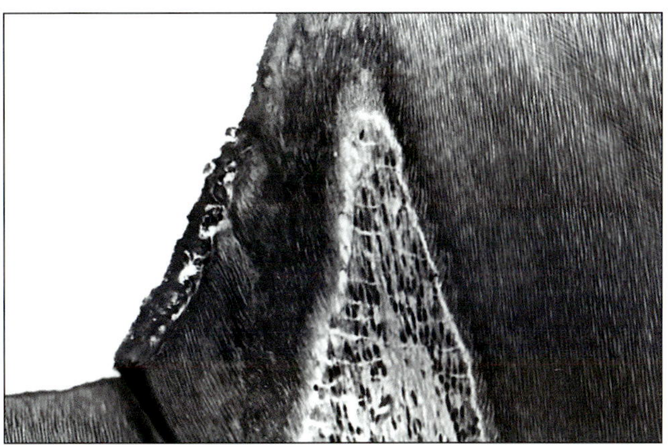

Fig 13-9 Example of a high-quality dentinal bridge exhibiting dentinal tubules without inclusion 67 days after the application of visible light-cured $Ca(OH)_2$ (H&E stain, original magnification ×200). (Reprinted from Stanley[36] with permission.)

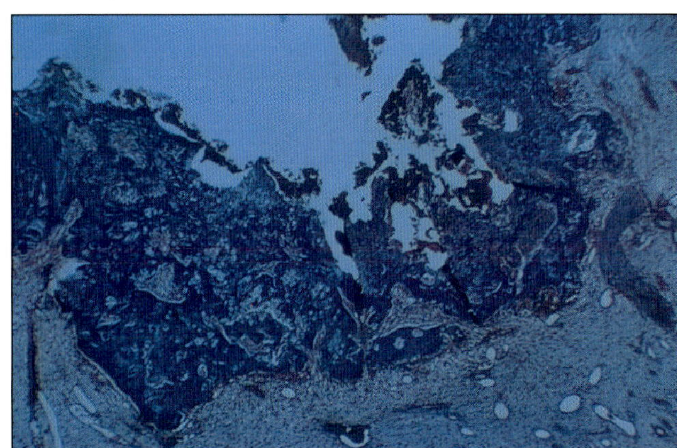

Fig 13-10 Example of a very porous dentinal bridge 4 weeks after a pulpotomy and treatment with Pulpdent paste (Pulpdent, Watertown, MA). (Masson stain, original magnification ×35). (Reprinted from Stanley[36] with permission.)

occurred was similar to that seen after treatment with $Ca(OH)_2$.

There are several limitations to this approach, however. First, long-term success of this seal has yet to be established.[18] Second, although a hybrid layer does form in artificial carious dentin, the bond strength is greatly reduced. Third, the most efficacious bonding technique has yet to be determined. Finally, the pH of the capping material must be considered, especially when using a preparation that causes a high-alkaline reaction. Two studies indicate that acidic materials may also elicit formation of dentinal bridges.[37,38]

Calcium Hydroxide Treatment

From a historical perspective, the introduction of $Ca(OH_2)$ products played an important role in the development of vital pulp therapy. The first materials to show promise as pulp-capping agents were dentinal chips and pastes utilizing $Ca(OH_2)$. Hermann's introduction of the material in 1920 marked a new era in pulp capping when he demonstrated that a $Ca(OH)_2$ formulation called Calxyl (OCO, Dirmstein, Germany) induced dentinal bridging of the exposed pulpal surface.[39-41] Numerous subsequent studies have demonstrated dentinal bridge formation in about 50% to 87% of cases treated with various $Ca(OH)_2$ formulations.[8,42-49] However, despite its long history, use of $Ca(OH)_2$ in vital pulp therapy remains controversial.

Part of this controversy concerns the caustic actions of $Ca(OH)_2$. When applied to dental pulp in the pure state, rather than functioning merely as a biologic dressing, $Ca(OH)_2$ actually destroys a certain amount of pulpal tissue. Numerous studies have shown that $Ca(OH)_2$ is also extremely toxic to cells in tissue culture. This destructive characteristic has triggered efforts to find a formula that can stimulate reparative dentinal bridging without the caustic effect.

Numerous studies have shown that $Ca(OH)_2$ is capable of promoting the formation of reparative dentin at the junction between the caustic zone and vital tissue in human subjects.[37,38] The caustic actions of the high-pH formulations of $Ca(OH)_2$ reduce the size of the subjacent dental pulp by up to 0.7 mm; the thickness of the resulting dentinal bridge has the same effect.[47-51] In contrast, the lower-pH formulations of $Ca(OH)_2$ have only a minor effect since only the thickness of the dentinal bridge reduces the bulk of the remaining vital pulp tissue.[36,52,53]

One advantage of $Ca(OH)_2$ is its antimicrobial property. Classic studies have demonstrated that bacteria represent the primary etiologic agent of pulpal necrosis[4,7] (see Figs 13-1 to 13-4), suggesting that antimicrobial properties may confer therapeutic advantages. Several pulp-capping studies have shown that $Ca(OH)_2$ products are effective in treating intentionally contaminated exposures.[8,36,46,50,54] In one study, canine pulps were exposed to *Streptococcus sanguis* for 2 days prior to placement of $Ca(OH)_2$; nonetheless, thick dentinal bridges formed 10 weeks later.[46] In a primate study with a 1- to 2-year follow-up, $Ca(OH)_2$-induced dentinal bridge formation occurred in 78 (85%) of 91 exposed and contaminated dental pulps, while 10% of the study sample became necrotic.[49] It is difficult, of course, to conduct well-controlled clinical trials evaluating this effect. However, one study has reported that asymptomatic teeth with carious exposures survived an average of 12 years after pulp-capping.[47]

Other studies have evaluated the ultrastructure of $Ca(OH)_2$-formed dentinal bridges, for example, to determine whether the structure was permeable and yet still provided satisfactory pulpal protection.[55] Another study employed scanning electron microscopy (SEM) to evaluate dentinal bridges formed 4 to 15 weeks after pulp-capping deliberately exposed human premolars and third molars with a $Ca(OH)_2$ paste (Pulpdent).[56] Results suggested complete bridging and increasing thickness over longer posttreatment periods. Cross sections of pulps treated for more than 6 weeks demonstrated a superior amorphous layer composed of tissue debris and $Ca(OH)_2$, a middle layer of a coarse meshwork of fibers identified as fibrodentin, and an inner layer showing tubular osteodentin. In a later study using microradiographic techniques, the same three layers in the dentinal bridge were observed, with the middle tubular layer exhibiting the highest mineral content.[57]

A subsequent study compared the hard tissue barrier formed following short-term (10- or 60-minute) applications of either cyanoacrylate or $Ca(OH)_2$ in pulpotomized monkey teeth. The application of $Ca(OH)_2$ increased the incidence of a continuous barrier and its location below the level of the original wound surface. The condition of the pulp was related to the presence of bacteria and the continuity of the hard tissue to the presence of inflammation, suggesting that low-grade irritation was responsible for hard tissue barrier formation.[58] Kirk and Meyer[59] compared $Ca(OH)_2$, zinc oxide–eugenol, and a cortisone and antibiotic combination (Ledermix [Wyeth Lederle, Glostrup, Denmark]) when used over pulpal exposures in rats. $Ca(OH)_2$ rapidly produced complete repair with remarkably regular formation of calcospherites. The other two preparations inhibited bridging of the defect. This study demonstrated qualitative and quantitative differences in the repair process resulting from chemical variations in the dressings used in the testing.

However, other studies have reported porosity in $Ca(OH)_2$-evoked dentinal bridges; in these, the term *tunneling* is used to describe incomplete dentinal bridge formation.[60] One group of investigators, summarizing the results of several primate studies involving direct pulp-capping with $Ca(OH)_2$, reported a number of inflamed and infected pulps after a follow-up period of 1 to 2 years.[61] They proposed that these findings resulted from deterioration of the overlying restorations and subsequent migration of microorganisms through tunnels within dentinal bridges, the latter resulting from $Ca(OH)_2$ placement. Of 192 dentinal bridges in primate teeth, they found that 172 (89%) contained tunnel defects. The authors also questioned the long-term efficacy of using commercially available $Ca(OH)_2$ bases, particularly in light of the potential for microleakage.

Comparison of $Ca(OH)_2$ with other materials for vital pulp therapy

Researchers have investigated the concept that the pulp-capping agent itself can serve as the equivalent of a reparative dentinal bridge, thereby reducing the loss of remaining vital pulp tissue.[36] This theory has been previously tested with dentinal chips,[23] synthetic hydroxyapatite,[62-68] osteogenic protein-1 and other proteins,[69-73] and Bioglass (USBiomaterials, Alachua, FL).[74-76] Several animal studies have shown that when bonding agents are placed directly on exposed pulpal tissue, some degree of pulpal repair and dentinal bridging occurs.[33,77] (For a more complete review, see chapter 14.) Given the present research interest in developing an optimal bonding system, it is possible that a technical spin-off could lead to another method of pulp-capping.

One primate study compared isobutyl cyanoacrylate with $Ca(OH)_2$ for pulp-capping.[58] The materials were left in place for only a short period of time (10 or 60 minutes). At 12 weeks after treatment, dentinal bridges were observed in 7 (78%) of 9 isobutyl cyanoacrylate cases and in 8 (80%) of 10 $Ca(OH)_2$ cases. However, histologic analysis indicated that tunnels through the dentinal bridges were observed in both treatment groups. The authors concluded that induction of bridge formation was caused by irritation factors, and not by the use of $Ca(OH)_2$ preparations, since the material was in contact with the pulp for very short time periods.

A rat molar study compared the effectiveness of hydroxyapatite (Osteogen [Impladent, Holliswood, NY]) to a $Ca(OH)_2$ formulation (Dycal; Dentsply) for pulp-capping.[63] At 7 days posttreatment, areas of acute inflammation and necrosis were more evident in the $Ca(OH)_2$-treated group, while hard tissue began to form around dental chips regardless of the materials used. At 28 days posttreatment, the $Ca(OH)_2$ group exhibited dense dentinal tissue, while the hydroxyapatite treatment produced globular dentin. In recommending the use of the $Ca(OH)_2$ preparation, the authors state that the use of hydroxyapatite products results in a generalized dystrophic calcification and renders subsequent endodontic treatment difficult. In a similar clinical study, mandibular molars scheduled for extraction (orthodontic indication) were pulp-capped with hydroxyapatite and $Ca(OH)_2$, then extracted at a later time. The histologic analyses indicated that $Ca(OH)_2$ stimulated dentinal bridge formation, whereas hydroxyapatite did not induce hard tissue formation.[66]

A subsequent canine dental pulp study compared different particle sizes of hydroxyapatite and beta-tricalcium phosphate.[67] Dentinal bridge formation was seen in 8 (47%) of 17 specimens treated with hydroxyapatite (300-µm particles) and in 11 (64%) of 17 specimens treated with tricalcium phosphate (300-µm particles). Smaller-sized (40-µm) particles of both preparations showed little, if any, bridge formation. Subsequent studies evaluated the calcified degenerative zones in amputated canine pulpal tissue.[68] Electron-dense spherical bodies were observed as early as the first day following the capping procedure in $Ca(OH)_2$ specimens. These bodies contained calcium and phosphorus. By the 14th day, differentiation of odontoblasts and tubular dentinal formation was observed, suggesting that the calcified degenerative zone has an important effect on the reparative process of pulpal tissue.

In a rat incisor model, three preparations (Pulpodent, zinc oxide–eugenol, and Ledermix) were compared after pulp-capping.[59] At 7 days posttreatment, the $Ca(OH)_2$ preparation produced rapid, complete repair, with a remarkably regular formation of calcospherites and a zone of relative inhibition perforated by canals at the periphery of each lesion. In contrast, both the zinc oxide–eugenol and Ledermix groups showed reduced bridging of the defect and reduced dentinal formation in the surrounding pulpal wall.

In a pulp-capping study using miniature swine, Bioglass was compared to autologous demineralized dentin matrix (DDM) and $Ca(OH)_2$ (Life [Kerr, Orange, CA]) in treating Class V pulpal exposures.[74,75] The preparations were restored with zinc oxide–eugenol after capping. At 90 days after treatment, all three groups induced dentinal formation, but the structure of the dentin and the condition of the pulpal tissue varied with the treatment group.

A study using adult miniature pigs compared recombinant human osteogenic protein-1 (hOP1) combined with collagen matrix, collagen matrix alone, and $Ca(OH)_2$ paste for pulp-capping.[69,70] At 5 weeks after treatment, the hOP1 group showed substantial amounts of hard tissue formation (osteodentin and tubular dentin) with complete bridging of the defects. The $Ca(OH)_2$ group displayed less dentinal formation. Collagen matrix failed to induce bridge formation.

A rat molar study compared bone sialoprotein (BSP) (another osteogenic protein) to sham carrier and $Ca(OH)_2$ treatment for pulp-capping.[72] Tissue was examined at 8- to 30-day intervals. In the $Ca(OH)_2$ group, a dentinal bridge was beginning to form by 8 days, a reparative osteodentinal bridge by 15 days. Treatment with BSP was characterized by the formation of a homogenous dentin-like deposit at 30 days, indicating a capacity for causing differentiation of cells that secrete an organized cellular matrix more efficiently than any other capping material.

Two more recent studies have evaluated adhesive systems for pulp-capping.[34,77] A recent review evaluated the literature on pulpal responses following total acid etching and application of adhesive resins on deep cavities or pulpal exposures in animals and concluded that these systems may be useful and safe when applied to dentin. In contrast, persistent inflammatory reactions as well as delays in pulpal healing and failure of dentin were seen in human pulps capped with these materials. The authors suggest that the results observed in animal teeth cannot be directly extrapolated to human clinical conditions.[78] Another evaluation of the literature on pulpal responses following total acid etching and application of adhesive resins in deep cavities and over pulpal exposures also concluded that animal experiments cannot be directly compared to human clinical conditions.[76] Further, the use of total-etch techniques for pulpal exposures in primary teeth resulted in attempted dentinal bridge formation in some samples and no bridge formation in other samples.[79] Some adhesives exhibited a severe histologic response, indicating that the total-etch technique was contraindicated in primary teeth. A recent study[77] mechanically exposed 33 sound human premolars and pulp-capped them with Clearfil Liner Bond 2 (Kuraray, Osaka, Japan) or $Ca(OH)_2$ and restored the teeth with a resin composite. The tissue was examined at 5, 30, and 120 to 300 days. Clearfil Liner Bond 2 elicited a mild to moderate inflammatory response. With time, macrophages and giant cells engulfed globules of resin and the chronic pulpal response did not allow pulpal repair. Pulps capped with $Ca(OH)_2$ exhibited an initial organization of elongated pulpal cells underneath a zone of coagulation necrosis. Pulpal repair and complete bridge formation were observed at the final evaluation periods.

Indirect Pulpal Treatment

Though not a new concept, indirect pulpal treatment continues to elicit a great deal of controversy. Many clinicians believe that the pulp may be

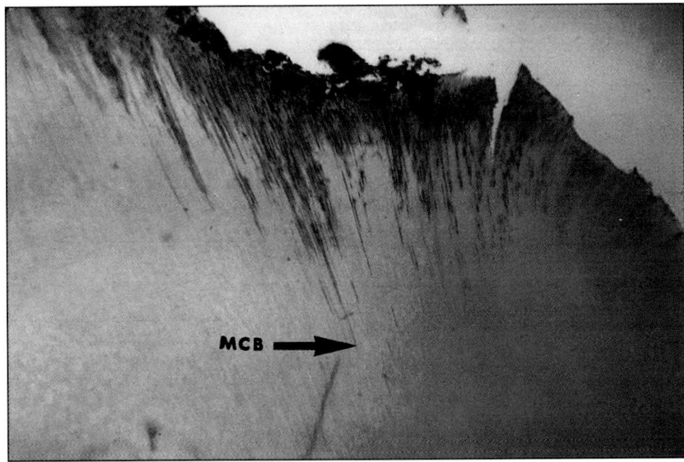

Fig 13-11a Brown and Brenn stain reveals that the closest distance between bacteria (MCB; *arrow*) and the pulp is 1.15 mm. At this level there is no pulpal lesion and no reparative dentin (original magnification ×25). (Reprinted from Reeves and Stanley[81] with permission.)

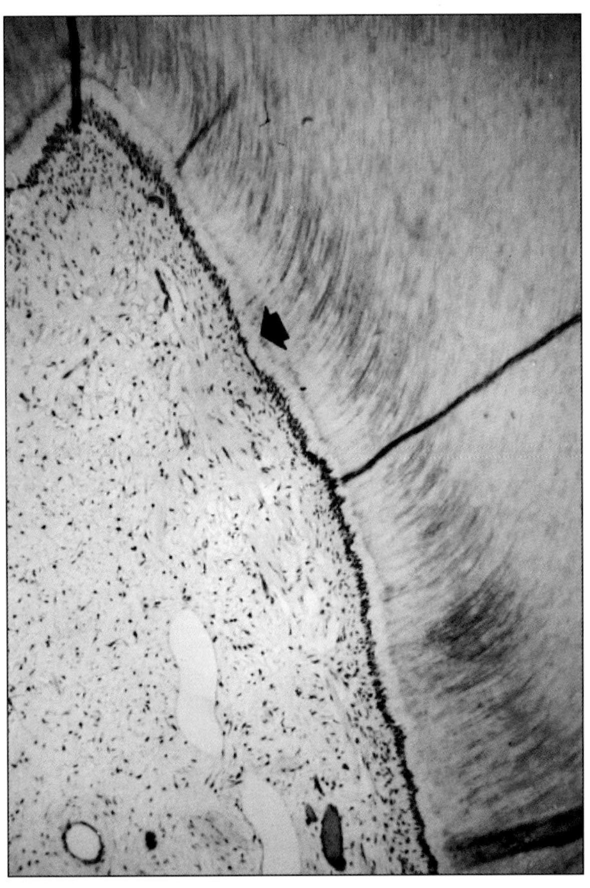

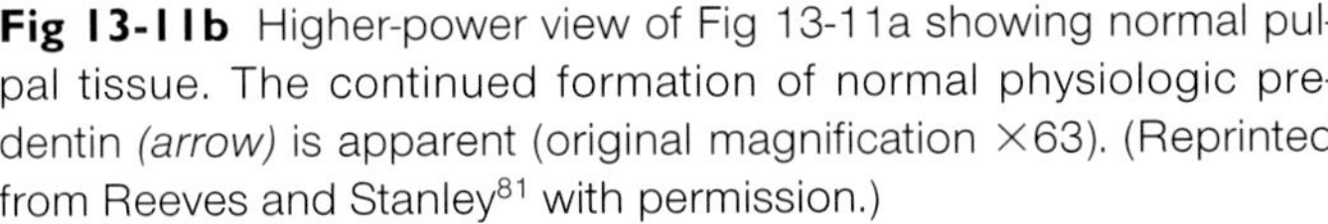

Fig 13-11b Higher-power view of Fig 13-11a showing normal pulpal tissue. The continued formation of normal physiologic predentin *(arrow)* is apparent (original magnification ×63). (Reprinted from Reeves and Stanley[81] with permission.)

so diseased beneath caries lesions that resolution of established lesions may not be possible. A review of the events occurring during development of caries is necessary to understand the histopathologic events involved in indirect pulp-capping (see also chapter 12).

In 1969, Keyes[80] described three groups of causative factors essential in the etiology of caries: a susceptible host, cariogenic microflora, and a suitable substrate. For caries to occur or progress, all groups must interact simultaneously. Reeves and Stanley[81] examined the relationship of bacterial penetration to caries and its effect on pulpal disease. A more recent study hypothesized that if the source of nutrition for the cariogenic bacteria could be eliminated, the organisms would die, thus arresting the carious process.[82]

Caries penetrates dentin at an average rate of approximately 1 mm every 6 months.[80] In untreated carious teeth, the relationship of bacterial penetration to pulpal pathosis is quite predictable. The intensity of the pulpal response to bacterial penetration of dentin is substantial, regardless of whether the penetration is 3 mm or 1 mm from the pulp. However, when the bacterial penetration comes within 0.75 mm of the pulp or when the bacteria invade previously formed reparative dentin, the degree of pulpal disease becomes extreme and, most likely, irreversible. In other words, although the practitioner cannot evaluate this measurement clinically, the pulp remains reasonably intact if there is at least 1 mm of intact bacteria-free dentin between the caries lesion and the pulp (Figs 13-11 to 13-13). The reason for this abrupt change in the intensity of the response in the last millimeter is that before the bacteria reach the pulp, their by-products (enzymes, toxins, and organic acids) can penetrate

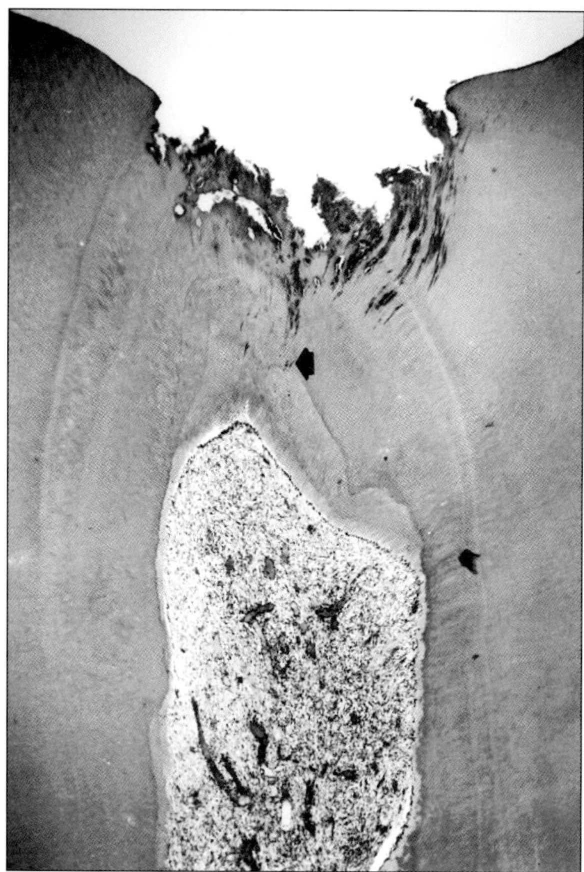

Fig 13-12 Generalized inflammatory response of the pulp to a caries lesion. As caries progresses into the bulk of the dentin, the pulp responds with inflammation. Here the cariogenic organisms *(arrow)* have reached within 0.15 mm of the pulp. In most cases, if the caries lesion is removed at this point, the pulp will return to normal. Nature has formed a layer of tertiary dentin to block the penetration of organisms and protect the pulp (original magnification ×25). (Reprinted from Reeves and Stanley[81] with permission.)

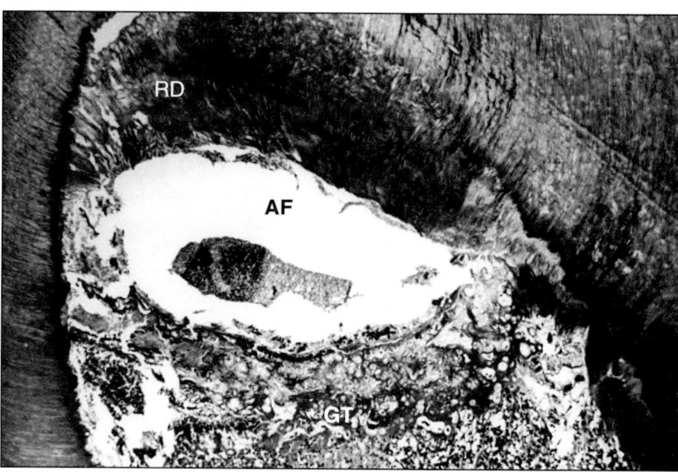

Fig 13-13 Severe response of dental pulp to intruding bacteria invading tertiary dentin (RD). Measurement of closest bacteria to pulp is 0.15 mm. Abscess formation (AF) and chronically inflamed granulation tissue (GT) also are shown (H&E stain, original magnification ×63). (Reprinted from Reeves and Stanley[81] with permission.)

the remaining tubular distance and cause pulpitis. Consequently, if all of the caries is removed except for the last deep layer overlying some intact, relatively bacteria-free primary, secondary, or reparative dentin, then the bulk of the lactic acid–producing complex is eliminated.

When the inflammation that previously prevented the continual formation of tertiary dentin has been eliminated, tertiary dentin can be formed by either the reactionary (via surviving postmitotic odontoblasts) or reparative mechanisms (via a new generation of odontoblast-like cells; see chapter 3). The few persisting cariogenic organisms that may filter through the remaining dentin are phagocytosed by neutrophils in the rejuvenated pulpal tissues. The process has shifted from favoring the caries lesion and a gradually dying pulp to one that favors the potential for complete resolution of the pulpal lesions, unless abscess formation has been established.

Although zinc oxide-eugenol has been proposed as an alternative to $Ca(OH)_2$ preparations, its use has been criticized because of its potential to diffuse through dentin and harm the underlying pulpal tissue. Studies indicate that it takes 2 to 3 hours for the eugenol component to reach the pulpal space and about 24 hours to achieve peak release.[83-85] Its peak release into dentin is 1,000 times less than its peak release into saline.[86] This slow and controlled release of eugenol toward pulp accounts for many of the beneficial effects (eg, antibacterial) of zinc oxide-eugenol when applied to intact dentin.

In an indirect pulpal treatment procedure, debridement of the carious layers in a manner that minimizes mechanical trauma is the first step toward pulpal recovery. Application of zinc oxide-eugenol, which is antibacterial and of low pulpal toxicity, reduces the bacterial threat. Its ability to seal the tooth from further ingress of bacteria is an important property. The last argument for its use is the possibility that the partially decalcified dentin would remineralize after depriving bacteria of a substrate, with subsequent return to normal tissue pH.[87]

An alternative method is to place resin composite systems directly on carious dentin or on pulpal tissue beneath deep cavity preparations. (For a more detailed review, see chapter 14.) The success of these materials depends on two events. The first is the ability of the pulp to respond to materials put in contact with or in close proximity to it. The second is the ability of the restorative materials to seal the interface between it and the preparation (hence the term *total etch, total seal*). Most reports of successful total seal occurrences appear to be empirical and/or anecdotal; therefore, more work is necessary to make valid determinations.[18] Some studies[88,89] support the occurrence of at least some of these conditions. However, a more extensive review is presented by Elledge[90] and others (see chapter 14).

A 10-year clinical trial compared the marginal integrity of three types of restorative preparations: *(1)* a conventional Class I preparation extended for prevention into noncarious fissures, with removal of all caries and placement of an amalgam restoration; *(2)* a more conservative preparation, with removal of all caries, restoration with amalgam, and use of pit and fissure sealant; and *(3)* preparation of a 45- to 60-degree bevel in the enamel surrounding a frank cavitated caries lesion; the deep soft portions of the caries remained untouched. The lesion extended no deeper than halfway into dentin between the dentinoenamel junction and the pulpal chamber, and resin-based composite was used.[87] At the 10-year follow-up period, open margins were found on 8% of the resin-based composite restorations, 9% of the sealed amalgam restorations, and 29% of the unsealed amalgam restorations. However, the most important result was that the caries lesions beneath the sealed resin-based composite restorations ceased to progress. Not one pulp became nonvital in the 10-year study. These results have contributed to a new understanding of the caries process and the value of indirect pulp-capping.

Conclusions

To improve the success rate of vital pulp therapy, a concerted effort must be made on the part of pulp biologists, dental researchers, and clinicians to recognize the progress that has been achieved in vital pulp therapy and to incorporate the newest information available into the teaching of these procedures. A review of the treatment techniques and other considerations associated with removing all caries (leading to an exposure) versus retaining a layer of carious dentin (indirect procedures) presents the dilemma most clinicians face in deciding how to treat these lesions (see also chapters 14 and 15).[91] Continued research and clinical trials are needed to develop the appropriate case selection guidelines, treatment approaches, and materials to maximize clinical success.

References

1. Rutherford B, Fitzgerald M. A new biological approach to vital pulp therapy. Crit Rev Oral Biol Med 1995;6: 218–229.
2. Tziafas D, Smith AJ, Lesot H. Designing new treatment strategies in vital pulp therapy. J Dent 2000;28:77–92.
3. Burke FM, Samarawickrama DY. Progressive changes in the pulpo-dentinal complex and their clinical consequences. Gerodontology 1995;12:57–66.
4. Kakehashi S, Stanley HR, Fitzgerald RJ. The effects of surgical exposures of dental pulps in germ-free and conventional laboratory rats. Oral Surg Oral Med Oral Pathol 1965;20:340.
5. Masterton JB. Inherent healing potential of the dental pulp. Br Dent J 1966;120:430–436.
6. Torneck CD, Moe H, Howley TP. The effect of calcium hydroxide on porcine pulp fibroblasts in vitio. J Endod 1983;9:131–136.
7. Kakehashi S, Stanley HR, Fitzgerald R. The exposed germ-free pulp: Effects of topical corticosteroid medication and restoration. Oral Surg Oral Med Oral Pathol 1969;27:60–67.
8. Cox CF, Bergenholtz G, Fitzgerald M, Heys DR, Avery JK, Baker JA. Capping of the dental pulp mechanically exposed to the oral microflora—A 5-week observation of wound healing in the monkey. J Oral Pathol 1982; 11:327–339.
9. Cox CF, Bergenholtz G, Baker JA. A 14-day observation of wound healing exposed/contaminated monkey pulps [abstract]. J Dent Res (special issue) 1983;62: 663.
10. Cox CF, Bergenholtz G, Syed SA, Heys DR, Fitzgerald MA. A 13-15 month observation of wound healing of exposed monkey pulps. J Dent Res 1983;62:250.
11. Cox CF, Subay RK, Suzuki S, Suzuksi SH, Ostro E. Biocompatiblity of various dental materials: Pulp healing with a surface seal. Int J Periodontics Restorative Dent 1996;16:240–251.
12. Cvek M. A clinical report on partial pulpotomy and capping with calcium hydroxide in permanent incisors with complicated crown fracture. J Endod 1978;4: 232–237.
13. Mejare I, Cvek M. Partial pulpotomy in young permanent teeth with deep carious lesions. Endod Dent Traumatol 1993;9:238–242.
14. Brännström M, Nyborg H. The presence of bacteria in cavities filled with silicate cement and composite resin materials. Sven Tandlak Tidskr 1971;64:149–155.
15. Brännström M, Vojinovic O. Response of the dental pulp to invasion of bacteria around three filling materials. ASDC J Dent Child 1976;43:83–89.
16. Bergenholtz G, Cox CE, Loesche WJ, Syed SA. Bacterial leakage around dental restorations: Its effect on the dental pulp. J Oral Pathol 1982;11:439–450.
17. Stanley HA. The relationship of bacterial penetration and pulpal lesions. In: Anusavice KJ (ed). Quality Evaluation of Dental Restorations: Criteria for Placement and Replacement [Proceedings of the International Symposium on Criteria for Placement and Replacement of Dental Restorations, 19–21 October 1987, Lake Buena Vista, Florida]. Chicago: Quintessence, 1989:303–323.
18. Bergenholtz G. Evidence for bacterial causation of adverse pulpal responses in resin-based dental restorations. Crit Rev Oral Biol Med 2000;11:467–480.
19. Schuurs AH, Gruythuysen RJ, Wesselink PR. Pulp capping with adhesive resin-based composite vs. calcium hydroxide: A review. Endod Dent Traumatol 2000;16: 240–250.
20. Isermann GT, Kaminski EJ. Pulpal response to minimal exposure in presence of bacteria and Dycal. J Endod 1979;5:322–327.
21. Cevk M, Cleaton-Jones PE, Austin JC, Andreasen JO. Pulp reactions to exposure after experimental crown fractures or grinding in adult monkeys. J Endod 1982;8:391–397.
22. Stanley HR, Pameijer CH. Conserving exposed pulp tissues—Capping agent becomes dentin bridge [abstract]. J Dent Res 1998;77(special issue):200.
23. Obersztyn A, Jedrzejczyk J, Smiechowska W. Application of lyophilized dentin chips, mixed with prednisolone and neomycin, on infected rat incisor pulp. J Dent Res 1968;47:374–380.
24. Horsted P, El Attar K, Langeland K. Capping of monkey pulps with Dycal and a Ca-eugenol cement. Oral Surg Oral Med Oral Pathol 1981;52:531–553.
25. Kitasako Y, Shibata S, Pereira PN, Tagami J. Short-term dentin bridging of mechanically-exposed pulps capped with adhesive resin systems. Oper Dent 2000;25: 155–162.
26. Turner C, Courts FJ, Stanley HR. A histological comparison of direct pulp capping agents in primary canines. ASDC J Dent Child 1987;54:423–428.
27. Marzouk MA, Van Huysen G. Pulp exposure without hemorrhage. J Dent Res 1966;45:405.
28. Heys DR, Heys RJ, Cox CF, Avery JK. The response of four calcium hydroxides on monkey pulps. J Oral Pathol 1980;9:372–379.
29. Heilig J, Yates J, Siskin M, McKnight J, Turner J. Calcium hydroxide pulpotomy for primary teeth: A clinical study. J Am Dent Assoc 1984;108:775–778.
30. Mjor IA, Dahl E, Cox CF. Healing of pulp exposures: An ultrastructural study. J Oral Pathol Med 1991;20: 496–501.

31. Chiego DJ Jr. An ultrastructural and autoradiographic analysis of primary and replacement odontoblasts following cavity preparation and wound healing in the rat molar. Proc Finn Dent Soc 1992;88(suppl 1): 243-256.
32. Stanley HR. The cells of the dental pulp. Oral Surg Oral Med Oral Pathol 1962;15:849-858.
33. Segura JJ, Llamas R, Rubio-Manzanares AJ, Jimenez-Planas A, Guerrero JM, Calvo JR. Calcium hydroxide inhibits substrate adherence capacity of macrophages. J Endod 1997;23:444-447.
34. Hebling J, Giro EM, Costa CA. Biocompatibility of an adhesive system applied to exposed human dental pulp. J Endod 1999;25:676-682.
35. Stanley HR, Pamcijer CH. Pulp capping with a new visible light-curing calcium hydroxide composition (Prisma VLC Dycal). Oper Dent 1985;10:156-163.
36. Stanley HR. Criteria for standardizing and increasing credibility of direct pulp capping studies. Am J Dent 1998;11(special issue):S17-S34.
37. Cox CF, Keall CL, Keall HJ, Ostro E, Bergenholtz G. Biocompatability of surface-sealed dental materials against exposed pulps. J Prosthet Dent 1987;57:1-8.
38. Snuggs HM, Cox CF, Powell CS, White KC. Pulpal healing and dentinal bridge formation in an acidic environment. Quintessence Int 1993;24:501-510.
39. Hermann BW. Calcium hydroxyd als mittelzurn behadeln und fullen von wurzelkanalen [thesis]. Würzburg, 1920.
40. Zander HA. Reaction of the pulp to calcium hydroxide. J Dent Res 1939;18:373-379.
41. Glass RL, Zander HA. Pulp healing. J Dent Res 1949;28: 97-107.
42. McWalter G, El-Kafrawy A, Mitchell D. Long-term study of pulp capping in monkeys with three agents. J Am Dent Assoc 1976;93:105-110.
43. Pitt Ford TR. Pulpal response to Procal for capping exposures in dog's teeth. J Br Endod Soc 1979;12: 67-72.
44. Isermann GT, Kaminski EJ. Pulpal response to minimal exposure in presence of bacteria and Dycal. J Endod 1979;5:322-327.
45. Pitt Ford TR. Pulpal response to a calcium hydroxide material for capping exposures. Oral Surg Oral Med Oral Pathol 1985;59:194-197.
46. Brännström M, Nyborg H, Stromberg T. Experiments with pulp capping. Oral Surg Oral Med Oral Pathol 1979;48:347-352.
47. Haskell EW, Stanley HR, Chellemi J, Stringfellow H. Direct pulp capping treatment: A long-term follow-up. J Am Dent Assoc 1978;97:607-612.
48. Heys DR, Cox CF, Heys RJ, Avery JK. Histological considerations of direct pulp capping agents. J Dent Res 1981;60:1371-1379.
49. Cox CF, Bergenholtz G, Heys DR, Syed SA, Fitzgerald M, Heys RJ. Pulp capping of dental pulp mechanically exposed to oral microflora: A 1-2 year observation of wound healing in the monkey. J Oral Pathol 1985;14: 156-168.
50. Heide S. The effect of pulp capping and pulpotomy on hard tissue bridges of contaminated pulps. Int Endod J 1991;24:126-134.
51. Staehle HJ, Pioch T. The alkalizing effect of calcium hydroxide-containing commercial preparations [in German]. Schweiz Monatsschr Zahnmed 1988;98: 1072-1077.
52. Ida K, Maseki T, Yamasaki M, Hirano S, Nakamura H. pH values of pulp-capping agents. J Endod 1989;15: 365-368.
53. Lombardi T, Di Felice R, Muhlhauser J. Analysis of pH variation of various calcium hydroxide compounds in vitro. Bull Group Int Rech Sci Stomatol Odontol 1991; 34:73-78.
54. Cotton WR. Bacterial contamination as a factor in healing of pulp exposures. Oral Surg Oral Med Oral Pathol 1974;38:441-450.
55. Holland R, de Souza V, de Mello W, Nery MJ, Bernabe PF, Otoboni Filho JA. Permeability of the hard tissue bridge formed after pulpotomy with calcium hydroxide: A histologic study. J Am Dent Assoc 1979;99: 472-475.
56. Franz FE, Holz J, Baume LJ. Ultrastructure (SEM) of dentine bridging in the human dental pulp. J Biol Buccale 1984;12:239-246.
57. Franz FE, Holz J, Baume LJ. Microradiographic assessment of neodentinal bridging following direct pulp capping in human teeth. J Endod 1985;11:6-10.
58. Cvek M, Granath L, Cleaton-Jones P, Austin J. Hard tissue barrier formation in pulpotomized monkey teeth capped with cyanoacrylate or calcium hydroxide for 10 and 60 minutes. J Dent Res 1987;66:1166-1174.
59. Kirk EE, Meyer MJ. Morphology of the mineralized front and observations of reparative dentine following induction and inhibition of dentinogenesis in the rat incisor. Endod Dent Traumatol 1992;8:195-201.
60. Walton RE, Langeland K. Migration of material in the dental pulp of monkeys. J Endod 1978;4:167-177.
61. Cox CF, Subay RK, Ostro E, Suzuki S, Suzuki SH. Tunnel defects in dentin bridges: Their formation following direct pulp capping. Oper Dent 1996;21:4-11.
62. Frank RM, Wiedemann P, Hemmerle J, Freymann M. Pulp capping with synthetic hydroxyapatite in human premolars. J Appl Biomater 1991;2:243.
63. Jaber L, Mascres C, Donahue WB. Electron microscope characteristics of dentin repair after hydroxylapatite direct pulp capping in rats. J Oral Pathol Med 1991;20: 502-508.

64. Subay RK, Asci S. Human pulpal response to hydroxyapatite and a calcium hydroxide material as direct capping agents. Oral Surg Oral Med Oral Pathol 1993;76:485–492.
65. Jaber L, Mascres C, Donohue WB. Reaction of the dental pulp to hydroxyapatite. Oral Surg Oral Med Oral Pathol 1992;73:92–98.
66. Higashi T, Okamoto H. Influence of particle size of hydroxyapatite as a capping agent on cell proliferation of cultured fibroblasts. J Endod 1996;22:236–239.
67. Higashi T, Okamoto H. Influence of particle size of calcium phosphate ceramics as a capping agent on the formation of a hard tissue barrier in amputated dental pulp. J Endod 1996;22:281–283.
68. Hayashi Y, Imai M, Yanagiguchi K, Viloria IL, Ikeda T. Hydroxyapaptite applied as direct pulp capping medicine substitutes for osteodentin. J Endod 1999;25:225–229.
69. Rutherford RB, Wahle J, Tucker M, Rueger D. Induction of reparative dentine formation in monkeys by recombinant human osteogenic protein-1. Arch Oral Biol 1993;38:571–576.
70. Rutherford RB, Spangberg L, Tucker M, Charette M. Osteogenic protein-1 stimulates reactionary dentin formation [abstract]. J Dent Res 1995;74(special issue):83.
71. Jepsen S, Albers HK, Fleiner B, Tucker M, Rueger D. Recombinant human osteogenic protein-1 induces dentin formation: An experimental study in miniature swine. J Endod 1997;23:378–382.
72. Decup S, Six N, Palmier B, Buch D, Lasfargues JJ, Salih E, Goldberg M. Bone sialoprotein-induced reparative dentinogenesis in the pulp of rat's molar. Clin Oral Investig 2000;4:110–119.
73. Zhang Q, Fan M, Bian Z, Chen Z, Zhu Q. Immunohistochemistry of bone sialoprotein and osteopontin during reparative dentinogenesis in vivo. Chin J Dent Res 2000;3:38–43.
74. Oguntebi BR, Clark A, Wilson J. Pulp capping with Bioglass and autologous demineralized dentin in miniature swine. J Dent Res 1993;72:484–489.
75. Oguntebi BR, Heaven T, Clark AE, Pink FE. Quantitative assessment of dentin bridge formation following pulp-capping in miniature swine. J Endod 1995;21:79–82.
76. Stanley HR, Clark AE, Pameijer CH, Louw NP. Pulp capping with a modified bioglass formula (#A68-modified). Am J Dent 2001;14:227–232.
77. De Souza Costa CA, Lopes do Nascimento AB, Teixeira HM, Fontana UF. Response of human pulps capped with a self-etching adhesive system. Dent Mater 2001;17:230–240.
78. Costa CA, Hebling J, Hanks CT. Current status of pulp capping with dentin adhesive systems: A review. Dent Mater 2000;16:188–197.
79. Cehreli ZC, Turgut M, Olmez S, Dagdeviren A, Atilla P. Short term human primary pulpal response after direct pulp capping with fourth-generation dentin adhesives. J Clin Pediatr Dent 2000;25:65–71.
80. Keyes PH. Present and future measures for dental caries control. J Am Dent Assoc 1969;79:1395–1404.
81. Reeves R, Stanley HR. The relationship of bacterial penetration of pulpal pathosis in carious teeth. Oral Surg Oral Med Oral Pathol 1966;22:59–65.
82. Mertz-Fairhurst EJ, Curtis JW Jr, Ergle JW, Rueggeberg FA, Adair SM. Ultraconservative and cariostatic sealed restorations: Results at 10 years. J Am Dent Assoc 1998;129:55–66.
83. Becker RM, Hume WR, Wolinsky LE. Release of eugenol from mixtures of ZOE in vitro. J Pedod 1983;8:71–77.
84. Hume WR. An analysis of the release and the diffusion through dentin of eugenol from zinc oxide-eugenol mixtures. J Dent Res 1984;63:881–884.
85. Hume WR. Effect of eugenol on respiration and division in human pulp, mouse fibroblasts, and liver cells in vitro. J Dent Res 1984;63:1262–1265.
86. Hume WR. Influence of dentine on the pulpward release of eugenol or acids from restorative materials. J Oral Rehabil 1994;21:469–473.
87. Hume WR, Massey WL. Keeping the pulp alive: The pharmacology and toxicology of agents applied to dentine. Aust Dent J 1990;35:32–37.
88. Cox CF, Hafez AA, Akimoto N, Otsuki M, Suzuki S, Tarim B. Biocompatibility of primer, adhesive and resin composite systems on non-exposed and exposed pulps on non-human primate teeth. Am J Dent 1998;11(special issue):S55–S63.
89. Tarim B, Hafez AA, Cox CF. Pulpal response to a resin-modified glass-ionomer material on nonexposed and exposed monkey pulps. Quintessence Int 1998;29:535–542.
90. Elledge DA. Multifunctional bases and liners. Dent Clin North Am 1998;42:739–754.
91. Dumsha T, Hovland E. Considerations and treatment of direct and indirect pulp-capping. Dent Clin North Am 1985;29:251–259.

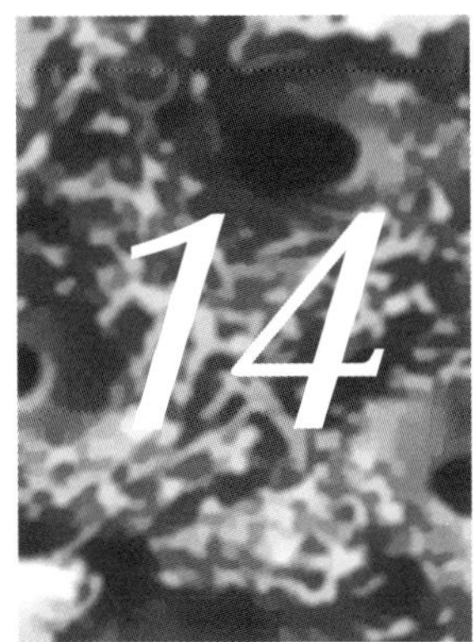

Repair of Pulpal Injury by Dental Materials

Charles F. Cox, DMD, PhD; George Bogen, DDS;
Hugh M. Kopel, DDS, MS; John D. Ruby, DMD, PhD

"How poor are they that have not patience! What wound did ever heal but by degrees?"

—Shakespeare, *Othello*

This chapter synthesizes the wide spectrum of information in dental material literature that relates to pulpal repair. Other aspects of pulpal repair are presented in chapters 3, 7, 8, 10, 13, 15, and 16. The challenge to clinicians is to apply this collective biologic knowledge to clinical practice, merging knowledge and critical experience to obtain optimal treatment decisions for patient care.

Treatment Decisions

Aside from traumatic emergencies that expose the vital pulp, traditional endodontic treatment generally involves canal debridement followed by obturation, a technique intended to provide a complete bacteriometic seal. Generally, this treatment is a consequence of irreversible pulpitis, nonvital (necrotic) pulp with or without periradicular radiolucency, or the need for elective removal of vital pulp for long-term success of a final restoration.

Other treatment options are indicated when caries excavation creates a mechanical pulp exposure, pushing bacteria-laden operative debris into the pulp, which can irritate a chronically inflamed pulp into a more acute condition leading to pulpitis and potential pain (see chapter 12). This occurrence generally presents the attending clinician with a choice of undertaking immediate biomechanical canal preparation and temporization or attempting a direct pulp-capping procedure after pulp vitality is carefully assessed. Each clinician must determine the most conservative treatment regimen for placing dental materials over the exposure: treatment of a carious mechanical pulp exposure or partial removal of a pulp and treatment with a material to allow pulp healing and continued root formation. The material must be biocompatible, nonresorbable, able to establish and maintain a bacteriometic seal, and able to promote pulpal repair. The importance of rubber dam isolation and optical magnification during clinical treatment cannot be overemphasized.

Commercially Available Pulp-Capping Materials

Today's market features only a small array of materials that can be used to predictably seal an exposed pulp, including various calcium hydroxide (Ca[OH]$_2$) agents, various resin-modified glass ionomers (RMGIs), various adhesive resins, and mineral trioxide aggregate (MTA). In the future we are sure to see hybrids of these materials in conjunction with certain growth or hormonal additives and delivery vehicles. These may feature autopolymerized or photopolymerized alternatives. The clinician's choice will be dependent on the clinical situation; his or her experience; and the material's efficacy, side-effect liability, and availability. Studies show mixed results with resins and RMGI. MTA is a rather new material that shows promise as a direct pulp-capping agent, and although longitudinal studies are not yet available, initial studies are very promising. MTA offers many desirable characteristics of an ideal pulp-capping agent with a compressive strength equal to that of zinc oxide-eugenol (ZnOE); in addition, MTA exhibits negligible solubility, sets in blood and serum fluids, prevents recontamination of the dental pulp, and promotes formation of the dentin bridge.

Do Dental Materials Stimulate Pulpal Repair?

Early dental literature[1] proposed that certain dental materials, specifically Ca(OH)$_2$, not only possessed a special capacity to provide an environment for pulp healing but, more important, also stimulated dentin bridge formation. Others also suggested that Ca(OH)$_2$ provided protection against postoperative pain following restorative treatment, and many clinicians continue to use this material today. However, a review of recent research data supports the potential of newer materials to stimulate pulpal repair after direct pulp capping, possibly reducing the need for immediate endodontic treatment after pulp exposure.

Several studies[2-5] have demonstrated that no particular dental material possesses a singular stimulating capacity for pulp repair, new odontoblastoid cell formation, or dentin bridge formation. Conversely, several bioactive agents and growth factors, ie, morphogenetic proteins (MPs) and osteogenic proteins (OPs), have been demonstrated to stimulate pulpal healing and dentinogenesis.[6-9] These are discussed in detail in chapter 3. In this chapter, we review available dental materials and evaluate whether any one material is uniquely stimulatory to pulp cells culminating in repair. However, before exploring these data, we will consider whether certain dental materials inhibit pulpal healing and repair or are in fact toxic to the pulp.

In vitro testing: The first biologic hurdle

In vitro research has shown that certain dental materials, ie, formocresol, glutaraldehyde, eugenol, hydroxyethyl methacrylate (HEMA), bisphenol glycidyl methacrylate (bis-GMA), and urethane dimethacrylate (UDMA), are toxic in cell culture,[9-14] both as single components and in mixtures. ZnOE cement is often used as the in vitro cell-culture control agent, producing cell toxicity, and acidic cements are often used as nonirritation control materials.

The intensity of the cell-culture response is generally dependent upon the concentration of the agent, the duration of the test, the possibility of an increased or decreased antagonistic response following polymerization,[15] and a host of other factors too numerous to discuss in this chapter. It has been suggested that the individual in vitro cytotoxicity of any single monomer is not adequate to determine if in vivo clinical use of any dental material with several components will be toxic, especially when cytotoxicity testing may release multiple components following mixing and placement.[16]

In vivo testing: An ISO hurdle

In vivo tests conforming to International Organization for Standardization (ISO) standards are generally performed after a dental material has passed the in vitro tests in development. A dental material is surgically implanted into the connective tissues of rats or rabbits and its biologic effects examined histologically at ISO-defined time intervals. Following histologic acceptance, the new dental material is placed in Class V cavities of nonhuman primates for ISO usage tests. Pulp responses are compared with accepted ISO control materials (ZnOE and phosphoric acid [H_3PO_4] -containing cement) at three time periods. ZnOE cement represents the nonirritating negative usage control materials, and acidic cements represent positive control materials, causing severe inflammation and necrosis due to the breakdown of the smear layer at the restoration interface from the acid component allowing bacterial invasion of the open dentinal tubules[5,17,18] (see also chapter 4). As illustrated in Fig 14-1, bacteria and their toxic products are the primary causes of pulp inflammation[3] (see also chapters 5, 12, and 13).

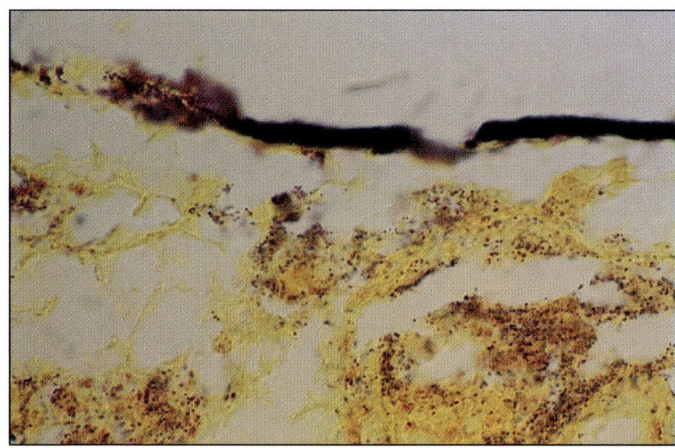

Fig 14-1 Histologic pulp section of an inflamed nonhuman primate pulp that was restored with zinc phosphate cement for 7 days with no bacteriometic seal. The acid demineralized the smear layer along the cement interface and allowed bacterial microleakage. Both gram-positive *(blue)* and gram-negative *(red)* bacteria are present among the yellow-stained pulp cells (modified McKay bacterial stain, original magnification ×500).

Clinical testing: The final hurdle

Following ISO in vivo tests, it is imperative to pursue independent clinical studies before any dental material reaches the marketplace. Several issues confound the process, and developers may bypass clinical testing by demonstrating that certain components of the new material have previous ISO acceptance. Another issue is that long-term clinical studies are often very expensive and difficult to conduct in university settings, as patient return rates are poor. Consequently, the rapid development process without clinical testing brings new dental materials to the marketplace quickly, only to disappear in a short time.

Is Pulpal Inflammation Caused by Dental Materials, Trauma, or Bacteria?

As reviewed in chapter 12, dental caries is related to several variables, including host factors, the bacterial ecosystem, and a fermentable diet. Miller's classic studies demonstrated that incubating teeth with saliva and carbohydrates results in local acid formation that dissolves the mineral portion of the tooth.[19] He then formulated the chemoparasitic hypothesis, proposing that dental caries is due to the effect of certain organic acids of oral bacteria that demineralize the mineral substrate. He suggested a high potential for remineralization when the collagen is not severely damaged. However, once other oral bacteria enter the dentinal tubule complex, they penetrate the tubules to the pulp, breaking down the collagen at the bacterial front (pioneer bacteria).[20,21] Once the pulpodentin complex becomes infiltrated with bacteria and their toxic factors, the pulp may develop a localized compartment of inflammation (see also chapters 10, 12, and 13). Cavities with 0.5 mm or less of remaining dentin on the floor showed subjacent edema, dilated blood vessels, and extravasated polymorphonuclear leukocytes. The deeper pulp would remain intact within normal limits.[22,23] Prolonged pulp inflammation generally resulted in increased inflammation and vascular changes, responding with more severe regional inflammation, often leading to regional or complete pulpal necrosis.

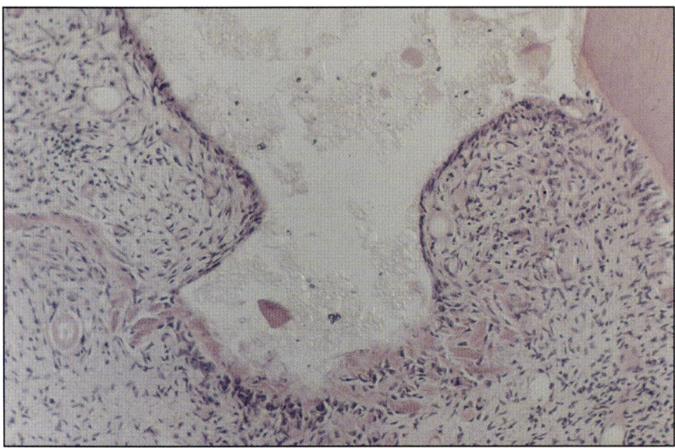

Fig 14-2 Histologic section from a 7-day nonhuman primate pulp that was direct capped with silicate. Particles are seen in the upper midfield. A new cell layer of odontoblastoid cells are adjacent to the material, with a new dentin bridge *(light pink)* adjacent to the silicate interface. The adjacent and deeper pulp is free of inflammation or silicate particles (H&E stain, original magnification ×100).

Infected dentin: The biologic culprit

Iatrogenic cavity preparation trauma, ultra-high versus low-speed frictional bur rotation, prolonged drying of the prepared surface with an air blast, and placement of organic solvents such as chloroform are all factors causing pulp inflammation.[2,3,24-29] However, it is difficult to distinguish reported dental material toxicity when used in nonexposed cavities from toxicity after usage in pulps exposed to caries. For example, no inflammatory changes occurred in nonhuman primate pulps into which four different materials were placed when a bacterial seal of ZnOE also was placed.[30] This finding is illustrated in Fig 14-2; the results emphasize the importance of bacterial leakage in evoking pulpal inflammation.

Since the early 1970s, investigators[4,26,31-33] have demonstrated that the presence of stained bacteria within the dentin tubules beneath the restorative material is positively correlated with pulpal inflammation. Additional histologic and culturing studies have confirmed that bacteria and their by-products play a direct role in pulpal inflammation.[34-38]

Bacterial growth: The real culprit

Following the original caries hypothesis,[19] our profession understands that bacteria are the primary cause of pulpal inflammation and eventual necrosis. Miller's thesis has been supported by numerous studies[26,28,31,35,39-41] that demonstrate that bacteria are responsible for recurrent caries and that treatment failure is a consequence of pulpal inflammation caused by bacterial invasion.

A classic in vivo germ-free study demonstrated that exposed dental pulps in rats proliferated against certain dental materials, and dentin bridge formation occurred in pulps where food debris was lodged (see Fig 13-1).[3] Control rats with normal bacterial flora showed pulpal inflammation and necrosis under the same material placement conditions. A later report[5] showed that exposed dental pulps in primates heal and permit the wound site to form a new reparative dentin bridge in the absence of bacterial influences, $Ca(OH)_2$ agents, or other inductive stimuli. This finding reinforces the important theory that the dental pulp possesses an inherent capacity to heal in the absence of bacteria. The molecular basis for this repair is described in detail in chapter 3.

Demonstration of a bacterial mechanism for pulpal inflammation implies that prevention of bacterial microleakage may prevent inflammation or necrosis. For example, there is a direct correlation between the presence of stained bacteria and anaerobically cultured samples from inflamed and necrotic pulps.[28] In addition, placing a bacterial cocktail on the cavity floor of a preparation resulted in pulp necrosis within 1 week.[42] These and other studies support the hypothesis that bacterial microleakage is the primary cause of pulp inflammation. Accordingly, by providing a bacteriometic seal along the entire restoration interface, we can predict the reduction of postoperative inflammation and recurrent caries.

Reparative and reactionary dentin are regarded as biologic responses of odontoblasts or odontoblast-like cells to pathologic or physiologic irritation.[6,43] In his classic paper, Fish[43] characterized the sclerotic front of hypermineralized dentin preceding caries as impervious to dyes. Contemporary investigators reported that reparative dentin is a localized area along the pulp-predentin interface below the external stimulus.[44] But what elicits this form of repair? Some investigators propose that placing $Ca(OH)_2$ or other dental materials stimulates formation of reparative dentin (see also chapter 13).[24,45-48] However, others suggest that preparation trauma and bacterial microleakage play the major role in stimulating reactionary and reparative dentin formation.[49] The following sections review the evidence presented in this debate in the context of discussing selected dental materials and their ability to promote pulpal healing.

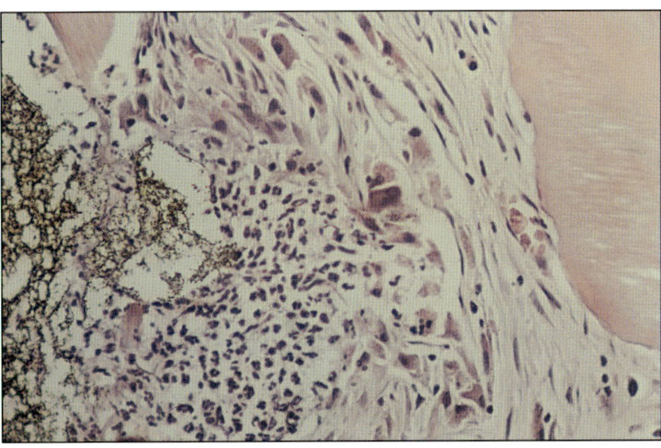

Fig 14-3 Histologic section from a nonhuman primate pulp exposure that was restored with Dycal and amalgam for 13 months. Dispersed $Ca(OH)_2$ particles are seen with many inflammatory cells in the subjacent pulp to the right. Bacteria are present in adjacent stained microslides, implying that $Ca(OH)_2$ has lost its capacity as a bacteriostatic agent (modified McKay bacterial stain, original magnification ×250).

Calcium Hydroxide: A Chimera?

$Ca(OH)_2$ agents have been used since the 1930s as a base or liner and are perhaps the most widely used dental restorative material around the world. Two-paste $Ca(OH)_2$ dental materials have been reported to have pulp-protection properties: a capacity to prevent patient postoperative sensitivity, to stimulate reactionary or reparative dentin deposition, to stimulate sclerosis of dentinal tubules, to provide an antimicrobial layer, and to stimulate odontoblastoid cell differentiation and eventual dentin bridge formation.[1,50-60] These and other studies have demonstrated that both nonexposed and exposed dental pulp have inherent capacity to repair and heal when treated with various two-paste $Ca(OH)_2$ systems and other dental materials (see also chapter 13).

Studies evaluating the physical properties of certain commercial $Ca(OH)_2$ liners and bases (eg, Dycal [Dentsply, York, PA], Hydrex [Henkel, Dusseldorf, Germany], Life [Kerr, Orange, CA], Reolit, Procal, and Renew) showed solubility in distilled water and in acidic or varnish solutions.[61-69] However, when placed in bulk, two-paste $Ca(OH)_2$ systems deform due to their low strength. Subsequent dissolution and disintegration reduces their supposed therapeutic and antimicrobial capacity (Fig 14-3) and eventually allows recurrent caries via bacterial microleakage. In addition, if not completely removed, dissolution particles may compromise the seal in adhesive hybridization treatments. Thus, the physical properties of $Ca(OH)_2$ systems confer substantial advantages and disadvantages.

Does $Ca(OH)_2$ provide a true seal?

Certain two-paste $Ca(OH)_2$ materials do provide in vivo antisepsis of carious dentin, an important property for indirect pulp protection.[62,70-72] However, this antimicrobial effect is transient, and there is no long-term mechanical seal of the restoration interface due to the material's nonadhesive property. Traditional $Ca(OH)_2$ bases and liners adhere to dentin by weak van der Waals forces, conferring no adhesive capacity. Moreover, currently available adhesives fail to bond to the interface of most two-paste $Ca(OH)_2$ agents. The placement of a two-paste $Ca(OH)_2$ liner or base to the cavity wall decreases the hybridization reaction,[17,38,39,73,74] reducing the formation of a seal against the dentin

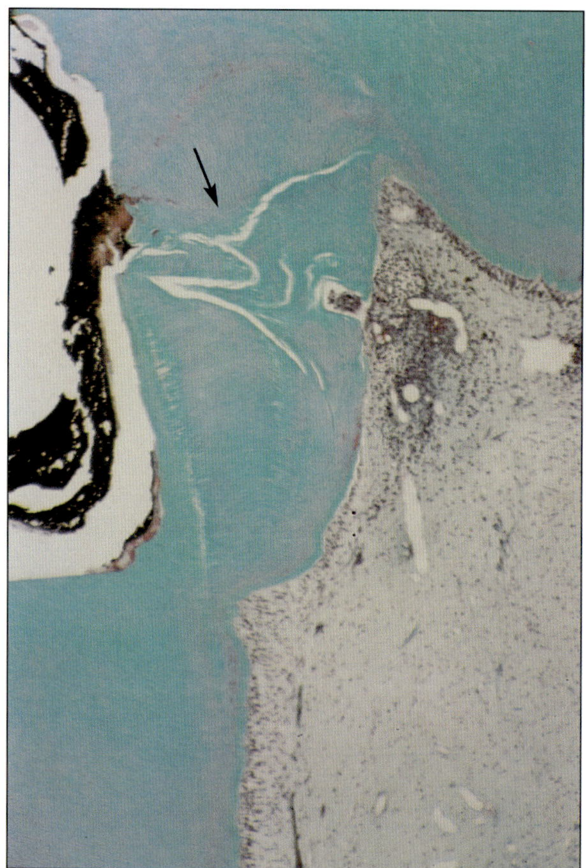

Fig 14-4 Histologic section from a nonhuman primate pulp that was direct capped with Dycal for 24 months. The dentin bridge *(upper left)* contains a tunnel defect *(arrow)* running from the restoration interface to the dental pulp, providing a route for bacteria and toxic products to migrate to the dental pulp and compromising the long-term health of the pulp. A focus of inflammation is seen in the pulp below the reparative dentin. The deeper pulp remains normal (Masson stain, original magnification ×40).

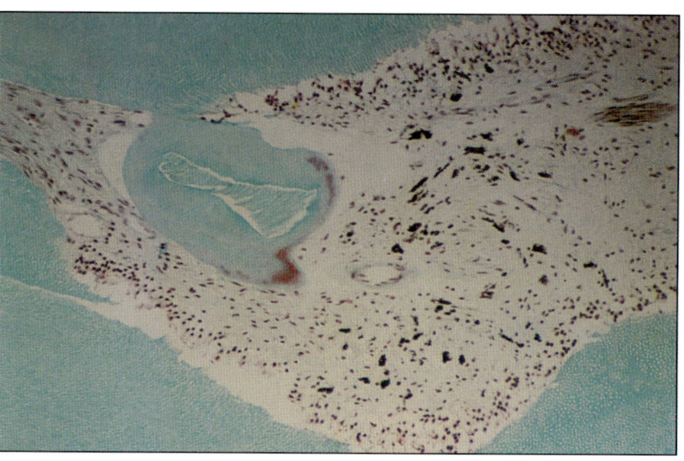

Fig 14-5 Histologic section of a nonhuman primate pulp showing the presence of $Ca(OH)_2$ particles in the dental pulp 24 months after capping. These particles do not appear to be physiologically cleared from the pulp but appear to be constantly reclaimed by new generations of pulp cells (fibroblasts, histiocytes, and macrophages) in repetitive fashion. An operative debris chip is present *(left)* with new reparative dentin around its periphery (Masson stain, original magnification ×100).

interface.[75] Other studies have shown that the ability of MTA or RMGI to form a seal over vital dentin and pulp tissue is not enhanced with the use of commercial $Ca(OH)_2$ agents.

$Ca(OH)_2$ and dentin bridge defects

$Ca(OH)_2$ materials have been popular due to their reported ability to stimulate reactionary or reparative dentin bridge formation.[76] However, the clinical utility of this property is reduced by the demonstration of incomplete dentin bridge formation. Defects in dentin bridges (Fig 14-4) permit an uncontrolled passage of bacteria and their by-products to the pulp. As described earlier (chapters 3, 10, 11, and 12), bacteria-related products and subsequent pulpal reactions elicit reparative dentin deposition and pulpal inflammation.[57,77-82] These defects permit the migration of dissolved $Ca(OH)_2$ particles into the underlying pulp (Fig 14-5), allowing constant percolation throughout the pulp, with particles remaining in pulpal fibroblasts for up to 2 years.[25,57,78-83]

$Ca(OH)_2$: Resorption versus stimulation

Pediatric dentists have reported that $Ca(OH)_2$ is responsible for causing resorption and early exfoliation of primary teeth.[52,84-86] Radiographic studies reported rates of root resorption equivalent to rates of dentin bridge formation,[52] which led to the suggestion that $Ca(OH)_2$ is singularly responsible for resorption, considered a contraindication for the use of $Ca(OH)_2$ in primary teeth.[86]

Endodontists utilize $Ca(OH)_2$ powder mixed with a sterile solution in adult teeth as a predictable interim procedure for the nonsurgical treatment of internal resorption, perforations, and canal antisepsis before obturation or final repair. On the other hand, restorative dentists often place two-paste $Ca(OH)_2$ materials for direct pulp-capping with confidence in their clinical success. Failures, when they occur, are often attributed to "other factors." It is important to realize that failure of the treatment in most direct pulp-capping studies is associated with the inability of the restorative material to maintain a long-term biologic or mechanical seal against microleakage of oral contaminants.[71]

Materials Containing Zinc Oxide–Eugenol

ZnOE is perhaps one of the must enduring dental materials. Eugenol provides an antimicrobial effect that facilitates the formation of a biologic seal against microleakage of bacteria or their toxins through dentin.[87] In addition, eugenol provides an anodyne effect against intradentinal nerve activity.[88] However, ZnOE with high concentrations of eugenol evokes chronic pulpal inflammation and necrosis when placed in direct contact with dental pulp in germ-free rats.[89] The use of ZnOE for pulpotomy or perforation repairs has been reported to be unsuccessful (ie, presenting with chronic inflammation) unless the tissue is first treated with formocresol.[90] Additional investigators have reported that ZnOE should not be placed for direct pulp-capping or pulpectomy, for it causes chronic inflammation and necrosis with time.[91] This toxicity is attributable to the concentration of eugenol in the mixture: a low concentration of eugenol caused minimal cell damage when placed in direct contact with dental pulp in monkeys.[29] Other ZnOE cements, such as intermediate restorative material (IRM) or base and temporary (B & T), are modified polymethyl methacrylate-reinforced ZnOE with supposedly superior characteristics. An in vivo study[92] has shown that IRM is only a slight irritant to primary odontoblasts and the subjacent cell-rich layer when placed in unlined cavities.

Materials Containing Formocresol

Gysi's triopaste was introduced in 1899 as the first material to combine creosote and formaldehyde to "fix" pulps. Later, formocresol therapy was suggested for clinical treatment of "putrescent pulps."[93] Sweet popularized the clinical use of formocresol for pulpotomy of vital primary teeth that were exposed by caries.[94] Additional studies reported clinical and histologic success after several months.[84,95-99]

However, concern has been raised about the toxicity of formocresol and its diffusion out of dental pulp. The reported toxicity profile of these compounds includes mutagenicity and carcinogenicity.[100,101] In addition, radiotracer studies indicate presence of C^{14}-labeled formocresol in the periodontal ligament and body fluids following pulpotomy procedures.[102,103] Consequently, if several formocresol pulpotomies were completed in the same individual, it is possible that systemic toxicity could result.

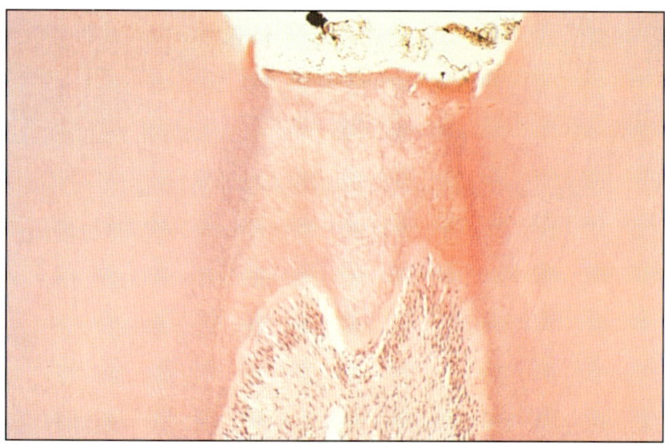

Fig 14-6 Histologic section of a nonhuman primate pulp that was direct capped with MTA for 5 months. A new dentin bridge is seen midfield directly below the MTA particles with new odontoblastoid cells along the pulp interface. The deeper pulp is free of operative debris chips and inflammation (H&E stain, original magnification ×50). (Reprinted from Pitt Ford et al[104] with permission.)

Mineral Trioxide Aggregate

The search over the last few decades for biocompatible agents that can induce in vivo pulp repair mechanisms has produced a variety of materials. Among these, the most promising material is mineral trioxide aggregate (MTA) because of its superior characteristics as a direct pulp-capping agent compared with $Ca(OH)_2$ controls in several animal models.[104-108] Results show reparative dentin bridge formation in the majority of samples with minimal inflammatory cell response.

MTA is a Portland cement derivative made primarily of fine hydrophilic particles whose main components are calcium phosphate and calcium oxide[109]; it is commercially available as ProRoot MTA (Tulsa Dental, Tulsa, OK). The material sets in approximately 3 to 4 hours and exhibits an initial pH of 10.2 and a set pH of 12.5, similar to that of $Ca(OH)_2$. MTA has been found to have a compressive set strength equal to that of IRM (approximately 70 MPa) and appears to be nonresorbable.

Studies indicate MTA exhibits high biocompatibility (Fig 14-6), minimal cytotoxicity, excellent marginal adaptation, and reliable cytokine production in human osteoblasts.[107-112] Placement of a wet cotton pellet over MTA induces a proper set,[109] and once set, the material is uninhibited by blood or moisture. It has been shown to have multiple clinical applications: in pulp-capping, root-end filling, perforation repair and internal resorption, promoting apexification, and recently in pulpotomy.[109,113-116] Current clinical studies are examining the use of MTA as a pulp-capping agent in conjunction with adhesion systems. The initial favorable findings indicate that MTA can be placed directly onto pulp tissue with negligible adverse response (G. Bogen and M. Torabinejad, personal communication, 2001).

Modified Glass Ionomers

Glass ionomer was developed as a silicate glass, modified to react with an aqueous solution of acrylic acid.[117] A photo-activated RMGI was developed (ie, Fuji II LC [GC America, Alsip IL]) by the addition of a light-hardened resin component, with the actual components differing among various products. In vitro tests measured through a disk of dentin showed the pH was reduced to neutrality with minimal to no cytoxicity.[118] Subsequent in vivo tests demonstrated only minimal pulp reactions when RMGI was evaluated in nonhuman usage models.[119] A recent in vivo study of direct capping showed pulp healing and dentin bridge formation (Fig 14-7) against an adhesive interface.[120] In contrast, the $Ca(OH)_2$ control showed various grades of inflammation associated with stained bacteria, suggesting the $Ca(OH)_2$ dissolved and created an avenue for bacteria to enter via microleakage and justifying the use of sodium hypochlorite (NaOCl) to control hemorrhage and remove the organic biofilm.

Recent studies have demonstrated that pulpotomy is successful when restored with an RMGI or adhesive.[121,122] Fewer stained bacteria were present in the RMGI and adhesive groups, suggesting that proper hemorrhage control and a definitive bacteriometic seal are prime factors to prevent microleakage and promote healing. RMGI has been used as a definitive restorative agent to decrease microleakage because of its capacity to bond to the tooth structure and its antimicrobial effects. The development of well-tolerated materials that provide excellent seal and good pulpal response represents a paradigm shift for our profession.

Adhesive Resin Systems

Although acid etching of vital dentin was originally thought to injure dental pulp,[123,124] many studies have shown excellent results with this method. For example, studies that conform to ISO usage standards report that adhesive resin systems are histologically comparable to $Ca(OH)_2$ controls. One important factor is the thickness of the remaining dentin.[125] In an in vitro model system, the diffusion rates of HEMA versus a triethylene glycol dimethacrylate (TEG-DMA) resin system were dependent upon the thickness of remaining dentin.[125] Based upon this factor, an intact vital dentin substrate of sufficient thickness has the potential to provide substantial protection against possible chemical toxicity of materials.[126] Other issues that relate to dentin permeability and the diffusion of substances through dentinal tubules are covered in chapter 4.

Nakabayashi introduced the term *hybrid layer* to describe the impregnation of vital etched dentin with an adhesive.[127] By posttreating the hybrid layer with hydrochloric acid and NaOCl in vitro, Nakabayashi demonstrated that the hybrid layer remains intact, suggesting it cohesively secures the entire enamel-dentin-resin interface with a continuous morphologic seal—a biometic barrier.

A number of ISO usage and clinical studies have reported that exposed nonhuman and human dental pulps and periapical tissues will heal when directly capped with various adhesives, glass ionomers, or MTA (Figs 14-8 and 14-9).[18,106,128-141] Most of these adhesive usage studies report lack of bacterial staining along the cavity walls or within the pulp tissue at long-term intervals. Their collective biologic assessment suggests that most of the adhesives are biologically compatible when directly capped onto exposed vital pulps, comparable to $Ca(OH)_2$ controls.

Others have suggested that pulpal inflammation is due primarily to the adhesive systems and not to bacterial inflammation.[123,124,142-144] These studies did not use NaOCl for pulp hemostasis, a critical component for antisepsis of the dentin-

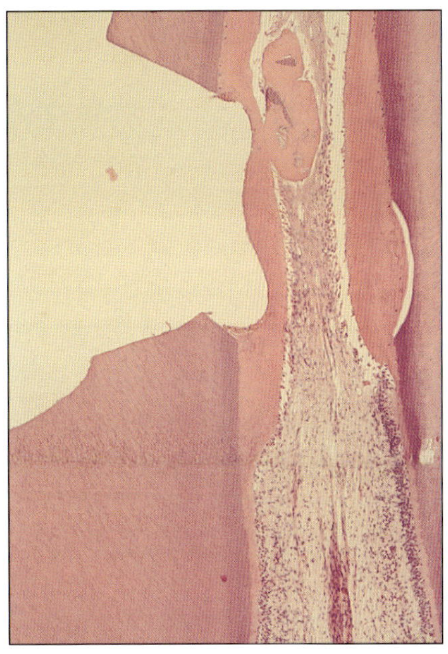

Fig 14-7 Histologic section of a nonhuman primate pulp. Following hemorrhage control, the exposure was direct pulp-capped with an Ultrablend system (Ultradent, South Jordan, UT) for 75 days. A new dentin bridge is seen at the resin interface and cavity space on the left. The new dentin bridge is continuous with the reparative and reactionary dentin along the canal walls. Reparative dentin is seen on the opposite pulpal wall. The deeper pulp is normal with no resin particles (H&E stain, original magnification ×50).

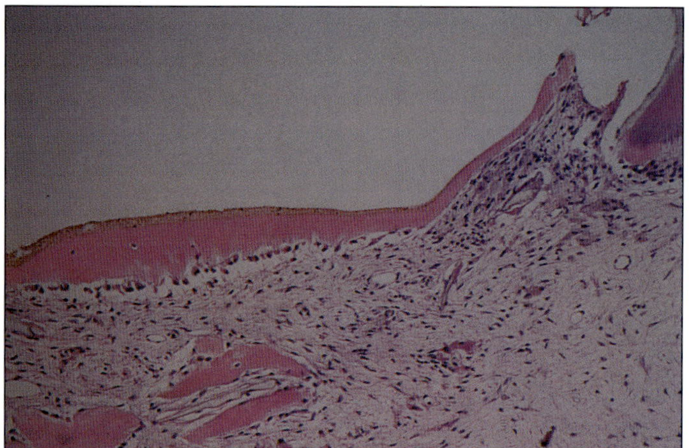

Fig 14-8 Histologic section of a nonhuman primate pulp exposure that was direct capped with Bisco Resinomer (Bisco, Schaumburg, IL) for 27 days. A new *(pink)* dentin bridge is seen directly at the material interface. New odontoblastoid cells are seen along thicker portions of the new dentin. Some operative debris chips remain in the lower left of the pulp. A thin mass of reparative dentin *(midright, light pink)* is seen at the pulp-dentin interface of the cavity wall. The deeper pulp is normal with no resin particles. No $Ca(OH)_2$ was employed in this procedure (H&E stain, original magnification ×125).

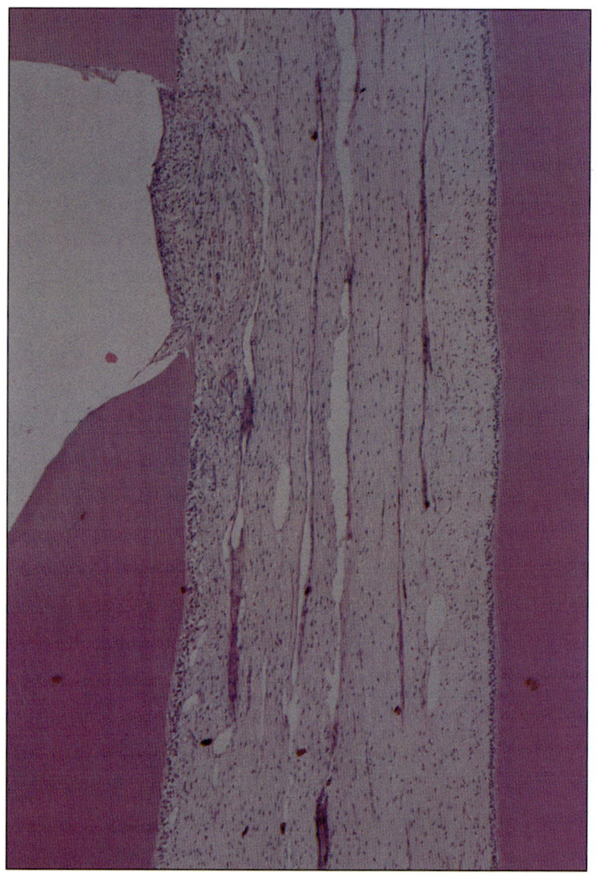

Fig 14-9 Histologic section of a non-human primate pulp exposure that was treated with 5% NaOCl for 30 seconds to remove operative debris and control hemorrhage. The exposure was capped with a Kuraray resin (Osaka, Japan) for 7 days. No clot, coagulum, or operative debris is present. The pulp has migrated to the clear interface on the left, previously filled with resin. There is only minimal presence of any inflammatory cells. Odontoblasts are present along the remaining dentin with a very thin zone of reactionary dentin having formed (H&E stain, original magnification ×50).

pulp interface.[41] A properly hybridized seal placed onto both vital dentin and pulp tissues will provide predictable results for immediate relief of postoperative sensitivity as well as long-term biologic success.

Certain studies of direct capping[141,145] report no pulp inflammation in adhesively capped pulps, whereas others[146,147] report presence of macrophages with adhesive particles, a consequence of morphologic or chemical factors. One remaining complicating factor may be biofilm contamination. If pulp cells protrude onto the cavity wall and cavity floor before material placement, there will be no hybridization and poor to no dentin bridge formation (Fig 14-10).[148] Consequently, failure occurs due to biofilm contamination on the dentin interface, causing loss of a complete bacteriometic seal and thus permitting bacterial microleakage to the pulp, resulting in inflammation and eventual necrosis.

Cavity Cleansing, Disinfection, and Hemorrage Control

A clinical review failed to support direct pulp-capping or pulpotomy procedures in teeth when a mechanical exposure pushes infected carious operative debris into the subjacent pulp.[79] Because of the stigma of long-term failures, our profession generally selects traditional endodontic treatment. Only in the treatment of pulp exposures in fractured young anterior teeth with open apices does the literature discuss pulpotomy or direct pulp-capping with $Ca(OH)_2$,[149,150] MTA,[114,116] or adhesives.[139,151] Recent studies demonstrate that a successful outcome requires absolute hemorrhage control, regardless of the dental material used for direct pulp-capping.[18,41,122] Traditional clinical teaching suggests that hemostasis may be achieved by mechanical pressure with a cotton pellet dampened with sterile saline, hydrogen peroxide, $Ca(OH)_2$, NaOCl, ferric sulfate, alcohol, or epinephrine; techniques such as electrocautery and laser energy application have also been reported with some success.

Healing Potential of the Pulp

A detailed review of pulpal healing is presented in chapter 3. In nonexposed usage studies, when cavities were placed to within 100 µm of the dental pulp and restored with adhesives, only slight or no pulpal responses were reported.[18,120] When caries is removed to avoid pulp exposures in deep caries lesions, reactionary or reparative dentin forms in teeth sealed with ZnOE and amalgam, maintaining pulp vitality for long periods. Generally, the primary odontoblastic layer below the cavities is lost through preparation trauma; however, reactionary dentin forms when a bacteriometic seal is developed.[152,153]

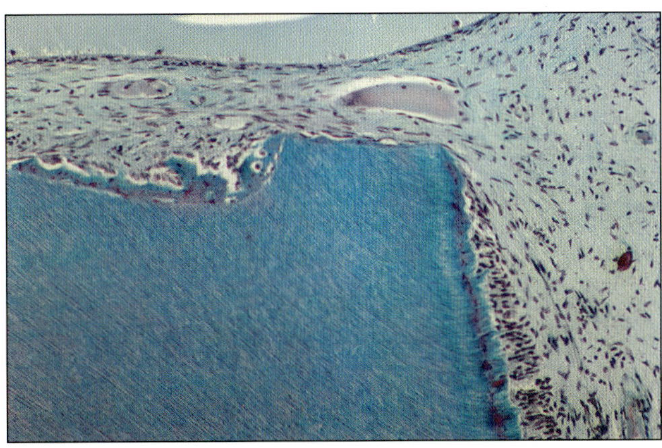

Fig 14-10 Histologic section of nonhuman primate pulp that was direct capped with Command resin (Kerr) for 21 days. Note the pulp has migrated into the area originally filled with clot and coagulum debris. Some reparative dentin with new odontoblastoid cells is seen on the cavity floor *(left)* and along the pulpal wall. Fibroblasts have stratified directly adjacent to the resin interface. No new dentin matrix is seen at this time and no inflammatory cells are present (Masson stain, original magnification ×100).

An Exudate-Free Interface

Successful pulp-capping has tended to focus on issues such as damage to the collagen of vital dentin and pulp tissues from acid etching and resin application. However, direct capping must be viewed as treating a surgical wound, following the principles of the medical model. Debridement of damaged tissues, removal of operative debris, aseptic management of the wound site, hemostasis, and proper bacteriometic sealing of all tissue interfaces are all important considerations for successful pulp therapy.

How might we reconcile hemorrhage control to our daily clinical practice? Generally, ISO usage studies require surgery and dental material placement under general anesthesia. Importantly, general anesthesia has little to no effect on pulp blood flow.[154] Consequently, complete hemorrhage control is more challenging in usage studies than in daily clinical practice, where local anesthetics are generally used.

NaOCl was introduced for clinical use after World War I.[155] Since then, NaOCl has gained bio-

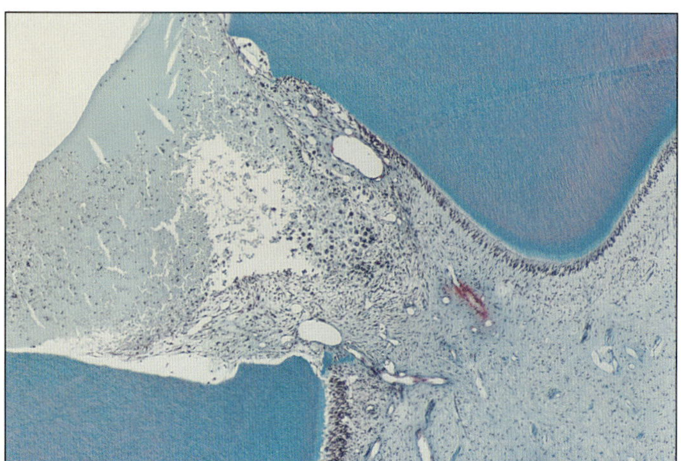

Fig 14-11 Histologic section of a nonhuman primate pulp exposure that was direct capped with an autocured resin for 7 days. No attempt was made to control hemorrhage or organic biofilm or to remove the operative debris. Due to a poor seal, the first line of inflammation (acute cells, ie, polymorphonuclear neutrophils [PMNs]) has migrated into the clot-coagulum space *(upper left)* ahead of the trailing pioneer pulp fibroblasts. Even with the lack of a biometic hybrid seal along the cavity wall, the deeper pulp is not yet showing traditional pulp inflammation or necrosis (Masson stain, original magnification ×40).

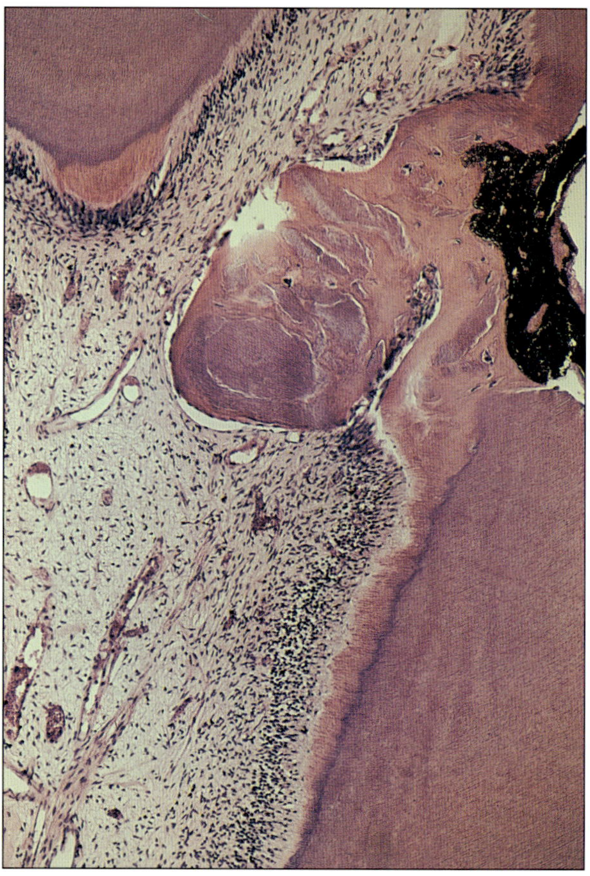

Fig 14-12 Histologic section of a nonhuman primate pulp that was direct capped with Dycal for 5 weeks. Dycal is seen on the right with a large dentin bridge mass incorporated with operative debris, a consequence of dentin chips being pushed into the subjacent pulp during the mechanical exposure. No hemorrhage control agents were employed (H&E stain, original magnification ×25).

logic acceptance as a suitable aseptic and hemostatic agent for clinical pulp treatment. Publications continue to demonstrate that concentrations of NaOCl provide ideal hemorrhage control when placed on an exposed pulp.[18,130,148,156–158] NaOCl in concentrations of 2.5% to 5.25% provides asepsis of the cavity interface, chemical amputation of the blood clot and fibrin, and removal of damaged cells and operative debris from the mechanical exposure and subjacent pulp. In general, agents with high pH (ie, NaOCl, $Ca[OH]_2$, MTA) all show improved histologic results due to their capacity to reduce or stop normal blood flow.

Recent in vivo usage studies employing adhesives for direct capping or pulpotomy report excellent hemostasis with NaOCl.[121,122] Until recently, no commercial dental material has shown consistent hemorrhage or biofilm control when general anesthesia is used for sedation; instead, studies show remaining operative debris with poor hemostasis and organic biofilm on the cavity walls[142,159] (Fig 14-11). This biofilm compromises hybridization of the underlying dentin, interfering with the formation of a uniform hybrid layer. Indeed, it has been suggested that the primary cause of pulp inflammation is incomplete control of homeostasis at the exposed pulp-dentin inter-

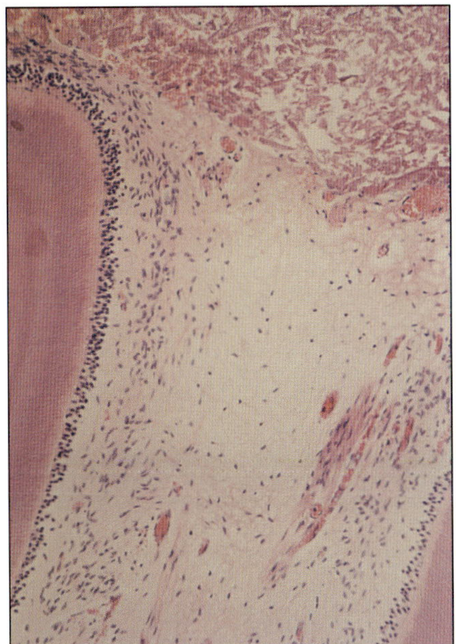

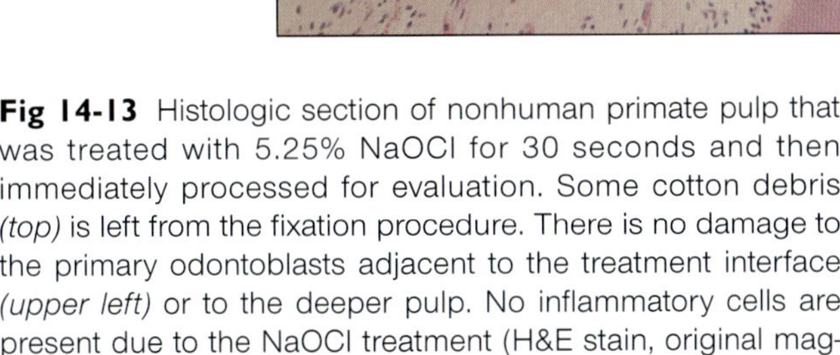

Fig 14-13 Histologic section of nonhuman primate pulp that was treated with 5.25% NaOCl for 30 seconds and then immediately processed for evaluation. Some cotton debris *(top)* is left from the fixation procedure. There is no damage to the primary odontoblasts adjacent to the treatment interface *(upper left)* or to the deeper pulp. No inflammatory cells are present due to the NaOCl treatment (H&E stain, original magnification ×100).

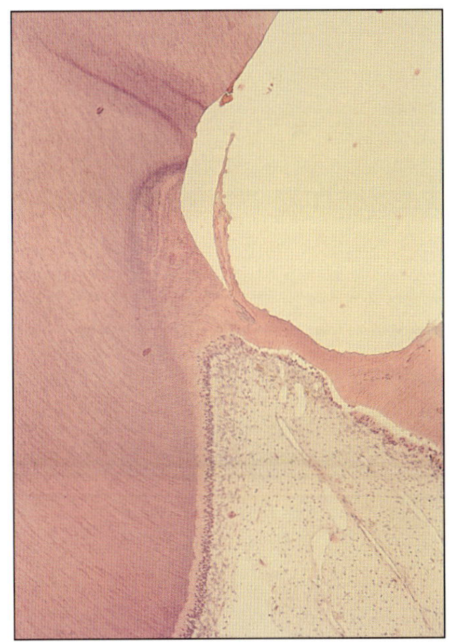

Fig 14-14 Histologic section of a nonhuman primate pulp that was treated with a 5% NaOCl for 30 seconds and then immediately restored with an Ultradent adhesive and resin composite system for 75 days. A new dentin bridge *(center below the cavity)* is continuous with the reparative dentin to the right. There is no operative debris within the reparative or dentin bridges or in the pulp below the exposure interface. The subjacent and deeper pulp is free of inflammation and resin particles (H&E stain, original magnification ×60).

face, leading to a poor bacteriometic seal and eventually to bacterial microleakage, inflammation, and necrosis.[158] Pushing operative debris from the mechanical exposure into the pulp immediately below the exposure site (Fig 14-12) (chipitis) has been reported to complicate healing and dentin bridging.[159] Consequently, complete removal of subjacent clot and operative debris is essential to promote unobstructed pulp healing.

Given these findings, it is evident that the ability to control hemorrhage and placement of any pulp-capping material on clean dentin is quintessential for long-term success of the clinical procedure. NaOCl solubilizes the biofilm more selectively than low-pH agents, which precipitate proteins rather than dissolve them. In nonexposed pulps, the volume of pulpal serum leakage and gingival fluid contamination onto the cavity preparation is minimal. The creation of a proper hybrid layer under these conditions is easily achieved, but apparently not an important factor when MTA is used. In exposed pulps where hemostasis is difficult to achieve, proper placement of hydrophilic primers on a clean dentin surface followed by hydrophobic systems is extremely technique sensitive. In fact, successful pulp-capping with any dental material is a technique-sensitive procedure, especially in a carious field.

Several important conclusions may be drawn with some confidence at this time. A recent study (C.F. Cox, unpublished data, 2001) has shown that use of NaOCl demonstrates no in vivo toxicity to pulp cells below the exposure interface (Fig 14-13), with no inhibition of pulp healing or the biologic mechanisms of odontoblastoid cell or dentin bridge formation. More important, there is a conspicuous absence of operative debris at the exposure interface with NaOCl use (Fig 14-14), and dentin bridge formation occurs directly adjacent to the adhesive interface.

Factors Leading to Success

In order to develop a proper understanding of the issue of direct pulp-capping with dental materials, it is imperative to consider the variables that may lead to failure or success. Age of the patient, history of previous restorations, symptomology, and assessment of pulp vitality must be considered during clinical application regardless of the material selection.[160] Assessment of radiographic evidence, thermal testing, dental history, physiologic mobility, and subjective symptomology are critical to predictable outcomes. Another consideration often overlooked is the use of propylene glycol-based caries-detector dyes, developed to preserve softened demineralized dentin subjacent to the pulp. Most clinicians elect to remove the affected dentin during subjective caries excavation. However, the preservation of inner carious dentin, identified by propylene glycol-based dyes, contributes to pulpal protection and remineralization in conjunction with a hybridized seal.[161,162] Data show that the inner carious layer, containing intact collagen fibers, will remineralize. Thus, preservation of this affected layer of softened dentin contributes to pulp protection, vitality, and increased prognosis for pulp longevity.[163-165]

Summary

In the past few decades, we have gained a much clearer understanding of pulp biology and initial repair mechanisms, providing an avenue for the development of techniques and materials to predictably repair the injured pulp. Strong histologic data demonstrate that repair of the vital pulp can occur against newly developed nonresorbable materials provided a true bacteriometic seal is developed at the dentin-pulp interface. These materials appear to possess favorable properties when applied in conjunction with proper tissue debridement, antisepsis, and hemorrhage control in the operative field.

Certain reservations must be placed on treatment protocols and dental materials of our past. Current knowledge and thinking, fueled by promising research and new dental materials, will enhance our selection of prospective materials with which to treat injured pulp in future clinical challenges.

References

1. Zander HA. Reaction of the pulp calcium hydroxide J Dent Res 1939;18:373-379.
2. Kozlov M, Massler M. Histologic effects of various drugs on amputated pulps of rat molars. Oral Surg 1966;13:455-469.
3. Kakahashi S, Stanley HS, Fitzgerald RJ. The effects of surgical exposures of dental pulps in germ-free and conventional laboratory rats. Oral Surg 1965;20:340-349.
4. Brännström M, Nyborg H. The presence of bacteria in cavities filled with silicate cement and composite resin materials. Swed Dent J 1971;64:149-158.
5. Snuggs HM, Cox CF, Powell CS, White KC. Pulpal healing and dentinal bridge formation in an acidic environment. Quintessence Int 1993;24:501-510.
6. Smith AJ, Cassidy N, Perry H. Reactionary dentinogenesis. Int J Dev Biol 1995;39:273-280.
7. Smith AJ, Sloan AJ, Matthews JB, Murray PE, Lumley P. Reparative processes in dentine and pulp. In: Addy M, Emberg G, Edger M, Orchardson R (eds). Tooth Wear and Sensitivity. London: Masters Durity, 1999:5-14.
8. Rutherford B, Spångberg L. Transdentinal stimulation of reparative dentine formation by osteogenic protein-1 in monkeys. Arch Oral Biol 1995;40:681-683.
9. Spångberg L. Kinetic and quantitative evaluation of material cytotoxicity in vitro. Oral Surg 1973;35:389-401.
10. Tyas MJ. A method for the in vitro toxicity testing of dental restorative materials. J Dent Res 1976;56:1285-1290.
11. Ruyter IE. Release of formaldehyde from denture base polymers. Acta Odontol Scand 1980;38:17-27.
12. Øysæd H, Ruyter IE, Kleven S. Release of formaldehyde from dental composites. J Dent Res 1988;67(10):1289-1294.

13. Wataha JC, Hanks CT, Craig RG. In vitro synergistic and duration of exposure effects of metal cations on eukaryotic cells. J Biomed Mater Res 1992;26: 1297–1309.
14. Noda M, Kaga M, Komatsu H, Sano H. Interaction between monomers related with dental filling materials and cell membrane of HeLa. In: Modern Trends in Adhesive Dentistry [Proceedings of the Adhesive Dentistry Forum, 1998, Sapporo Japan]. Osaka, Japan: Kuraray, 1998:102–106.
15. Hashieh IA, Cosset A, Franquin JC. In vitro cytotoxicity of one-step dentin bonding systems. J Endod 1999;25: 89–92.
16. Ratanasathien S, Wataha JC, Hanks CT, Dennison JB. Cytotoxic interactive effects of dentin bonding components on mouse fibroblasts. J Dent Res 1995;74: 1602–1606.
17. Brännström M, Nyborg H. Points in the experimental study of pulpal response to restorative materials. Odont Tidsk 1969;77:42142–146.
18. Akimoto N, Momoi Y, Kohno A, Otsuki M, Cox CF. Biocompatibility of Clearfil Liner Bond 2 and Clearfil AP-X system on nonexposed and exposed primate teeth. Quintessence Int 1998;29:177–188.
19. Miller WD. The Micro-organisms of the Human Mouth: The Local and General Diseases Which Are Caused By Them. Philadelphia: SS White Dental, 1890:119–144.
20. Fusayama T, Okuse K, Hosoda H. Relationship between hardness, discoloration, and microbial invasion in carious dentin. J Dent Res 1966;45:1033–1047.
21. Ohgushi K, Fusayama T. Electron microscopic structure of the two layers of carious dentin. J Dent Res 1975;54: 1019–1026.
22. Reeves R, Stanley HR. The relationship of bacterial penetration and pulpal pathosis in carious teeth. Oral Surg 1966;22:59–65.
23. Eidelman E, Ulmansky M. Histopathology of the pulp with deep dentinal caries. Pediatr Dent 1992;14: 372–375.
24. Shroff FR. The effects of filling materials on the dental pulp: An histological experimental study with special reference to synthetic porcelain, part II. N Zealand Dent J 1947;43:35–58.
25. Langeland K, Tronstad L, Langeland LE. Human pulp changes of iatrogenic origin. Oral Surg 1971;32: 943–980.
26. Brännström M, Vojinovic O. Response of the dental pulp to invasion of bacteria around three filling materials. J Dent Child 1976;43:15–21.
27. Cotton WR. Bacterial contamination as a factor in healing of pulp exposures. Oral Surg 1974;38:441–450.
28. Bergenholtz G, Cox CF, Loesche WJ, Syed SA. Bacterial leakage around dental restorations: Its effect on the dental pulp. J Oral Pathol 1982;11:439–450.
29. Cox CF, Keall CL, Keall HJ, Ostro E, Bergenholtz G. Biocompatibility of surface-sealed dental materials against exposed dental pulps. J Prosthet Dent 1987;57:1–8.
30. Cox CF, Sübay RK, Ostro E. Biocompatibility of various dental materials: Pulp healing with a surface seal. Int J Periodontics Restorative Dent 1996, 16:241–251.
31. Qvist V. Pulp reactions in human teeth to tooth colored filling materials. Scand J Dent Res 1975;83:54–66.
32. Watts A. Bacterial contamination and the toxicity of silicate and zinc phosphate cements. Br Dent J 1979;146: 7–13.
33. Torstenson B, Nordenvall KJ, Brännström M. Pulpal reaction and microorganisms under Clearfil composite resin in deep cavities with acid etched dentin. Swed Dent J 1982;6:167–176.
34. Bergenholtz G, Lindhe J. Effect of soluble plaque factors on inflammatory reactions in the dental pulp. Scand J Dent Res 1975;83:153–158.
35. Mejáre B, Mejáre L, Edwardsson S. Bacteria beneath composite restorations: A culturing and histo-bacteriological study. Acta Odontol Scand 1979;37:267–275.
36. Bergenholtz G. Inflammatory response of the dental pulp to bacterial irritation. J Endod 1981;7:100–104.
37. Meryon SD. The influence of dentine on the in vitro toxicity testing of dentinal restorative materials. J Biomed Mater Res 1984;18:771–779.
38. Fusayama T. Factors and prevention of pulp irritation by adhesive composite resin restorations. Quintessence Int 1987;18:633–641.
39. Kidd E. Microleakage: A review. J Dent 1976;4:199–206.
40. Fujitani M, Inokishi S, Hosoda H. Effect of acid etching on the dental pulp in adhesive composite restorations. Int Dent J 1992;43:3–11.
41. Matsuo T, Nakanishi T, Shimizu H, Ebisu S. A clinical study of direct pulp capping applied to cariously exposed pulps. J Endod 1996;22:551–556.
42. Warfvinge J, Bergenholtz G. Healing capacity of human and monkey dental pulps following experimentally induced pulpitis. Endod Dent Traumatol 1986;2: 256–262.
43. Fish EW. The pathology of the dentine and dental pulp. Br Dent J 1932;53:351–353.
44. Beust TB. Physiologic changes in the dentin. J Dent Res 1931;11:267–275.
45. Weider SR, Schour I, Mohammed CI. Reparative dentine following cavity and fillings in the rat molar. Oral Surg 1956;9:221–222.
46. Millsop RC, Stanley HR. Human pulp response to mechanical condensation [abstract]. J Dent Res 1967;46:573.
47. Goto G, Jordan RE. Pulpal response to composite-resin materials [abstract]. J Prosthet Dent 1972;28:601–606.
48. Seelig A, Doyle JI. Pulp reactions to anterior restorative materials [abstract]. J Dent Res 1974;555:193.

49. Murray PE, About I, Franquin J-C, Remsuat M, Smith AJ. Restorative pulpal and repair responses. J Am Dent Assoc 2001;132:482–490.
50. Hermann BW. Dentinobliteration der Wurzelkanale nach Behandlung mit Calcium. Zahnärztl Rdsch 1930;39:887–899.
51. Marmasse A. Pulp exposures closed by secondary dentin. Northwest Dent 1948;24:38–41.
52. Via WF. Evaluation of deciduous molars treated by pulpotomy and calcium hydroxide. J Am Dent Assoc 1955;50:34–43.
53. Nyborg H. Healing process in the pulp on capping. Acta Odontol Scand 955;13(16):129–130.
54. Berman DS, Massler M. Experimental pulpotomies in dental pulps. J Dent Res 1958;37:229–272.
55. Kapur KK, Shaporo S, Shklar D. Response of the human dental pulp to various physical and chemical agents: A correlated clinical and histopathologic study. Oral Surg 1964;17:640–649.
56. Sayegh FA, Reed AJ. Correlated and histological evaluation of Hydrex in pulp therapy. J Dent Child 1967;34: 471–477.
57. Ulmansky M, Sela J, Sela M. Scanning electron microscopy of calcium hydroxide induced bridges. J Oral Pathol 1972;1:244–248.
58. Ichikawa T. Light and electron microscopic studies of the dentin bridge formation following vital pulpotomy in dog's teeth. Shikwa Gakuho 1976;76:391–439.
59. Pitt Ford TR, Roberts GJ. Immediate and delayed direct pulp capping with the use of a new visible light-cured $Ca(OH)_2$ preparation. Oral Surg 1991;71:338–342.
60. Stanley HR. Trashing the dental literature—Misleading the general practitioners: A point of view. J Dent Res 1996;75(9):1624–626.
61. Chong WF, Swartz ML, Philips RW. Displacement of cement bases by amalgam condensation. J Am Dent Assoc 1967;74:97–110.
62. Fischer FJ. The effect of three proprietary lining materials on micro-organisms in carious dentine. Br Dent J 1977;143:231–235.
63. Bryant RW, Wing G. The effect of manipulative variables on base forming materials for amalgam restorations. Aust Dent J 1976;21:211–216.
64. Lloyd CH, Anderson JN. The strength and fracture toughness of calcium hydroxide preparations. J Oral Rehabil 1980;7:155–165.
65. Reinhardt JW, Chalkey Y. Softening effects of bases on composite resins. Clin Prev Dent 1983;5:9–12.
66. McComb D. Comparison of physical properties of commercial calcium hydroxide lining cements. J Am Dent Assoc 1983;95:601–613.
67. Hwas M, Sandrick JL. Acid and water solubility and strength of calcium hydroxide bases. J Am Dent Assoc 1984;108:46–48.
68. Burke FJT, Watts DC. Weight loss of four calcium hydroxide-based materials following a phosphoric acid and washing cycle. J Dent 1986;14:226–227.
69. Titus HW, Draheim RN, Murrey AJ. The effect of enamel etchant on the solubility of three calcium hydroxide bases. J Prosthet Dent 1988;60:178–180.
70. Fisher FJ. The effect of a calcium hydroxide/water paste on micro-organisms in carious dentin. Br Dent J 1972;133:19–21.
71. Paterson RC. Bacterial contamination and the exposed pulp. Br Dent J 1976;140:231–236.
72. Barkhordar RA, Kempler D. Antimicrobial activity of calcium hydroxide liners on S. mutans and S. sanguis. J Prosthet Dent 1989;61:314–316.
73. Schröder U, Granath LE. Scanning electron microscopy of hard tissue barrier following experimental pulpotomy in intact human teeth and capped with calcium hydroxide Odontol Rev 1972;23:211–220.
74. Feilzer AJ, de Gee AJ, Davidson CL. Setting stresses in composites for two different curing modes. Dent Mater 1993;9:2–5.
75. Goracci G, Mori G. Scanning electron micrographic evaluation of resin-dentin and calcium hydroxide-dentin interface with resin composite restorations. Quintessence Int 1996;27:129–135.
76. Ranly D. Pulp therapy at the turn of the century. Am Acad Pediatr Dent 1999;21:384–386.
77. Rowe AH. Reaction of the rat molar pulp to various materials. Br Dent J 1967;122:291–300.
78. Watts A, Paterson RC. Simple metallic compounds as pulp-capping agents. Oral Surg 1979;48:561–563.
79. Walton RE, Langeland K. Migration of materials in the dental pulp of monkeys. J Endod 1978;4:167–177.
80. Russo MC, Holland R, de Souza V. Radiographic and histological evaluation of the treatment of inflamed dental pulps. Int Endod J 1982;15:137–142.
81. Goldberg F, Massone EJ, Spielberg C. Evaluation of the dentinal bridge after pulpotomy and calcium hydroxide dressing. J Endod 1984;10:318–320.
82. Cox CF, Bergenholtz G. Tunnel defects in dentin bridges: Long-term direct capping evaluation [abstract 1445]. J Dent Res 1984;63:331.
83. Tronstad L, Barnett F, Flax M. Solubility and biocompatibility of calcium hydroxide-containing root canal sealers. Endod Dent Traumatol 1988;4:152–159.
84. Doyle WA. A Comparison of the Formocresol Pulpotomy Technique with the Calcium Hydroxide Technique [master's thesis]. Bloomington: Indiana Univ School of Dentistry, 1961:1–55.
85. Doyle WA, McDonald RE, Mitchell DF. Formocresol versus calcium hydroxide in pulpotomy. J Dent Child 1962;2:86–79.
86. Cabrini RI, Maisto OA, Manfredi EE. Internal resorption of dentine: Histopathologic control of eight cases after pulp amputation and capping with calcium hydroxide. Oral Surg 1957;10:90–96.

87. Hume RW. Are restorative materials and procedures harmful to the pulp? Trans Acad Dent Mater 1998;12: 105–119.
88. Trowbridge HO, Edwall L, Panopoulas P. Effect of zinc oxide-eugenol and calcium hydroxide on intradental nerve activity. J Endod 1982;8:403–406.
89. Watts A, Paterson R. Migration of materials and microorganisms in the dental pulp of dogs and rats. J Endod 1982;8:53–58.
90. Bramante CM, Berbert A. Root perforations dressed with calcium hydroxide or zinc oxide and eugenol. J Endod 1987;13:392–395.
91. Hendry JA, Jeansonne BG, Dummett CO, Burrell WA. Comparison of calcium hydroxide and zinc oxide and eugenol pulpectomies in primary teeth of dogs. Oral Surg 1982;54:445–449.
92. Brännström M, Nordenvall K, Torstenson B. Pulpal reaction to IRM cement: An intermediate restorative material containing eugenol. ASDC J Dent Child 1981;48: 259–263.
93. Buckley JP. The chemistry of pulp decomposition with rational treatment for this condition and its sequelae. J Am Dent Assoc 1904;3:764–771.
94. Sweet CA. Procedure for treatment of exposed and pulpless deciduous teeth. J Am Dent Assoc 1930;17: 1150–1153.
95. Strange EM. Is vital pulpotomy worthwhile? J Dent Child 1953;20:38–42.
96. Wong KC. Effects of Paraformaldehyde Preparation on the Periapical Tissues in Non-vital Pulpotomy Procedures [master's thesis]. Evanston, IL: Northwestern Univ School of Dentistry, 1958:1–122.
97. Mansuhkani N, Massler M. Effects of formocresol on the dental pulp. J Dent Child 1959;26:277–297.
98. Emmerson CC, Miyamoto O, Sweet CA, Bhatia HO. Pulpal changes following formocresol applications on rat molars and human primary teeth. SC Dent Am J 1959;27:309–323.
99. Spedding RH. The Effects of Formocresol and Calcium Hydroxide on the Dental Pulps of Rhesus Monkeys [master's thesis]. Bloomington: Indiana Univ School of Dentistry, 1963:1–73.
100. Lewis B. Formaldehyde in dentistry: Review for the millennium. J Clin Paediatr Dent 1998;22:167–177.
101. Ranly D, Garcia-Godoy F. Current and potential pulp therapies for primary and young permanent teeth. J Dent 2000;28:153–161.
102. Myers DR, Shoa FHK, Dirksen TR, Pashley DH, Whitford GM, Reynolds KE. Distribution of 14C-formaldehyde after pulpotomy with formocresol. J Am Dent Assoc 1978;96:805–813.
103. Pashley EL, Myers DR, Pashley DH, Whitford GM. Systemic distribution of 14C-formaldehyde from formocresol-treated pulpotomy sites. J Dent Res 1980;59:603–608.
104. Pitt Ford TR, Torabinejad M, Abedi HR, Bakland LK, Kariyawasam SP. Using mineral trioxide aggregate as a pulp-capping material. J Am Dent Assoc 1996;127: 1491–1494.
105. Abedi HR, Torabinejad M, Pitt Ford TR, Bakland LK. The use of mineral trioxide aggregate cement (MTA) as a direct pulp capping agent [abstract 44]. J Endod 1996;22:199–209.
106. Junn DJ, McMillan P, Bakland LK, Torabinejad M. Quantitative assessment of dentin bridge formation following pulp capping with mineral trioxide aggregate (MTA). J Endod 1998;24:278–288.
107. Koh ET, Pitt Ford TR, Torabinejad M, MacDonald F. Mineral trioxide aggreagate stimulate cytokine production in human osteoblasts [abstract]. J Bone Res 1995;10 (suppl):S406.
108. Koh ET, McDonald R, Pitt Ford TR, Torabinejad M. Cellular response to mineral trioxide aggregate. J Endod 1998;24:543–547.
109. Torabinejad M, Higa RK, McKendry DJ, Pitt Ford TR. Dye leakage of four root-end filling materials: Effects of blood contamination. J Endod 1995;21:109–121.
110. Kettering JD, Torabinejad M. Investigation of mutagenicity of mineral trioxide aggregate and other commonly used root-end filling materials. J Endod 1995;21: 537–539.
111. Zhu Q, Haglund R, Safave KE, Spångberg LSW. Adhesion of human osteoblasts on root-end filling materials. J Endod 2000;26(7):404–406.
112. Torabinejad M, Wilder Smith P, Pitt Ford TR. Comparative investigation of marginal adaptation of mineral trioxide aggregate and other commonly used root-end filling materials. J Endod 1995;21:295–299.
113. Osorio RM, Hefti A, Vertucci FJ, Shawley AL. Cytotoxicity of endodontic materials. J Endod 1998;21:91–96.
114. Torabinejad M, Chivian N. Clinical applications of mineral trioxide aggregate. J Endod 1999;25:197–205.
115. Holland R, Filho JAO, de Souza V, Nery MJ, Bernabé PFE, Junior ED. Mineral trioxide aggregate repair of lateral root perforations. J Endod 2001;27:281–284.
116. Eidelman E, Holan G, Fuks AB. Mineral trioxide aggregate vs. formocresol in pulpotomized primary molars: A preliminary report. Pediatr Dent 2001;23:15–18.
117. Wilson A, Kent B. A new translucent cement for dentistry: The glass ionomer cement. Br Dent J 1972;132: 133–135.
118. Hume WR. A new technique for screening chemical toxicity to the pulp from dental restorative materials and procedures. J Dent Res 1985;64:1322–1325.
119. Felton D, Cox CF, Odom M, Kanoy B. Pulpal response to chemically cured and experimental light-cured glass ionomer cavity liner. J Prosthet Dent 1991;65:704–712.

120. Tarim B, Hafez AA, Suzuki SH, Cox CF. Biocompatibility of Optibond and XR-Bond adhesive systems in nonhuman primate teeth. Int J Periodontics Restorative Dent 1998;18:87–99.
121. Hafez AA, Kopel HM, Cox CF. Pulpotomy reconsidered: Application of an adhesive system to pulpotomized permanent primate pulps. Quintessence Int 2000;31: 579–589.
122. Hafez AA, Cox CF, Tarim B, Otsuki M, Akimoto N. An in vivo evaluation of hemorrhage control using NaOCl in exposed non-human primate pulps and direct capping with Bisco All Bond 2, or One Step adhesive systems. Quintessence Int 2002;33:737–748.
123. Pameijer CH, Stanley HR. Pulp reactions to resin cements. Am J Dent 1992;5:81–87.
124. Stanley HR, Pameijer CH. Sequential death of exposed pulps with "total etch" bonding treatments [abstract]. J Dent Res 1997;76:305.
125. Hamid A, Hume WR. Diffusion of resin monomers through human carious dentin in vitro. Endod Dent Traumatol 1997;13:1–5.
126. Hume RW. Are restorative materials and procedures harmful to the pulp? Trans Acad Dent Mater 1998;12: 105–109.
127. Nakabayashi N. Resin reinforced dentine due to the infiltration of monomers into the dentine at the adhesive interface. J Jpn Soc Dent Mat Dev 1982;1:78–81.
128. Inokoshi S, Iwaku M, Fusayama T. Pulpal response to a new adhesive restorative resin. J Dent Res 1982;61: 1014–1019.
129. Fusayama T. Pulp capping following removal of infected dentin using Caries Detector. Phillip J Restaur Zahnmed 1988;5:105–107.
130. Otsuki M, Tagami J, Kanca J III, Akimoto N, Cox CF. Histologic evaluation of two Bisco adhesive systems on exposed pulps. J Dent Res 1997;76:78.
131. Harnirattisai C, Hosoda H. Pulpal responses to various dentin bonding systems to dentin cavities. Dent Mater J 1991;10:149–164.
132. Andreasen JO, Munksgaard EC, Fredebo L, Rud J. Periodontal tissue regeneration including cementogenesis adjacent to dentin-bonded retrograde composite fillings in humans. J Endod 1993;19:151–153.
133. Al-Ajam AD, McGregor AJ. Comparison of the sealing capabilities of Ketac silver and extra-high copper alloy amalgam when used as retrograde root canal filling. J Endod 1993;19:353–356.
134. Inoue T, Miyakoshi S, Shimono M. Dentin pulp/adhesive resin interface: Biological view from basic science to clinic. Quintessence Int 1966(special issue):217–220.
135. Ebihara T, Katoh Y. Histopathological study on the development of adhesive resinous material containing calcium hydroxide as direct pulp capping agent. Jpn J Conserv Dent 1996;39:1288–1295.
136. Demirci M, Üçok M, Küçükkeles N, Soydan N. Pulp reaction to a tri-cure resin-modified glass ionomer. Oral Surg 1998;85:712–719.
137. Mannocci F, Ferrari M. Apical seal of roots obturated with laterally condensed gutta-percha, epoxy resin cement, and dentin bonding agent. J Endod 1998;24: 41–44.
138. Ölmez A, Özlas N, Basak F, Sabuncuoglu B. A histopathologic study of direct pulp-capping with adhesive resins. Oral Surg Oral Med Oral Pathol Oral Radiol Endod 1998;86:98–103.
139. Baratieri LN, Junior SM, Caldeira de Andrada MA, Vieira LCC, Cardoso AC, Ritter AV. Esthetics: Direct Adhesive Restoration on Fractured Anterior Teeth. Chicago: Quintessence, 1998:137–205.
140. Maeda H, Hashiguchi I, Nakamuta H, Toriya Y, Wada N, Akamine A. Histological study of periapical tissue healing in the rat molar after retrofilling with various materials. J Endod 1999;25:38–42.
141. Kitasako Y, Inokishi S, Tagami J. Effects of direct resin pulp capping techniques on short-term response of mechanically exposed pulps. J Dent 1999a;27:257–263.
142. De Costa CAS, Hebling J, Teixeira MF. Preliminary study of biocompatibility of All Bond 2 and Scotchbond MP adhesive systems: Histological evaluation on subcutaneous implants in rats. Rev Odont USP 1997;11:11–18.
143. Pereira JC, Segala AD, de Costa CAS. Human pulp response to direct capping with an adhesive system: Histologic study [abstract]. J Dent Res 1997;76:180.
144. Hebling J, Giro EMA, Costa CA. Biocompatibility of an adhesive system applied to exposed human dental pulp. J Endod 1999;25:676–682.
145. Kitasako Y, Inokishi S, Fujitani M, Otsuki M, Tagami J. Short-term reaction of exposed monkey pulp beneath adhesive resins. Oper Dent 1999b;23:308–317.
146. Gwinnett AJ, Tay FR. Early and intermediate time response of the dental pulp to an acid etch technique in vivo. Am J Dent 1998;11:35–44.
147. Shimono M, Inoue T. Pathology of Wound Healing: Clinical Aspects of Endodontic Treatments. Osaka, Japan: Ishiyaku, 1993:195–200.
148. Cox CF, Hafez AA, Akimoto N, Otsuki M, Tarim B. Biocompatibility of primer, adhesive and resin composite systems on non-exposed and exposed pulps of nonhuman primate teeth. Am J Dent 1998;10:55–63.
149. Cvek M. A clinical report on partial pulpotomy and capping with calcium hydroxide in permanent incisors with complicated fractures. J Endod 1978;4:232–237.
150. Mejáre B, Cvek M. Partial pulpotomy in young permanent teeth with deep carious lesions. Endod Dent Traumatol 1993;9:238–242.
151. Kanca J III. An alternative hypothesis to the cause of pulpal inflammation in teeth treated with phosphoric acid on the dentin. Quintessence Int 1990;21:83–86.
152. Jordan RE, Suzuki M. Conservative treatment of deep carious lesions. J Can Dent Assoc 1971;37:337–342.

153. Jordan RE, Suzuli M, Skinner DH. Indirect pulp-capping of carious teeth with periapical lesions. J Am Dent Assoc 1978;97:37–43.

154. Heyeraas K, Myking A. Pulpal blood flow in immature permanent dog teeth after replantation. Scand J Dent Res 1985;93:227–238.

155. Gutmann J. History. In: Cohen S, Burns R (eds). Pathways of the Pulp, ed 4. St. Louis: Mosby, 1987:766–782.

156. Sudo C. A study on partial pulp removal (pulpotomy) using NaOCl (sodium hypochlorite). J Jpn Stomatol Soc 1959;26:1012–1024.

157. Hiroto K. A study on partial pulp removal (pulpotomy) using four different tissue solvents. J Jpn Stomatol Soc 1959;26:1588–1603.

158. Katoh M, Kidokoro S, Kurosu K. A study on the amputation of pulp using sodium hypochlorite (NaOCl). Jpn J Pediatr Dent 1978;16:107–116.

159. Pameijer CH, Stanley H. The disastrous effects of the "total etch" technique in vital pulp capping in primates. Am J Dent 1998;11(special issue):S45–S54 [erratum 11:S148].

160. Abou-Rass M. The stressed pulp condition: An endodontic-restorative diagnostic concept. J Prosthet Dent 1982;48:264–267.

161. Katao S, Fusayama T. Recalcification of artificially decalcified dog dentin in vitro. J Dent Res 1970;49:1061–1067.

162. Tatsumi T. Physiological remineralization of artificially decalcified monkey dentin under adhesive composite resin. J Jpn Stomatol Soc 1989;56:47–74.

163. Fusayama T, Terachima S. Differentiation of two layers of carious dentin by staining. J Dent Res 1972;51:866.

164. Fusayama T, Nakamura M, Kurosaki N, Iwaku M. Non-pressure adhesion of a new adhesive restorative system. J Dent Res 1979;58:1364–1370.

165. Fusayama T, Yamada T, Inokishi S. The use of a caries detector dye during cavity preparation [comment]. Br Dent J 1993;175:312–313.

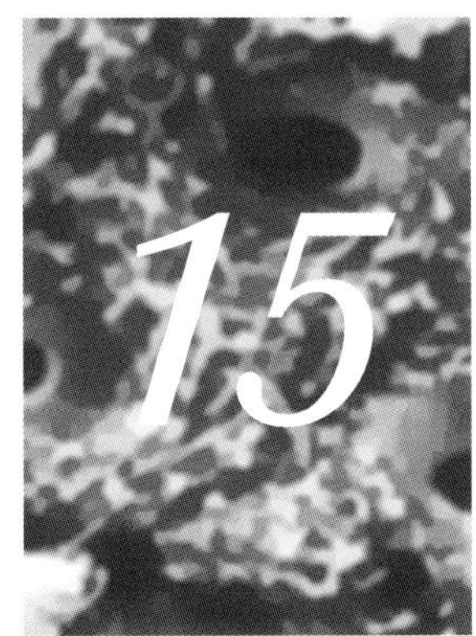

Permanent Restorations and the Dental Pulp

Harold H. Messer, DDS, PhD

Restorative dentistry is in a period of rapid change. The advent of methods providing adhesion to enamel and dentin has resulted in more conservative cavity preparations and a more effective seal against bacterial microleakage. Toward the more adventurous limits of adhesive dentistry, the possibility of preserving carious dentin and even of placing restorative materials directly over exposed pulps is receiving serious attention. The "post-amalgam age" of restorative dentistry promises not only better protection of the pulp against injury but also promotion of the healing of damaged pulps.[1] At the same time, preservation of intact dentitions into old age has led to an increased demand for complex restorative procedures. A cumulative history of caries and repeated restoration means that the aging dental pulp is subjected to increasing injury.

Every aspect of restorative dentistry potentially has an effect on the pulp. Most of these effects are indirect, mediated via diffusion across the underlying dentin. The healthy pulp is also able to mount a protective response, and the effects of restorative procedures on the pulp are for the most part minor and transient (Fig 15-1). This chapter first considers in general terms those restorative procedures that affect the dental pulp and the pulpal response, then reviews in detail specific materials and procedures. The biomechanics of restored teeth, including endodontically treated teeth, is also considered.

Role of Dentin in Mediating Effects of Restorative Procedures

Effects of restorative procedures on the pulp can be understood only within the context of the role of intervening dentin and, more specifically, that of dentinal tubules (see chapter 4). Acute effects of cavity preparation and material placement result from a hydrodynamic effect of fluid flow within tubules. Diffusion of toxic components of restorative materials and bacterial toxins occurs via fluid-filled tubules, and part of the protective response of the pulp involves occlusion of tubules and a reduction in dentinal permeability.

In human teeth, dentin is, on average, approximately 3 mm thick. The highly mineralized matrix is traversed by fluid-filled dentinal tubules, ranging from less than 1 μm in diameter close to the dentinoenamel junction (DEJ) to 2 to 3 μm at the

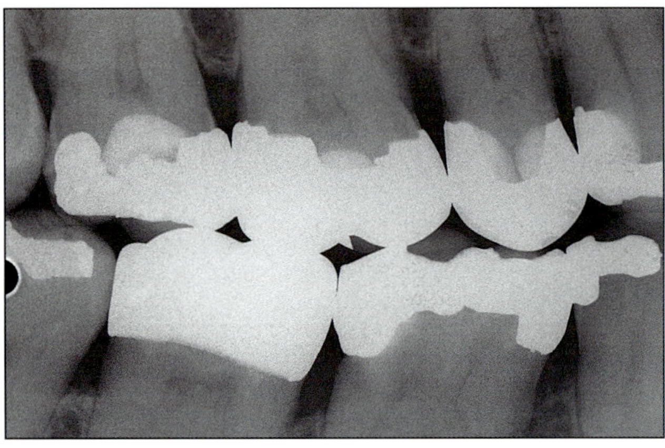

Fig 15-1 A heavily restored dentition in a mature adult. Despite repeated cycles of extensive restoration, all pulps remain vital.

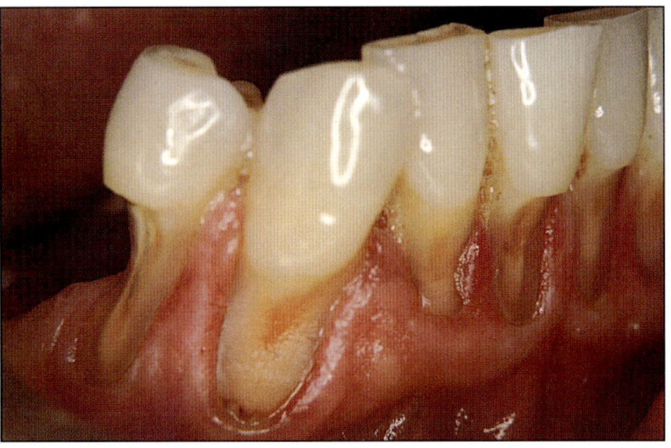

Fig 15-2a Cervical noncaries lesions. Loss of tooth structure extends through the original canal space, but dentinal sclerosis and tertiary dentinal deposition have protected the pulp from injury.

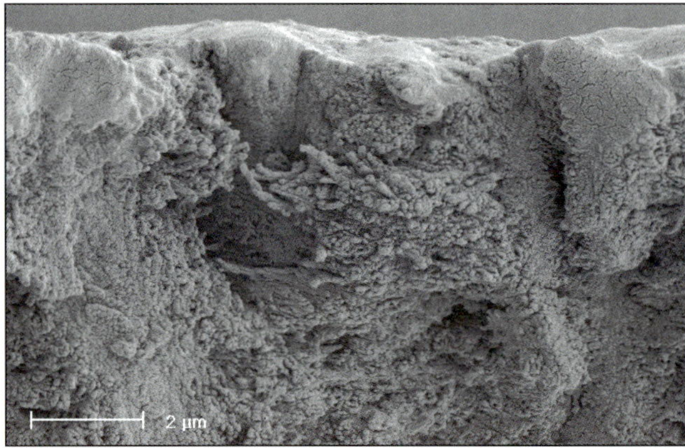

Fig 15-2b Fractured section of a cervical noncaries lesion, showing the surface hypermineralized zone and tubule obliteration. (Courtesy of Dr M. Burrow.)

pulpal surface. Tubules converge as they approach the pulp, increasing in density from approximately 20,000/mm^2 in outer dentin to 45,000/mm^2 adjacent to the pulp. The cross-sectional area of dentin occupied by tubules varies from less than 1% near the dentinoenamel junction to more than 20% close to the pulp. Hence, when dentin is cut, permeability to noxious agents is much greater close to the pulp than in outer dentin. Permeability is not uniform throughout the tooth, but is greater overlying pulpal horns and on axial walls than on the occlusal surface (see chapter 4).[2,3]

A positive hydrostatic pressure from pulpal circulation results in outward fluid flow when tubules are exposed. Outward fluid flow may contribute to pulpal protection because, as a transudate of plasma, it contains proteins (immunoglobulins, fibrinogen) and minerals (calcium, phosphate). Outward fluid flow also limits the rate of diffusion of noxious agents in a pulpal direction.[2] Tubules also contain odontoblast processes, which may be severed by preparations cut deeply into intact dentin, damaging the underlying odontoblast cell bodies within the pulp.

Dental history

When subjected to a gradually progressive injury, a major part of the pulp's response is the deposition of mineral within dentinal tubules, occluding the tubule against further ingress of noxious stimuli (see chapter 3). With increasing age, peritubular dentinal deposition increases and may completely obliterate dentinal tubules. Cervical noncaries lesions ("abrasion" or "abfraction" lesions) also show occluded dentinal tubules as well as a surface hypermineralized zone (Fig 15-2).[4] Dentin affected by caries is frequently classified into two layers: demineralized, bacteria-containing "infected" dentin and a deeper "affected" layer that includes a "transparent" zone with tubules occluded by mineral deposits.[5,6] Regardless of the stimulus, occlusion of tubules reduces dentinal permeability. From a clinical perspective, it is important to preserve this layer because it protects the pulp against injury from restorative materials or procedures. At the same time, acid etching of this layer is less effective than on normal dentin, making dentin bonding (and hence a durable marginal seal) more difficult.[4,7]

Prepared dentinal surface

Techniques of cavity preparation now include chemical means of caries removal, airborne particle abrasion, laser irradiation, and minimal surface preparation (cervical noncaries lesions). Following these techniques, the dentinal surface may be very different from that after cutting with rotary instruments, and with adhesive techniques it is often further modified by etching or "conditioning" with strong acids. Rotary or hand instruments create a smear layer, typically 1 to 2 μm thick and consisting primarily of debris from cutting the underlying dentin, with smear plugs extending into the cut dentinal tubules.[8-10] The smear layer and smear plugs reduce dentinal permeability by approximately 85% and serve as a barrier to bacterial penetration of dentinal tubules.[3,9] Airborne particle abrasion results in a relatively featureless surface layer that occludes tubule orifices[11]; it is thought to consist of superficial debris as well as embedded abrasive particles, with uncertain consequences for permeability or subsequent restoration. Chemical removal of caries by means of a high-pH gel (eg, Carisolv [MediTeam, Sävedalen, Sweden], initial pH 11) combined with gentle hand excavation produces a minimal smear layer and numerous areas with exposed dentinal tubules.[11] The extreme variability in the prepared dentinal surface and the permeability of the underlying dentin makes it difficult to make generalizations regarding the response of the pulp to a restorative procedure or material.

Box 15-1 Restorative factors contributing to pulpal injury

- Effects of cavity preparation:
  - Frictional heat
  - Desiccation
  - Exposure of dentinal tubules
  - Direct damage to odontoblast processes
  - Chemical treatment of the exposed dentinal surface
- Factors associated with the restorative material and its placement:
  - Material toxicity
  - Insertion pressures
  - Thermal effects
  - Induced stresses
- Effects subsequent to restoration:
  - Marginal leakage
  - Cuspal flexure

Impact of Restorative Procedures and Materials on the Pulp

The net effect of a restorative procedure on the pulp is the result of a complex interaction among many factors: health of the underlying pulp, thickness and permeability of intervening dentin, mechanical injury during cavity preparation, toxicity of the restorative material, and microbial leakage (microleakage). As indicated in Box 15-1, the sources of pulpal injury associated with restorative procedures can be conveniently grouped into three categories: those occurring during cavity preparation, those associated with the restorative material and its placement, and those occurring subsequent to restoration of the tooth. We should not, however, lose sight of the fact that most restorative procedures result in relatively mild, reversible effects on the pulp.

Effects of cavity preparation

Cutting dentin exposes dentinal tubules. If cavity preparations could always be limited to the extent of affected dentin, the pulpal effects of restorative procedures would probably be minimal[3]: tubules occluded by mineral deposition are less permeable to bacterial products and diffusible components of restorative materials; the hydrodynamic response to cutting, heating, and drying is likely to be reduced; and the risk of mechanical damage to odontoblast processes, which recede toward the pulp as tubules are occluded peripherally, is minimized. Despite the more conservative cavity preparations recommended in contemporary restorative dentistry, cutting of intact unaffected dentin is still necessary in instances such as full-crown preparations.

Thermal effects on the pulp of cutting dentin were well documented many years ago[12] and are considered in detail in chapters 4 and 16. The low thermal diffusivity of dentin tends to minimize direct elevation of intrapulpal temperature unless the preparation is cut deep in dentin without effective cooling. There appears to be a "critical range" for intrapulpal temperature, with an increase of approximately 6°C required before irreversible pulpal injury occurs.[12] This extent of temperature increase occurs after about 25 seconds of dry cutting with either high- or low-speed burs. In contrast, the use of water cooling led to a transient decrease in intrapulpal temperature of 6°C to 7°C.

Much more frequently encountered is a hydrodynamic effect, in which heat generated by frictional effects at the dentinal surface results in rapid inward fluid movement in exposed tubules.[13] Desiccation of the exposed dentinal surface, for example, from a stream of air used to dry the cavity preparation, leads to an outward fluid flow. If the stimulus is severe enough, injury to the odontoblast layer may result, causing disruption of junctional complexes and displacement of odontoblast cell bodies into the dentinal tubules.[2]

Direct trauma to odontoblast processes will occur with deep cutting of intact dentin. In mature dentin, odontoblast processes extend into dentinal tubules a distance of 0.1 to 1.0 mm. Importantly, odontoblast cell numbers were unaffected by cavity preparations as close as 0.5 mm to the pulp, indicating absence of an irreversible level of injury.[14,15] Deeper cutting (less than 0.3 mm from the pulp) resulted in direct odontoblast injury and cell death.[16]

Factors associated with the restorative material and its placement

Toxicity of restorative materials

In addition to replacing lost or damaged tissue and restoring function, a restorative material should be biocompatible, ie, it should not elicit an adverse reaction either in the tissues with which it comes into contact or systemically.[17] Traditionally, the ideal material is "biologically neutral," which implies that it is insoluble and inert.[17] Current trends in restorative materials include attempts to incorporate therapeutic agents that may promote pulpal healing.[18,19]

The International Standards Organization (ISO) in 1997 promulgated ISO standard 7405 to regulate the preclinical evaluation of dental material biocompatibility under standardized conditions. Three levels of testing are prescribed: cytotoxicity, using cell culture techniques; tissue toxicity assessed by implantation in subcutaneous tissue or muscle; and "usage tests." Excellent reviews of systemic effects and cytotoxicity of dental materials are available[20-22] and need not be considered here. Of greater relevance is the effect on the underlying pulp, assessed in experimental animals or humans under conditions simulating normal clinical use. Little correlation has been noted between the results of cytotoxicity testing and clinical usage tests.[23]

For restorative materials, the usage test involves placement in prepared cavities of permanent teeth for intervals of up to 3 months. The ISO standard 7405 stipulates that materials should be tested in cervical (Class 5) cavity preparations,[24] which has been widespread practice for many years. The coronal margin is within enamel while the gingival margin is typically in dentin (or cementum). This location provides a rigorous test of the marginal seal of a restoration (Fig 15-3). Bonding to dentin is more difficult than it is to enamel, and tooth flexure during normal function imposes large stresses on the gingival margin. Microleakage is greater at the gingival (dentinal) margin than the coronal (enamel) margin and greater in teeth in functional occlusion than in those that are unstressed.[25] Histologic sections are scored for pulpal inflammation and for the presence of bacteria.

In the absence of bacteria, the extent of pulpal inflammation will be a function of the toxicity of the material itself, modulated by the rate and extent of diffusion through underlying dentin, buffering or binding as the material diffuses through the tubules, outward fluid flow, and the rate of clearance by the pulpal circulation.[2,3] Particulate materials entering the pulp, such as polymerized resin globules, may evoke a foreign body reaction.[26,27] Toxicity of the material must also be distinguished from damage resulting from the cavity preparation (through use of appropriate controls) and, much more importantly, the effects of bacterial microleakage (see chapter 14). The extent of pulpal inflammation is closely correlated with the presence of bacteria at the tooth-restorative material interface, while most materials provoke only a slight pulpal response if bacteria are absent (see next section).

Although most effects of commonly used materials are considered mild and transient,[28] material toxicity per se should not be underestimated,[20] particularly when the material is placed in deep cavities or directly onto the pulpal surface. As one example, in a human study involving more than 300 teeth restored with a range of resin composite and glass-ionomer restorations, the frequency of moderate or severe inflammation in teeth where no bacteria were detected was greater than 50%.[29]

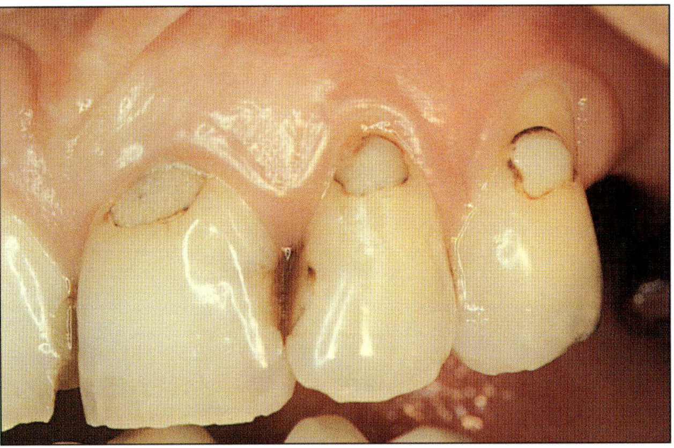

Fig 15-3 Cervical restorations (an early-generation resin composite) with marginal staining indicative of extensive marginal leakage.

Effects of material placement

Amalgam is condensed under sufficient pressure to cause measurable strain in cusps.[30] Moreover, a transient neutrophil infiltration between the odontoblast layer and predentin following amalgam placement was attributed to condensation pressures.[31] Crown cementation also involves substantial pulpal pressures to the extent that components of luting cements and bacterial toxins can be forced into the pulp.[13,32,33] Heat generated during polymerization of resin composite materials may cause hydrodynamic effects (inward fluid movement), while polymerization shrinkage results in permanent stresses in the tooth, accompanied by postoperative sensitivity.[34,35] The long-term consequences of such stresses in teeth are not well understood.

Effects subsequent to restoration

Microleakage

The significance of an inadequate marginal seal between the restorative material and cavity wall, permitting bacterial ingress, is well recognized

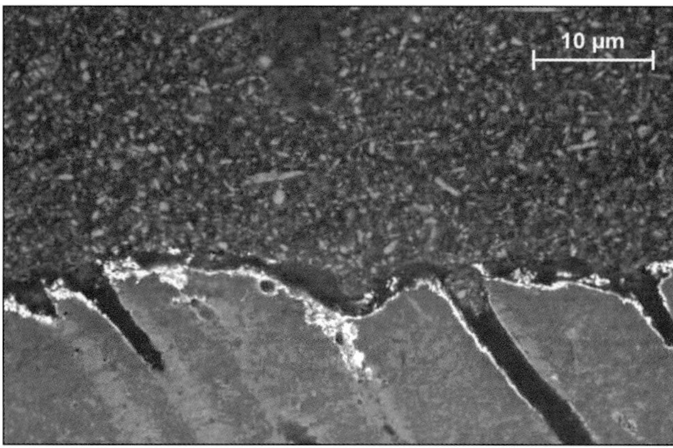

Fig 15-4 Backscatter scanning electron micrograph demonstrating nanoleakage between the hybrid layer and dentin in a bonded composite restoration. Silver particles (appearing as white dots) are seen within, deep to the hybrid layer and extending into resin-filled dentinal tubules. (Courtesy of Dr M. Burrow.)

(see chapters 12 and 14). Beginning with the work of Brännström and Nyborg in the early 1970s,[36] numerous studies have shown that bacteria are commonly present at the material-cavity interface, often penetrating dentinal tubules beneath the cavity floor but not invading the pulp.[37,38] Bacteria enter the space between the material and cavity wall after the restoration has been placed; they do not result from contamination during the cavity preparation stage.[38,39] Bacterial toxins have been shown to diffuse through dentin and even to penetrate the smear layer and smear plugs (chapters 4 and 12).[40] The underlying pulp typically shows moderate to severe inflammation, which historically was attributed to the toxicity of the filling material. If bacterial ingress is prevented (eg, by placing a zinc oxide-eugenol "surface seal" over the test material), or if the material possesses antibacterial properties (eg, zinc oxide-eugenol, calcium hydroxide), the underlying pulpal response tends to be greatly reduced and of shorter duration.[37,41] Even when applied directly to exposed pulps, many commonly used materials are well tolerated when bacteria are excluded by a surface seal.[41,42] Hence, many investigators have concluded that microleakage rather than material toxicity is the primary factor in an inflammatory pulpal response.[13,29,39]

If this is the case, a fundamental question arises: How effectively do contemporary restorative materials and procedures prevent microleakage? The presence of bacteria as determined by a bacterial stain has ranged from 60% or more for conventional (nonadhesive) restorative materials[37,42] to no recorded bacterial penetration with a dentin bonding agent and resin composite restoration.[43] Extremely variable results have been reported with adhesive materials, ranging up to approximately 20% for bonded amalgams[44] and more than 30% for resin composites and glass ionomers.[29,45] The rapid progress of bonding systems offers a very real prospect for a reliable (and durable) marginal seal, although it has not been achieved to date.

On the other hand, some have questioned the primacy of microleakage in promoting pulpal inflammation unless leakage is "extreme," such as that associated with a defective restoration predisposing to secondary caries.[20] Dentinal permeability decreases with time, and the pulp is capable of mounting a protective response. The severity of pulpal inflammation associated with microleakage also decreases with time,[29,46] and pulpal recovery with hard tissue repair is the most commonly encountered outcome.[46]

Interestingly, ISO standard 7405 does not stipulate the use of a surface seal for the evaluation of pulpal effects of materials in the pulp and dentin usage test.[24] Rather, it specifies that materials should be placed according to the manufacturer's directions, including (when recommended) the use of a lining material or cavity treatment agent such as a dentinal adhesive. The standard does, however, prescribe the use of a bacterial stain to detect the presence of bacterial microleakage. Given the contribution of bacterial leakage to pulpal inflammation, the ISO standard procedure may be more a measure of marginal leakage than of material toxicity,[47-49] or at least a combination of the two (plus mechanical injury during cavity preparation).[20]

Nanoleakage refers to leakage within the hybrid layer of resin bonded to dentin,[50,51] and is unrelated to gaps between the restorative material and cavity walls. Incomplete penetration by resin of the etched dentinal surface results in a porous zone that can be penetrated by tracers, such as silver nitrate, or dyes, providing a pathway into dentinal tubules (Fig 15-4). Spaces 20 to 100 nm in width[50] will not permit the penetration of bacteria, but may allow passage of water, acids, and bacterial products (including proteolytic enzymes[52]) that ultimately weaken the bond. Thus, even in the absence of a marginal gap between the restoration and dentin, bonded restorations do not necessarily provide a complete and enduring seal. Nanoleakage appears to occur with all types of bonding systems and dentinal surface treatments. The clinical significance of nanoleakage is not known. Bond strength ultimately may be affected and pathways for the diffusion of bacterial products into dentinal tubules established.

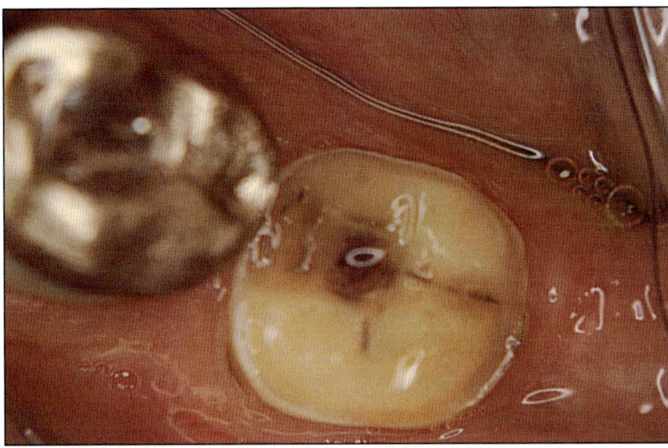

Fig 15-5 Incomplete fracture of the disto-occlusal aspect of a mandibular second molar without pulpal involvement. The tooth has been prepared for a crown to minimize cuspal flexure and to prevent further crack propagation.

Biomechanical factors

The effect of occlusal forces on the clinical behavior of restorations has been largely ignored, certainly with respect to pulpal effects. By analogy with the behavior of bone under stress, Pashley[53] speculated that the fluid-filled dentinal tubules might be important in the hydraulic transfer of occlusal stresses within the tooth. Again, by analogy with bone behavior, the fluid-filled dentinal tubules may contribute to time-dependent (viscoelastic) properties of dentin. Cuspal flexure is known to occur during occlusal function, although the extent of flexure tends to be small in the intact tooth.[54,55] Cavity preparations increase markedly the extent of cuspal flexure under occlusal load.[54,56] Depending on the type of restorative material used, this increased cuspal flexure may persist following restoration of the tooth. Lee and Eakle[57] proposed that the entire tooth flexes during normal occlusal function, and this idea serves as the basis for the "abfraction" theory of cervical noncaries lesions.[58]

Fluid movement in response to occlusal loading has only recently been measured, using intact extracted teeth.[59] The magnitude of fluid flow was similar to hydrodynamic effects accompanying cavity preparation (thermal, desiccation) or osmotic stress. The authors speculated that dentinal fluid flow, in association with pulpal mechanoreceptors, might serve primarily to monitor the magnitude and direction of occlusal forces on teeth (as opposed to a pain-sensing mechanism in exposed dentin). The effects of cuspal or tooth flexure on dentinal fluid flow have not been measured experimentally but are likely to be great, particularly if the tubules are exposed because of cavity preparation. The magnitude of cuspal flexure in response to clinically realistic occlusal loads under experimental conditions (up to 25 μm) is sufficient to result in marginal leakage if the restoration does not protect the cusps.[60,61] Incomplete cuspal or crown fracture (Fig 15-5) results in a sudden marked sensitivity to occlusal load and thermal stimuli that has been attributed to increased dentinal fluid flow.[62] The role of biomechanical factors in pulpal responses to cavity design and restoration merits much greater attention. One study attempted to measure dentinal fluid flow in response to loads applied to occlusal restorations in extracted teeth, but the technical difficulties are considerable.[63]

Putting it all together: Restorative injury to the pulp

Prevailing opinion is that bacterial microleakage is the dominant factor in injury to the pulp associated with restorations. In a large study of human teeth involving more than 300 restorations placed under controlled conditions, Camps and colleagues[29] attempted to rank the effects of different components of the restorative procedure on pulpal inflammation. They concluded that presence of bacteria was the main factor, followed by remaining dentinal thickness and postoperative interval. They did not include material toxicity in their ranking. This is a generalization that should be accepted with caution, especially in terms of clinical practice. The net effect on the pulp is the sum of all of the steps involved in preparation and restoration, modulated by the permeability of underlying dentin and the health of the pulp before restoration. In the study mentioned above, 100% of pulps showed severe inflammation soon after restoration, when the remaining dentinal thickness was less than 500 μm, regardless of bacterial status or type of restorative material.[29] This result implies that initially the trauma of deep cavity preparation is dominant. In experimental studies, bacterial leakage is scored simply as present or absent without assessment of severity. Clinically, the variability of each step in a restorative procedure, including the extent of microleakage, indicates that the major source of injury may vary from case to case.

Pulpal Response to Restorative Procedures

Odontoblast responses

Dentin and pulp are generally considered to function pathophysiologically as a single unit (the pulpodentin complex).[2] It is convenient for descriptive purposes to consider the response of odontoblasts separately from the pulpal inflammatory response to restorative procedures. Odontoblasts, with processes extending into dentinal tubules, are the first cells contacted by an external stimulus applied to the tooth and may be directly injured during cavity preparation. An odontoblast response, in the form of tubule occlusion and tertiary dentinal formation, can be detected in the absence of underlying pulpal inflammation (see chapter 3). Fundamentally, however, the two are an integral part of the same process.

Odontoblasts, dentinal sclerosis, and tertiary dentinal deposition

Odontoblasts show a gradation in their response to injury. With a gradual, progressive injury that does not directly involve the odontoblast process (caries, abrasion), tubules become progressively occluded by mineral deposits, which serve to wall off the underlying pulp. (In the case of caries, it is uncertain whether tubule occlusion is the result of an active defense mechanism or the reprecipitation of mineral dissolved during the caries process.[6]) Additional dentin that also may be deposited on the pulpal surface underlying the injury is commonly termed *tertiary dentin* and can be further classified into *reactionary* or *reparative dentin* (see chapter 3). Depending on the severity of injury, the odontoblasts may survive to deposit reactionary dentin, the tubules of which are continuous with those of overlying primary and secondary dentin. If odontoblasts are irreversibly damaged, reparative dentin is laid down following the differentiation of new odontoblast-like cells from the dental pulp.[64,65]

The most important determinant of the severity of odontoblast injury and the extent of tertiary dentinal deposition appears to be the trauma of the cavity preparation rather than the effects of restorative materials.[64,65] In experimental studies involving cavity preparations in sound dentin of previously intact teeth, the concept of "remaining dentinal thickness" (RDT) as a factor in restorative injury to the pulp has been investigated extensively. RDT may well be a surrogate for direct injury to odontoblast processes, although it is recognized that dentinal permeability also increases with decreasing RDT (see chapter 4). Mature dentin is normally approximately 3 mm thick, and odontoblast processes extend from 0.1 to 1.0 mm into tubules.[2] RDT of 2 mm or more effectively precludes restorative damage to the pulp.[20] In support of this point, odontoblast cell numbers were unaffected by deeper cavity preparations with as little as 0.5 mm RDT, while the quantity of tertiary dentin increased with decreasing RDT.[64,65] The response was also brief, with reactionary dentin deposition ceasing within 28 days.[65] Deeper cutting (less than 0.3 mm from the pulp) results in direct odontoblast injury,[16] including displacement of cell bodies into tubules and cell death, necessitating the differentiation of new odontoblast-like cells before reparative dentinal deposition can begin.

Neurovascular response and pulpal inflammation

Exposure of dentinal tubules during cavity preparation initiates a sequence of hydrodynamic fluid shifts that are capable of disrupting the odontoblast layer, triggering the firing of sensory nerves and initiating neurogenic inflammation via release of neuropeptides. The exposed tubules also serve as the pathway for bacterial products and toxic materials to diffuse into the pulp, which, under experimental conditions, can occur within hours.[40] The early pulpal inflammatory response may be triggered by mediators such as the neuropeptides released from stimulated sensory nerves and in response to bacterial toxins diffusing through tubules.[66] The pulp responds rapidly to tubule exposure, with a reduction in permeability occurring within hours by precipitation of plasma proteins such as fibrinogen and possibly immune complexes within tubules.[2,66] Histologically, the pulpal response to injury involves increasing levels of odontoblast layer disruption, underlying vascular changes and hemorrhage, inflammatory cell infiltration, and abscess formation.

In clinical usage tests, pulpal inflammation is scored as *none*, *mild*, *moderate*, or *severe*; there is also a category of abscess formation or extended lesions.[24] A mild inflammatory response involves localized subodontoblastic hemostasis and hemorrhage with an intact odontoblast layer; moderate inflammation is characterized by accumulations of acute or chronic inflammatory cells depending on the postoperative interval, with vasodilation and an irregular odontoblast layer; a severe response is indicated by complete disruption of the odontoblast layer, localized microabscess formation, and more widespread inflammatory cell infiltration in the pulpal core.[64,67]

Resolution or progression to pulpal death

Both histologically and clinically, pulpal responses to restorative procedures generally decline over time. Postoperative sensitivity, which can affect a high percentage of teeth soon after the procedure and is generally attributed to the effect of cavity preparation rather than the restorative material, declines within days or weeks and is infrequent beyond 30 days.[68,69] Reactionary dentinal deposition is also complete within this time,[65] and it appears that dentinal permeability is reduced to the point at which pulpal defense mechanisms begin to dominate. When pulps do succumb, they tend to do so after prolonged periods.

Experimental studies have focused on acute pulpal injury and relatively short-term pulpal responses. The pulp will normally survive an injury sufficient to provoke reactionary and even reparative dentinal deposition (involving death of primary odontoblasts), as well as a moderate inflammatory cell infiltration.[14,70] Resolution may be accompanied by fibrosis and premature "aging" of the pulp.[67] Damage to underlying cells of the subodontoblastic zone and deeper pulp with abscess formation constitutes the point of no return for ultimate pulpal death.[70] Cell death may be by apoptosis rather than necrosis.[14,67] Clinical-

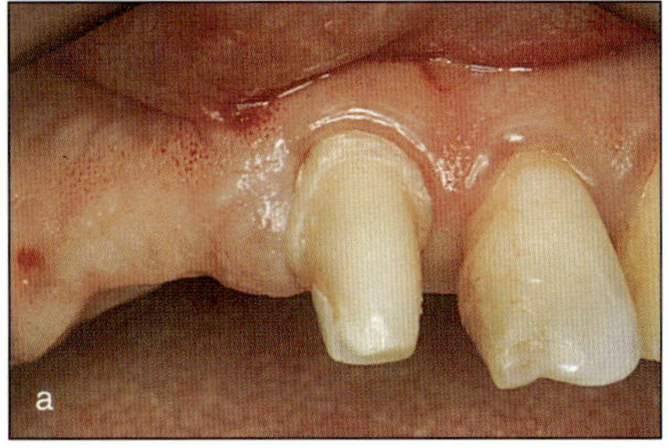

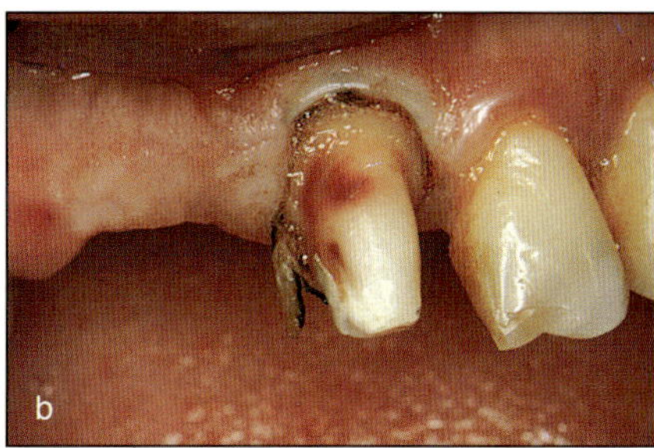

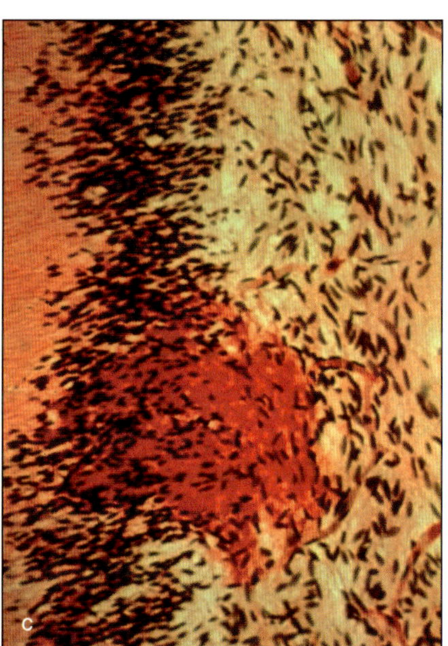

Fig 15-6 Pulpal hemorrhage associated with crown preparation. *(a)* Maxillary central incisor immediately after crown preparation. *(b)* One week later, showing dentinal discoloration as a result of intrapulpal hemorrhage. *(c)* Histologically, displacement of odontoblast cell bodies into tubules and intrapulpal hemorrhage indicate irreversible pulpal damage (H&E stain, original magnification ×250).

ly, there is no reliable way of judging when irreversible injury has occurred, other than by symptoms of irreversible pulpitis, or, rarely, by discoloration of dentin resulting from extensive intrapulpal hemorrhage (Fig 15-6).

Specific Materials and Procedures

Metallic restorations and ceramics

Its long clinical history and the exhaustive analysis of its local and systemic effects set amalgam apart as the most thoroughly evaluated of all dental materials. Concerns regarding toxicity are directed to systemic effects of mercury rather than to direct effects on dental pulp. Experimental studies over a period of almost 60 years (beginning well before the recognition of microbial leakage as a factor in apparent toxicity or of the protective effect of the smear layer) have shown that amalgam is very well tolerated by the pulp.[20] A recent study of high-copper amalgam, placed in deep cavities of human teeth (RDT 0.15 to 0.5 mm) in conjunction with a zinc oxide–eugenol outer seal, showed no inflammation or only slight inflammatory cell infiltration.[71] Amalgam undergoes corrosion in the mouth, and the accumulation of corrosion products in marginal spaces between the cavity wall and the restoration is considered responsible for a progressive reduction in marginal leakage. Mercury from amalgam restorations does not penetrate dentin, while zinc and tin ions have been found in high concentrations in dentin beneath amalgam restorations.[72] These metals do not appear to exert an effect on the pulp, although the inflammation accompanying direct placement of amalgam over exposed pulps was tentatively attributed to zinc toxicity.[71]

Other, generally short-lived pulpal effects of amalgam have been described. For example, neutrophils transiently migrate between the odontoblast layer and predentin; this has been attributed to condensation pressures during amalgam placement.[31] The high thermal conductivity of amalgam results in postoperative sensitivity unless a liner or base is used, except in shallow cavities.[73,74] The smear layer, which is normally left intact with amalgam restorations, may serve to reduce postoperative sensitivity because of its ability to occlude dentinal tubules.[68] At the same time, its presence on the cavity wall appears to promote marginal leakage.[10] The use of a copal varnish minimizes marginal gaps initially, but the varnish gradually dissolves upon exposure to oral fluids.[10] More recently, dentin bonding agents have been proposed as an alternative to copal varnish, either with or without bonding to amalgam. The technique involves removal of the smear layer and bonding to dentin, with a resin layer occluding tubules (see below). Microleakage is reduced with the use of these agents, but the durability of the bond has been questioned. Histologically, the pulpal response is dictated by the etching procedure and the bonding agent, as well as bacterial microleakage, rather than by the amalgam. In a human study, approximately one third of bonded amalgam restorations had pulpal inflammation regardless of the presence or absence of bacterial leakage.[44] Clinically, the frequency and severity of postoperative sensitivity with bonded amalgams is not markedly different from those with no liner or copal varnish (with the smear layer intact).[68,69,75] The clinical benefit of bonded amalgams has yet to be demonstrated.

Pulpal responses to cast metals and ceramics (inlays, crowns) are related to the luting cement used rather than to the material itself or leachable breakdown products.[20] Corrosion products are released from alloys commonly used in cast restorations,[76] but pulpal effects are insignificant in comparison with effects of cement constituents or bacterial products that penetrate the dentinal tubules during cementation. Hydraulic pressures generated during cementation and their adverse effects on the pulp are considered in more detail below.

Resin composites and glass ionomers

Despite differences in chemistry and bonding mechanisms, resin composites and glass ionomers are conveniently considered together as adhesive restorative materials. Clinical applications of various formulations include restorative materials, luting cements, and cavity liners.

Conventional resin composites consist of an organic resin matrix and inorganic filler particles, with a silane coupling agent. The organic matrix is usually methacrylate-based, and polymerization may be activated chemically or by exposure to light. The composition of commercially available materials is complex, with a wide range of monomers, comonomers, and additives. Because polymerization is never complete, unreacted monomers and other components can be leached from the set materials, and they should not be considered inert.[21,22,77] Glass ionomers (glass polyalkenoates) consist of an ion-leachable glass and an aqueous polyalkenoic acid such as polyacrylic acid. A calcium fluoro-aluminosilicate glass powder is mixed with a solution of the polyacid, which commonly consists of a copolymer of acrylic acid and a di- or tri-carboxylic acid such as itaconic or maleic acid. Setting occurs by an acid-base reaction in which calcium and aluminum ions are released from the glass surface and cross-link the polyacid chains.[78] Bonding of glass ionomers to enamel and dentin appears to occur by ionic bonding between carboxyl groups of the polyalkenoic acid and calcium ions in hydroxyapatite. An important property of glass ionomers is release of fluoride, with its caries-protective effects on surrounding enamel and dentin. To take advantage of the better physical and working properties of resin composites and the fluoride-releasing benefits of glass ionomers, the two technologies have converged. A light-curable resin component (frequently including hydroxyethyl methacrylate [HEMA]) has been added to resin-modified glass ionomers, while ion-releasing glasses have been incorporated into polyacid-modified resin composites, or compomers. An expanding range of materials with diverse clinical applications is available commercially.[79,80]

Pulpal effects of these materials (other than those secondary to microleakage) can potentially arise from etching or conditioning of the dentinal surface as well as from material constituents or breakdown products. Glass ionomers have a low pH by virtue of their aqueous polyalkenoic acid content, which is enhanced by the inclusion of tartaric acid to control setting rate as well as the addition of dry polyacrylic or polymaleic acid powder to the glass powder.[81] After mixing, the pH tends to remain low for a longer period than with zinc phosphate cements.[82] Conditioning the dentinal surface with 10% or 20% polyacrylic acid removes the smear layer but leaves smear plugs intact within the dentinal tubules.[80] Glass ionomers are generally regarded as having excellent biocompatibility with minimal pulpal effects even in deep cavities, as long as bacterial leakage does not occur.[20,21,81] Hence, glass ionomers and resin-modified glass ionomers are widely used as cavity liners and bases.[28] Postoperative sensitivity when glass ionomer is used as a luting agent has been reported, and has been attributed to the hydraulic effect of crown cementation forcing unreacted acid through dentinal tubules into the pulp.[81] Others have reported only slight pulpal reactions that subsided within 90 days.[83-85] Moreover, even direct placement of a resin modified glass ionomer onto exposed pulps of monkey teeth produced pulpal healing similar to that observed with calcium hydroxide, including dentinal bridge formation.[86] In view of the potential toxicity of resin components[22] and the acidic effects of unset material,[21] little advantage is gained by the direct application of these materials to dental pulp.

Numerous leachable compounds from resin-based restorative materials (unreacted monomers and additives, breakdown products) have been identified as having cytotoxic or bioactive effects with potentially important clinical consequences.[22] No compelling argument can be made that all or even many pulpal effects of resin composites are the result of microleakage. In any case, as Schmalz has pointed out, bacterial penetration remains a significant clinical problem despite improvements in adhesive techniques, and there is some evidence that components of resins actually promote bacterial growth.[21] Direct toxicity of resin composites to the underlying pulp has been well documented[22] but is more of an issue in association with acid etching of deep dentin and dentin bonding.[77]

Dentin bonding agents

Clinically reliable adhesion to dentin has become feasible within the last decade, and techniques and materials continue to develop rapidly. Thus, there is a paucity of information on the pulpal effects of dentin bonding, and much of what is known may be rapidly superseded by subsequent developments. In addition to the ongoing development of materials and techniques, clinical applications of dentin bonding are being extended, somewhat controversially, to include procedures such as direct pulp-capping and bonding to retained carious dentin.

Dentin bonding consists essentially of three steps: acid demineralization of the dentinal surface to expose the collagen matrix (etching or conditioning), infiltration of the exposed collagen meshwork with a primer, and application and polymerization of the adhesive resin.[87,88] To simplify the procedure and to reduce technique sensitivity, the etchant and primer, the primer and adhesive, or all three components have been combined in a variety of commercially available or experimental systems.[43,88] The formation of a hybrid layer of resin matrix and demineralized collagen (see Fig 15-4) provides the bond strength and sealing ability of the restoration.

Three aspects of dentin bonding may affect the underlying pulp: acid etching, which increases dentinal permeability; cytotoxic effects of resin components diffusing through exposed tubules; and bacteria or microbial products (microleakage or nanoleakage).[22] Etching with strong acid removes the smear layer and demineralizes the cut dentinal surface (intertubular dentin) to a depth of 2 to 5 μm.[7] In addition, smear plugs are dissolved from within tubules, and tubules are enlarged as peritubular dentin is etched to a variable depth. Hence, dentinal permeability is increased, at least temporarily, until the resin penetrates and polymerizes. Diffusion of resin components toward the pulp is increased as a result, although the extent of diffusion is strongly influenced by dentinal thickness. Highest bond strength and lowest leakage are achieved when resin tags are present within tubules and bonded to tubule walls, in addition to the hybrid layer on the intertubular surface.[7]

Material toxicity to the underlying pulp becomes an issue only when the remaining dentinal thickness is less than approximately 300 μm.[77] The hydrophilic priming agent 2-HEMA has received a great deal of attention because it is applied directly to the etched dentinal surface. HEMA diffuses readily across etched dentin even against a positive hydrostatic pressure,[32] with the possibility of acute cytotoxicity and other cellular effects.[89] Several clinical studies involving human teeth have evaluated the pulpal response to dentin bonding agents applied to etched deep dentin in association with resin composite restorations.[26,90,91] A persistent chronic inflammatory response with only infrequent evidence of hard tissue repair was noted. Resin globules within the dentinal tubules, extending into predentin and even into the odontoblast layer and pulp, appeared to provoke a foreign-body reaction, characterized by the presence of macrophages and multinucleated giant cells.

The pulpal response is exacerbated by the application of bonding agents directly over experimental pulpal exposures. Despite favorable reports of direct pulp capping with bonding agents in monkeys,[86] the pattern in human teeth is typically a persistent chronic inflammation and a foreign-body reaction with macrophages and giant cells surrounding particles of resin dispersed within the pulpal tissue.[26,27] Some investigators have stressed the difference in pulpal responses between monkey and human teeth and caution against the use of bonding techniques in the clinical management of pulpal exposures.[77,92]

Dentin bonding should reduce microleakage because the hybrid layer provides continuity between the restorative material and underlying dentin. While one recent study reported no evidence of bacterial contamination in any teeth restored with a one-application dentin bonding system,[43] others have reported bacterial leakage in more than 30% of experimental teeth.[29,45] The gingival margin of cervical lesions, placed in cementum or dentin and subjected to cyclic stresses associated with occlusal loading, provides a rigorous test of dentin bonding. The cervical margin of proximal restorations is also recognized as an area that requires meticulous technique to achieve a good marginal seal. While dentin bonding agents have developed enormously in a short time, it is premature to imagine that they routinely provide a reliable barrier to microbial penetration.

Extensive restorative procedures

Except in cases of trauma, teeth requiring extensive restorations generally have a long history of pulpal injury and diminished repair potential. Full-crown preparations, probably the greatest restorative injury to which the pulp is subjected, have been estimated to involve up to 1 cm^2 of cut dentin, exposing 2×10^6 or more tubules.[93] Nonetheless, extensive restorative procedures result in a low rate of pulpal necrosis, variously estimated in long-term clinical studies at approximately 1% per year for crowns[94] and 2% to 3% per year for complex amalgam restorations.[95]

Pins

Complex amalgam restorations in teeth with vital pulps may rely on auxiliary retention such as pins inserted into dentin.[96] Threaded pins pose a significant hazard to the pulp, including placement into the pulp. Pin placement within 0.5 mm of the pulp of monkey teeth provoked a severe inflammatory response, while placement at a distance greater than 1 mm had little effect.[97] In addition to the risk of perforation, self-threading pins pose two potential problems: heat generation and stresses within adjacent dentin. Substantial heat is generated during pin hole preparation, placement of the pin, and even during reduction of pin height following placement.[98,99] Localized temperature increases in dentin during pin hole preparation (in extracted teeth) reached approximately

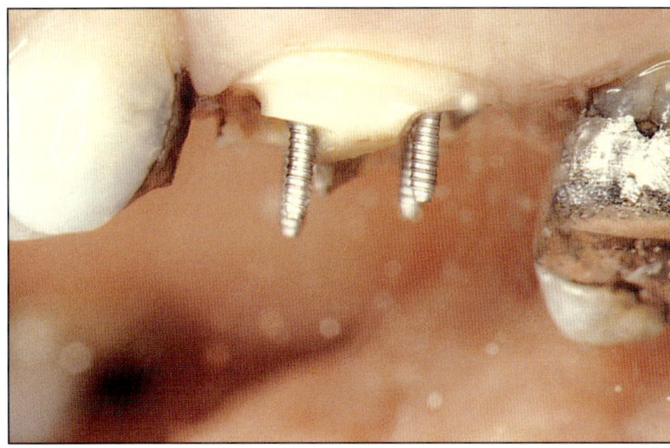

Fig 15-7a Pins used to retain a large restoration in a tooth with little remaining coronal structure but with a vital pulp.

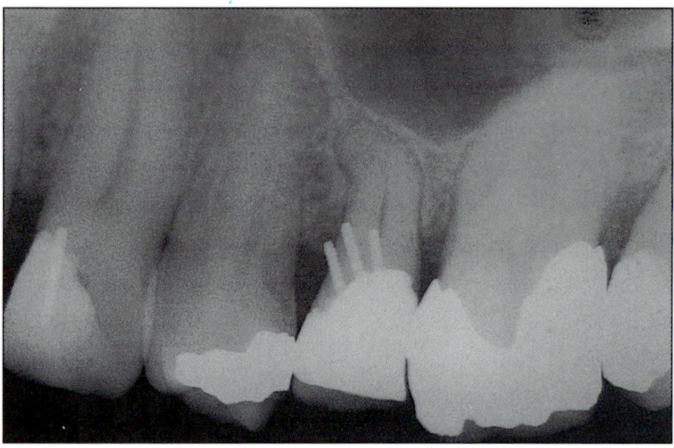

Fig 15-7b Inappropriate pin placement presents danger to the pulp and periodontal ligament.

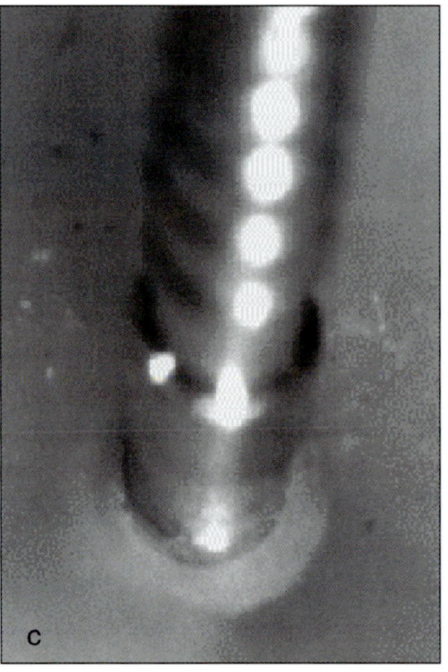

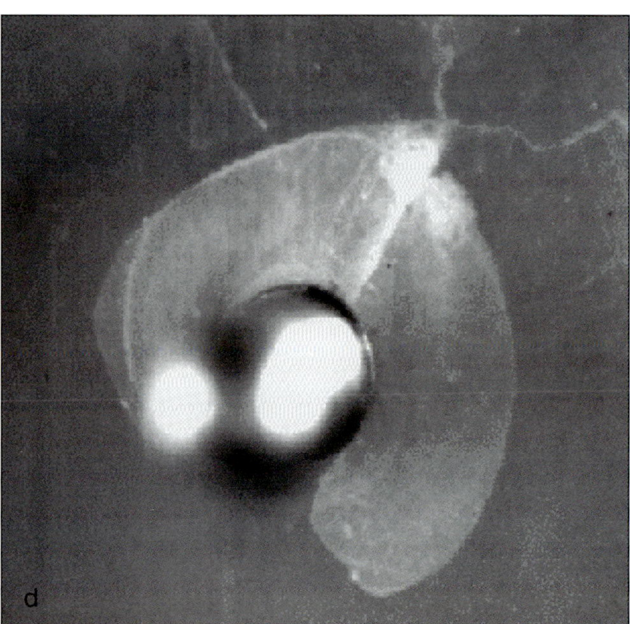

Figs 15-7c and 15-7d Crazing and flaking (conchoid fracture) of dentin associated with threaded pin placement. In Fig 15-7d, the pin is perpendicular to the plane of the photograph.

70°C and more than 30°C during pin placement.[98] The low thermal diffusivity of dentin means that the temperature increase on the pulpal surface would be much less and was estimated at only 1°C to 2°C. Localized effects on underlying odontoblasts, mediated by thermally induced dentinal fluid flow, are likely to occur, and the risk is increased as pins are placed close to the pulp. Self-threading pins generate considerable stresses within adjacent dentin when they are inserted, resulting in crazing of dentin that may extend onto the pulpal surface (Fig 15-7).[100] The sudden generation of stresses in dentin during pin placement is also likely to result in rapid dentinal fluid flow; dye placed into a pin hole before pin insertion spreads throughout adjacent dentin and even into the pulpal space of extracted teeth.[101] Slots and "amalgapins" (shallow, round holes in dentin into which amalgam is condensed) appear less damaging to pulp and provide comparable retention.[75,97] The use of bonded amalgam, possibly in association with retentive features such as amalgapins, has recently been suggested as a more dentin-conserving approach than self-threading pins for complex amalgam restorations.[75]

Crowns

Placement of crowns is associated with a high rate (23%) of postcementation sensitivity[102] and a small but significant loss (approximately 1% per year) of pulpal vitality. Pulpal death following crown placement appears to occur at a steady rate over many years (Fig 15-8),[94,95] implying a progressive degenerative response of the pulp.[70] Pulpal injury can occur at almost every stage of crown preparation and placement. The extensive cutting during crown preparation exposes a large number of highly permeable dentinal tubules, many of them intact and previously unaffected by caries or restorative procedures.[93] Desiccation, thermal injury, and bacterial contamination have all been implicated in the injury associated with tooth preparation.[13,103] At the same time, formation of a smear layer markedly reduces the transmission of pressure toward the pulp that occurs during cementation.[104,105]

Cementation of crowns is potentially highly traumatic to pulps. Crowns are typically seated with substantial force,[106,107] generating a pressure pulse transmitted toward pulp via dentinal tubules.[108] In association with the pressure pulse, components of luting cements and bacterial toxins may be forced into the pulp.[13,33,109] Despite the low pH of cements such as zinc phosphate and glass ionomer, material toxicity appears to be less of a factor in subsequent pulpal sensitivity than desiccation before crown seating or bacterial contamination.[110] Marginal leakage of crowns in clinical function, with bacterial penetration, may be the greatest ongoing injury to the pulp.[13,111]

The placement of a well-sealed coronal restoration is thought to be a major factor in the clinical success of the endodontically treated tooth. In an epidemiologic study using an insurance database of 44,613 endodontically treated teeth with a minimum 2-year follow-up, teeth with no subsequent restorative code had an 11.2% incidence of extractions whereas teeth restored with a crown had a 2.5% incidence of subsequent extractions.[112] In two radiographic survey studies, each evaluating more than 1,000 patients, the teeth determined to have poor restoration and poor endodontic treatment had an increase of 1.4 to 5.0 times the rate of periradicular radiolucency as compared to teeth determined to have good restoration and good endodontic treatment.[113,114] Both studies concluded that teeth with good restorations had significantly better radiographic outcomes as compared to teeth judged to have poor restorations.

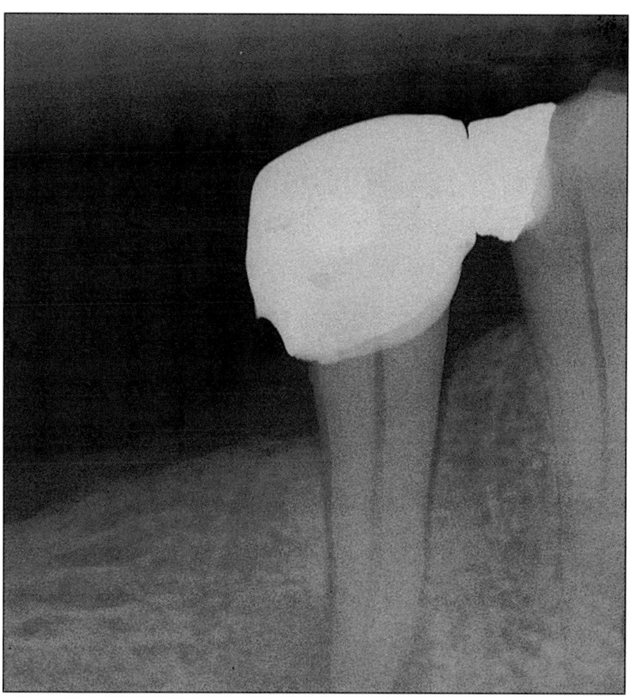

Fig 15-8 Periapical and surrounding bone radiolucency 7 years after crown placement.

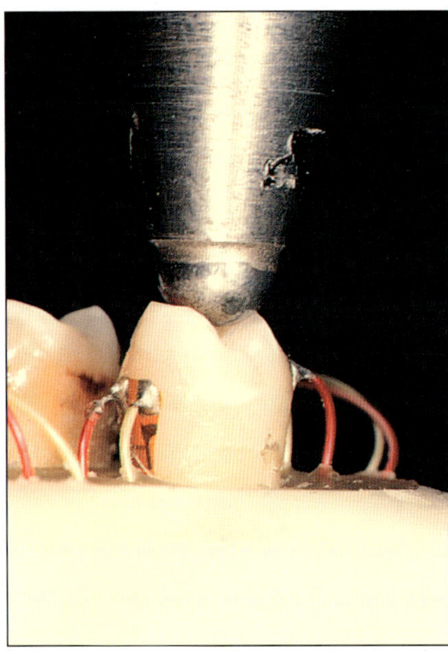

Fig 15-9 Extracted maxillary premolar with strain gauges bonded to the buccal and palatal cusps, subjected to experimental cuspal loading. Nondestructive sequential testing of the effects of cavity preparation and restoration on cuspal flexure is possible with this approach.

Biomechanical Considerations: Cuspal Flexure and Its Consequences

Teeth deform under occlusal load. While the intact tooth is very stiff, any breach in the continuity of enamel weakens the tooth and increases cuspal flexure. The potential effects of cuspal and tooth flexure on dentinal fluid flow have already been considered. In this section we consider factors influencing the extent of cuspal flexure, clinical consequences of excessive flexure, and the role of the restoration in protecting against cuspal flexure. Hood[56] has emphasized the importance of avoiding differential movement between the tooth and restoration in the ultimate success or failure of the restored tooth. We will also consider briefly the biomechanics of endodontically treated teeth in relation to prevention of crown or root fracture.

A brief review of terminology and of experimental methods is in order. The extent to which cusps are weakened (or reinforced) by restorative procedures can be expressed in terms of *cuspal stiffness* or *cuspal flexure*. Both refer to experimental measurement of cuspal bending in response to an applied load. Nondestructive techniques permit repetitive testing on the same tooth; in this way, changes in stiffness can be related to each step of a restorative procedure. Stiffness is commonly measured using strain gauges bonded to the enamel surface (Fig 15-9), and the strain under experimental conditions is expressed in relation to the strain measured in the intact tooth, or *relative stiffness*.[54,55] Linear measurement devices (such as an extensometer or a linear variable differential transformer) measure actual cuspal displacement, often with an accuracy of 0.1 μm.[56,115] Cuspal flexure increases as cuspal stiffness declines (though not necessarily in direct proportion to each other).[115] Destructive testing techniques lead to the fracture of a tooth or cusp and hence measure the ultimate strength of a tooth. Loading to fracture by means of a gradually increasing load is the easiest technique experimentally, but impact testing or cyclic loading resulting in fatigue fracture more closely resembles clinical conditions of tooth failure.[56] These experimental techniques using extracted teeth are often supplemented by numeric methods of analysis (finite element analysis) or by photoelastic stress analysis.

Restorative factors influencing cuspal flexure

Beginning with the work of Vale,[116] numerous investigators have studied the effects of cavity preparations on cuspal flexure or resistance to fracture. Vale demonstrated that an isthmus width of one third the intercuspal width or greater was associated with a lower fracture strength, a finding confirmed by numerous investigators.[116] Moreover, loss of one or both marginal ridges results in a major reduction in cuspal stiffness.[55] Others have shown that the depth of the cavity floor may be more important than width in reducing resistance to fracture, as well as predisposing to unrestorable fracture.[117-119] Hood[56] has integrated these observations into the cantilever beam hypothesis of cuspal flexure, with the unsupported cusp functioning as a cantilever beam and the floor of the cavity preparation serving as the fulcrum. Beam deflection is a function of both the length and the width raised to the third power. If the length of the beam is doubled or the thickness of the beam reduced by one half, then the deflection in response to the same load will increase by a factor of 8. Depending on the tooth type, a mesio-occlusodistal (MOD) cavity preparation reduces cuspal stiffness and fracture resistance by 50% or more.[55,56,61,120]

The greatest loss of coronal tooth structure is encountered in teeth undergoing endodontic treatment, which often will have suffered from extensive caries and repeated cycles of restoration, resulting in weakened and undermined cusps. If the access cavity is confined to the occlusal floor of the cavity preparation, it has only a small effect on cuspal flexure.[55] More extensive access preparation extending into the proximal boxes results in much greater cuspal flexure.[61] Individual cusps flex outward by up to 25 μm under simulated occlusal loading within a physiologic range. Clinically, excessive coronal flaring of canals resulted in a much higher frequency of cuspal fractures.[121]

Consequences of increased cuspal flexure

Dentinal fluid flow and tooth sensitivity

Only one study has attempted to measure dentinal fluid flow in association with occlusal loading of restored teeth.[63] The authors reported increased fluid flow in extracted teeth restored with resin composites relative to intact or amalgam-restored teeth. They attempted to relate the increased fluid flow to the sensitivity often encountered clinically following placement of resin composite restorations.[122]

Marginal leakage and its sequelae

Unless the restoration reduces the cuspal flexure or bonds to the tooth, the possibility exists for a marginal gap to open up with every occlusal load cycle. A tooth in normal function will be subjected to more than a million chewing and swallowing cycles per year. Granath and Svensson[119] concluded that a conservative MOD cavity preparation in combination with average chewing forces did not constitute an "imminent risk" of marginal leakage, but more extensive preparations expose teeth to the danger of salivary leakage, ingress of bacteria, and consequent pulpal inflammation and secondary caries. The much greater cuspal flexure associated with extensive preparations plus endodontic access[60,61] potentially puts the tooth at even greater risk, with consequences for coronal leakage and endodontic failure.[123] Of greater concern for endodontically treated teeth, however, is the risk that extensive cuspal flexure will lead to cuspal or tooth fracture.

Cuspal and tooth fracture

Cuspal or tooth fracture is a significant clinical problem, often resulting in extraction.[124] A large majority of teeth undergoing fracture have been previously restored, mostly with Class 2 amalgams.[125,126] Cuspal flexure, which is not reduced by a conventional intracoronal amalgam restoration, has been implicated in this association (Fig 15-10).[56] Fracture may result from a high-impact force that exceeds the strength of the cusp[124] or, more commonly, from fatigue produced by repeated flexure of the cusp.[56,127] Both clinically and experimentally, cuspal fracture characteristically occurs from the base of the cavity preparation (pulpoaxial line angle) obliquely toward the buccal or lingual cervical area.[128] The pulpoaxial line angle is the region of greatest stress during cuspal loading.[129] It should be emphasized that nonendodontically treated teeth restored with conventional Class 2 amalgams, including complex restorations, have very high survival rates[95,130]; the frequent association of amalgam with cuspal fractures reflects the dominant use of the material for posterior tooth restoration. There are, however,

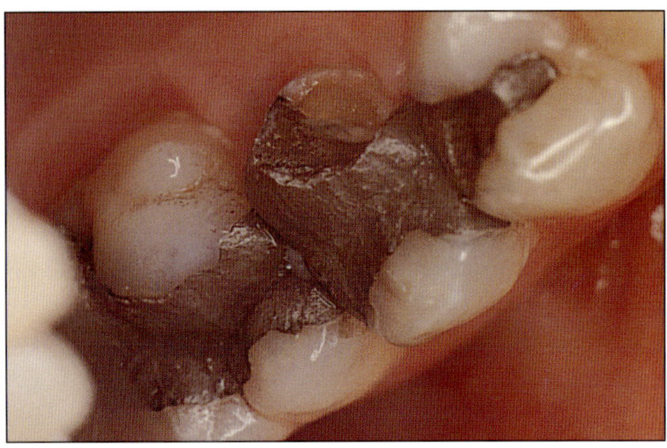

Fig 15-10a Palatal cuspal fracture in a maxillary premolar restored with an extensive MOD amalgam without cuspal protection.

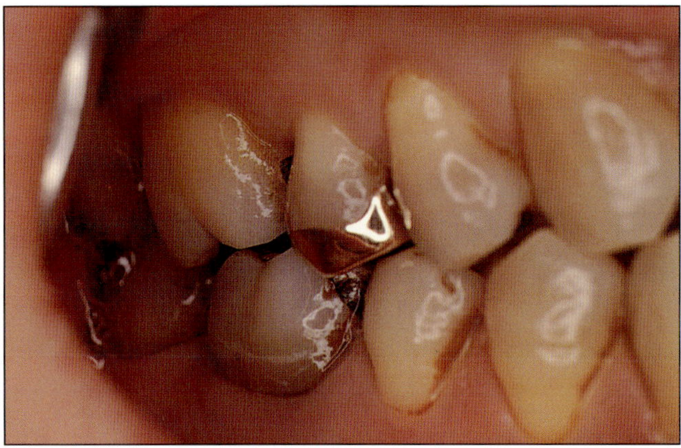

Fig 15-10b Cast gold restoration with buccal cuspal overlay provides a very strong restoration but may not satisfy esthetic requirements for many patients.

limits to its successful use without cuspal protection.

Restoration to minimize cuspal flexure

In view of the adverse consequences of excessive cuspal flexure, large restorations should incorporate features that reinforce the cusps. This is essential for endodontically treated posterior teeth with lost marginal ridges, which have a high failure rate when a routine intracoronal amalgam is placed.[131,132] Metallic restorations (amalgam, cast gold) can be used to overlay cusps, resulting in a marked reduction in cuspal flexure and an increase in fracture strength often exceeding that of the intact tooth (Fig 15-11; see also Fig 15-10b).[120,133,134]

The advent of adhesive dentistry, and particularly bonding to dentin, has led to recommendations that bonded restorations be used as an alternative to cuspal coverage. Theoretically, bonding between the restorative material and the cavity wall shifts the greatest stresses during cuspal loading from the pulpoaxial line angle (ie, the base of the cusp) to the interface between the restorative material and enamel at the cavity surface.[129] Thus, bonding should reduce cuspal flexure, which has been demonstrated in resin composites[54,135] and bonded amalgams[128,136] in extracted teeth. Results demonstrating the effect of bonded restorations on fracture resistance have been extremely variable. Bonded amalgam restorations have been said to increase fracture resistance by up to 72%, depending on materials, tooth type, and cavity preparation, while other studies have shown no benefit.[128] Adhesive resin restorations have also performed inconsistently with respect to fracture resistance.[133,137,138] Two other considerations must be taken into account with regard to bonded restorations: the creation of stresses within the tooth during placement of the restoration and failure of the bond after repeated occlusal loading.

Condensation forces during the placement of amalgam generate transient cuspal strains, followed by immediate elastic recovery.[30] Depending on the setting expansion of amalgam, a small, permanent outward cuspal deformation may also occur.[30,139] Polymerization shrinkage of resin composites bonded to tooth structure results in transfer of stresses to the tooth with inward deflection of cusps, causing permanent stress on the tooth.[35]

While incremental placement techniques have been advocated to reduce cuspal deformation and have become accepted clinical procedure, they do not reduce the shrinkage stresses accompanying polymerization.[35] The clinical consequences of such permanent stresses are adverse: postoperative sensitivity, cracking of enamel, and ultimate failure of the bond, leading to marginal leakage and the risk of secondary caries.

Clinical correlations of cuspal flexure

Bond failure in bonded amalgam restorations

Bonded amalgam restorations offer many potential advantages: more conservative preparations with less reliance on mechanical retention, reduced cuspal flexure, increased fracture resistance, and decreased marginal leakage and postoperative sensitivity.[128,140] Clinically, Mahler and Engle[140] found no effect of bonding on postoperative sensitivity or marginal integrity in Class 1 and 2 restorations after 3 years. Davis and Overton[75] reported reduced cold sensitivity after 3 and 12 months in teeth with incomplete fractures restored with bonded cuspal overlay amalgams.

It is tempting to use bonded amalgams for large restorations (including endodontically treated teeth) and to rely on the bond rather than cuspal coverage to protect against cuspal flexure and tooth fracture. No long-term clinical studies of the effectiveness of bonded amalgam restorations in protecting against fracture have been published. Experimental studies using extracted teeth have shown an initial partial improvement in cuspal stiffness and fracture resistance.[128,141,142] The benefit was rapidly lost, however, after storage (as little as 7 days in water), thermocycling, or load cycling.[142] Once the bond is lost, the tooth behaves biomechanically as if it were unrestored, with potentially catastrophic consequences. While amalgam bonding may have some benefits in terms of retention (though probably not reduced sensitivity), it should be used only in association with other forms of cuspal protection to guard against fracture.

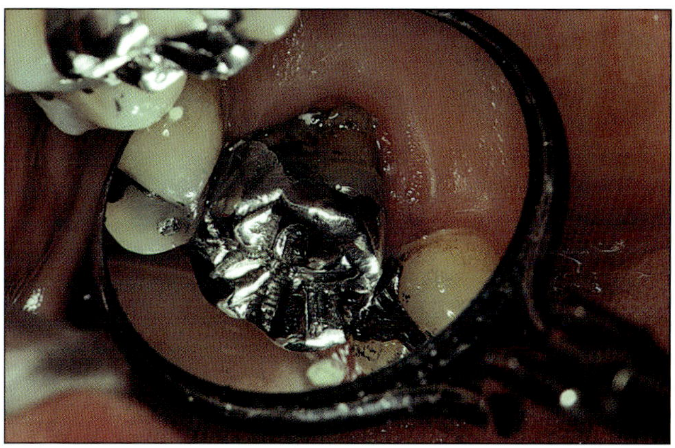

Fig 15-11 Cuspal overlay amalgam serves as a durable interim restoration following endodontic treatment and provides good protection against cuspal flexure.

Incomplete cuspal fracture

Incomplete cuspal or tooth fracture ("cracked tooth syndrome") is characterized by the sudden onset of sharp pain upon biting and thermal (typically cold) sensitivity. The sensitivity is considered to result from increased dentinal fluid flow accompanying the increased cuspal movement.[62] Careful diagnosis and prompt restorative intervention to minimize cuspal flexure and prevent crack propagation are often sufficient to resolve symptoms rapidly and permanently. Without intervention, the problem is likely to result in complete cuspal fracture or, depending on the path of fracture, pulpal involvement and vertical fracture. Palliative treatment (such as a provisional zinc oxide–eugenol restoration) without control of excessive cuspal movement is ineffective. Excellent recent reviews of diagnosis and management are available.[75,143]

The restoration should include all involved cusps, which should be reduced in height and overlaid with the restorative material. A cast restoration has the advantage of antiflexure features, such as a reverse bevel, that are readily incorporated into the restoration design; cuspal stiffness and fracture resistance can exceed that

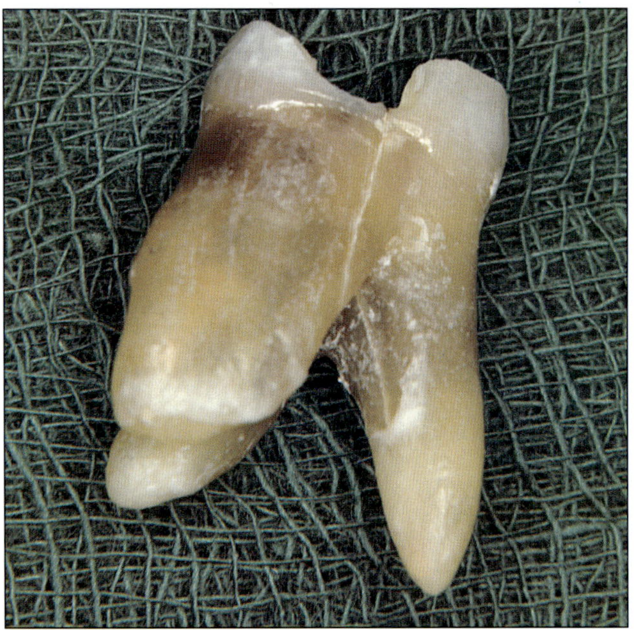

Fig 15-12 Incomplete fracture extending from a proximal box, across the floor of the pulpal chamber, and partially along the buccal surface of the palatal root of a maxillary molar. Pulpal necrosis and periodontal ligament breakdown necessitated extraction of the tooth.

of intact teeth.[133] Complex amalgam restorations with at least a 2-mm reduction of the affected cusps also appear to be satisfactory restorations, providing prompt resolution of symptoms.[75,143] This may be one clinical situation where the use of an amalgam bonding agent is appropriate.[75,143] It must be emphasized, however, that bonding should be used in conjunction with cuspal reduction and overlay, not as an alternative to cuspal coverage. Long-term clinical studies are needed to confirm its durability.

Delayed management severely compromises health of the pulp because a crack penetrating to the pulpal chamber provides a pathway for bacterial invasion, pulpal inflammation, and necrosis. Extension of the crack to the pulpal floor or below the gingival margin generally results in a hopeless prognosis, as does complete separation of the fractured parts (Fig 15-12).

Restoration of endodontically treated teeth

A comprehensive coverage of restoration of endodontically treated teeth is beyond the scope of this chapter, and indeed is only peripherally related to the central theme of permanent restorations and the dental pulp. Many aspects of restoring endodontically treated teeth are only an extension of the same principles as discussed above—the endpoint is preserving the tooth as a functional unit rather than preserving the pulp. As considered earlier, the major concern is cuspal flexure and its consequences of marginal leakage and tooth fracture.

For many years the emphasis in restoration of endodontically treated teeth was on reinforcement to prevent fracture, primarily with the use of a large post. With the recognition that posts do not reinforce the root and commonly weaken it, emphasis has changed to conservation and protection of remaining tooth structure. Conserving tooth structure should not come at the expense of protecting the tooth from fracture. Intracoronal amalgam restorations have been shown in both clinical and experimental studies to be susceptible to failure and should not be used.[120,121,131-133] As a general guideline, cusps adjacent to a lost marginal ridge should be overlaid, with sufficient bulk of amalgam (usually 3 to 4 mm) to resist occlusal forces. The amalgam should extend into the pulpal chamber and canal orifices to aid retention. Longevity of extensive amalgams is similar to that of cast restorations,[95] and the amalgam may subsequently serve as a core for full coronal coverage if indicated. Bonded amalgams do not increase fracture resistance and should not be used as a substitute for cuspal overlays.[138,144] Bonded resin composite restorations should also be used with caution. Experimental data on fracture resistance are conflicting,[138,144] and concerns related to the long-term effects of stresses resulting from polymerization shrinkage and of bond failure from fatigue need to be addressed. Bonded restorations (both amalgam and composite) will almost certainly become more widely used as bonding materials and techniques continue to improve. Cast restorations provide the greatest occlusal protection, and the strength of gold allows conservative tooth reduction and a reverse bevel for greater cuspal reinforcement.[56,120,133]

A full crown needs to be used only when remaining coronal tooth structure is insufficient for a more conservative restoration, or where occlusal stresses require the splinting effect of full coronal coverage. Full-crown preparation requires further tooth reduction and often leaves little remaining coronal dentin. To retain the crown, a core, and occasionally a post to retain the core, must be placed. When a post is required, the minimum post space (in terms of diameter and taper) consistent with that need should be prepared. The role of posts, as well as the bond between post and tooth, are undergoing substantial rethinking, and long-term clinical trials will be needed to provide better answers to the question of the ideal post.[145] Stiffer (gold or titanium) posts may lead to root fracture, whereas more flexible (carbon fiber) posts deform with the tooth and tend to fail without fracturing the tooth.[146,147]

References

1. Lutz F. The postamalgam age. Oper Dent 1995;20: 218-222.
2. Pashley DH. Dynamics of the pulpo-dentin complex. Crit Rev Oral Biol Med 1996;7:104-133.
3. Pashley DH, Pashley EL. Dentin permeability and restorative dentistry: A status report for the American Journal of Dentistry. Am J Dent 1991;4:5-9.
4. Duke ES, Lindemuth J. Variability of clinical dentin substrates. Am J Dent 1991;4:241-246.
5. Ogawa K, Yamashita Y, Ichijo T, Fusayama T. The ultrastructure and hardness of the transparent layer of human carious dentin. J Dent Res 1983;62:7-10.
6. Marshall GW, Chang YJ, Gansky SA, Marshall SJ. Demineralization of caries-affected transparent dentin by citric acid: An atomic force microscopy study. Dent Mater 2001;17: 45-52.
7. Pashley DH, Carvalho RM. Dentine permeability and dentine adhesion. J Dent 1997;25:355-372.
8. Dippel HW, Borggreven JMPM, Hoppenbrouwers PMM. Morphology and permeability of the dentinal smear layer. J Prosthet Dent 1984;52:657-662.
9. Pashley DH. Smear layer: Physiological considerations. Oper Dent 1984;3(suppl):13-29.
10. Pashley DH. Interactions of dental materials with dentin. Trans Acad Dent Mater 1990;3:55-73.
11. Banerjee A, Kidd EAM, Watson TF. Scanning electron microscope observations of human dentine after mechanical caries excavation. J Dent 2000;28:179-86.
12. Zach L, Cohen G. Pulp response to externally applied heat. Oral Surg Oral Med Oral Pathol 1965;19:5155-30.
13. Brännström M. Reducing the risk of sensitivity and pulpal complications after the placement of crowns and fixed partial dentures. Quintessence Int 1996;27: 673-678.
14. Murray PE, About I, Lumley PJ, Franquin JC, Remusat M, Smith AJ. Human odontoblast cell numbers after dental injury. J Dent 2000;28:277-285.
15. Murray PE, About I, Lumley PJ, Smith G, Franquin JC, Smith AJ. Postoperative pulpal and repair responses. J Am Dent Assoc 2000;131:321-329.
16. Lee S-J, Walton RE, Osborne JW. Pulp response to bases and cavity depths. Am J Dent 1992;5:64-68.
17. Mjör IA. Problems and benefits associated with restorative materials: Side effects and long-term cost. Adv Dent Res 1992;6:7-16.
18. Rutherford RB, Fitzgerald M. A new biological approach to vital pulp therapy. Crit Rev Oral Biol Med 1995;6: 218-229.
19. Sloan AJ, Rutherford RB, Smith AJ. Stimulation of the rat dentine-pulp complex by bone morphogenetic protein-7 in vitro. Arch Oral Biol 2000;45:173-177.
20. Stanley HR. Local and systemic responses to dental composites and glass ionomers. Adv Dent Res 1992; 6:55-64.
21. Schmalz G. The biocompatibility of non-amalgam dental filling materials. Eur J Oral Sci 1998;106:696-706.
22. Geurtsen W. Biocompatibility of resin-modified filling materials. Crit Rev Oral Biol Med 2000;11:333-355.
23. Wennberg A, Mjör IA, Hensten-Pettersen A. Biological evaluation of dental restorative materials—A comparison of different test methods. J Biomed Mater Res 1983;17:23-36.
24. International Standards Organization. International Standard ISO 7405. Dentistry—Preclinical evaluation of biocompatibility of medical devices used in dentistry—Test methods for dental materials. Geneva: International Standards Organization, 1997.
25. Qvist V. The effect of mastication on marginal adaptation of composite resins in vivo. J Dent Res 1983;62: 904-906.
26. Gwinnett AJ, Tay FR. Early and intermediate time response of the dental pulp to an acid etch technique in vivo. Am J Dent 1998;11:535-544.
27. Hebling J, Giro EMA, Costa CAS. Human pulp response after an adhesive system application in deep cavities. J Dent 1999;27:557-564.

28. Hilton TJ. Cavity sealers, liners and bases: Current philosophies and indications for use. Oper Dent 1990; 21:34–46.
29. Camps J, Dejou J, Remusat M, About I. Factors influencing pulpal response to cavity restorations. Dent Mater 2000;16:432–440.
30. Assif D, Marshak BL, Pilo R. Cuspal flexure associated with amalgam restorations. J Prosthet Dent 1990;63: 258–262.
31. Swerdlow H, Stanley HR. Response of the human pulp to amalgam restoration. Oral Surg Oral Med Oral Pathol 1962;15:499–508.
32. Gerzina TM, Hume WR. Effect of hydrostatic pressure on the diffusion of monomers through dentin in vitro. J Dent Res 1995;74:369–373.
33. Al-Fawaz A, Gerzina TM, Hume WR. Movement of resin cement components through acid-treated dentin during crown cementation in vitro. J Endod 1993;19: 219–223.
34. Hussey DL, Biagioni PA, Lamey P-J. Thermographic measurement of temperature change during resin composite polymerization in vivo. J Dent 1995;23:267–271.
35. Versluis A, Douglas WH, Cross M, Sakaguchi RL. Does an incremental filling technique reduce polymerization shrinkage stresses? J Dent Res 1996;75:871–878.
36. Brännström M, Nyborg H. The presence of bacteria in cavities filled with silicate cement and resin composite material. Sven Tandlak Tidskr 1971;64:149–155.
37. Bergenholtz G, Cox CF, Loesche WJ, Syed SA. Bacterial leakage around dental restorations: Its effect on the dental pulp. J Oral Pathol 1982;11:439–450.
38. Browne RM, Tobias RS, Crombie IK, Plant CG. Bacterial microleakage and pulpal inflammation in experimental cavities. Int Endod J 1983;16:147–155.
39. Browne RM. Animal tests for biocompatibility of dental materials—Relevance, advantages and limitations. J Dent 1994;22(suppl 2):S21–S24.
40. Nissan R, Segal H, Pashley DH, Stevens R, Trowbridge H. Ability of bacterial endotoxin to diffuse through dentin. J Endod 1995;21:62–64.
41. Cox CF, Keall CL, Keall HJ, Ostro E, Bergenholtz G. Biocompatibility of surface-sealed dental materials against exposed pulps. J Prosthet Dent 1987;57:1–8.
42. Cox CF, Sübay RK, Suzuki S, Suzuki SH, Ostro E. Biocompatibility of various dental materials: Pulp healing with a surface seal. Int J Periodontics Restorative Dent 1996; 16:240–251.
43. Kitasako Y, Nakajima M, Pereira PN, Okuda M, Sonoda H, Otsuki M, Tagami J. Monkey pulpal response and microtensile bond strength beneath a one-application resin bonding system in vivo. J Dent 2000;28:193–198.
44. Sübay RK, Cox CF, Kaya H, Tarim B, Subay AA, Nayir M. Human pulp reaction to dentine bonded amalgam restorations: A histologic study. J Dent 2000;28: 327–332.
45. Tarim B, Hafez AA, Suzuki SH, Suzuki S, Cox CF. Biocomaptibility of compomer restorative systems of nonexposed dental pulps of primate teeth. Oper Dent 1997;22:49–58.
46. Robertson A, Andreasen FM, Bergenholtz G, Andreasen JO, Munksgaard C. Pulp reactions to restoration of experimentally induced crown fractures. J Dent 1998;26:409–416.
47. Kanca J. Pulpal studies: Biocompatibility or effectiveness of marginal seal? Quintessence Int 1990;21: 775–779.
48. Cox CF. Interactions of dental materials with pulp tissues: Old ideas—New perspectives. Trans Acad Dent Mater 1990;3:74–95.
49. Cox CF. Evaluation and treatment of bacterial microleakage. Am J Dent 1994;7:293–295.
50. Sano H, Takatsu T, Ciucchi B, Horner JA, Matthews WG, Pashley DH. Nanoleakage: leakage within the hybrid layer. Oper Dent 1995;20:18–25.
51. Dörfer CE, Staehle HJ, Wurst MW, Duschner H, Pioch T. The nanoleakage phenomenon: Influence of different dentin bonding agents, thermocycling and etching time. Eur J Oral Sci 2000;108:346–351.
52. Spencer, Swafford JR. Unprotected protein at the dentin-adhesive interface. Quintessence Int 1999;30:501–507.
53. Pashley DH. Dentin permeability: Theory and practice. In: Spangberg L (ed). Experimental Endodontics. Boca Raton, FL: CRC Press, 1990:19–49.
54. Morin DL, Douglas WH, Cross M, DeLong R. Biophysical stress analysis of restored teeth: Experimental strain measurement. Dent Mater 1988;4:41–48.
55. Reeh ES, Messer HH, Douglas WH. Reduction in tooth stiffness as a result of endodontic and restorative procedures. J Endod 1989;15:512–516.
56. Hood JAA. Biomechanics of the intact, prepared and restored tooth: Some clinical implications. Int Dent J 1991;41:25–32.
57. Lee WC, Eakle WS. Possible role of tensile stress in the etiology of cervical erosive lesions of teeth. J Prosthet Dent 1984;52:374–380.
58. Grippo JO. Abfractions: A new classification of hard tissue lesions of teeth. J Esthet Dent 1991;3:14–19.
59. Paphangkorakit J, Osborn JW. The effect of normal occlusal forces on fluid movement through human dentine in vitro. Arch Oral Biol 2000;45:1033–1041.
60. Grimaldi JR, Hood JAA. Lateral deformation of the tooth crown under axial cuspal loading [abstract]. J Dent Res 1973;52:584.
61. Panitvisai P, Messer HH. Cuspal deflection in relation to restorative and endodontic procedures. J Endod 1995; 21:57–61.
62. Brännström M, Aström A. The hydrodynamics of dentin. Its possible relationship to dentinal pain. Int Dent J 1972;22:219–227.

63. Hirata K, Nakashima M, Sekine I, Mukouyama Y, Kimura K. Dentinal fluid movement associated with loading of restorations. J Dent Res 1991;70:975–978.
64. Murray PE, About I, Lumley PJ, Franquin JC, Remusat M, Smith AJ. Human odontoblast cell numbers after dental injury. J Dent 2000;28:277–285.
65. Murray PE, About I, Lumley PJ, Smith G, Franquin JC, Smith AJ. Postoperative pulpal and repair responses. J Am Dent Assoc 2000;131:321–329.
66. Bergenholtz G. Pathogenic mechanisms in pulpal disease. J Endod 1990;16:98–101.
67. Goldberg M, Lasfargues JJ, Legrand JM. Clinical testing of dental materials—Histological considerations. J Dent 1994;22(suppl 2):S25–S28.
68. Gordan VV, Mjör IA, Hucke RD, Smith GE. Effect of different liner treatments on postoperative sensitivity of amalgam restorations. Quintessence Int 1999;30:55–59.
69. Gordan VV, Mjör IA, Moorhead JE. Amalgam restorations: Postoperative sensitivity as a function of liner treatment and cavity depth. Oper Dent 1999;24:377–383.
70. Zöllner A, Gängler P. Pulp reactions to different preparation techniques on teeth exhibiting periodontal disease. J Oral Rehabil 2000;27:93–102.
71. Torstenson B, Brännström M. Pulpal response to restoration of deep cavities with high-copper amalgam. Swed Dent J 1992;16:93–99.
72. Halse A. Metals in dentinal tubules beneath amalgam fillings in human teeth. Arch Oral Biol 1975;20:87–88.
73. Harper RH, Schnell RJ, Swartz ML, Phillips RW. In vivo measurements of thermal diffusion through restorations of various materials. J Prosthet Dent 1980;43:180–185.
74. Craig RG. Restorative Dental Materials, ed 9. St Louis: Mosby, 1993.
75. Davis R, Overton JD. Efficacy of bonded and nonbonded amalgam in the treatment of teeth with incomplete fractures. J Am Dent Assoc 2000;131:469–478.
76. Lucas LC, Lemons JE. Biodegradation of restorative metallic systems. Adv Dent Res 1992;6:32–37.
77. Carvalho RM, Lanza LD, Mondelli J, Tay FR, Pashley DH. Side effects of resin-based materials. In: Tagami J, Toledano M, Prati C (eds). Advanced Adhesive Dentistry. Osaka: Kuraray, 2000:241–257.
78. Smith DC. Composition and characteristics of glass ionomer cements. J Am Dent Assoc 1990;120:20–22.
79. Leyhausen G, Abtahi M, Karbakhsch M, Sapotnick A, Geurtsen W. Biocompatibility of various light-curing and one conventional glass-ionomer cement. Biomaterials 1998;19:559–564.
80. Tyas MJ. Adhesive properties of glass ionomer cements: Laboratory and clinical studies. In: Momoi Y, Akimoto N, Kohno A (eds). Modern Trends in Adhesive Dentistry. Osaka: Kuraray, 2000.
81. Stanley HR. Pulpal responses to ionomer cements—Biological characteristics. J Am Dent Assoc 1990;120:25–29.
82. Smith DC, Ruse ND. Acidity of glass ionomer cements during setting and its relation to pulp sensitivity. J Am Dent Assoc 1986;112:654–657.
83. Heys RJ, Mark F, Heys D, Charbeneau GT. An evaluation of a glass ionomer luting agent: Pulpal histological response. J Am Dent Assoc 1987;114:607–611.
84. Mjör IA, Nordahl I, Tronstad L. Glass ionomer cements and dental pulp. Endod Dent Traumatol 1991;7:59–64.
85. Inokoshi S, Fujitani M, Otsuki M, Sonoda H, Kitasako Y, Shimada Y, Tagami J. Monkey pulpal responses to conventional and adhesive luting cements. Oper Dent 1998;23:21–29.
86. Tarim B, Hafez AA, Cox CF. Pulpal response to a resin-modified glass-ionomer material on nonexposed and exposed monkey pulps. Quintessence Int 1998;29:535–542.
87. Eick JD, Gwinnett AJ, Pashley DH, Robinson SJ. Current concepts of adhesion to dentin. Crit Rev Oral Biol Med 1997;8:306–335.
88. Swift EJ. Bonding systems for restorative materials—A comprehensive review. Pediatr Dent 1998;20:80–84.
89. Schuster GS, Caughman GB, Rueggeberg FA. Changes in cell phospholipid metabolism in vitro in the presence of HEMA and its degradation products. Dent Mater 2000;16:297–302.
90. Tay FR, Pang WR, Gwinnett AJ, Wei SHY. A scanning electron microscopic study of the extent of resin penetration into human coronal dentin following a total etch technique in vivo. Cell Mater 1994;4:317–329.
91. Hebling J, Giro EMA, Costa CAS. Biocompatibility of an adhesive resin system applied to exposed human dental pulp. J Endod 1999;25:676–682.
92. Costa CA, Hebling J, Hanks CT. Current status of pulp capping with dentin adhesive systems: A review. Dent Mater 2000;16:188–197.
93. Richardson D, Tao L, Pashley DH. Dentin permeability: Effects of crown preparation. Int J Prosthodont 1991;4:219–225.
94. Valderhaug J, Jokstad A, Ambjornsen E, Norheim PW. Assessment of the periapical and clinical status of crowned teeth over 25 years. J Dent 1997;25:97–105.
95. Martin JA, Bader JD. Five-year treatment outcomes for teeth with large amalgams and crowns. Oper Dent 1997;22:72–78.
96. Papa J, Wilson PR, Tyas MJ. Pins for direct restorations. J Dent 1993;21:259–264.
97. Felton DA, Webb EL, Kanoy BE, Cox CF. Pulpal response to threaded pin and retentive slot techniques: A pilot investigation. J Prosthet Dent 1991;66:597–602.
98. Biagioni PA, Hussey D, Mitchell CA, Russell DM, Lamey PJ. Thermographic assessment of dentine pin placement. J Dent 1996;24:443–447.

99. Knight JS, Smith HB. The heat sink and its relationship to reducing heat during pin-reduction procedures. Oper Dent 1998;23:299–302.
100. Webb EL, Straka WF, Phillips CL. Tooth crazing associated with threaded pins: A three-dimensional model. J Prosthet Dent 1989;61:624–628.
101. Hummert T, Kaiser D. In vitro evaluation of dynamic fluid displacement in dentinal tubules activated on pin placement. J Prosthet Dent 1992;68:248–255.
102. Johnson G, Powell L, Derouen T. Evaluation and control of post-cementation pulpal sensitivity: Zinc phosphate and glass ionomer luting cements. J Am Dent Assoc 1993;124:38–46.
103. Yuen TWH, Wilson PR. The effect of venting on pulpward pressure transmission and seating on crown cementation: A laboratory study. J Oral Rehabil 2000;27:958–966.
104. Ahlquist M, Franzen O, Coffey J, Pashley D. Dental pain evoked by hydrostatic pressures applied to exposed dentin in man: A test of the hydrodynamic theory of dentin sensitivity. J Endod 1994;20:130–134.
105. Lam CW, Wilson PR. The effect of dentine surface treatment on pulpward pressure transmission during crown cementation: A laboratory study. Int Dent J 1998;48:196–202.
106. Hoard RJ, Caputo AA, Contion RM, Koenig ME. Intracoronal pressure during crown cementation. J Prosthet Dent 1978;40:520–525.
107. Black S, Amoore JN. Measurement of forces applied during the clinical cementation of dental crowns. Physiol Meas 1993;14:387–392.
108. Wylie SG, Wilson PR. An investigation into the pressure transmitted to the pulp chamber on crown cementation: A laboratory study. J Dent Res 1994;73:1684–1689.
109. Gerzina TM, Hume WR. Movement of glass ionomer through human dentin during crown cementation in vitro. J Dent Res 1990;69:934.
110. Rosenstiel SF, Land MF, Crispin BJ. Dental luting agents: A review of the current literature. J Prosthet Dent 1998;80:280–301.
111. Goldman M, Laosonthorn P, White RR. Microleakage—Full crowns and the dental pulp. J Endod 1992;18: 473–475.
112. Lazarski M, Walker W, Flores C, Schindler W, Hargreaves K. Epidemiologic evaluation of the outcomes of nonsurgical root canal treatment in a large cohort of insured dental patients. J Endod (in press).
113. Ray H, Trope M. Periapical status of endodontically treated teeth in relation to the technical quality of the roofilling and the coronal restoration. Int Endod J 1995;28:12–18.
114. Tronstad L, Asbjornsen K, Doving L, Pederson J, Erickson H. Influence of coronal restorations on the periapical health of endodontically treated teeth. Endod Dent Traumatol 2000;16:218–221.
115. Jantarat J, Panitvisai P, Palamara JEA, Messer HH. Comparison of methods for measuring deformation in teeth: LVDTs vs strain gauges. J Dent 2001;29:75–82.
116. Vale WA. Cavity preparation. Ir Dent Rev 1956;2:33–41.
117. Blaser PK, Lund MR, Cochran MA, Potter RH. Effects of designs of Class 2 preparations on resistance of teeth to fracture. Oper Dent 1983;8:6–10.
118. Re GJ, Norling BK, Draheim RN. Fracture resistance of lower molars with varying faciocclusolingual amalgam restorations. J Prosthet Dent 1982;47:518–521.
119. Granath L, Svensson A. Elastic outward bending of loaded buccal and lingual premolar walls in relation to cavity size and form. Scand J Dent Res 1991;99:1–7.
120. Linn J, Messer HH. The effect of restorative procedures on the strength of endodontically treated molars. J Endod 1994;20:479–485.
121. Hansen EK, Asmussen E. Cusp fracture of endodontically treated posterior teeth restored with amalgam. Teeth restored in Denmark before 1975 versus after 1979. Acta Odontol Scand 1993;51:73–77.
122. Eick JD, Welch FH. Polymerization shrinkage of posterior composite resins and its possible influence on postoperative sensitivity. Quintessence Int 1986;17:103–111.
123. Saunders WP, Saunders EM. Coronal leakage as a cause of failure in root-canal therapy: A review. Endod Dent Traumatol 1994;10:105–108.
124. Burke FJT. Tooth fracture in vivo and in vitro. J Dent 1992;20:131–139.
125. Eakle WS, Maxwell EH, Braly BV. Fractures of posterior teeth in adults. J Am Dent Assoc 1986;112:215–218.
126. Gher ME, Dunlap RM, Anderson MH, Kuhl LV. Clinical survey of fractured teeth. J Am Dent Assoc 1987;114: 174–177.
127. Arola D, Huang MP, Sultan MB. The failure of amalgam restorations due to cyclic fatigue crack growth. J Mater Sci 1999;10:319–327.
128. Pilo R, Brosh T, Chweidan H. Cusp reinforcement by bonding of amalgam restorations. J Dent 1998;26: 467–472.
129. Arola D, Galles LA, Sarubin MF. A comparison of the mechanical behavior of posterior teeth with amalgam and composite MOD restorations. J Dent 2001;29: 63–73.
130. Plasmans PJJM, Creugers NHJ, Mulder J. Long-term survival of extensive amalgam restorations. J Dent Res 1998;77:453–460.
131. Sorensen JA, Martinoff JT. Intracoronal reinforcement and coronal coverage: A study of endodontically treated teeth. J Prosthet Dent 1984;51:780–784.
132. Hansen EK, Asmussen E, Christiansesn NC. In vivo fractures of endodontically treated posterior teeth restored with amalgam. Endod Dent Traumatol 1990;6:49–55.
133. Reeh ES, Douglas WH, Messer HH. Stiffness of endodontically treated teeth related to restoration technique. J Dent Res 1989;68:1540–1544.

134. Mondelli RF, Barbosa WF, Mondelli J, Franco EB, Carvalho RM. Fracture strength of weakened human premolars restored with amalgam and without cusp coverage. Am J Dent 1998;11:181-184.
135. Meredith N, Setchell DJ. In vitro measurement of cuspal strain and displacement in composite restored teeth. J Dent 1997;25:331-337.
136. El-Badrawy WA. Cuspal deflection of maxillary premolars restored with bonded amalgam. Oper Dent 1999; 24:337-343.
137. Trope M, Tronstad L. Resistance to fracture of endodontically treated premolars restored with glass ionomer cement or acid etch composite resin. J Endod 1991;6: 257-259.
138. Ausiello P, De Gee AJ, Rengo S, Davidson CL. Fracture resistance of endodontically-treated premolars adhesively restored. Am J Dent 1997;10:237-241.
139. Shimizu A, Hasegawa M, Kishimoto H, Yoshioka W. An in vitro investigation of the tooth strains associated with four different restorations in Class II cavity. J Prosthet Dent 1996;76:309-314.
140. Mahler DB, Engle JH. Clinical evaluation of amalgam bonding in class I and II restorations. J Am Dent Assoc 2000;131:43-49.
141. Eakle WS, Staninec M, Lacy AM. Effect of bonded amalgam on the fracture resistance of teeth. J Prosthet Dent 1992;68:257-260.
142. Bonilla E, White SN. Fatigue of resin-bonded amalgam restorations. Oper Dent 1996;21:122-126.
143. Ailor JE. Managing incomplete tooth fractures. J Am Dent Assoc 2000;131:1168-1174.
144. Steele A, Johnson BR. In vitro fracture strength of endodontically treated premolars. J Endod 1999;25:6-8.
145. Asmussen E, Peutzfeld A, Heitmann T. Stiffness, elastic limit, and strength of newer types of endodontic posts. J Dent 1999;27:275-278.
146. Christensen GJ. Posts and cores. State of the art. J Am Dent Assoc 1998;129:96-97.
147. Martinez-Insua A, da Silva L, Santana U. Comparison of the fracture resistances of pulpless teeth restored with a cast post and core or carbon-fiber post with a composite core. J Prosthet Dent 1998;80:527-532.

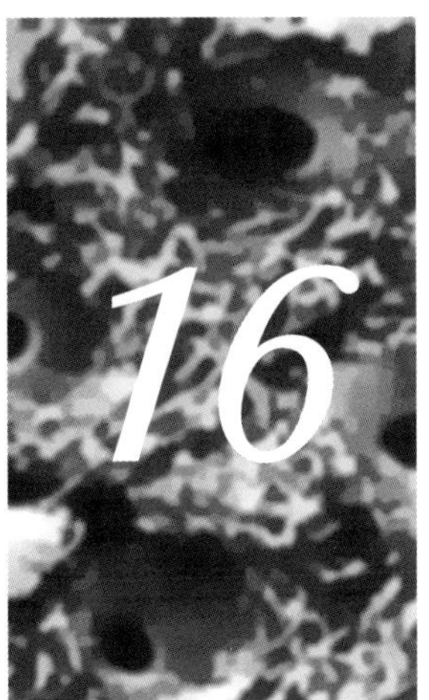

Pulpal Effects of Thermal and Mechanical Irritants

Harold E. Goodis, DDS; David Pashley, DMD, PhD; Adam Stabholtz, DDS

Clinical dental procedures often generate thermal and mechanical stimuli of sufficient magnitude to injure dental pulp or surrounding tissues. This chapter reviews the physical properties of these stimuli; the thermal properties of the pulpodentin complex; the ways in which stimuli are transmitted to the dental pulp or surrounding tissues; and the pathophysiologic processes that occur in response to stimuli. It is important for the clinician to understand these factors in order to provide minimally traumatic restorative or endodontic dental care. Other physical properties of the pulpodentin complex are reviewed in chapter 4, and the circulatory responses to thermal and mechanical stimuli are reviewed in chapter 6.

Physical Properties

For an understanding of the thermal dynamics that occur in the pulpal and periodontal tissues, it is necessary to review the physical properties of dental materials. Thermal changes occur during dental treatment in response to heat generated by restorative procedures or by laser treatment and in the root canal and surrounding tissues during the application of thermoplasticized gutta percha. One important thermal property, *thermal conductivity* (κ), is defined as the quantity of heat in calories or joules that passes per second through a body 1 cm thick, with a cross-sectional area of 1 cm^2, when the temperature gradient is 1°C.[1] Thermal conductivity is measured in units of cal sec^{-1} cm^{-2}/°C per cm. Materials with thermal conductivities greater than 0.1, which includes most metals, are considered good thermal conductors. Materials with low thermal conductivities, such as enamel, dentin, porcelain, cements, resins, and gutta-percha, are considered poor thermal conductors or, conversely, excellent insulators. Dentin is an excellent insulator because it is a poor thermal conductor (Table 16-1).[2,3]

A second important thermal property is the *specific heat* of a material. This is the amount of heat, in calories, necessary to raise the temperature of 1 g of substance by 1°C. Water is the preferred reference standard, and hence 1 calorie is defined as the heat required to raise 1 g of water from 15°C to 16°C. Water is unique in that it has very high heat capacity. In general, the specific heat of liquids is higher than that of solids, and metals have specific heats that are less than 10%

Table 16-1 Thermal properties of teeth, gutta-percha, and selected materials

Materials	Thermal conductivity (cal cm sec^{-1} cm^{-2} $°C^{-1}$)	Specific heat (cal g^{-1} $°C^{-1}$)	Thermal diffusivity (cm^2/sec^{-1})
Gold	0.710	0.031	0.119
Amalgam	0.055	–	0.0096
Zinc phosphate cement	0.0028	–	0.0023
Acrylic resin	0.0005	0.35	0.00123
Enamel	0.0022	0.18	0.00469
Dentin	0.0015	0.28	0.00183
Water	0.0014	1.00	–

that of water (see Table 16-1). The higher specific heat of dentin over that of enamel is largely due to its greater water content. The low specific heat of metals, combined with their high thermal conductivity, means that they can be heated and cooled rapidly compared to dentin. This property has clear clinical implications when polishing or removing metallic restorations with mechanical friction (ie, handpiece and bur).

The third important thermal property is the *thermal diffusivity* (Δ) that determines the transient heat flow.[1] It is defined as the thermal conductivity (κ) divided by the product of the specific heat of a material times its density (ρ). It is measured in units of cm^2/second. The thermal diffusivity of a material describes the rate at which a body of nonuniform temperature approaches equilibrium.[1] The thermal diffusivity of metals is more than 100-fold higher than that of dentin (see Table 16-1). The flow of heat across dentin obeys Fickian diffusion theory. The diffusion coefficient for heat has the same units as thermal diffusivity (cm^2/second). In bulk dentin, this value is between 1.8×10^{-3} cm^2/second and 2.3×10^{-3} cm^2/second.[2,4]

Pulpal Responses to Thermal Stimuli During Cavity Preparation

Early studies on pulpal reactions to thermal challenges were performed by Zach and Cohen[5] using rather crude instruments. They were concerned about heat generated during cavity preparation or finishing procedures. Their histopathologic assessment of the subsequent pulpal reactions to application of heat to enamel in intact teeth indicated that pulpal temperature increases of 5°C to 17°C would cause progressively more severe pulpal necrosis. A study by Nyborg and Brännström[6] applied heat to the dentinal floor of Class 5 cavities in human volunteers. They applied a 150°C stimulus for 30 seconds to dentin that had remaining dentinal thickness (RDT) of 0.5 mm. Histologic examination of the pulps of these teeth showed loss of odontoblasts on the side of the pulp containing the cavity. After 1 month, the pulpal reaction beneath the heated dentin exhibited excessive collagen matrix formation that occasionally contained cells and capillaries but did not mineralize. Of the 20 test teeth, 14 were free of inflammation. The patients had no painful sensations in the heated teeth over the 30-day period.

Many authors have assumed that 5°C to 10°C elevations in external root temperatures would produce damage to the periodontal tissues similar to that produced in pulpal tissues. However, the higher blood flow in the periodontal ligament per mg of tissue relative to the pulp may influence the outcome.[7]

In their classic study of pulpal reactions to cavity preparation, Zach and Cohen[5] demonstrated that cavity preparations with high-speed handpieces using air-water spray actually lowered pulp-

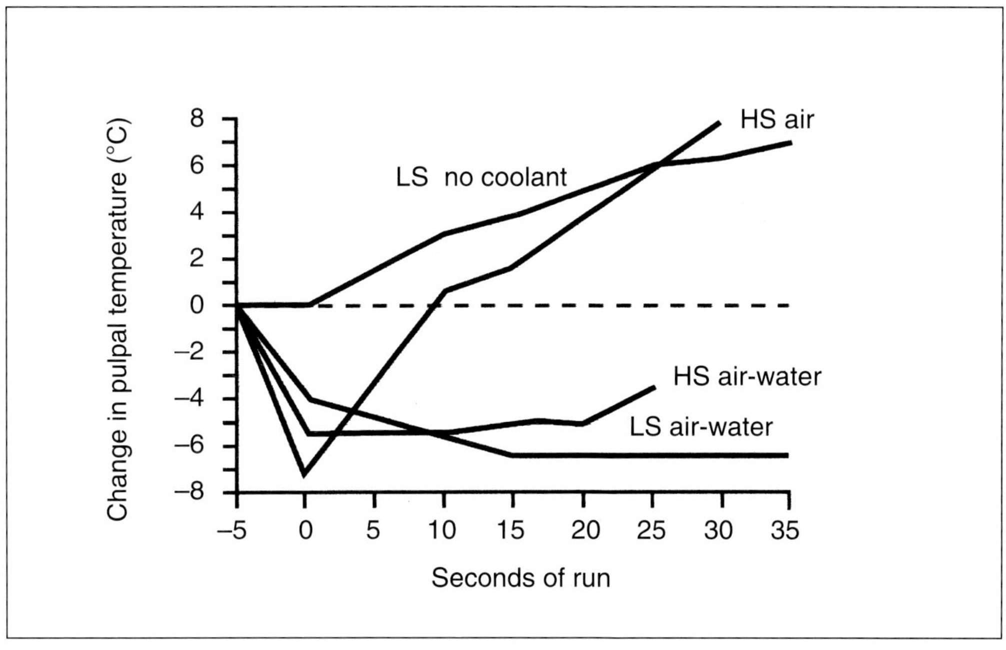

Fig 16-1 Summary of the changes in pulpal temperature during low- (LS) and high-speed (HS) cavity preparation with and without cooling. (Modified from Zach and Cohen[5] with permission.)

al temperature because the water spray was cooler than the temperature of the pulp and because of the high heat capacity of water. They recommended what they called the "washed-field" technique of tooth reduction in which the tooth surface is exposed to the air-water spray for 5 seconds before cutting. After initial cutting, the bur is lifted off the surface for 1 second following every 4 seconds of cutting. Consequently, the pulpal temperature never rises above basal temperatures (Fig 16-1). Cutting at high speeds with air alone as a coolant lowered pulpal temperature prior to cavity preparation; however, the pulpal temperature rapidly rose as much as 8°C above normal during the procedure.[5] This observation has been confirmed by others.[8-10] The frictional heat production will depend on rotational speed and torque,[11] the amount of force applied to the bur,[12] the cooling efficiency of the irrigant, and the prior wear and design of the bur (eg, cutting blades such as carbide fissure burs or grinding surface such as diamond burs).[13]

Collectively, these results indicate that pulpal reactions to various restorative procedures[12,14-17] are not necessarily caused by excessive heat production. However, it is difficult to precisely position temperature sensors to detect heat generated during cutting. In addition, the poor thermal conductivity of dentin can result in thermal burns to surface dentin without much change in pulpal temperature.[18]

Pulpal reactions to restorative procedures may in part be caused indirectly. It is possible that a high surface temperature can thermally expand the dentinal fluid in the tubules immediately beneath poorly irrigated burs. If the rate of expansion of dentinal fluid is high, the fluid flow across odontoblast processes, especially where the odontoblast cell body fills the tubules in predentin, may create shear forces sufficiently large[19] to tear the cell membrane and induce calcium entry into the cell,[20] possibly leading to cell death. This hypothesis suggests that thermally induced fluid shifts across tubules serve as the transduction mecha-

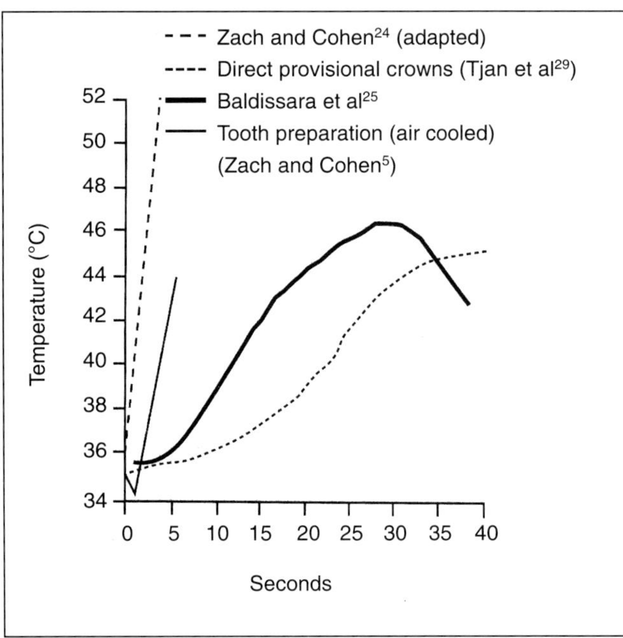

Fig 16-2 Summary of increases in pulpal temperature following a variety of experimental procedures. (Modified from Baldissara et al[25] with permission.)

nism for pulpal cell injury without causing much change in pulpal temperature.

An additional factor that can cause pulpal irritation is evaporative fluid flow.[21] Blowing air on dentin causes rapid outward fluid flows that can induce the same cell injury as the inward fluid flow caused by heat. This is why dry cutting with air is not recommended. Although air lowers pulpal temperature,[5,8,10,13] it induces very rapid outward fluid flow in dentinal tubules[22,23] that would create shear stress across odontoblasts and subodontoblastic cells and may tear their membranes.

Recent studies have not been able to confirm the earlier reports of pulpal damage from thermal stress. Since many dental procedures can elevate pulpal temperatures by 9°C to 15°C, Baldissara et al[25] evaluated the pulpal response to these temperature changes in normal young premolars scheduled for extraction for orthodontic purposes. They placed custom-fabricated metal plates on the teeth. Thermoresistors were attached to the plates to produce controlled heat flows. The surface temperature of the test teeth was measured before and during controlled heating in nonanesthetized patients who were able to record both prepain and pain sensations during these procedures. The rate of heat application in this study was much lower than that used by Zach and Cohen[24] and was selected based on the rate of heating reported in the literature from a variety of restorative procedures (Fig 16-2). In monkeys, Zach and Cohen[24] found that pulpal temperature of 40.5°C produced pulpal necrosis in 60% of the teeth. In the human study conducted by Baldissara et al,[25] heating teeth to 39.5°C to 50.4°C (average 44.5°C) caused pain. This was perceived first as a "swelling" of the tooth, but as the thermal stimulus continued, the pain became more intense in magnitude, dull in perceptual character, and poorly localized. These symptoms are hallmarks of unmyelinated C nociceptor pain (see chapters 7 and 8). The occurence of any postoperative symptoms were followed for 63 to 91 days, during which time none of the patients reported any spontaneous tooth pain. Histologic examination of the teeth failed to demonstrate any signs of inflammation, reparative dentin, etc. Similar in vitro studies were done on extracted human teeth with thermocouples placed at the pulpodentin border, immersed to the cemento-enamel junction (CEJ) in 37°C.[25] When the same electric currents were applied to the teeth in vitro, the authors could follow the rate and duration of changes in pulpal temperature (see Fig 16-2). This study concluded that young premolars could withstand increases in pulpal temperature between 8.9°C and 14.7°C without any histologic evidence of pulpal damage. Their rate of heat application was less than that used in the studies by Zach and Cohen.[5,24] Thus, the rate of delivery of heat is probably more important than the absolute rise in pulpal temperature.

This temperature range is similar to that measured in pulpal chambers during finishing or polishing of restorations.[26,27] Even higher increases in pulpal temperature have been measured during self-curing of temporary crowns[28-30] and from visible light-cured crowns. These studies need to be repeated using the turbo-tips that concentrate light on smaller surfaces and using new high-intensity light sources.

Pulpal Responses to Mechanical Stimuli During Cavity Preparation

Several studies have reported on the release of enzymes and other immunoreactive substances in the dental pulp during mechanical tooth-preparation procedures. The release of these substances may be due to temperature increases, to the mechanical stimuli of tooth preparation, or to both. Since temperature effects were discussed above, this section will review only the mechanical nontemperature causes of release of these substances.

Many enzymes and other immunoreactive substances are normally present in the pulp under nonstimulated conditions. When the pulp is stimulated mechanically, these substances are released by physiologic mechanisms (eg, exocytosis) or by disruption of cellular membranes. An early study in monkey teeth examined the effect of cavity preparation on pulpal enzyme release (alkaline-acid phosphatases and others).[31] Tooth preparation by air turbine and adequate water cooling did not affect enzyme activity, nor did the application of corticosteroids. When calcium hydroxide ($Ca[OH_2]$) was applied to the cavity floor, however, enzyme activity was increased after 24 hours in the odontoblastic and subodontoblastic cell layers adjacent to the $Ca(OH)_2$-covered dentin. Fifteen days later, slight dentinal formation was found, possibly indicating a role for these enzymes in stimulated hard tissue formation.[32]

Neuropeptides such as substance P and calcitonin gene-related peptide (CGRP) are present in dental pulp in relatively high concentrations (see also chapters 7 and 8). Rat molar dentin was prepared with a high-speed handpiece and bur to determine injury-related changes in the levels of immunoreactivity of both of these substances.[33] Pulpal exposures caused massive decreases of immunoreactive substance P (10% of baseline levels) and moderate decreases in immunoreactive CGRP levels (45% of baseline levels). Preparation and acid etching without exposure caused decreases of 10% to 20% and 60%, respectively, of baseline levels.

This study indicated that pulpal neuropeptides undergo dynamic injury-specific and peptide-specific responses following pulpal trauma (see also chapters 7 and 8). Other changes may occur in the trigeminal ganglion (see also chapter 8). For example, dental injuries affect the presence and distribution of neuropeptide Y-like immunoreactivity.[34] In normal trigeminal ganglion, some perivascular nerves displayed neuropeptide Y-like immunoreactivity, but there were no immunoreactive ganglionic cells. After dental injury (extraction, pulp exposure), neuropeptide Y-like immunoreactive cells appeared in the ganglion, indicating a change in the primary sensory neurons of the ganglion.

When dentin is exposed, plasma proteins such as albumin, IgG, and fibrinogen are released by the process of plasma extravasation (chapter 6). Data were compared to relative concentrations of these proteins in the dental pulp.[35] Albumin and IgG were found in all dentinal samples and were similar to fluid samples from exposed pulpal tissue. Fibrinogen was found in all pulpal samples but in only 25% of dentinal samples. The results indicated varying responses of plasma protein release in reaction to mechanical injuries. Another study examined changes in distribution of fibrinogen/fibrin and fibronectin in the pulpodentin complex after Class 5 cavity preparation in maxillary rat molars.[36] Fibrinogen was detected in the exudates and dentinal tubules at various times after preparation. Fibronectin staining showed a similar pattern in the exudates. At 3 days, the irregularly shaped dentin under the preparation showed strong fibronectin staining. The results indicated that these substances are present during the healing process after mechanical injury.

Mechanically induced injury to pulp elicits a number of responses of immunocompetent Class II, major histocompatibility complex (MHC) antigen-expressing cells (see also chapters 5, 10, and 11). Cavity preparations in rat maxillary first molars caused an acute edematous reaction between injured odontoblasts and the predentin, and most of the OX6-immunopositive cells normally present in uninjured teeth shifted away from the pulpodentin junction.[37] At 24 to 72 hours after injury, many of these cells accumulated along this border and newly differentiated odontoblasts appeared, indicating that Class II MHC antigen-expressing cells in the pulp participate in the initial defense reaction and may serve as a biologic sensor for external stimuli. Collectively, these studies indicate that substances and cells normally found in healthy dental pulp play a role in events occurring when the pulp is adversely stimulated.

A later study measured the response of $OX6^+$ and $ED1^+$ cells (Class II MHC cells) and macrophages to mechanical preparation and a resin-bonding agent.[38] Preparations were made and immediately restored in maxillary rat molars, with unrestored and nontreated teeth serving as positive and negative controls. The teeth were evaluated at 3 and 28 days posttreatment using anti-Class II antisera (OX6) and antimacrophage antisera (ED1). In the restored teeth at 3 days, densities of both cells were significantly higher than in the intact group. At 28 days, sound reparative dentin was seen, and the density of immunocompetent cells was comparable to that of the intact teeth. Pulpal abscesses were observed in 14 of the 16 samples in the teeth without resin, indicating that the resin-bonding agent reduced transdentinal antigenic challenges.

In vitro studies into the dynamics of events occurring due to dentin/pulp injury using cultured dental pulp cells are able to express typical markers of cell differentiation, but have not been able to recreate pulpal response to dentin preparation. However, a report of the behavior of thick slices of human dentin drilled immediately after extraction attempted to develop a model correlated to tissue healing.[39] This study showed that the damaged pulp beneath the preparation demonstrated cell proliferation, neovascularization, and presence of functional cuboidal cells close to the injured area. After 30 days of culture, elongated spindle-shaped cells were aligned along the edges of the prepared dentin, which may indicate formation of odontoblasts and the onset of odontogenesis. This model may be useful for testing factors regulating pulpal repair.

Bone morphogenetic proteins (BMPs) affect the differentiation of pulp cells to odontoblast-like cells after injury during reparative dentinogenesis (see chapter 3). The effect of BMPs on the expression of nuclear proto-oncogenes (c-jun, jun-B) was evaluated after injury and during repair in rat molars.[40] While both are co-expressed in tooth germs, only c-jun was expressed in the odontoblast layer of adult molars, whereas jun-B expression was absent in all pulp cells. After injury, both were co-expressed in cells beneath cavities, and their levels greatly increased during early repair. At 14 days, both were seen only in pulp cells lining the surface of thick reparative dentin. The results indicate a role for active formation of dentin matrix during primary and reparative dentinogenesis.

Several other chemical mediators are released during pulpal injury. Nitric oxide, produced by nitric oxide synthase (NOS) (several isozymes have been discovered) has been implicated in multiple inflammatory processes, and the level of NOS can be used as a marker of tooth pulpal insult. Therefore, relative distributions of NOS in uninflamed and inflamed rat pulp were examined.[41] Tissue levels of both macrophage NOS (macNOS) and neuronal NOS (nNOS) in normal and inflamed rat molar pulp were determined at multiple time points. Deep cavity preparation produced a time-dependent inflammatory response that was acute in nature early, later progressing to a chronic, granulomatous response with necrosis, and spreading down the root adjacent to the preparation. Nonprepared teeth showed a faint homogenous distribution of NADPH-d and macNOS, but no discernible nNOS reactivity. Similar changes were seen around the inflamed areas. The results indicate a role for nitric oxide in mediating pulpal inflammation after an injury.

Odontoblasts are formative cells that are responsible for dentin matrix formation and mineralization. Studies indicate that they display dynamic responses to injurious mechanical stimuli. Recent studies have examined injury to the pulp cells responsible for hard tissue formation. One study measured the changes in odontoblast cell numbers in response to injury due to cavity restoration variables and patient factors and the effect those factors had on tertiary dentin repair.[42] Class 5 cavity preparations and restorations were placed in premolars of patients between the ages of 9 and 17 years. After removal (28 to 163 days later), the area of reactionary dentin and the area of the odontoblasts were measured histomorphometrically. Only the age of the subject appeared to have an effect on odontoblast dentinal secretory capacity, with the older subjects demonstrating fewer odontoblasts per unit area. The area of reactionary dentin formation increased in proportion to subject age. Since preparations were made into dentin leaving 0.5 mm of dentin over the pulp, the repair capacity of the pulpodentin complex would appear to be age dependent. A companion study found that RDT was the one variable determining reactive dentin formation.[43] RDT below 0.25 mm caused a 23% decrease in odontoblasts with minimal reactionary dentin repair observed.

It is apparent from these studies that multiple levels of responses and interactions occur in reaction to mechanical injuries of the dental pulp. Responses include inflammatory changes mediated by release of various neuropeptides and changes that are defensive in nature and responsible for genesis of new hard tissue to replace the tissue injured by caries and typically removed by traumatic methods. The pulp is a complex tissue that reacts much as other body tissues react and must be protected in its environment to extend the life of the tooth.

As will be discussed later, various types of lasers can increase pulpal temperatures when they are used to irradiate enamel or dentin surfaces. White et al[44] published the only available report that compared the increase in pulpal temperature induced by pulsed Nd:YAG laser irradiation with that of a high-speed bur operated with only air spray for 20 seconds (Fig 16-3). They obtained a 4.7°C rise in pulpal temperature across 1.0 mm of RDT, similar to that induced by the 0.7 W (10 Hz) of Nd:YAG laser irradiation.

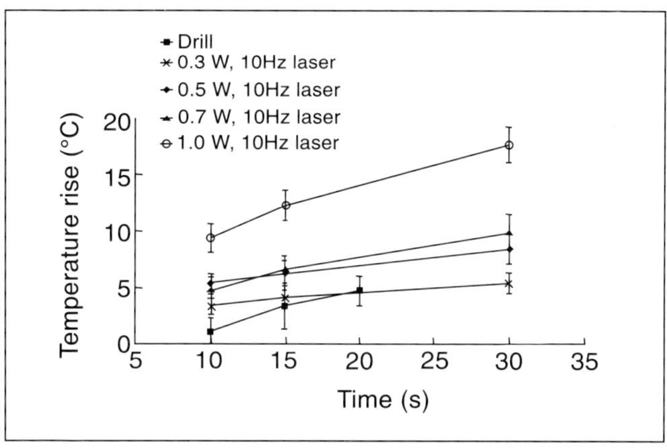

Fig 16-3 Comparison of high-speed drill vs Nd:YAG laser irradiation on pulpal temperature. No significant differences were found between the drill and the 0.3, 0.5, and 0.7 W (10Hz) lasers ($P \leq .05$). (Reprinted from White et al[44] with permission.)

Responses to Thermoplasticized Gutta-Percha Obturation Techniques

The clinical technique of warm vertical condensation procedures relies on a combination of fortuitous properties. The high thermal conductivity and low heat capacity of stainless steel means that it can be rapidly heated and can deliver that heat quickly. This permits thermoplasticization of gutta-percha, thereby softening it, lowering its stiffness,[45,46] reducing its viscosity, and allowing it to flow within a cylinder made up of a good thermal insulator (ie, root dentin). The use of metallic carriers at temperatures heated to 321°C[47] would seem extreme, but the mass (and hence the specific heat) of stainless steel times the mass of the metallic heat carrier determines how many calories of heat energy can be transferred into the root canal.

The development of the split-root model containing an array of 16 thermocouples has provided a convenient method for evaluating changes in pulpal and periodontal surface temperatures during various endodontic procedures.[48] The introduction of electrically heated carriers such as the Touch 'N Heat (Karr, Redmond, WA) and the System B (Analytic Technology, Redmond, WA) has made it much more convenient to deliver large amounts of heat to gutta-percha in the root canal space. These devices can generate tip temperatures between 250°C and 600°C. There was concern that such high temperatures could cause thermal damage to periodontal[49] and/or periapical tissues.[50,51]

Recently, electronic heat sources that can generate heat of up to 600°C have been used to plasticize gutta-percha, offering the potential for delivering excessive heat to the periodontal ligament. However, when the temperature at the external surface of the root was measured over an intracanal temperature range of 200°C to 600°C (using a System B heat source), the measured increases in root surface temperature were only 1.04°C to 5.78°C regardless of the internal root temperature. The authors speculated that this was due to brief but profound heat loss from the hot gutta-percha back up to the inactivated heat carrier that served as a heat sink.[52]

The use of heat to plasticize gutta-percha during obturation of root canals raises the risk of overheating the periodontal ligament[49] or the surrounding bone.[53] The warm vertical condensation technique was shown to increase apical temperature by only 4°C and cervical temperatures by only 12.5°C in an in vitro study.[54] These low temperatures were probably due to the low thermal conductivity of gutta-percha and the small size of the heat carriers used with that technique. In vivo studies of the histologic response to the periodontal ligament and surrounding bone to obturation with thermoplasticized gutta-percha found little adverse response.[55,56] The high external root temperatures produced by the thermomechanical compaction technique (27°C increase by Hardie[57]; 31°C increase by Fors et al[58]) have made clinicians wary of potential periodontal injury.

Thermal Responses to Laser Treatment

The search for alternative methods for removing enamel and dentin has led to the development of techniques such as lasers and air abrasion devices.[59] The word *laser* is an acronym for *light amplification by the stimulated emission of radiation*. Dental lasers used today for clinical procedures and research operate at the infrared, visible, or ultraviolet range of the electromagnetic spectrum (Figs 16-4 and 16-5). While *l* stands for *light*, the actual physical process that occurs within a laser device is amplification by stimulated emission of radiation. The laser beam (re-stimulated emission of radiation) differs from conventional light sources in three ways: *(1)* it is a single wavelength (monochromatic); *(2)* it is collimated (very low divergence); and *(3)* the photons are in phase (referred to as *coherence*).

The medium producing the beam is what identifies the laser and distinguishes one from another. Different types of lasers used in dentistry, such as carbon dioxide (CO_2), erbium (Er), and neodymium (Nd), various other substances used in the medium (eg, yttrium, aluminum, garnet [YAG]), and argon, diode and excimer types, all produce light of a specific wavelength. The CO_2, Er:YAG, and Nd:YAG lasers emit invisible beams in the infrared range. These lasers are coupled with a nonabsorbing light source (often red, green, or white) that serves as a pointer for the working laser. The argon laser emits a visible light beam at either 488 or 514 nm, while the

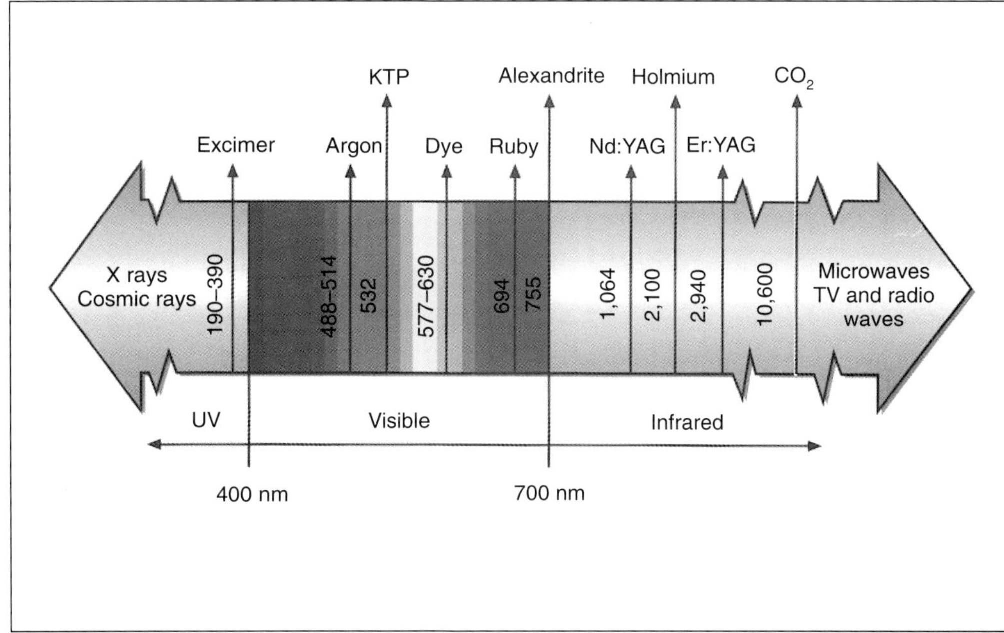

Fig 16-4 The wavelengths of different types of lasers according to their emission spectrum. Laser types differ in wavelength, beam characteristics, and available energies. (Courtesy of Opus Dent.)

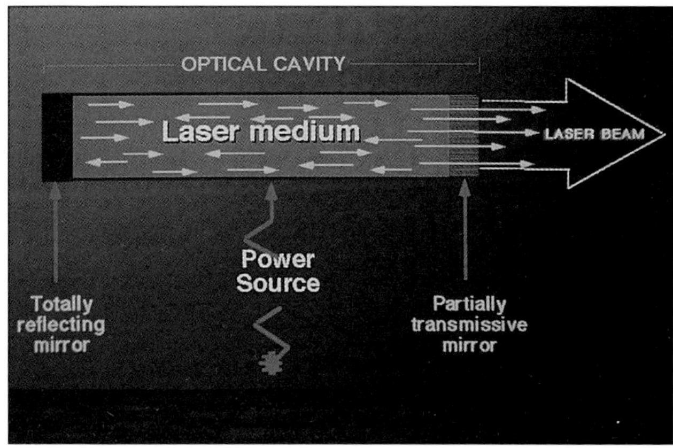

Fig 16-5 Schematic diagram of a laser.

excimer lasers emit invisible ultraviolet light beams at various predetermined wavelengths.

Laser photons interact with tissue in one of four general ways: they are transmitted through tissue, reflected from tissue, scattered within tissue, or absorbed by tissue. Transmission of light passes energy through the tissue without interaction and thus causes no effect or injury (Fig 16-6). When scattered, light travels in different directions and energy is absorbed over a greater surface area, producing a less intense and less precise thermal effect. When absorbed, light energy is converted into thermal energy. In general, a single laser device cannot perform all possible functions since the beam is absorbed or reflected according to its wavelength and the color of the object impacted.[60]

The particular properties of each type of laser and the specific target tissue make them suitable for different procedures. The CO_2 laser is most effective on tissues with high water content and is highly absorbed by all biologic hard and soft tissues. This results in thermal absorption and may damage pulp. Argon lasers are more effective on pigmented or highly vascular tissues. The photons of the Nd:YAG laser are transmitted through tissues by water and interact well with vascularized tissues such as the dental pulp. The

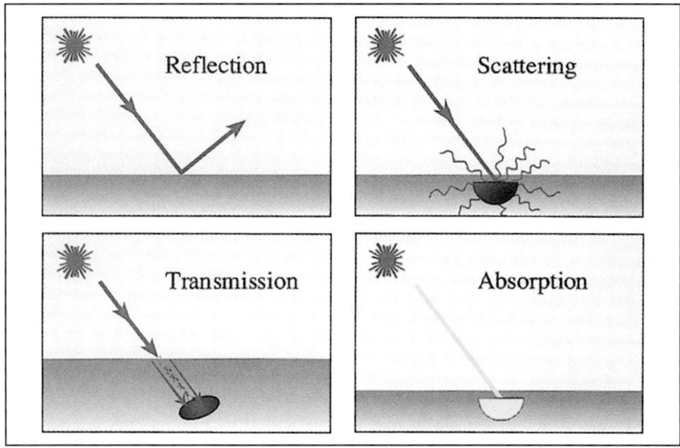

Fig 16-6 Four basic types of laser interaction occur when light hits matter or tissue: reflection, scattering, transmission, and absorption. (Courtesy of Opus Dent.)

excimer lasers generate light in the ultraviolet range of the electromagnetic spectrum and function by breaking molecular bonds. The Nd:YAG, argon, and excimer lasers may have utility for cleaning and shaping root canal systems due mainly to their use in a contact mode.

The extent of the interaction of laser energy with tissue will generally be determined by two dependent variables: the specific wavelength of the laser emission and the optical characteristics of the particular target tissue.[61-63] These variables dictate absorption (ie, ability to affect tissue changes, generation of heat, etc) and are important for pulpal tissue safety. The clinician controls four parameters when operating the laser: *(1)* the level of applied power (power density); *(2)* the total energy delivered over a given surface area (energy density); *(3)* the rate and duration of the exposure (pulse repetition); and *(4)* the mode of delivery of the energy to the target tissue (ie, continuous versus pulsed energy and direct contact or no contact with target tissue).

The pulpal responses to laser application have been adequately described.[64-70] Depending on the experimental conditions, pulpal responses to lasing include altering the presence and position of odontoblastic nuclei, destroying odontoblasts, and changing the consistency and composition of the intercellular matrices. The threshold response for pulpal reactions through intact enamel and dentin is thought to occur at energy densities somewhat less than 60 J/cm^2, although remaining dentinal thickness is an important variable.[64] Several studies have measured laser-induced increases in pulpal temperature,[39,65,66,71,72] although results from in vitro studies may overestimate pulpal temperature responses since blood flow is not available to moderate temperature changes.[67,68]

At least four approaches have been developed to reduce laser-induced increases in pulpal temperature. First, the use of an air and water spray provides pulpal protection equivalent to that of the common dental drill.[5,69,70] Second, the development of extremely brief pulsed laser systems (ie, nanosecond or picosecond pulses) permits heat to dissipate from the site of irradiation before a second pulse impacts the tissue. Third, the development of excimer lasers that operate in the ultraviolet range with short (15-nanosecond) pulses minimizes the transfer of heat compared to earlier lasers, while still forming plasma at high enough temperatures for hard tissue destruction.[73] Fourth, patent dentinal tubules have been recognized as potential pathways for direct transference of light energy to the pulp.[74] This has led to the suggestion that dentinal tubules should be closed or occluded by lasers or conventional methods.[75,76] Both the Nd:YAG laser and the excimer laser have been shown to reduce dentinal permeability or sensitivity.[77,78]

Numerous studies have evaluated the effects of lasers on enamel and dentin. Ruby lasers, one of the first types used, produced cratering in enamel, particularly at higher energy densities or when applied to dark or decayed enamel.[79,80] In one study of the use of ruby lasers on hamster teeth, application of 55 J of energy produced complete pulpal necrosis at 3 days, while 35 J produced pulpal inflammation that was reversible in some cases.[81] In the first report of a laser application in humans, two 1-millisecond pulses of 17 J produced no pain sensation in spite of the destruction of some enamel.[82] In a comprehensive study on ruby lasers applied to dog incisors, it was con-

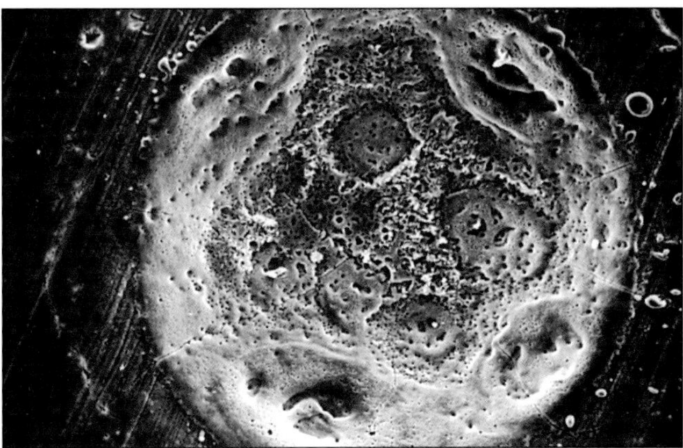

Fig 16-7 Scanning electron micrograph (SEM) of CO_2-irradiated dentin at an energy density of 113 J/cm^2. Much of the crater walls appear to be glazed, but the floor is covered with pits (original magnification ×100). (Reprinted from Pashley et al[96] with permission.)

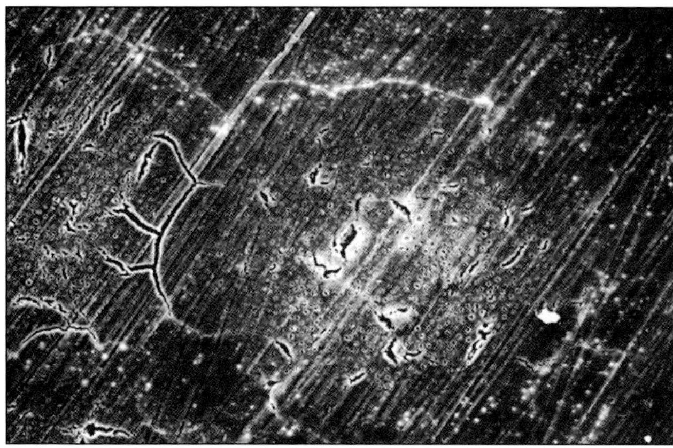

Fig 16-8 SEM of CO_2-irradiated dentin at an energy density of 566 J/cm^2. Most of the crater surface is glazed, although numerous pits remain. Inner halo devoid of smear layer of smear plugs; outer halo shows more tubulocclusion (original magnification ×120). (Reprinted from Pashley et al[96] with permission.)

cluded that the amount of energy required for hard tissue removal caused pulpal necrosis, leading the investigators to consider alternative therapies.[83] Under certain conditions, use of lasers increases the acid resistance of enamel or dentin. Thus, it is not surprising to find that laser-treated dentin may produce lower resin-dentin bond strengths than untreated acid-etched dentin.[84,85]

Several lasers have been used inside root canals to clean and shape the canal, to remove smear layers, or to sterilize the canal.[86–88] There are several limitations to intracanal use of lasers: the guidelight is emitted at the end instead of the side, it must be very small (approximately 0.2 mm), and it must be stiff but not brittle to permit easy manipulation within the canal. It is almost impossible to obtain uniform coverage of the canal surface using a laser. Further, bacteria often invade the tubules and remain viable below the surface, where they can multiply back into the canal. The potential for thermal damage to the periapical tissues remains a concern with lasers operated in the nanosecond to millisecond pulse width. The intracanal use of a KTP/532 laser (an Nd:YAG beam based through a potassium titanyl phosphate crystal to change the wavelength from invisible infrared to visible green light) increased the permeability of ethylenediaminetetraacetic acid (EDTA)–etched root dentin by removing organic material, as was definitively shown by the elegant Fouier transform infrared (FTIR) photoacoustic spectroscopy studies of Spencer et al.[89] The authors used pulse widths of 0.2 to 1 second. When pulse widths were decreased to 100 picoseconds, Serafetinides et al[90] obtained very different results with the same wavelength laser in that thermal damage was minimized. Even less thermal damage was obtained at 1,064 nm for 100-picosecond pulses, confirming the earlier work of Willms et al.[91]

CO_2 lasers represent an alternative to ruby lasers since the infrared wavelength produces significantly different thermal effects, permitting fusion of pits and fissures, conversion of hydroxyapatite to the more insoluble calcium orthophosphate, stimulation of new dentin formation, and reduced pulpal responses.[92–94] In a study measuring hydraulic conductance (Lp) across dentin disks, CO_2 lasers increased dentin permeability 1.4- to 24-fold by such mechanisms as removal of smear layer and smear plugs, cratering, and cracking in the glazed surface of the crater (Figs 16-7 and 16-8).[95,96] However, there is a major limitation

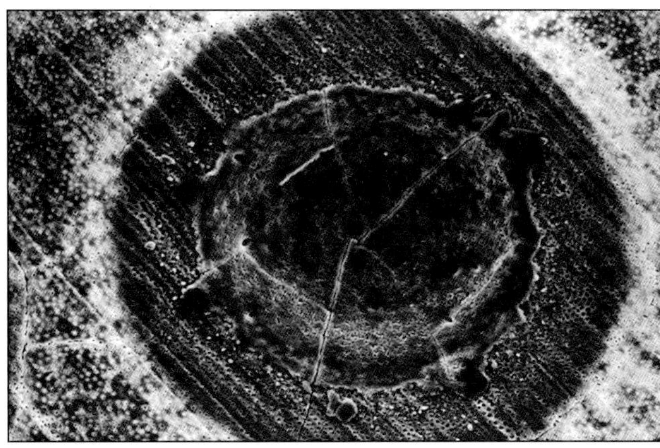

Fig 16-9 SEM of CO_2-irradiated dentin at an energy density of 11 J/cm^2 single impact crater. Large cracks were not present when the hydraulic conductance of the sample was measured (original magnification ×100). (Reprinted from Pashley et al[96] with permission.)

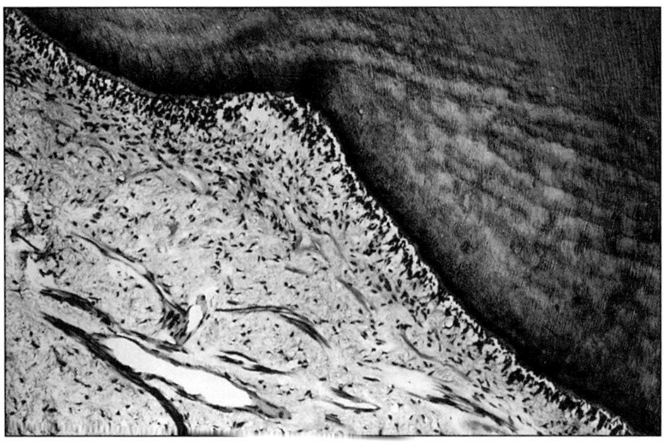

Fig 16-10a Er:YAG laser cavity preparation in dentin in monkey teeth (H&E stain, original magnification ×40).

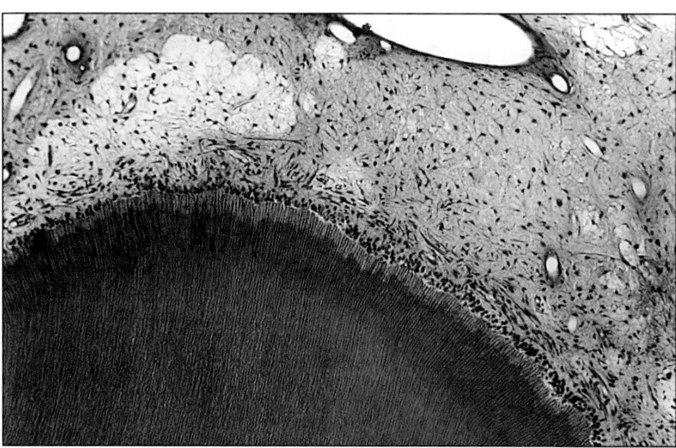

Fig 16-10b CO_2 laser cavity preparation in monkey teeth (H&E stain, original magnification ×25).

to the CO_2 laser: when used to prepare cavities, it creates high thermal damage to dentin due to the strong absorption of the emitted photons by water (Fig 16-9).[96-99] In a clinical trial with CO_2 lasers, the increase in pulpal temperature never exceeded 10.5°C, although the odontoblast destruction was inversely related to remaining dentinal thickness.[99] Others have demonstrated that as little as 3.5 J of CO_2 laser irradiation may produce pulpal damage in vivo, and concern has been raised using levels as low as 1.0 J.[100,101]

Several studies have evaluated the properties of the Er:YAG laser. The depth and diameter of Er:YAG laser-drilled holes are a function of pulse number and the amount of exposure to energy parameters.[102,103] Using various wavelengths, Wigdor et al[104] compared the histologic response of the dental pulp to dentinal ablation in dog teeth and suggested that the thermal effect might be lower than that of the other lasers tested. Others (Goodis et al, unpublished data, 1993) found that when used in cavity preparation, the Er:YAG produced no detectable pulpal damage at energy levels of 3W and 10 to 30 Hz (Fig 16-10). In 1997, the US Food and Drug Administration approved the use of the Er:YAG laser for caries removal, tooth preparations, and modification of dentin and enamel. As to pulpal tissue effects, the Er:YAG laser and the turbine handpiece were judged to be equivalent.[105] However,

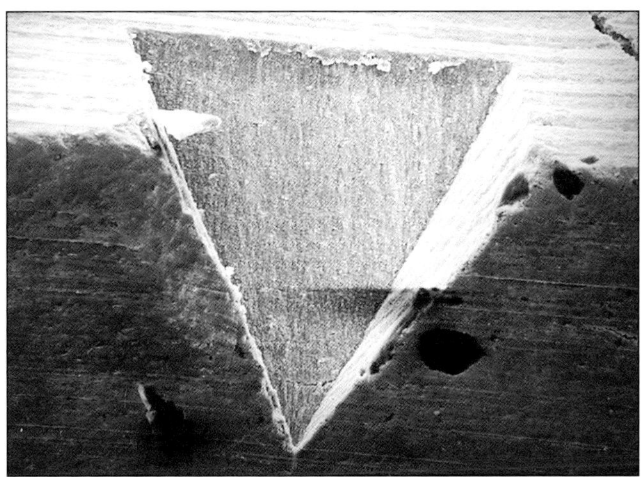

Fig 16-11a SEM of enamel irradiated with excimer laser to show the precise removal of hard tissue at 248 nm using 15-nanosecond pulses. (Reprinted from Pearson and McDonald[112] with permission.)

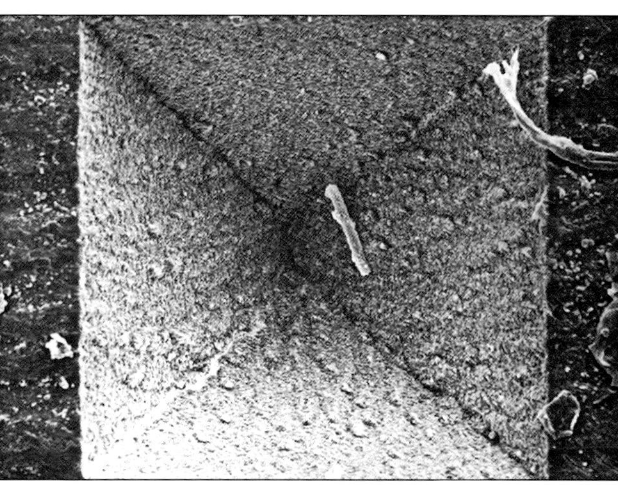

Fig 16-11b SEM of dentin irradiated at 248 nm using an excimer laser with 15-nanosecond pulse widths. (Reprinted from Pearson and McDonald[112] with permission.)

a general impression among clinicians is that the speed of preparation in dentin and especially in enamel is much slower with the Er:YAG laser than with the conventional high-speed drill.

Other studies have focused on the use of Nd:YAG lasers. In a 2-week clinical trial, hypersensitive teeth treated with Nd:YAG lasers were significantly less sensitive to air blasts than were nontreated control teeth.[77] During treatment, the power was increased either until the patient detected the laser energy or until a maximum of 100 mJ was reached. While it is unlikely that this relatively low energy would have sealed exposed dentinal tubules, it might have altered A-delta nerve thresholds.[106-108] Thus, although more research is indicated, there seems to be some potential for use of the Nd:YAG laser as a method for obtaining temporary analgesia. The lack of thermal damage but improved "cutting efficiency" of picosecond pulses of Nd:YAG laser irradiation is thought to be due to the fact that the energy per single photon emission is only 1.18 eV, which is insufficient to break molecular bonds or destroy ionic crystalline lattices. Although the photon absorption of 1,064 nm energy by dentin is low,[109] Nd:YAG energy absorption by water is relatively high, allowing vaporization to occur so rapidly as to create microexplosions that cause mechanical ablation.[103]

According to Niemz,[110] mechanical disruption can be of two types: "plasma-mediated ablation" results when the laser energy ionizes enough tissue components and heats it to a plasma state, whereas a "photodisruption" type of ablation is due largely to acoustical shock waves from rapid vaporization of water.

Excimers, lasers that emit photons in the ultraviolet range, offer the potential advantage of reduced heat absorption that may promote cracking by establishing extremely high thermal gradients. Both the ArF excimer (193 nm) and the XeCl excimer (308 nm) melted dentin but did not occlude dentinal tubules.[78,111] Although permeability of the dentin was not measured, subsurface deposits that may have reduced dentinal permeability were unlikely. The use of excimer lasers as a method for cutting enamel and dentin without generating excess thermal stress looks very promising. Operating at 248 nm, the excimer laser can preferentially remove intertubular dentin without creating a smear layer; the dentinal surfaces are so clean, they appear as if they were fractured (Fig 16-11).[112] The photon energy in excimer lasers operating at 193 and 248 nm is higher than the molecular bond energies holding collagen together. This results in photoacoustic destruction of dentin without melting. However, reductions in the pulse length from millisecond to picosecond have been shown to reduce thermal damage for both excimer and Nd:YAG[113] or Nd:YSF lasers.[114] This is thought to be because picosecond pulse durations are less than the thermal relaxation times of dentin, thus minimizing any thermal effects.[103,115-117]

Two mechanisms have been proposed for laser-induced reduction in dentinal hypersensitivity. First, lasers may occlude dentinal tubules by melting and fusing dentin or the smear layer, or by coagulating proteins in dentinal tubules.[117] Second, lasers may directly reduce neuronal activity.[106-108]

While the use of lasers for laser-induced hard tissue procedures is increasing, they have been approved for use for soft tissue procedures, such as periodontal pocket elimination, closure of oral surgical wounds, frenectomy, and operculum excisions, for approximately the last 10 years. Their use for contouring of bone or removal of bone lesions is questionable at best, but they have been examined for root canal cleaning and shaping procedures and for use in obturation. Further study must be carried out before their use can be fully recommended. As their use in dentistry increases, there will be a continuing need to evaluate pulpal responses following laser application to teeth.

Pulpal Responses to Airborne Particle Abrasion (Kinetic Cavity Preparation)

Another technology, airborne particle abrasion, has recently been re-introduced for caries removal and cavity preparation. Airborne particle abrasion had fallen into disuse because the stream of particles used in tooth preparation procedures could not be controlled, resulting in pitting and abrasion of adjacent teeth and injury to gingival tissues. It was easily replaced with high-speed, air-driven turbine handpieces, which are more efficient and can construct a more precisely defined tooth preparation.[119-122]

Airborne particle-abrasion technology has recently been refined and used as a method to produce "kinetic cavity preparations."[123] Its potential for pulpal damage has not been fully investigated, but its use has been suggested due to newer restorative materials and their direct placement in altered preparations, sometimes referred to as *micropreparation*. Advances in microabrasion technology allow for more precise removal of enamel and dentin than the older systems.

Laurell et al[122] examined the pulpal responses of an air-abrasion system in 120 molars and premolars of dogs. Two pressures (80 and 160 psi) were used with two aluminum oxide particle sizes (27 and 50 μm). Class 5 cavity preparations were made and then restored with an intermediate restorative material, and the teeth were removed in 72 hours. Sections were examined for odontoblast displacement, disruption of cell layers, inflammatory infiltrate, and necrosis and compared to preparations made with a high-speed turbine handpiece. They found that higher pressures and smaller particles had significantly fewer pulpal effects than the high-speed treated teeth. This study represents the only controlled pulpal injury study to date in the literature. While other papers in proprietary (commercial) journals report similar results, they are anecdotal in nature. The ever-increasing popularity of such technology indicates that more studies are needed to be certain of the safety of these devices.

References

1. Craig RC. Restorative Dental Materials, ed 10. St. Louis: Mosby, 1997.
2. Braden M. Heat conduction in normal human teeth. Arch Oral Biol 1964;9:479–486.
3. Spierings TA, Peters MC, Bosman F, Plasschaert AJ. Verification of theoretical modeling of heat transmission in teeth by in vitro experiments. J Dent Res 1987;66: 1336–1339.

4. Brown WS, Dewey WA, Jacobs HR. Thermal properties of teeth. J Dent Res 1970;49:752–755.
5. Zach L, Cohen G. Thermogenesis in operative dentistry: Comparison of four methods. J Prosthet Dent 1962;12: 977–984.
6. Nyborg H, Brännström M. Pulp reaction to heat. J Prosthet Dent 1968;19:605–612.
7. Sasano T, Kuriwada S, Sanjo D, Izumi H, Tabata T, Karita K. Acute response of periodontal ligament blood flow to external force application. J Periodontal Res 1992;27(4 pt 1):301–304.
8. Bhasker SN, Lilly GE. Intrapulpal temperature during cavity preparation. J Dent Res 1965;44:644–647.
9. Carson J, Rider T, Nash D. A thermographic study of heat distribution during ultra-speed cavity preparation. J Dent Res 1979;58:1681–1684.
10. Goodis HE, Schein B, Stauffer P. Temperature changes measured in vivo at the dentinoenamel junction and pulpodentin junction during cavity preparation in the Macsaca fascicularis monkey. J Endod 1988;14: 336–339.
11. Schuchard AD, Watkins EC. Temperature response to increased rotational speeds. J Prosthet Dent 1961;11: 313–317.
12. Stanley HR, Swerdlow H. Biologic effects of various cutting methods in cavity preparation: The part pressure plays in pulpal response. J Am Dent Assoc 1960;61: 450–456.
13. Harnett J, Smith W. The production of heat in the dental pulp by use of the air turbine. J Am Dent Assoc 1961;63:210–214.
14. Langeland K. Tissue Changes in the Dental Pulp. An Experimental Study [thesis]. Oslo: Univ of Oslo, 1957.
15. Langeland K. Histologic evaluation of pulpal reactions to operative procedures. Oral Surg 1959;1235–1249.
16. Stanley HR, Swerdlow H. Reaction of the human pulp to cavity preparation: Results produced by eight different operative grinding techniques. J Am Dent Assoc 1959;58:49–59.
17. Stanley HR. Traumatic capacity of high-speed and ultrasonic dental instrumentation. J Am Dent Assoc 1961;63: 749–766.
18. Stanley HR. Human Pulp Response to Restorative Dental Procedures. Gainesville: Storter, 1981.
19. Evans EA. New membrane concept applied to analysis of fluid shear- and micropipette-deformed red blood cells. Biophys J 1973;13:941–954.
20. Hung CT, Allen FD, Pollack SR, Brighton CT. Intracellular Ca^{2+} stores and extracellular Ca^{2+} are required for the real-time Ca^{2+} response of bone cells experiencing fluid flow. J Biomech 1996; 29:1411–1417.
21. Pashley DH. Dynamics of the pulpodentin complex. Crit Rev Oral Biol Med 1996;7:104–133.
22. Goodis HE, Tao L, Pashley DH. Evaporative water loss from human dentine in vitro. Arch Oral Biol 1990;35: 523–527.
23. Matthews WG, Showman CD, Pashley DH. Air blast-induced evaporative water loss from human dentine, in vitro. Arch Oral Biol 1993;38:517–523.
24. Zach L, Cohen G. Pulp response to externally applied heat. Oral Surg 1965;19:515–530.
25. Baldissara P, Catapano S, Scotti R. Clinical and histological evaluation of thermal injury thresholds in human teeth: A preliminary study. J Oral Rehabil 1997;24: 791–801.
26. Stewart GP, Bachman TA, Hatton JF. Temperature rise due to finishing of direct restorative materials. Am J Dent 1991;4:23–28.
27. Hatton JF, Holtzmann DJ, Ferrillo PJ Jr, Stewart GP. Effect of handpiece pressure and speed on intrapulpal temperature rise. Am J Dent 1994;7:108–110.
28. Grajower R, Shaharbani S, Kaufman E. Temperature rise in pulp chamber during fabrication of temporary self-curing resin crowns. J Prosthet Dent 1979;41:535–540.
29. Tjan AH, Grant BE, Godfrey MF. Temperature rise in the pulp during fabrication of provisional crown. J Prosthet Dent 1989;62:622–626.
30. Goodis HE, White JM, Gamm B, Watanabe L. Pulp chamber temperature changes with visible-light-cured composites in vitro. Dent Mater 1990; 6:99–102.
31. Haug SR, Berggreen E, Heyeraas KJ. The effect of unilateral sympathectomy and cavity preparation on peptidergic nerves and immune cells in rat dental pulp. Exp Neurol 2001;169:182–190.
32. Hasselgren G, Tronstad L. Enzyme activity in the pulp following preparation of cavities and insertion of medicaments in cavities in monkey teeth. Acta Odontol Scand 1977;35:289–295.
33. Grutzner EH, Garry MG, Hargreaves KN. Effect of injury on pulpal levels of immunoreactive substance P and immunoreactive calcitonin-gene-related peptide. J Endod 1992;11:553–557.
34. Wakisaka S, Youn SH, Maeda T, Kurisu K. Neuropeptide Y-like immunoreactive primary afferents in the periodontal tissues following dental injury in the rat. Regul Pept 1996;63:163–169.
35. Knutsson G, Jontell M, Bergenholtz G. Determination of plasma proteins in dentinal fluid from cavities prepared in healthy young human teeth. Arch Oral Biol 1994;39:185–190.
36. Izumi T, Yamada K, Inoue H, Watanabe K, Nishigawa Y. Fibrinogen/fibrin and fibronectin in the dentin-pulp complex after cavity preparation in rat molars. Oral Surg Oral Med Oral Pathol Oral Radiol Endod 1998;86: 587–591.

37. Ohshima H, Sato O, Kawahara I, Maeda T, Takano Y. Responses of immunocompetent cells to cavity preparation in rat molars: An immunohistochemical study using OX6-monoclonal antibody. Connect Tissue Res 1995;32:303-311.
38. Kamal AM, Okiji T, Suda H. Response of Class II molecular-expressing cells and macrophages to cavity preparation and restoration with 4-META/MMA-TBB resin. Int Endod J 2000;33:367-373.
39. Magloire H, Joffre A, Bleicher F. An in vitro model of human dental pulp repair. J Dent Res 1996;75:1971-1978.
40. Kitamura C, Kimura K, Nakayama T, Terashita M. Temporal and spatial expression of c-jun and jun-B proto-oncogenes in pulp cells involved with reparative dentinogenesis after cavity preparation of rat molars. J Dent Res 1999;78:673-680.
41. Law AS, Baumgardner KR, Meller ST, Gebhart GF. Localization and changes in NADPH-diaphorase reactivity and nitric oxide synthase immunoreactivity in rat pulp following tooth preparation. J Dent Res 1999;78:1585-1595.
42. Murray PE, About I, Lumley PJ, Franquin J-C, Remusat M, Smith AJ. Human odontoblast cell numbers after dental injury. J Dent 2000;28:277-285.
43. About I, Murray PE, Franquin J-C, Remusat M, Smith AJ. The effect of cavity restoration variables on odontoblast cell number and dental repair. J Dent 2001;29:109-117.
44. White JM, Fagan MC, Goodis HE. Intrapulpal temperatures during pulsed Nd:YAG laser treatment of dentin, in vitro. J Periodontol 1994;65:255-259.
45. Marciano J, Michailesco P, Charpentier E, Carrera LC, Abadie MJM. Thermomechanical analysis of dental gutta-percha. J Endod 1992;18:263-270.
46. Camps JJ, Pertot WJ, Escavy JY, Pravaz M. Young's modulus of warm and cold gutta-percha. Endod Dent Traumatol 1996;12:50-53.
47. Marciano J, Michailesco PM. Dental gutta-percha: Chemical composition, x-ray identification, enthalpic studies and clinical implications. J Endod 1989;15:149-153.
48. Weller RN, Jurcak JJ, Donley Dl, Kulild JC. A new model system for measuring intracanal temperatures. J Endod 1991;17:491-494.
49. Barkhordar R, Goodis HE. Evaluation of temperature rise on the outer surface of teeth during root canal obturation techniques. Quintessence Int 1990;21:585-588.
50. Weller RN, Koch KA. In vitro temperatures produced by a new heated injectable gutta-percha system. Int Endod J 1994;27:299-303.
51. Weller RN, Koch KA. In vitro radicular temperatures produced by injectable thermoplasticized gutta percha. Int Endod J 1995;28:86-90.
52. Floren JW, Weller RN, Pashley DH, Kimbrough WF. Changes in root surface temperatures with in vitro use of the System B HeatSource. J Endod 1999;25:593-595.
53. Atrizadeh F, Kennedy J, Zander H. Ankylosis of teeth following thermal injury. J Periodontal Res 1971;6:159-167.
54. Martin J, Schilder H. Physical properties of gutta-percha when subjected to heat and vertical condensation. Oral Surg 1973;36:872-879.
55. Hand RE, Huget EF, Tsaknis PJ. Effects of warm gutta-percha technique on the lateral periodontium. Oral Surg 1976;42:395-401.
56. Gutmann JL, Rakusin H, Powe R, Bowles WH. Evaluation of heat transfer during root canal obturation with thermoplasticized gutta-percha. Part II. In vivo response to heat levels generated. J Endod 1987;13:441-448.
57. Hardie EM. Heat transmission to the outer surface of the tooth during the thermo-mechanical compaction technique of root canal obturation. Int Endod J 1986;19:73-77.
58. Fors U, Jonasson E, Bergquist A, Berg JO. Measurements of root surface temperature during thermo-mechanical root canal filling in vitro. Int Endod J 1985;18:199-202.
59. Christiansen GJ. Cavity preparation: Cutting or abrasion. J Am Dent Assoc 1996;127:1651-1654.
60. Nelson SJ, Berns MW. Basic laser physics and tissue interactions. Contemp Dermatol 1988;2:1-15.
61. Dederich DN. Laser tissue interaction. Alpha Omegan 1991;84:33-36.
62. Maiman TH. Stimulated optical radiation in ruby. Nature 1960;187:493-494.
63. Stern RH, Sognnaes RF. Laser beam effect on dental hard tissues. J Dent Res 1964;43:873.
64. Arcoria CJ, Miserendino LJ. Laser effects on the dental pulp. In: Miserendino LJ, Pick RM (eds). Lasers in Dentistry. Chicago: Quintessence, 1995.
65. Yu D, Powell GL, Higuchi WI, Fox JL. Comparison of three lasers on dental pulp chamber temperature change. J Clin Laser Med Surg 1993;11:119-122.
66. White JM, Goodis HE, Setcos JC, Eakle S, Hulscher BE, Rose CL. Effects of pulsed Nd:YAG laser energy on human teeth: A three-year follow up study. J Am Dent Assoc 1993;124:45-51.
67. Friedman S, Liu M, Izawa T, Moynihan M, Dörscher-Kim J, Kim S. Effects of CO_2 laser irradiation on pulpal blood flow. Proc Finn Dent Soc 1992;88(Supp 1):167-171.
68. Raab WH. Temperature related changes in pulpal microcirculation. Proc Finn Dent Soc 1992;88(Supp 1):469.

69. Abt E, Miserendino LJ, Levy GC. Histologic effects of Nd:YAG and Er:YAG on dentin, pulp and bone [abstract]. In: Proceedings of Third International Congress on Lasers in Dentistry. International Society for Lasers in Dentistry Meeting, Salt Lake City, UT, 1992. Salt Lake City: Univ of Utah, 1992.
70. Miserendino LJ, Levy GC, Abt E, Rizoiu IM. Histologic effects of thermally cooled Nd:YAG laser on the dental pulp and supporting structures of rabbit teeth. Oral Surg 1994;78:93–100.
71. Gow AM, McDonald AV, Pearson GL, Setchell DJ. An in vitro investigation of the temperature rises produced in dentine by Nd:YAG laser light with and without cooling. Eur J Prosthodont Restorative Dent 1999;7:71–77.
72. Leighty SM, Pogrel MA, Goodis HE, Marshall GW, White JM. Thermal effects of the carbon dioxide laser on teeth. Lasers Life Sci 1991;4:93.
73. Srinivasan R. Ablation of polymers and biological tissue by ultraviolet. Science 1986;234:559–565.
74. Walton RE, Outhwaite WC, Pashley DH. Magnification–An interesting optical property of dentin. J Dent Res 1976;55:639–642.
75. Addy M, Dowell P. Dentin hypersensitivity. A review. II. Clinical and in vitro evaluation for treatment agents. J Clin Periodontol 1977;10:351.
76. Kerns DG, Scheidt MJ, Pashley DH, Horner AJ, Strong SL, Van Dyke TE. Dentinal tubule occlusion and root hypersensitivity. J Periodontol 1991;62:421–428.
77. Renton-Harper P, Midda M. Nd:YAG laser treatment of dentinal hypersensitivity. Brit Dent J 1992;172:13–16.
78. Stabholtz A, Neer J, Liaw LH, Stabholz A, Khayet A, Torabinejad M. Sealing of human dentinal tubules by XeCl 308-nm excimer laser. J Endod 1993b;19:267.
79. Kinersly T, Jarabak JP, Phatak NM, DeMent J. Lasers effects on tissue and materials related to dentistry. J Am Dent Assoc 1965;70:592–600.
80. Gordon TE. Some effects of laser impacts on extracted teeth. J Dent Res 1966;42:372–375.
81. Taylor R, Shklar G, Roeber F. The effects of laser radiation on teeth, dental pulp, and oral mucosa of experimental animals. Oral Surg Oral Med Oral Pathol 1965; 19:786–795.
82. Stern RH, Sognnaes RF. Laser inhibition of dental caries suggested by first tests in vivo. J Am Dent Assoc 1972; 85:1087–1090.
83. Adrian JC, Bernier JL, Sprauge WG. Laser and the dental pulp. J Am Dent Assoc 1971;83:113–117.
84. Armengol V, Jean A, Weiss P, Hamel H. Comparative in vitro study of the bond strength of composite to enamel and dentine obtained with laser irradiation or acid-etch. Lasers Med Sci 1999;14:207.
85. Kameyama A, Kawada E, Takizawa M, Oda Y, Hirai Y. Influence of different acid conditioners on the tensile bond strength of 4-META/MMA-TBB resin to Er:YAG laser-irradiated bovine dentine. J Adhes Dent 2000;2:297–304.
86. Goodis HE, White JM, Marshall SJ, Marshall GW Jr. Scanning electron microscopic examination of intracanal wall dentin: Hand versus laser treatment. Scanning Microsc 1993;7:979–987.
87. Önal B, Ertl T, Siebert G, Müller G. Preliminary report on the application of pulsed CO_2 laser radiation on root canals with AgCl fibers: A scanning and transmission electron microscopic study. J Endod 1993;19:272–276.
88. Tewfik HM, Pashley DH, Horner JA, Sharawy MM. Structural and functional changes in root dentin following exposure to KTP/532 laser. J Endod 1993;19:492–497.
89. Spencer P, Cobb CM, McCollum MH, Wieliczka DM. The effects of CO_2 laser and Nd:YAG with and without water/air surface cooling on tooth root structure: Correlation between FTIR spectroscopy and histology. J Periodontal Res 1996;31:453–462.
90. Serafetinides AA, Khabbaz MG, Makropoulou MI, Kar AK. Picosecond laser ablation of dentine in endodontics. Lasers Med Sci 1999;14:168.
91. Willms L, Herschel A, Niemz M. Preparation of dental hard tissues with picosecond laser pulses. Lasers Med Sci 1996;11:45.
92. Lobene RR, Rhussry BR, Fine S. Interaction of carbon dioxide laser radiation with enamel and dentin. J Dent Res 1968;47:311–317.
93. Kantola S. Laser induced effects on tooth structure. VII. X-ray diffraction study of dentin exposed to carbon dioxide laser. Acta Odontol Scand 1973;31:311–317.
94. Melcer J, Chaumette MT, Melcer F. Dental pulp exposed to the CO_2 laser beam. Lasers Surg Med 1987;7: 347–352.
95. Read RP, Baumgartner JC, Clark SM. Effects of a carbon dioxide laser on human root dentin. J Endod 1995;21: 4–8.
96. Pashley EL, Horner JA, Liu M, Kim S, Pashley DH. Effects of CO_2 laser energy on dentin permeability. J Endod 1992;18:257–262.
97. Jeffrey IW, Lawrenson B, Longbottom C, Saunders EM. CO_2 laser application to the mineralized dental tissues—The possibility of iatrogenic sequelae. J Dent 1990;18:24–30.
98. Jeffrey IW, Lawrenson B, Saunders EM, Longbottom C. Dentinal temperature transients caused by exposure to CO_2 laser irradiation and possible pulpal damage. J Dent 1990;18:31–36.
99. Melcer J, Chaumette MT, Zeboulon S, Melcer F, Hasson R, Merard R, et al. Preliminary report on the effect of CO_2 laser beam on the dental pulp of Macaca mulatta primate and the beagle dog. J Endod 1985;11:1–5.

100. Powell GL, Whisenant BK, Morton TH. Carbon dioxide laser oral safety parameters for teeth. Lasers Surg Med 1990;10:389–392.
101. Bonin P, Boivin R, Poulard J. Dentinal permeability of the dog canine after exposure to a cervical cavity to the beam of a CO_2 laser. J Endod 1991;17:116–118.
102. Paghdiwala AF. Application of the Er-YAG laser on hard dental tissue: Measurements of the temperature changes and depth of cut. Proc ICALEO 88. Laser Institute of America 1989;64:192.
103. Hibst R, Keller U. Experimental studies of the application of the Er:YAG laser on dental hard substances: I. Measurement of the ablation rate. Lasers Surg Med 1989;9:338–344.
104. Wigdor H, Abt E, Ashraft S, Walsh JT. The effect of lasers on dental hard tissues. J Am Dent Assoc 1993;124: 65–70.
105. Cozean C, Arcoria CJ, Pelagalli J, Powell GI. Dentistry for the 21st century? Erbium: YAG laser for teeth. J Am Dent Assoc 1997;128:1080–1087.
106. Orchardson R, Peacock JM, Whitters CJ. Effect of pulsed Nd:YAG laser radiation on action potential conduction in isolated mammalian spinal nerves. Lasers Surg Med 1997;21:142–148.
107. Orchardson R, Peacock JM, Whitters CJ. Effects of pulsed Nd:YAG laser radiation on action potential conduction in nerve fibers inside teeth *in vitro*. J Dent 1998;26:421–426.
108. Whitters CJ, Hall A, Creanor SL, Moseley H, Gilmour WH, Strang R, et al. A clinical study of pulsed Nd:YAG laser-induced analgesia. J Dent 1995;23:145–150.
109. White JM, Goodis HE. Laser interactions with dental hard tissues—Effects on the pulp/dentin complex. In: Shimono M, Maeda T, Suda H, Takahashi K (eds). Dentin/Pulp Complex. Tokyo: Quintessence, 1996: 41–50.
110. Niemz M. Investigation and spectral analysis of the plasma-induced ablation mechanism of dental hydroxyapatite. Appl Phys 1994;B58:273.
111. Stabholz A, Neev J, Liaw LH, Stabholz A, Khayet A, Torabinejad M. Effect of ArF-193 nm excimer laser on human dentinal tubules. A scanning electron microscopic study. Oral Surg Oral Med Oral Pathol 1993;75: 90–94.
112. Pearson GJ, McDonald AV. Use of infra-red and ultra-violet lasers in the removal of dental hard tissues. Lasers Med Sci 1994;9:227.
113. McDonald A, Claffey N, Pearson G, Blau W, Setchell D. The effect of Nd:YAG pulse duration on dentine crater depth. J Dent 2001;29:43–53.
114. Niemz MH. Cavity preparations with the Nd:YLF picosecond laser. J Dent Res 1995;74:1194–1199.
115. Partovi F, Izatt JA, Cothren RM, Kittrell C, Thomas JE, Strikwerda S, et al. A model for thermal ablation of biological tissue using laser radiation. Lasers Surg Med 1987;7:141–154.
116. McCormack SM, Fried D, Featherstone JD, Glena RE, Seka W. Scanning electron microscope observations of CO_2 laser effects on dental enamel. J Dent Res 1995;74: 1702–1708.
117. McKenzie AL. Physics of thermal processes in laser-tissue interactions. Phys Med Biol 1990;35:1175–1209.
118. Goodis HE, White JM, Marshall GW Jr, Yee K, Fuller N, Gee L, Marshall SJ. Effects of Nd: and Ho:yttrium-aluminium-garnet lasers on human dentine fluid flow and dental pulp chamber temperature *in vitro*. Arch Oral Biol 1997;42:845–854.
119. Black RB. Technique for nonmechanical preparation of cavities and prophylaxis. J Am Dent Assoc 1945;32:953.
120. Black RB. Application and re-evaluation of the air abrasion technique. J Am Dent Assoc 1955;50:408.
121. Morrison AH, Berham I. Evaluation of the airdent unit: Preliminary report. J Am Dent Assoc 1953;46:298.
122. Myers GE. The airbrasive technique. Br Dent J 1954;97: 291.
123. Laurell KA, Carpenter W, Daughtery D, Beck M. Histopathologic effects of kinetic cavity preparation for the removal of enamel and dentin. Oral Surg Oral Med Oral Pathol Oral Radiol Endod 1995;80:214–225.

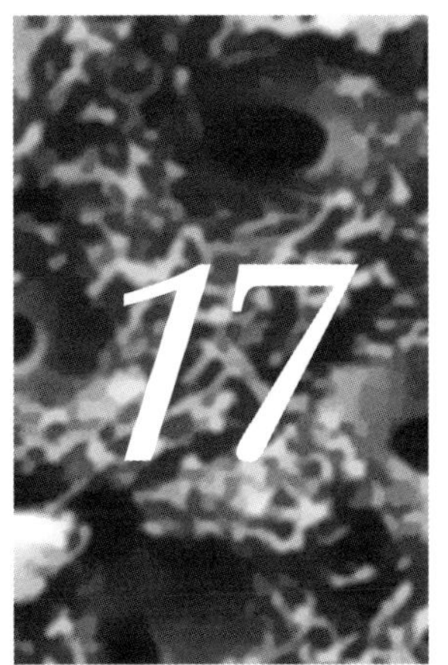

Interrelationship of Dental Pulp and Apical Periodontitis

Philip Stashenko, DMD, PhD

Infections of the dental pulp occur as a consequence of caries, operative dental procedures, and trauma, and involve a mixed, predominantly gram-negative, anaerobic bacterial flora.[1] These infections initially elicit an immune response in the dental pulp, which very often is ineffective in eliminating the invading microorganisms (see chapters 11 and 12). Consequently, these infections often cause total pulpal necrosis and subsequently stimulate a secondary immune response in the periapical region. The latter is commonly referred to as a periapical "lesion," but in fact it represents a protective response to the bacteria in the necrotic pulp and root canal system.

Both pulpal and periapical immune responses initially involve *innate immunity*, particularly the influx of phagocytic leukocytes and the production of proinflammatory cytokines. As infections become more chronic, *adaptive immune elements* are also activated and become superimposed on the innate response, including T and B cells, leading to a typical "mixed" inflammatory cell response. In this milieu, a complex array of immunologic mechanisms is activated, some of which act primarily to protect the pulp and periapical region, while others mediate tissue destruction, particularly periapical bone resorption. The latter include the expression of a plethora of host-derived factors, including cytokines, arachidonic acid metabolites, and neuropeptides that contribute to or modulate apical periodontitis.

Although many gaps in knowledge still remain, understanding of these processes is rapidly expanding through the application of new biologic tools such as recombinant proteins, knockout mice, and new model systems. In this chapter, we review the immune mechanisms that protect the host against pulpal infections, as well as those that primarily contribute to periapical tissue destruction. The ultimate goal is to better understand the immunobiology of apical periodontitis that occurs due to pulpal infection, and ultimately to use this knowledge in the rational design of improved clinical procedures.

Pulpal and Periapical Immune Responses

Pulpal responses

The dental pulp, similar to most connective tissues, has certain immunocompetencies that facili-

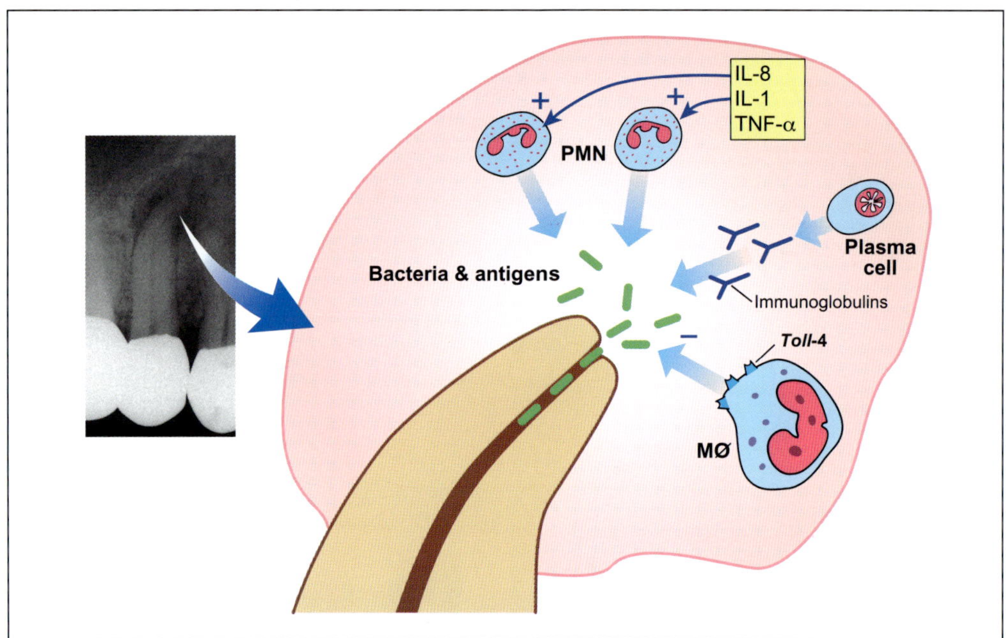

Fig 17-1 Schematic illustration of the major immunologic mechanisms that result in killing and eliminating microorganisms or antigens derived from the root canal system. Specific experiments and references supporting this network are described in the text. IL, interleukin; MØ, macrophage; TNF, tumor necrosis factor.

tate the host response to noxious stimuli, including bacteria (see also chapter 11). For example, antigen-presenting dendritic cells are present in the odontoblast layer, and macrophage-like cells are found centrally in the pulp.[2-4] A small number of T cells are present in the normal pulp, primarily in blood vessels, which likely represent recirculating T cells that serve an immunosurveillance function. In contrast, B cells are extremely rare or undetectable,[2,5] and plasma cells are absent.[6]

The earliest pulpal response to frank bacterial infection, or to the diffusion of bacterial antigens through dentinal tubules, includes the infiltration of polymorphonuclear neutrophils (PMNs) and monocytes.[7-9] The cellular infiltrate intensifies as the infection progresses provoking elements of the adaptive response, including T-helper and T-cytotoxic/suppressor cells, B cells, and in later stages, antibody-producing plasma cells. Nonspecific elements, including PMNs, monocytes, and natural killer (NK) cells, continue to be present.[5,6] The levels of locally produced immunoglobulin[5] (IgG and IgA) are elevated,[10] and antibodies are present that react with microorganisms isolated from deep caries.[11] As noted, these mechanisms are usually unable to clear the infection. Tissue destruction subsequently proceeds, beginning with the formation of small abscesses and necrotic foci in the pulp and eventually resulting in total pulpal necrosis.[5]

Periapical responses

Periapical immune responses (also known as *apical periodontitis* or *periapical lesion*) may be viewed as a second line of defense, the purpose of which appears to be to localize the infection within the confines of the root canal system and prevent its egress and systemization[12-15] (Fig 17-1). Periapical responses to bacterial infection essen-

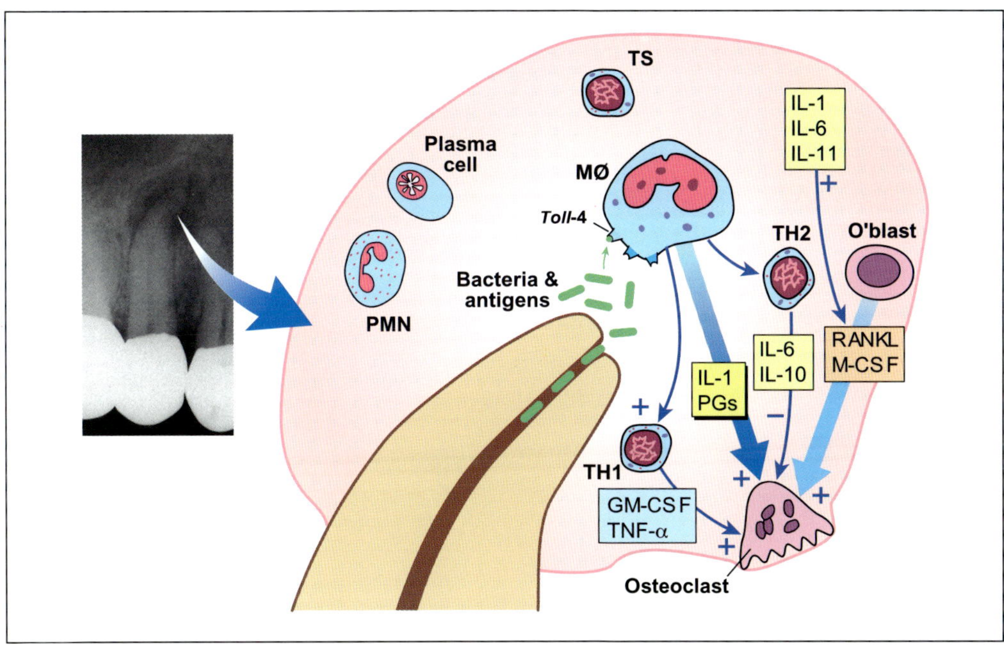

Fig 17-2 Schematic illustration of the major immunologic mechanisms that mediate the development of apical periodontitis elicited by microorganisms or antigens from the root canal system. Specific experiments and references supporting this network are described in the text. PGs, prostaglandins; GM-CSF, granulocyte-macrophage colony-stimulating factor; M-CSF, macrophage colony-stimulating factor; RANKL, receptor activator of NF-κB ligand.

tially recapitulate the pulpal response described above, with the additional feature that periapical bone is destroyed (Fig 17-2).

In experimental models such as the rat, where the timing of pulpal infection is controlled, the earliest periapical response involves an influx of PMNs and monocytes 3 days after pulpal exposure (Fig 17-3).[4,16,17] Periapical inflammatory cell infiltration, increased numbers of osteoclasts, and bone destruction are apparent well in advance of total pulpal necrosis (Fig 17-4), at a time when vital pulp is still present in the apical root canal.[18,19] These data explain the clinical observation that vital tissue (and pain) is often present even in teeth with periapical radiolucencies. A further implication is that pulpal infections cause periapical tissue destruction indirectly and from a distance via stimulation of soluble host-derived mediators rather than by the direct effects of bacteria on bone.

The inflammatory cell infiltrate in chronic periapical lesions in both humans and animals has been extensively studied and characterized. As with pulpal responses, a mixed infiltrate of T and B lymphocytes, PMNs, macrophages, plasma cells, NK cells, eosinophils, and mast cells is present.[17,20-28] There remains some disagreement about the predominant infiltrating cell type in periapical lesions: lymphocytes[21,22,29-31] or macrophages[17,20,26] are variously reported to be the more numerous. Large numbers of PMNs are present,[30,31] while T cells consistently outnumber B cells.[24,30,31] Among the T lymphocytes, both T-helper (TH) and T-suppressor (TS) cells have been identified.[22,25-27,30,32-35] In several studies, a lower TH-to-TS ratio than that seen in peripheral blood (< 2.0) has been reported in chronic lesions.[24,27,30]

Kinetic studies suggest that after the first days of infection, few temporal differences in the cell

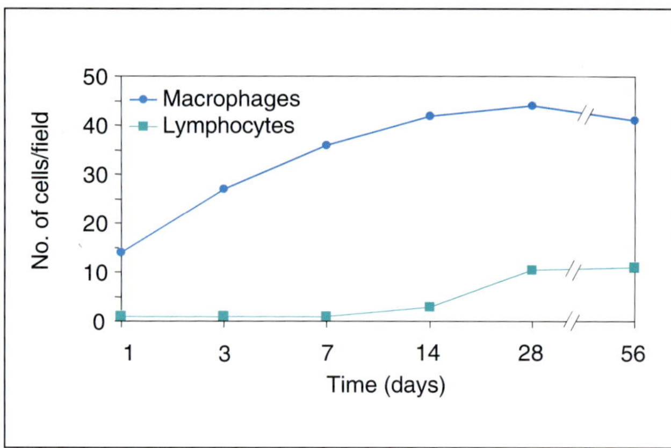

Fig 17-3 Effects of pulpal inflammation and necrosis on accumulation of macrophages and other phagocytic cells (labeled with ED1 antibody) and T lymphocytes (labeled with OX-19 anatisera) into periapical tissue of rats. The dental pulp underwent total necrosis by 14 to 28 days after pulpal exposure. (Redrawn from Kawashima et al[17] with permission.)

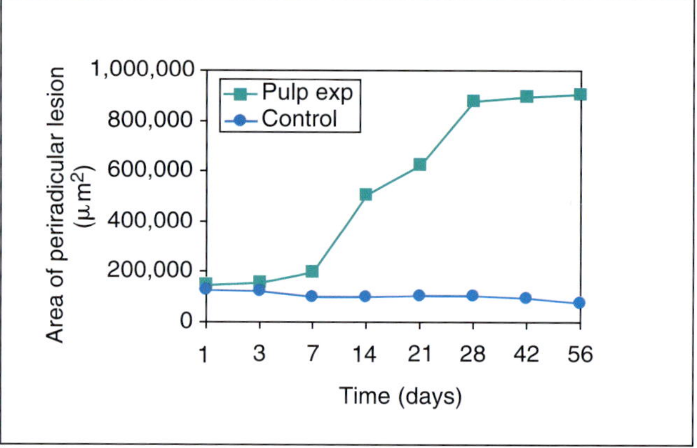

Fig 17-4 Effect of pulpal inflammation and necrosis on area of periradicular lesion in rats after pulpal exposure *(squares)* or no-treatment controls *(circles)*. The dental pulp underwent total necrosis by 28 days after pulpal exposure. (Redrawn from Yamasaki et al[18] with permission.)

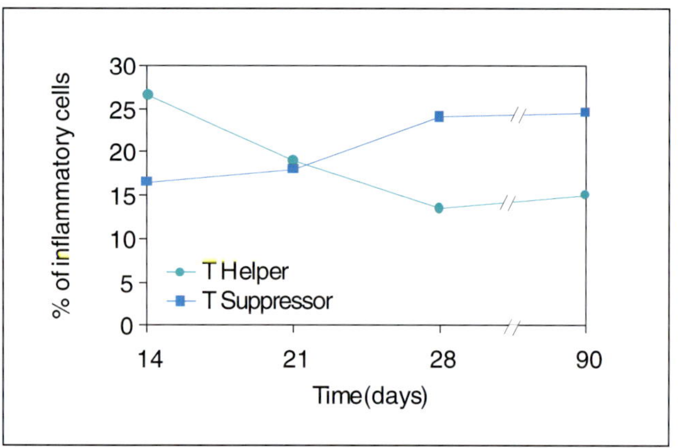

Fig 17-5 Effect of pulpal inflammation and necrosis on subpopulations of T lymphocytes in rat periradicular lesions after pulpal exposure. Tissue levels of T-helper and T-suppressor lymphocytes were determined by immunohistochemical markers. (Redrawn from Stashenko and Yu[27] with permission.)

infiltrate remain after pulp exposure. One notable exception is an increase in TS cells as the lesion becomes more chronic (Fig 17-5).[17,27] This may reflect the evolution of a specific T-cell response; TH cells are initially activated to proliferate by exposure to antigen and subsequently induce TS cells that may dampen excessive immunoreactivity in periapical lesions.[36]

Periapical lesions contain immunoglobulin-producing cells. Of these, IgG-positive cells are most prominent (70%), followed by IgA (14%), IgE (10%), and IgM (4%).[20,35,37-39] Of the IgG subclasses, IgG1 is produced in largest quantity, followed by IgG2 > IgG3 = IgG4.[40] Some of the antibody produced in lesions is reactive with infecting microorganisms.[41,42] Explant cultures of periapical tissues produce antibody against common endodontic pathogens, including *Prevotella intermedia*, *P endodontalis*, *P gingivalis*, *P micros*, *Actinomyces israelii*, *Staphylococcus intermedius*, and *Fusobacterium nucleatum*. It has long been known that antigens within the root canal are also capable of stimulating a systemic antibody response. Introduction of bovine serum albumin and sheep erythrocytes into the root canals of monkeys stimulated systemic antibody

Box 17-1	Functions mediated by cells that infiltrate periapical lesions	
Neutrophils:	Phagocytosis (bacterial killing); cytokine production (IL-1, TNF-α)	
Monocytes:	Phagocytosis (bacterial killing); immune induction; cytokine production (IL-1, TNF-α, IL-6, IL-10, IL-12); prostaglandin E (PGE) production	
Eosinophils:	Histamine release, immediate-type (anaphylactic) hypersensitivity	
B cells:	Differentiate to plasma cells; low-level antibody production	
Plasma cells:	Large-scale antibody production:	
		IgM: Complement-mediated lysis; chemotaxis stimulated by C3a, C5a
		IgG: Opsonization; immune complex formation; complement-mediated lysis; chemotaxis
		IgA: Inhibition of adhesion
T cells:	CD4⁺:	TH1: Delayed-type hypersensitivity; interferon-γ (IFN-γ), IL-12, TNF-α
		TH2: "Help" for antibody production; anti-inflammatory modulation (IL-4, IL-5, IL-6, IL-10, IL-13)
	CD8⁺:	Cytotoxicity; suppression

formation against both antigens.[43] Systemic antibody responses have been shown against lipopolysaccharide (LPS) and other bacterial antigens.[44,45] These observations suggest that both locally and systemically produced antibacterial antibodies could protect the host against bacterial egress from the root canal into the circulation via opsonization or complement-mediated lysis.

It has also been suggested that antibody-mediated mechanisms could actually contribute to periapical bone destruction. However, there is at present no direct evidence that these mechanisms actually stimulate bone resorption in vivo. These mechanisms include the binding of antibodies to bacterial antigens to form antigen-antibody complexes that are capable of stimulating periapical bone destruction in experimental systems.[46] Complement components are present in lesions.[37,38] Complement fixation and the generation of cleavage products (C3a, C5a) may stimulate PMN chemotaxis. Potentially destructive byproducts of PMNs include elastase, cathepsin-G, and leukotriene B4, all of which are elevated in inflamed pulps.[47,48] The presence of mast cells in combination with IgE suggests that anaphylactic hypersensitivity reactions may also occur periapically.[28,37,49,50]

Arguing against a role for antibody-mediated phenomena in the pathogenesis of apical periodontitis is the lack of correlation between the number of antibody-producing cells and periapical lesion expansion.[16,31] More importantly, antibody protects against disseminating dentoalveolar infections in immunocompromised animals and reduces bone resorption in animals that develop abscesses.[13-15]

Protective Immunity to Pulpal Infections

From the foregoing discussion, it is apparent that the mixed inflammatory cell infiltrate in both the dental pulp and in periapical lesions is potentially capable of mediating the entire spectrum of immunologic responses. Summarized in Box 17-1, these include antibody-mediated phenomena (antigen-antibody complex formation, complement-dependent cell lysis and chemotaxis, immediate-type hypersensitivity); delayed-type hypersensitivity; cytotoxicity; and cytokine and prostaglandin production. However, the critical question is not which antibacterial responses

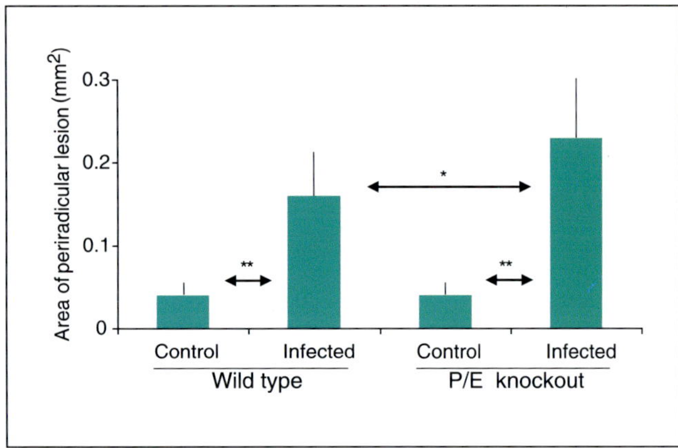

Fig 17-6 Effect of deletion of the P- and E-selectin genes on size of periradicular lesions after pulp exposure in mice. The endothelium of P/E$^{-/-}$ mice lacks the constitutive P selectin and the inducible E selectin and therefore lacks the critical initial step of rolling adhesion of leukocytes to endothelium in inflamed tissue. $^{*}P < .05$ and $^{**}P < .01$. (Redrawn from Kawashima et al[74] with permission.)

are present, but rather which antibacterial responses actually function to protect pulpal/periapical tissues. To answer this question, animals with various immunodeficiencies have been studied to identify which immune functions are critical in reducing or preventing infection and periapical bone resorption.

Immunodeficiencies fall into two broad categories depending on whether they primarily affect *nonspecific* or *specific* immune responses. In general, individuals with defects in nonspecific phagocytes, including neutrophils and monocytes, have increased susceptibility to bacterial infections. Although the effect of these deficiencies on pulpal infections has not been reported, they clearly increase the severity of marginal periodontitis.[51,52] In contrast, patients with defects in specific immunity and/or diminished T- or B-cell numbers or function exhibit marginal periodontitis that is similar to or less than that seen in normal age-matched individuals.[53-57] An exception may be the marginal periodontitis that occurs in some HIV-infected individuals, although the disease appears to be somewhat atypical and may not be identical to other periodontal diseases.[58]

Deficiencies in innate responses

Individuals with PMN defects, including chronic granulomatous disease, cyclic neutropenia, Papillon-Lefèvre syndrome, Chediak-Higashi syndrome, and leukocyte adhesion deficiencies, have an increased incidence and severity of bacterial infection, including oral (periodontal) infections.[59-61] Best studied are the leukocyte adhesion deficiencies (LAD), of which there are currently two recognized types.[62-64] LAD-I is due to a genetic defect in the β chain of integrins, which are important for leukocyte transmigration across the blood vessel wall. LAD-II is due to a defect in the Lewis sialyl-X ligand on leukocytes to which P and E selectins on endothelial cells bind, an interaction that mediates the initial "rolling adhesion" of leukocytes to the blood vessel wall (see Fig 11-2). In both conditions, the adhesion deficiency results in a significantly reduced ability of PMNs to migrate from the vascular system into tissues. Patients present with severe infections and elevated numbers of circulating PMNs and macrophages (leukocytosis), yet no pus is formed. In addition, they exhibit early-onset or prepubertal marginal periodontitis.[64-68] Based on these considerations, it is not surprising that a recent case report of a patient with an LAD-I immunodeficiency described numerous examples of infected necrotic teeth with apical periodontitis.[69] Others have provided case reports of patients with cyclic neutropenia showing increased prevalence of apical periodontitis.[70]

Older studies have attempted to determine the role of innate immune cells such as PMNs and monocyte/macrophages in periapical responses to infection. The administration of cyclophosphamide, which causes severe neutropenia, was reported to increase periapical bone destruction.[71] In cyclophosphamide-treated animals, bacteria were observed both in the pulp and in the periapical lesion, suggesting increased bacterial invasion in the absence of PMNs. However, in another study, methotrexate treatment, which also causes neutropenia, was reported to inhibit the development of apical periodontitis.[72]

The reason for these differences is unclear; however, it must be kept in mind that although the effects of the immunosuppressive agents were correlated with neutropenia, both cyclophosphamide and methotrexate also profoundly affect the production and responses of lymphocytes, so these effects could not be solely attributed to PMNs.

More recently, so-called knockout mice deficient in both P and E selectins ($P/E^{-/-}$) have been developed as a model of human LAD-II. $P/E^{-/-}$ mice have defective rolling adhesion and leukocytosis, increased susceptibility to various infections, and few reported defects in adaptive immunity.[73] Interestingly, $P/E^{-/-}$ mice were shown to develop larger periapical lesions than their normal, wild-type counterparts (Fig 17-6), which correlated both with decreased PMN infiltration into periapical tissues and increased periapical expression of the bone-resorptive cytokine, interleukin-1 (IL-1).[74]

Another experimental approach has been to increase the function of innate immune cells using immunomodulators and to determine the effect on pulpal and periapical resistance to infection. Poly-beta-1-6-glucotriosyl-beta-1-3-glucopranose (PGG) glucan is a biologic response modifier derived from yeast that effectively increases host antibacterial responses without inducing inflammation, including a complete lack of pro-inflammatory cytokine production (IL-1, tumor necrosis factor [TNF] -α) by macrophages and other cells.[75-77] Systemic administration of PGG glucan increases PMN production and primes phagocytic and bactericidal activity in vivo.[78] It also prevents postsurgical infections in humans.[79] In the pulp exposure model, PGG glucan reduced periapical bone destruction by 40% (Fig 17-7).[19] Animals in which PGG glucan was administered had increased numbers of circulating PMNs and monocytes, which showed enhanced phagocytic activity ex vivo. The protective effect on periapical bone was secondary to decreased pulpal necrosis, with only 3% of pulps exhibiting complete pulpal necrosis in PGG glucan–treated animals compared with 41% of controls. These results clearly indicate that PMNs are predominantly protective against pulpal infections and reduce periapical bone destruction.

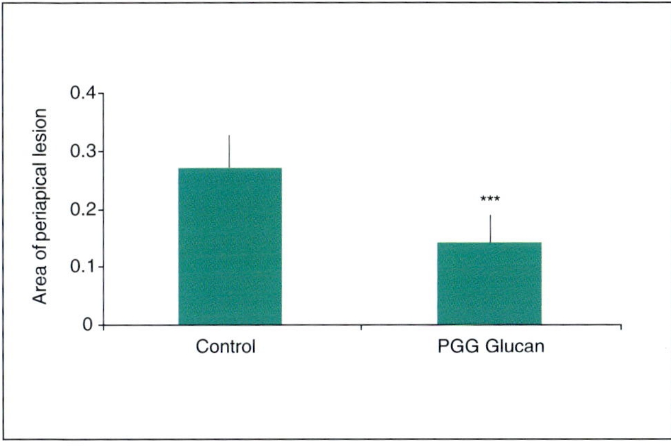

Fig 17-7 Effect of the biologic response modifier PGG glucan on size of periapical lesions after pulp exposure in rats. Animals were administered PGG glucan or a vehicle starting 1 day before pulp exposure. PGG glucan increases host immunologic responsiveness by increasing neutrophil production and by priming phagocytic and bactericidal activity. $^{***}P < .001$. (Redrawn from Stashenko et al[19] with permission.)

Deficiencies in specific responses

A number of human immunodeficiency diseases affect specific immunity. These include severe combined immunodeficiency (SCID), DiGeorge syndrome (thymic aplasia resulting in a decrease or absence of T cells), hypogammaglobulinemias, and selective IgA and IgG deficiencies.

SCID is characterized by profound defects in both humoral and cellular immunity. Because most patients do not survive into adulthood, reports of oral manifestations are limited. Although no studies are available on the effects of SCID on periapical destruction in humans, some potentially important data have been derived from studies in genetically engineered SCID mice.[13,80,81] In these animals, functional T and B lymphocytes are totally absent, whereas cells involved in nonspecific immunity, including neutrophils and monocytes,

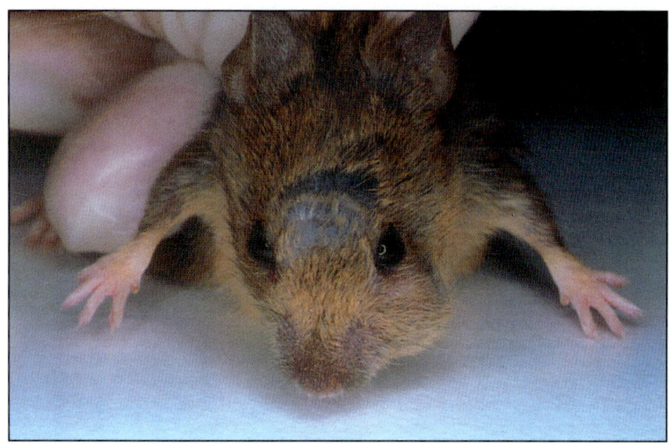

Fig 17-8 The development of an orofacial abscess of endodontic origin after pulp exposure in a RAG-2 mouse. RAG-2 animals are genetic knockouts for the recombination activator 2 gene (RAG-2) and are thus unable to generate immunoglobulins or T-cell receptors. RAG-2 knockouts are a model of SCID because they have substantial defects in both humoral and cellular immunity. (Reprinted from Teles et al[13] with permission.)

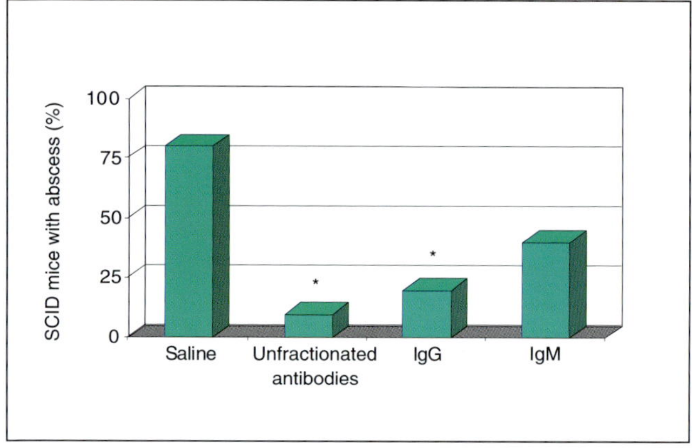

Fig 17-9 Effect of intravenous administration of saline, an unfractionated mixture of antibodies, or purified IgG or IgM antiserum on the incidence of disseminated orofacial abscesses in SCID mice after pulpal exposure. *$P < .05$ vs saline (chi-square test). N = 10–11 per group.

are intact. Following pulpal exposure in this model, approximately one third of SCID mice developed gross orofacial abscesses, splenomegaly, weight loss, and in some cases septic shock, whereas normal animals were always able to localize the infection to the root canal system (Fig 17-8).[13] Abscessed SCID mice had more local periapical bone destruction than nonabscessed SCID mice or normal controls. Fouad[81] also found that SCID mice displayed bone resorption similar to that of controls but did not observe abscess formation. These findings are similar to those in immunized monkeys with periapical lesions, which, although not different in size, were more circumscribed than those in nonimmunized animals.[82] Furthermore, nonimmunized animals had an inflammatory infiltrate resembling osteomyelitis that extended into the trabecular system of the bone.[82]

More recently, studies have shown that B cell–deficient, but not T cell–deficient or complement-deficient, mice are susceptible to disseminating infections.[14] Infection dissemination could be largely prevented by the transfer of antibody against infecting endodontic pathogens in SCID mice, with IgG being more effective than IgM. In contrast, the transfer of T cells had no protective effect. The finding that complement-deficient animals were not susceptible to infection dissemination suggests that opsonization rather than complement-mediated lysis of bacteria is involved in protection.

This was shown more directly in experiments in which antibody against infecting endodontic pathogens was transferred intravenously to SCID mice prior to pulp exposure. The dissemination of the pulpal infection to orofacial tissues (see Fig 17-8), was found to be largely prevented by antibody transfer, leading to a reduction in frequency of orofacial abscess formation from 73% to 25% ($P < .05$). When the antibodies were fractionated into IgG- and IgM-enriched preparations, IgG was found to be more effective in preventing orofacial abscess formation than IgM (Fig 17-9). This finding further indicates that IgG antibody probably exerts protection by opsonizing bacteria, leading to their more efficient phagocytosis and killing by neutrophils and macrophages in the pulp and periapical lesion (see Fig 17-1).

The results of these studies are consistent with studies of the effect of pure T-cell deficiencies on pulpal and periapical destruction. Congenital thymic aplasia (DiGeorge syndrome) results in drastically reduced or absent T cells and decreased antibody levels, secondary to a lack of TH activity for B cells. Affected individuals mount normal immune responses against common bacterial infections but are extremely susceptible to viral, protozoan, and fungal infection.[83] There are as yet no reports of increased susceptibility to oral infections in DiGeorge patients. In animal models that mimic DiGeorge syndrome, athymic *nu/nu* animals have yielded conflicting results, with one study indicating no effect of T-cell deficiency on periapical destruction[84] but a second study reporting decreased destruction.[85]

In progressive HIV infection, there is a profound depression in $CD4^+$ T cells and a lack of cell-mediated immunity. Several infections affect the periodontium in such individuals, resulting in a wide range of clinical presentations.[86,87] However, several cross-sectional studies have failed to find an increase in the frequency of endodontic complications after root canal treatment in HIV-infected individuals.[88,89]

Individuals with pure antibody deficiencies are not at an increased risk of developing marginal periodontitis or dental caries compared with age- and sex-matched controls.[54,57,90] Little is known about the effects of pure antibody deficiencies on periapical pathogenesis. Because most hypogammaglobulinemic patients also receive long-term administration of antibiotics and/or gamma globulins, the oral flora may be significantly suppressed, resulting in reduced inflammation.[57,91]

Taken together, these data suggest that specific immune responses mediated by B cells and antibodies protect against systemic spread of endodontic infections but may otherwise have relatively minor effects on localized periapical bone destruction, whereas T cells have only a marginal effect on the extent and severity of periapical inflammation.

Mediators of Periapical Inflammation

Most evidence suggests that periapical inflammation and bone destruction are stimulated primarily by host-derived mediators that are induced by infection rather than by direct interaction of bacteria with osteoclasts and other host cells. These mediators help to combat infection but appear to do so at the price of stimulating concomitant tissue degradation. In this section, the activity of various mediators of periapical inflammation and destruction is discussed.

Proinflammatory cytokines

As noted, the earliest periapical responses to pulpal infection involve the migration of PMNs and monocytes. Chemokines, including interleukin-8 (IL-8) and monocyte chemoattractant peptide-1 (MCP-1), are produced locally and are likely to be involved in regulating PMN and monocyte infiltration.[92-94] IL-8 also helps to "prime" PMNs for an elevated oxidative burst that is important in bacterial killing.

Once activated by bacterial components, macrophages and PMNs express a cascade of proinflammatory cytokines (see Fig 17-2). The proximal members of this cascade include IL-1α, IL-1β, and TNF-α. IL-1α and TNF-α may further stimulate each other's expression in an autoregulatory fashion. Downstream, cytokines IL-6, IL-8, and granulocyte-macrophage colony-stimulating factor (GM-CSF) are induced as secondary mediators. GM-CSF stimulates bone marrow production of PMNs and monocytes and also primes PMN activation. As will be discussed later, IL-6 can synergize with prostaglandin E_2 (PGE_2) to increase some inflam-

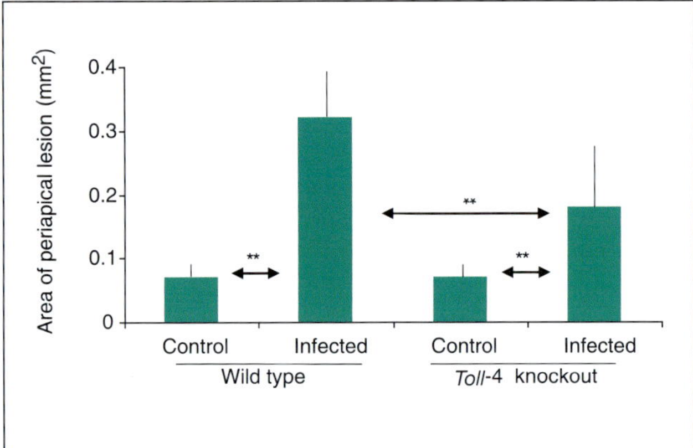

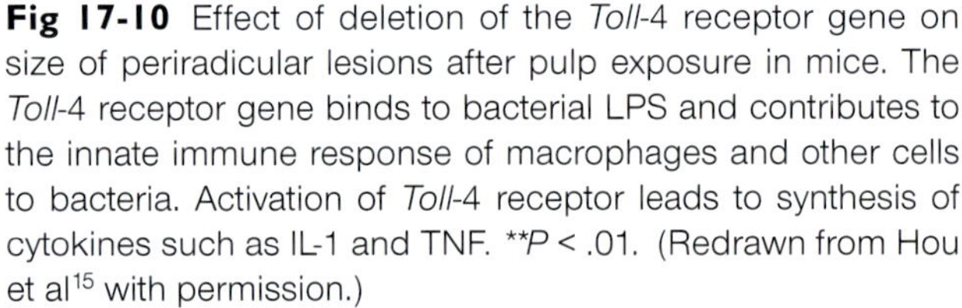
Fig 17-10 Effect of deletion of the *Toll*-4 receptor gene on size of periradicular lesions after pulp exposure in mice. The *Toll*-4 receptor gene binds to bacterial LPS and contributes to the innate immune response of macrophages and other cells to bacteria. Activation of *Toll*-4 receptor leads to synthesis of cytokines such as IL-1 and TNF. $^{**}P < .01$. (Redrawn from Hou et al[15] with permission.)

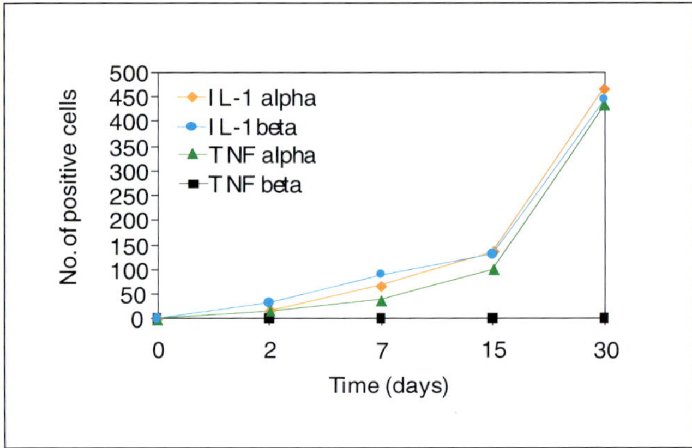

Fig 17-11 Effect of pulpal inflammation and necrosis on number of cytokine-expressing cells in periradicular tissue of rats following pulp exposure. (Redrawn from Tani-Ishii et al[111] with permission.)

matory responses, but its predominant action overall is anti-inflammatory.

Macrophages and other types of cells express an evolutionarily conserved family of recently described *Toll*-like receptors that recognize bacterial structures including LPS, peptidoglycans, and lipoteichoic acid.[95] Activation of *Toll*-like receptors triggers signaling pathways that result in the expression of IL-1, TNF-α, and perhaps other cytokines (see Fig 17-2). Thus, *Toll*-like receptor activation explains the observation that IL-1 and TNF-α are induced in periapical lesions in the absence of T or B cells.[81] Recently, it has been shown that mice deficient in *Toll*-like receptor 4, the primary receptor for LPS,[96,97] have reduced inflammatory cytokine responses and decreased periapical bone resorption (Fig 17-10).[15]

IL-1α, IL-1β, TNF-α, and TNF-β stimulate bone resorption by osteoclasts. Collectively these mediators comprise the activity formerly termed *osteoclast-activating factor* (OAF).[98-101] IL-6 and IL-11 have also been reported to increase bone resorption, but this effect is probably secondary to their ability to stimulate osteoclast formation from precursor stem cells rather than to activate pre-existing osteoclasts. In humans, IL-1β constitutes most OAF activity, reflecting both its high level of expression and its pharmacologic potency.[98,102,103] In this regard, IL-1 has been shown to be approximately 500-fold more potent than TNF in stimulating bone resorption.[104] Both IL-1 and TNF-α are produced in large quantities by macrophages and other cells, including fibroblasts,[105] keratinocytes,[106] osteoblasts,[107] and osteoclasts.[108] In addition to bone resorption, IL-1 and TNF-α possess overlapping activities relevant to periapical tissue destruction, including induction of PGE_2,[109] proteinase production,[110] and inhibition of bone formation.[99,102]

At sites of pulpal and periapical inflammation, IL-1α, IL-1β, and TNF-α mRNA and protein are expressed in the first few days following infection (Fig 17-11).[111-114] These mediators are largely derived from macrophages and PMNs.[111] IL-1β is present in inflamed human pulp,[115] periapical lesions,[116] and cysts.[117] Higher levels of IL-1β are present in periapical lesions from more severely affected, symptomatic teeth.[118,119] The level of IL-

1β in human periapical exudates was twice that of IL-1α.[120] Interestingly, IL-1β declined following treatment, whereas IL-1α increased, suggesting that IL-1β may be primarily associated with pathogenesis. TNF-α has been identified in periapical exudates.[121] IL-6, which induces osteoclast formation but does not appear to stimulate activation, is expressed by macrophages, PMNs, and T cells and has been detected in periapical tissue and radicular cysts.[122-126] IL-11 is present in periapical lesions, but its role is unclear.[74]

IL-1 appears to play a central role in stimulating periapical bone resorption by osteoclasts. Bone-resorbing activity is present in extracts of both human and rat periapical tissues.[127,128] In experimental models such as the rat, in which the timing of lesion induction can be controlled,[129] the highest levels of resorbing activity are present in periapical tissues during the active phase of lesion expansion (3 to 14 days after pulp exposure). Most of this activity can be resolved to a peak molecular weight of 15,000 to 20,000, consistent with the size of IL-1. Moreover, this activity is neutralized primarily by anti-IL-1 but not by anti-TNF-α antibodies.[129,130] Thus, despite its fairly high level of expression in periapical lesions, TNF-α did not exert significant resorptive activity due to its lower potency in stimulating osteoclasts. By comparison, only 10% to 15% of resorptive activity in lesions was due to the action of PGE_2.

Specific inhibition of IL-1 in vivo by infusion of rats with IL-1 receptor antagonist (IL-1ra)[131] over a 14-day period decreased lesion size by approximately 60% (Fig 17-12).[108] IL-1ra, another member of the IL-1 family induced during inflammatory responses, binds to IL-1 receptors but fails to activate cellular responses. Consequently, it acts as a competitive inhibitor of both IL-1α and IL-1β. The expression of endogenous IL-1ra is induced following infection and has been found in periapical lesions.[132] Interestingly, the ratio of IL-1ra to IL-1β was three-fold lower in periapical exudates from symptomatic than from asymptomatic lesions, suggesting that the balance between inhibitor and agonist may determine lesion progression. The central role of IL-1 in infection-stimulated bone

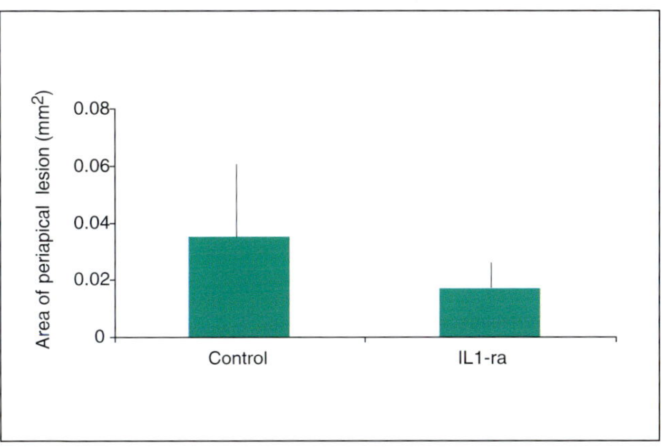

Fig 17-12 Effects of administration of an IL-1 receptor antagonist (IL1-ra) or a vehicle on size of periapical lesions after pulp exposure in rats. (Redrawn from Stashenko et al[108] with permission.)

resorption is further underscored by findings in models of periodontal disease. Thus, treatment of monkeys with soluble IL-1 receptors (which block IL-1 activity) reduces periodontal bone loss by 60% to 70%.[133]

Recently, the effect of a lack of IL-1 and/or TNF receptor signaling has been studied with respect to periapical destruction. Surprisingly, mice deficient in the primary receptor for IL-1 (IL-1 type I receptor [IL-1RI]) or for both receptors for TNF-α (TNFR), p55 and p75, were reported to have greater periapical bone resorption than wild-type controls.[134] Mice deficient in both IL-1RI and TNFR p55 exhibited even more bone resorption. This increase correlated with more rapid bacterial penetration through the radicular pulp and increased pulpal destruction. Mice deficient in IL-1RI, but not TNFR, p55 and p75, also exhibited soft tissue abscess formation and increased mortality.[135] Although not yet confirmed, these results suggest that some functions mediated by IL-1 and TNF-α may in fact contribute to pulpal and periapical protection, particularly early after infection. As lesions progress,

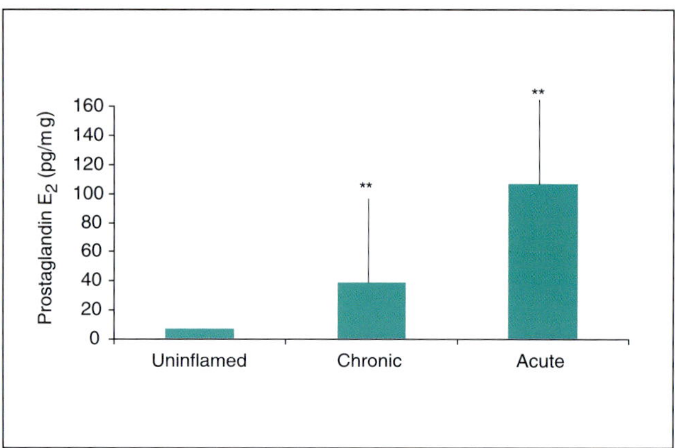

Fig 17-13 Prostaglandin levels in periapical tissue collected from endodontic surgery patients. Uninflamed tissue samples consisted of periapical tissue from clinically normal unerupted third molars. Chronic inflamed tissue was taken from teeth diagnosed as having chronic apical periodontitis. Acutely inflamed tissue was taken from teeth diagnosed as having acute apical lesions. $^{**}P < .01$ versus uninflamed tissue. N = 16. (Redrawn from McNicholas et al[139] with permission.)

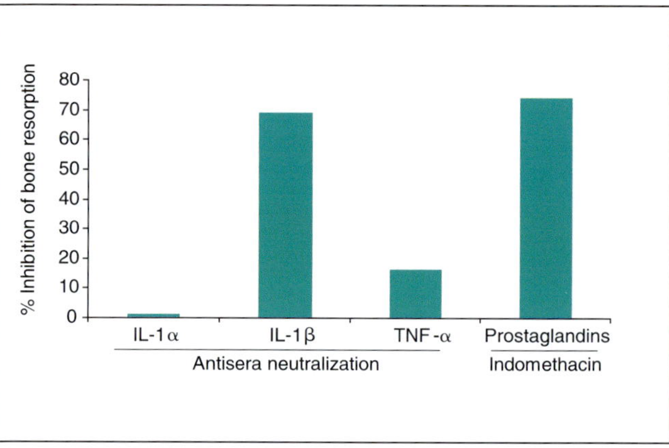

Fig 17-14 Inhibition of the bone-resorbing activity of extracts taken from human periradicular lesions. Cytokine activity was blocked by immunoneutralization with antisera to IL-1α, IL-1β, TNF-α, or TNF-β. Prostaglandin activity was blocked with indomethacin. (Redrawn from Wang and Stashenko[128] with permission.)

however, the effect of IL-1 is clearly destructive, as discussed earlier. One possible mechanism underlying a protective effect is that both IL-1 and TNF-α can stimulate PMN migration to sites of infection and prime PMNs for increased bacteriocidal responses.[136, 137] However, in the experiments described above, infiltrating PMNs and monocytes were actually increased in animals deficient in both IL-1 and TNF receptors.[134] Thus, the mechanism that underlies these observations is presently unclear and requires further study.

Arachidonic acid metabolites

Products of arachidonic acid metabolism have also been correlated with pulpal and periapical inflammation. PGE_2 has been shown to be present in higher concentrations in symptomatic than in asymptomatic pulps[138] and in acute periapical lesions (Fig 17-13),[139] and PGE_2 levels of periapical exudates decrease following root canal treatment.[140] Experimentally induced inflammation of dental pulp increases the production of 6-keto-PGF1α, thromboxane B2, and leukotriene C4.[141] Similarly the application of bacterial LPS to pulps increases production of all arachidonic acid metabolites.[142] The prostaglandins increase vascular permeability[143] and stimulate bone resorption, and as previously noted, PGE_2 is directly responsible for 10% to 15% of total bone-resorbing activity in extracts of rat periapical tissues.[128] However, approximately 60% of the bone-resorbing activity stimulated by IL-1 is inhibited by indomethacin. This finding reflects the fact that IL-1–induced resorption is partly dependent on PGE_2 synthesis by cells present at inflammatory sites (Fig 17-14).

IL-1 and PGE_2 have been shown to synergize with respect to bone resorption.[104,144,145] Indomethacin was found to block the progression of periapical bone destruction in experiments in which the deposition of immune complexes into root canals of cats induced such lesions.[46] The participation of PGE_2 in periapical destruction in vivo is also supported by the finding that indomethacin-treated rats displayed milder inflammation and less bone resorption than controls.[146] This finding also concurs with periodontal disease studies in which long-term administration of the cyclo-oxygenase inhibitor flurbiprofen suppressed naturally occurring periodontal destruction in beagles by 60% to 70%.[147]

Paradoxically, infusion of PGE_2 in vivo has actually been found to increase bone formation rather than to stimulate bone resorption,[148] and inhibitors of PGE_2 production (such as ibuprofen) inhibit fracture repair.[149] PGE_1 has been shown to induce regeneration of cementum, alveolar bone, and periodontal ligament in dogs.[150] Because prostaglandins appear to act largely through synergy with other mediators, it may be that their primary effect is to increase the sensitivity of osteoblasts and osteoclasts to other signals, regardless of whether they stimulate bone resorption, such as proinflammatory cytokines, or bone formation, such as growth factors.

Regulation of proinflammatory cytokines: The cytokine network

The expression and action of pro-inflammatory/bone resorptive mediators is modulated by a network of regulatory cytokines. Although complex, this network is best understood in the context of the two major subpopulations of T-helper cells. TH1 and TH2 cells represent distinct subsets that may be distinguished both by gene expression profile and by function.[151-154] TH1 cells produce interferon-γ (IFN-γ), IL-2, and TNF-α; mediate delayed-type hypersensitivity reactions through the activation of macrophages by IFN-γ; increase inflammation; and inhibit the responses of TH2 cells. Conversely, TH2 cells produce IL-4, IL-5, IL-6, IL-10, and IL-13; stimulate the production of most subclasses of antibody by B cells; decrease inflammation; and inhibit the responses of TH1 cells.

These T-cell subsets derive from nonpolarized precursor cells (THp), which may be directed toward a TH1 rather than a TH2 pathway of differentiation in the cytokine milieu. In many cases, the cytokines that determine TH1/TH2 commitment are produced by macrophages following their stimulation by bacteria. The macrophage-derived cytokines IL-12 and IL-18 favor the development of a TH1 response,[155] whereas IL-10 promotes TH2 responses.[156-159] However, IL-4 and IL-13 derived from other T cells, basophils, and NK cells are also important determinants of TH2 commitment.

As previously noted, TH1 and TH2 cells are *cross-regulatory* and their cytokines are antagonistic, acting to inhibit the proliferation and cytokine production of the opposing subset.[160] Data from periodontal disease models suggest that inflammation and bone resorption are increased by TH1 responses and decreased by TH2 responses. Thus, transfer of TH1 clones exacerbates periodontal bone resorption while TH2 clones are protective.[161,162] A model for the operation of such a network in periapical inflammation predicts that the TH1 subset increases IL-1 and other pro-inflammatory cytokines, whereas inhibitors of IL-1 are related to the TH2 subset (see Fig 17-2). Many of these regulatory cytokines have been identified in mouse periapical lesions, including IFN-γ, IL-2, IL-4, IL-6, IL-10, IL-12, IL-13, and transforming growth factor (TGF) -β.[163] TH1-type cytokines IL-2, IL-12, and IFN-γ showed a linear increase in periapical lesions up to day 28. In contrast, TH2-type cytokines IL-4, IL-6, and IL-10 were increased following pulp exposure, but levels declined by day 28, suggesting possible inhibition by TH1-type mediators. Significant correlations were observed between levels of IL-1 and TH1 cytokines in periapical tissues, whereas there was a lack of correlation between IL-1 and TH2-type mediators. These results demonstrate that a cytokine network is activated in the periapex in response to infection and that TH1-modulated pro-inflammatory pathways predominate in early pathogenesis.

In chronic human lesions, IFN-γ, IL-2, IL-4, IL-6, and IL-10 have been identified by immunohistochemistry.[164] In contrast to findings in the mouse, human lesions exhibited greater expression of IL-4, IL-6, and IL-10 than IL-2 and IFN-γ, which suggests that TH2-type mediators predominate and may act to stabilize the size of chronic lesions.

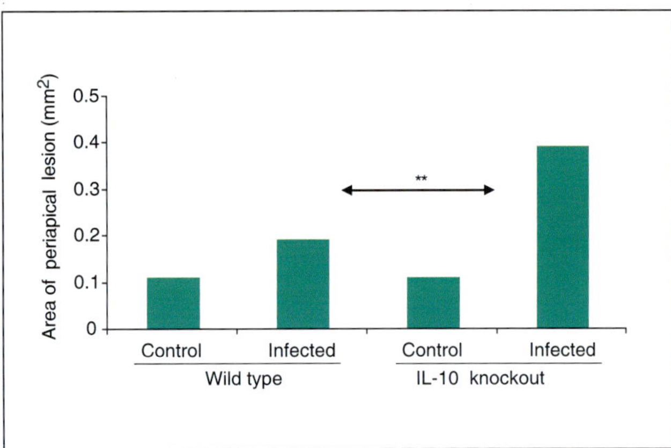

Fig 17-15 Effect of deletion of anti-inflammatory cytokines on the size of periapical lesions in mice after pulp exposure. Mice were engineered to have knockouts of the IL-10 gene. The cytokine IL-10 promotes the anti-inflammatory TH2 response of lymphocytes and inhibits osteoclast activity. $^{**}P < .01$. (Redrawn from Sasaki et al[165] with permission.)

Functional studies of regulatory cytokines

The hypothesis that emerges from these findings is that regulation of periapical bone resorption is mediated principally through the effects of a mediator on IL-1 expression by macrophages and other cell types. This scenario is clearly an oversimplification, however, because a number of cytokines, including IFN-γ, IL-4, IL-8, IL-10, and IL-18, have been reported to directly inhibit osteoclasts. Again, we must ask what these cytokines actually do functionally within developing periapical lesions rather than what they can do in other systems. Experiments to address this question have either employed genetic "knockouts" of individual cytokines or inhibition of cytokines with specific inhibitors, antagonists, or neutralizing antibodies. Such analyses have now been carried out for many of the key regulatory cytokines expressed in periapical lesions.

Using knockout animals, the effect of a lack of the prototype TH2 anti-inflammatory cytokines IL-4, IL-6, and IL-10 has been determined.[165,166] The results demonstrated that IL-10-deficient mice had dramatically increased periapical bone destruction (> 250%) (Fig 17-15), whereas, surprisingly, IL-4-deficient animals had bone loss similar to that of controls .[165] IL-$6^{-/-}$ and animals treated with anti-IL-6 antibodies also had increased resorption, but this increase was moderate (approximately 50%) compared to that seen in IL-$10^{-/-}$.[166] The increased bone destruction in the IL-10 knockouts correlated with a ten-fold elevation in the periapical levels of IL-1α, whereas IL-1α was increased by two-fold in IL-$6^{-/-}$ but not increased in IL-$4^{-/-}$. Macrophage IL-1α expression was inhibited to a significant degree by IL-10 and IL-6, but not by IL-4 in vitro. These data demonstrate that endogenous IL-10 has a strong (and nonredundant) inhibitory effect on periapical bone destruction and that pro-inflammatory pathways predominate in its absence. IL-4, although a potent inhibitor of inflammation in other systems, has no effect on bone resorption in vivo. This finding also contrasts with its reported inhibition of bone resorption in organ culture.[167] The role of IL-6 is interesting because it is often considered to be pro-inflammatory. Part of this misconception is due to the fact that IL-6 increases osteoclastogenesis, and its absence might be expected to decrease osteoclast formation as well as resorption. However, IL-6 also possesses many anti-inflammatory effects. These include the induction of acute phase proteins, many of which are themselves anti-inflammatory, as well as a weak inhibition of IL-1 expression. Thus, the predominant actions of IL-6 are anti-inflammnatory, consistent with its categorization as a TH2 cytokine.

TGF-β is produced by many cell types, including macrophages and epithelial cells. Although not a TH subset-related cytokine, TGF-β is also a powerful negative regulator of inflammation. Thus, animals lacking TGF-β have multifocal inflammation and exhibit severe pulpal and periapical inflammation.[153,168,169] The role of TGF-β in periapical resorption induced by infection has not been determined.

Prototype TH1-type cytokines IL-12 and IFN-γ, which may be expected to increase IL-1 expression and resorption, have also been analyzed.[165] However, neither IFN-$\gamma^{-/-}$ nor IL-$12^{-/-}$ showed decreased resorption compared with untreated wild-type controls. IL-1α levels were not significantly altered in lesions of any of these animals. These findings indicate that endogenous expression of TH1-type cytokines IL-12 and IFN-γ has at most only minor effects on IL-1 expression and IL-1-mediated bone destruction, perhaps because innate mechanisms operating through *Toll*-like receptors are already maximally stimulated in these infections.

A number of other cytokines with potential modulating activity on periapical resorption have not yet been assessed in these in vivo systems. These include the macrophage-derived TH1-inductive mediators IL-15 and IL-18 and the TH2 cytokine IL-13, which is also produced by NK cells. Other soluble cytokine receptors (eg, sIL-4R) may affect the network by antagonizing regulatory cytokines.[170,171]

Several clinical implications arise from this review of the pathogenesis of apical periodontitis. First, patients with diseases or taking drugs that suppress immune fuction may experience a greater risk of developing apical periodontits or exhibit apical periodontitis that is more resistant to endodontic treatment, as compared to healthy patients. The known effects of certain immunodeficiencies have been noted previously in this chapter (see also chapter 21). Second, the primary etiologic factor for apical periodontitis is pulpal bacterial infection and the resulting immune response. Accordingly, those endodontic procedures that have the greatest effect in reducing bacteria and antigens in root canal systems are likely to hae greater success in resolving apical periodontits. To date, thorough chemomechanical debredement with NaOCl irrigation, followed by intracanal administration of Ca $(OH)_2$ for at least 7 days has the best evidence for reduction of pulpal bacteria.

Conclusions

There has been significant progress in recent years in our understanding of the pathogenesis of apical periodontitis, particularly with respect to its modulation by the immune system. The elements of innate and specific immunity that protect against pulpal infections and prevent their dissemination have been defined, at least in broad terms. A number of the key mediators of periapical bone resorption have been elucidated. Future studies will seek, first, to completely characterize the protective versus destructive components in this system and, second, to learn how to control them through immunotherapy.

Several clinical implications arise from this review of the pathogenesis of apical periodontitis. First, patients with diseases or taking drugs that suppress immune function may experience a greater risk of developing apical periodontitis or exhibit apical periodontitis that is more resistant to endodontic treatment, as compared to healthy patients. The known effects of certain immunodeficiencies have been noted previously in this chapter (see also chapter 21). Second, the primary etiologic factor for apical periodontitis is pulpal bacterial infection and the resulting immune response. Accordingly, those endodontic procedures that have the greatest effect in reducing bacteria and antigens in root canal systems are likely to have greater success in resolving apical periodontitis. To date, thorough chemomechanical debridement with NaOCl irrigation, followed by intracanal administration of $Ca(OH)_2$ for at least 7 days has the best evidence for reduction of pulpal bacteria.

References

1. Sundqvist G. Taxonomy, ecology, and pathogenicity of the root canal flora [review]. Oral Surg Oral Med Oral Pathol 1994;78:522-530.
2. Jontell M, Gunraj M, Bergenholtz G. Immunocompetent cells in the normal dental pulp. J Dent Res 1987;66: 1149-1153.

3. Jontell M, Bergenholtz G, Scheynius A, Ambrose W. Dendritic cells and macrophages expressing Class II antigens in the normal rat incisor pulp. J Dent Res 1988; 67:1263–1266.
4. Okiji T, Kawashima N, Kosaka T, Kobayashi C, Suda H. Distribution of Ia antigen-expressing nonlymphoid cells in various stages of induced periapical lesions in rat molars. J Endod 1994;20:27–31.
5. Hahn CL, Falkler WA Jr, Siegel MA. A study of T and B cells in pulpal pathosis. J Endod 1989;15:20–26.
6. Pulver WH, Taubman MA, Smith DJ. Immune components in normal and inflamed human dental pulp. Arch Oral Biol 1977;22:103–111.
7. Bergenholtz G, Lindhe J. Effect of soluble plaque factors on inflammatory reactions in the dental pulp. Scand J Dent Res 1975;83:153–158.
8. Warfvinge J, Dahlen G, Bergenholtz G. Dental pulp response to bacterial cell wall material. J Dent Res 1985;64:1046–1050.
9. Bergenholtz G, Nagaoka S, Jontell M. Class II antigen presenting cells in experimentally induced pulpitis. Int Endod J 1991;24:8–14.
10. Speer ML, Madonia JV, Heuer MA. Quantitative evaluation of the immunocompetence of the dental pulp. J Endod 1977;3:418–423.
11. Hahn CL, Falkler WA Jr. Antibodies in normal and diseased pulps reactive with microorganisms isolated from deep caries. J Endod 1992;18:28–31.
12. Stashenko P. Role of immune cytokines in the pathogenesis of periapical lesions [review]. Endod Dent Traumatol 1990;6:89–96.
13. Teles R, Wang CY, Stashenko P. Increased susceptibility of RAG-2 SCID mice to dissemination of endodontic infections. Infect Immun 1997;65:3781–3787.
14. Hou L, Sasaki H, Stashenko P. B cell deficiency predisposes to disseminating anaerobic infections: Protection by passive antibody transfer. Infect Immun 2000;68:5645–5651.
15. Hou L, Sasaki H, Stashenko P. TLR4 deficient mice have reduced bone destruction following mixed anaerobic infection. Infect Immun 2000;68:4681–4687.
16. Akamine A, Hashiguchi I, Toriya Y, Maeda K. Immunohistochemical examination on the localization of macrophages and plasma cells in induced rat periapical lesions. Endod Dent Traumatol 1994;10:121–128.
17. Kawashima N, Okiji T, Kosaka T, Suda H. Kinetics of macrophages and lymphoid cells during the development of experimentally induced periapical lesions in rat molars: A quantitative immunohistochemical study. J Endod 1996;22:311–316.
18. Yamasaki M, Kumazawa M, Kohsaka T, Nakamura H, Kameyama Y. Pulpal and periapical tissue reactions after experimental pulpal exposure in rats. J Endod 1994;20:13–17.
19. Stashenko P, Wang CY, Riley E, Wu Y, Ostroff G, Niederman R. Reduction of infection-stimulated periapical bone resorption by the biological response modifier PGG glucan. J Dent Res 1995;74:323–330.
20. Stern MH, Dreizen S, Mackler BF, Selbst AG, Levy BM. Quantitative analysis of cellular composition of human periapical granulomas. J Endod 1981;7:117–122.
21. Stern MH, Dreizen S, Mackler BF, Selbst AG, Levy BM. Isolation and characterization of inflammatory cells from the human periapical granuloma. J Dent Res 1982;61:1408–1412.
22. Nilsen R, Johannessen AC, Skaug N, Matre R. In situ characterization of mononuclear cells in human dental periapical inflammatory lesions using monoclonal antibodies. Oral Surg Oral Med Oral Pathol 1984;58: 160–165.
23. Cymerman JJ, Cymerman DH, Walters J, Nevins AJ. Human T lymphocyte subpopulations in chronic periapical lesions. J Endod 1984;10:9–11.
24. Torabinejad M, Kettering JD. Identification and relative concentration of B and T lymphocytes in human chronic periapical lesions. J Endod 1985;11:122–125.
25. Gao Z, Mackenzie IC, Rittman BR, Korszun AK, Williams DM, Cruchley AT. Immunocytochemical examination of immune cells in periapical granulomata and odontogenic cysts. J Oral Pathol 1988;17:84–90.
26. Kopp W, Schwarting R. Differentiation of T lymphocyte subpopulations, macrophages, and HLA-DR-restricted cells of apical granulation tissue. J Endod 1989;15: 72–75.
27. Stashenko P, Yu SM. T helper and T suppressor cell reversal during the development of induced rat periapical lesions. J Dent Res 1989;68:830–834.
28. Marton IJ, Kiss C. Characterization of inflammatory cell infiltrate in dental periapical lesions. Int Endod J 1993; 26:131–136.
29. Bergenholtz G, Lekholm U, Liljenberg B, Lindhe J. Morphometric analysis of chronic inflammatory periapical lesions in root-filled teeth. Oral Surg Oral Med Oral Pathol 1983;55:295–301.
30. Kontianen S, Ranta H, Lautenschlager I. Cells infiltrating human periapical inflammatory lesions. J Oral Pathol 1986;15:544–546.
31. Yu SM, Stashenko P. Identification of inflammatory cells in developing rat periapical lesions. J Endod 1987;13: 535–540.
32. Matthews JB, Browne RM. An immunocytochemical study of the inflammatory cell infiltrate and epithelial expression of HLA-DR in odontogenic cysts. J Oral Pathol 1987;16:112–117.
33. Barkhordar RA, Desouza YG. Human T-lymphocyte subpopulations in periapical lesions. Oral Surg Oral Med Oral Pathol 1988;65:763–766.

34. Lukic A, Arsenijevic N, Vujanic G, Ramic Z. Quantitative analysis of the immunocompetent cells in periapical granuloma: Correlation with the histological characteristics of the lesions. J Endod 1990;16:119–122.

35. Matsuo T, Ebisu S, Shimabukuro Y, Ohtake T, Okada H. Quantitative analysis of immunocompetent cells in human periapical lesions: Correlations with clinical findings of the involved teeth. J Endod 1992;18: 497–500.

36. Morimoto C, Letvin NL, Distaso JA, Aldrich WR, Schlossman SF. The isolation and characterization of the human suppressor-inducer T cell subset. J Immunol 1985;134:1508–1515.

37. Pulver WH, Taubman MA, Smith DJ. Immune components in human dental periapical lesions. Arch Oral Biol 1978;23:435–443.

38. Yanigisawa S. Pathologic study of periapical lesions I. Periapical granulomas: Clinical, histopathologic and immunohistopathologic studies. J Oral Pathol 1980;9: 288–300.

39. Matthews JB, Mason GI. Immunoglobulin producing cells in human periapical granulomas. Br J Oral Surg 1983;21:192–197.

40. Takahashi K, Lappin DF, MacDonald GD, Kinane DF. Relative distribution of plasma cells expressing immunoglobulin G subclass mRNA in human dental periapical lesions using in situ hybridization. J Endod 1998;24: 164–167.

41. Baumgartner JC, Falkler WA Jr. Reactivity of IgG from explant cultures of periapical lesions with implicated microorganisms. J Endod 1991;17:207–212.

42. Kettering JD, Torabinejad M, Jones SL. Specificity of antibodies present in human periapical lesions. J Endod 1991;17:213–216.

43. Barnes GW, Langeland K. Antibody formation in primates following introduction of antigens into the root canal. J Dent Res 1966;45:1111–1114.

44. Dahlen G. Immune response in rats against lipopolysaccharides of *Fusobacterium nucleatum* and *Bacteroides oralis* administered in the root canal. Scand J Dent Res 1980;88:122–129.

45. Dahlen G, Fabricius L, Holm SE, Moller AJ. Circulating antibodies after experimental chronic infection in the root canal of teeth in monkeys. Scand J Dent Res 1982; 90:338–344.

46. Torabinejad M, Kiger RD. Experimentally induced alterations in periapical tissues of the cat. J Dent Res 1980; 59:87–96.

47. Cootauco CJ, Rauschenberger CR, Nauman RK. Immunocytochemical distribution of human PMN elastase and cathepsin-G in dental pulp. J Dent Res 1993; 72:1485–1490.

48. Okiji T, Morita I, Suda H, Murota S. Pathophysiological roles of arachidonic acid metabolites in rat dental pulp. Proc Finn Dent Soc 1992;1(suppl):433–438.

49. Mathiesen A. Preservation and demonstration of mast cells in human apical granulomas and radicular cysts. Scand J Dent Res 1973;81:218–229.

50. Perrini N, Fonzi L. Mast cells in human periapical lesions: Ultrastructural aspects and their possible physiopathological implications. J Endod 1985;11:197–202.

51. Van Dyke TE, Hoop GA. Neutrophil function and oral disease. Crit Rev Oral Biol Med 1990;1:117–33.

52. Crawford JM, Watanabe K. Cell adhesion molecules in inflammation and immunity: Relevance to periodontal diseases. Crit Rev Oral Biol Med 1994;5:91–123.

53. Tollefson T, Saltvedt E, Koppang HS. The effect of immunosuppressive agents on periodontal disease in man. J Periodontal Res 1978;13:240–250.

54. Robertson PB, Mackler BF, Wright TE, Levy BM. Periodontal status of patients with abnormalities of the immune system II. Observations over a 2-year period. J Periodontol 1980;51:70–73.

55. Sutton RBO, Smales FC. Cross-sectional study of the effects of immunosuppressive drugs on chronic periodontal disease in man. J Clin Periodontol 1983;10: 317–326.

56. Leggot PJ, Robertson PB, Greenspan D, Wara KW, Greenspan JS. Oral manifestations of primary and acquired immunodeficiency diseases in children. Pediatr Dent 1987;2:98–104.

57. Dahlen G, Bjorkander J, Gahnberg L, Slots J, Hanson LA. Periodontal disease and dental caries in relation to primary IgG subclass and other humoral immunodeficiencies. J Clin Periodontol 1993;20:7–13.

58. Winkler JR, Murray PA. Periodontal disease: Potential intraoral expression of AIDS may be a rapidly progressive periodontitis. Calif Dent Assoc J 1987;15:20–24.

59. Van Dyke TE, Taubman MA, Ebersole JL, Haffajee AD, Socransky SS, Smith DJ, Genco RJ. The Papillon-LeFevre syndrome: Neutrophil dysfunction with severe periodontal disease. Clin Immunol Immunopathol 1984;31 (3):419–429.

60. Cohen MS, Leong PA, Simpson DM. Phagocytic cells in periodontal defense: Periodontal status of patients with chronic granulomatous disease of childhood. J Periodontol 1985b;56:611–617.

61. Waldrop TC, Anderson DC, Hallmon WW, Schmalsteig FC, Jacobs RL. Periodontal manifestations of the heritable Mac-1, LFA-1, deficiency syndrome. J Periodontol 1987;58:400–416.

62. Springer TA, Thompson WS, Miller LJ, Schmalstieg FC, Anderson DC. Inherited deficiency of the Mac-1, LFA-1, p150,95 glycoprotein family and its molecular basis. J Exp Med 1984;160:1901–1918.

63. Anderson DC, Springer TA. Leukocyte adhesion deficiency: An inherited defect in the Mac-1, LFA-1 and p150,95 glycoproteins. Ann Rev Med 1987;38:175–94.

64. Von Andrian UH, Chambers JD, Berg EL, Michie SA, Brown DA, Karolak D, et al. L-selectin mediates neutrophil rolling in inflamed venules through sialyl lewis x-dependent and independent recognition pathways. Blood 1993;82:182–191.
65. Bowen TJ, Ochs HD, Altman LC. Severe recurrent bacterial infections associated with defective adherence and chemotaxis in two patients with neutrophils deficient in a cell-associated glycoprotein. J Pediatr 1982;101: 932–940.
66. Page RC, Bowen TJ, Altman. Prepubertal periodontitis I. Definition of a clinical disease entity. J Periodontol 1983;54:257–271.
67. Etzioni A, Frydman M, Pollack S, Avidor I, Phillips ML, Paulson JC, Gershoni-Baruch R. Recurrent severe infections caused by a novel leukocyte adhesion deficiency. N Engl J Med 1992;327:1789–1792.
68. Schenkein H, Van Dyke T. Early onset periodontitis: Systemic aspects of etiology and pathogenesis. Periodontol 2000 1994;6:7–25.
69. Majorana A, Notarangelo LD, Savoldi E, Gastaldi G, Lozada-Nur F. Leukocyte adhesion deficiency in a child with severe oral involvement. Oral Surg Oral Med Oral Pathol Oral Radiol Endod 1999; 87: 691–694.
70. Pernu HE, Pajari UH, Lanning M. The importance of regular dental treatment in patients with cyclic neutropenia; follow-up of 2 cases. J Periodontol 1996;67: 454–459.
71. Kawashima N, Okiji T, Kosaka T, Suda H. Effects of cyclophosphamide on the development of experimentally induced periapical lesions in the rat. Jpn J Conserv Dent 1993;36:1388–1396.
72. Yamasaki M, Kumazawa M, Kohsaka T, Nakamura H. Effect of methotrexate-induced neutropenia on rat periapical lesions. Oral Surg Oral Med Oral Pathol 1994b;77:655–661.
73. Frenette PS, Mayadas TN, Rayburn H, Hynes RO. Susceptibility to infection and altered hematopoiesis in mice deficient in both P- and E-selectins. Cell 1996;84: 563–569.
74. Kawashima N, Niederman R, Hynes RO, Ullmann-Cullere M, Stashenko P. Infection-stimulated infraosseus inflammation and bone destruction is increased in P-/E-selectin knockout mice. Immunology 1999;97:117–123.
75. Jamas S, Easson DD Jr, Ostroff GR. PGG: A novel class of macrophage activating immunomodulators [abstract 698]. In: Proceedings of the International Congress on Infectious Diseases. Munich: MMV Medizin Verlag, 1990:143.
76. Dinarello CA. PGG, a glucan polymer, primes interleukin-1 and tumor necrosis factor production in human peripheral blood mononuclear cells in vitro [abstract 697]. In: Proceedings of the International Congress on Infectious Diseases. Munich: MMV Medizin Verlag, 1990:52–56.
77. Onderdonk AB, Cisneros RL, Hinkson P, Ostroff GR. Anti-infective effect of poly-b1-6-glucotriosyl-b1-3-glucopyranose glucan in vivo. Infect Immun 1992;60:1642–1647.
78. Shah PM, Interweis EW, Nzeramasanga P, Stille W. Influence of PGG on the phagocytosis of *Staphylococcus aureus* or *Escherichia coli* by human granulocytes or human peritoneal macrophages [abstract 504]. In: Proceedings of the International Congress on Infectious Diseases. Munich: MMV Medizin Verlag, 1990:171.
79. Babineau T, Marcello P, Swails W, Kenler A, Wakshull E, Oldman F. Randomized phase I/II trial of a macrophage-specific immunomodulator (PGG-glucan) in high risk surgical patients. Surg Forum 1993;44:51–53.
80. Shinkai Y, Rathbun G, Lam KP, Oltz EM, Stewart V, Mendelsohn M, et al. RAG-2-deficient mice lack mature lymphocytes owing to inability to initiate V(D)J rearrangement. Cell 1992;68:855–867.
81. Fouad AF. IL-1 alpha and TNF-alpha expression in early periapical lesions of normal and immunodeficient mice. J Dent Res 1997;76:1548–1554.
82. Dahlen G, Fabricius L, Heyden G, Holm SE, Moller AJ. Apical periodontitis induced by selected bacterial strains in root canals of immunized and nonimmunized monkeys. Scand J Dent Res 1982b;90:207–216.
83. Kuby J. Immunodeficiency diseases. In: Kuby J (ed). Immunology. New York: Freeman, 1992:443–456.
84. Wallstrom JB, Torabinejad M, Kettering J, McMillan P. Role of T cells in the pathogenesis of periapical lesions: A preliminary report. Oral Surg Oral Med Oral Pathol 1993;76:213–218.
85. Tani N, Kuchiba K, Osada T, Watanabe Y, Umemoto T. Effect of T cell deficiency on the formation of periapical lesions in mice: Histological comparison between periapical lesion formation in BALB/c and BALB/c nu/nu mice. J Endod 1995;21:195–199.
86. Winkler JR, Robertson, PB. Periodontal disease associated with HIV infection [review]. Oral Surg Oral Med Oral Pathol 1992;73:145–150.
87. Holmstrup P, Westergaard J. Periodontal diseases in HIV-infected patients [review]. J Clin Periodontol 1994;21:270–280.
88. Cooper H. Root canal treatment in patients with HIV infection. Int Endod J 1993;26:369–371.
89. Glick M, Abel SN, Muzyka BC, DeLorenzo M. Dental complications after treating patients with AIDS. J Am Dent Assoc 1994;125:296–301.
90. Engstrom GN, Engstrom PE, Hammarstrom L, Smith CI. Oral conditions in individuals with selective immunoglobulin A deficiency and common variable immunodeficiency. J Periodontol 1992;63:984–989.
91. Loesche WJ, Syed SA, Morrison EC, Laughon B, Grossman NS. Treatment of periodontal infections due to anaerobic bacteria with short-term treatment with metronidazole. J Clin Periodontol 1981;8:29–44.

92. Rahimi P, Wang CY, Stashenko P, Lee SK, Lorenzo JA, Graves DT. Monocyte chemoattractant protein-1 expression and monocyte recruitment in osseus inflammation in the mouse. Endocrinol 1995;136: 2752–2759.
93. Jiang Y, Russell TR, Schilder H, Graves DT. Endodontic pathogens stimulated monocyte chemoattractant protein-1 and interleukin-8 in mononuclear cells. J Endod 1998;24:86–90.
94. Matsushita K, Tajima T, Tomita K, Takada H, Nagaoka S, Torii M. Inflammatory cytokine production and specific antibody responses to lipopolysaccharide from endodontopathic black-pigmented bacteria in patients with multilesional periapical periodontitis. J Endod 1999;25:795–799.
95. Kopp EB, Medzhitov R. The *Toll*-receptor family and control of innate immunity. Curr Opin Immunol 1999;11:13–18.
96. Hoshino K, Takeuchi O, Kawai T, Sanjo H, Ogawa T, Takeda Y, et al. Toll-like receptor 4 (TLR4)-deficient mice are hyporesponsive to lipopolysaccharide: evidence for TLR4 as the *Lps* gene product. J Immunol 1999;162:3749–3752.
97. Qureshi S, Lariviere L, Leveque G, Clermont S, Moore KJ, Gros P, Malo D. Endotoxin-tolerant mice have mutations in Toll-like receptor 4 (*Tlr4*). J Exp Med 1999;189: 615–625.
98. Dewhirst FE, Stashenko P, Mole JM, Tsurumachi T. Purification and partial sequence of human osteoclast-activating factor: Identity with interleukin-1β. J Immunol 1985;135:2562–2568.
99. Bertolini DR, Nedwin GE, Bringman TS, Smith DD, Mundy GR. Stimulation of bone resorption and inhibition of bone formation in vitro by human tumor necrosis factors. Nature 1986;319:516–518.
100. Ishimi YC, Miyaura CH, Jin T, Akatsu T, Abe E, Nakamura Y, et al. IL-6 is produced by osteoblasts and induces bone resorption. J Immunol 1990;145:3297–3302.
101. Girasole G, Passeri G, Jilka RL, Manlagos SC. Interleukin-11: A new cytokine critical for osteoclast development. J Clin Invest 1994;93:1516–1524.
102. Stashenko P, Peros WJ, DesJardins L, Rooney M, Dewhirst FE. Interleukin 1β is a potent inhibitor of bone formation in vitro. J Bone Miner Res 1987;2: 559–565.
103. Lorenzo JA, Sousa SL, Alander C, Raisz LG, Dinarello CA. Comparison of the bone resorbing activity in the supernatants from PHA-stimulated human peripheral blood mononuclear cells with that of cytokines through the use of an antiserum to interleukin-1. Endocrinol 1987;121:1164–1170.
104. Stashenko P, Dewhirst FE, Peros WJ, Kent RL, Ago JM. Synergistic interactions between interleukin-1, tumor necrosis factor, and lymphotoxin in bone resorption. J Immunol 1987;138:1464–1468.
105. Del Pozo V, DeAndres B, Martin E, Maruri N, Zubeldia JM, Palomino P, Lahoz C. Murine eosinophils and IL-1: Alpha IL-1 mRNA detection by in situ hybridization. J Immunol 1990;144:3117–3122.
106. Auron PE, Warner SJC, Webb AC, Cannon JG, Bernheim HA, McAdam KJ, et al. Studies on the molecular nature of human interleukin 1. J Immunol 1987;138:1447–1456.
107. Dinarello CA. Interleukin-1 [review]. Adv Immunol 1988;44:153–195.
108. Stashenko P, Wang CY, Tani-Ishii N, Yu SM. Pathogenesis of induced rat periapical lesions. Oral Surg Oral Med Oral Pathol 1994;78:494–502.
109. Saito S, Ngan P, Saito M, Kim K, Lanese R, Shanfeld J, Davidovitch Z. Effects of cytokines on prostaglandin E and cAMP levels in human periodontal ligament fibroblasts in vitro. Arch Oral Biol 1990;35:387–395.
110. Meikle MC, Atkinson SJ, Ward RV, Murphy G, Reynolds JJ. Gingival fibroblasts degrade type I collagen films when stimulated with tumor necrosis factor and interleukin-1: Evidence that breakdown is mediated by metalloproteinases. J Periodont Res 1989;24:207–213.
111. Tani-Ishii N, Wang CY, Stashenko P. Immunolocalization of bone resorptive cytokines in rat pulp and periapical lesions following surgical pulp exposure. Oral Microbiol Immunol 1995;10:213–219.
112. Hamachi T, Anan H, Akamine A, Fujise O, Maeda K. Detection of interleukin-1βmRNA in rat periapical lesions. J Endod 1995;1:118–121.
113. Wang CY, Tani-Ishii N, Stashenko P. Bone resorptive cytokine gene expression in developing rat periapical lesions. Oral Microbiol Immunol 1997;12:65–71.
114. Matsumoto A, Anan H, Maeda K. An immunohistochemical study of the behavior of cells expressing interleukin-1α and interleukin-1β within experimentally induced periapical lesions in rats. J Endod 1998;24: 811–816.
115. D'Souza R, Brown LR, Newland JR, Levy BM, Lachman LB. Detection and characterization of interleukin-1 in human dental pulps. Arch Oral Biol 1989;34:307–313.
116. Barkhorder RA, Hussain MZ, Hayashi C. Detection of interleukin-1 beta in human periapical lesions. Oral Surg Oral Med Oral Pathol 1992;73:334–336.
117. Meghji S, Harvery W, Harris M. Interleukin-1-like activity in cystic lesions of the jaw. Br J Oral Maxillofac Surg 1989;27:1–11.
118. Lim GC, Torabinejad M, Kettering J, Linkhardt TA, Finkelman RD. Interleukin-1 beta in symptomatic and asymptomatic human periradicular lesions. J Endod 1994;20:225–227.
119. Kuo ML, Lamster IB, Hasselgren G. Host mediators in endodontic exudates I. Indicators of inflammation and humoral immunity. J Endod 1998;24:598–603.

120. Matsuo T, Ebisu S, Nakanishi T, Yonemura K, Harada Y, Okada H. Interleukin-1 alpha and interleukin-1 beta in periapical exudates of infected root canals: Correlations with the clinical findings of the involved teeth. J Endod 1994;20:432–435.
121. Safavi KE, Rossomando EF. Tumor necrosis factor identified in periapical tissue exudates of teeth with apical periodontitis. J Endod 1991;17:12–14.
122. Bando Y, Henderson B, Meghji S, Poole S, Harris M. Immunocytochemical localization of inflammatory cytokines and vascular adhesion receptors in radicular cysts. J Oral Pathol Med 1993;22:221–227.
123. Formigli L, Orlandini SZ, Tonelli P, Gianelli M, Martini M, Brandi M. Osteolytic processes in human radicular cysts: morphological and biochemical results. J Oral Pathol Med 1995;24:216–220.
124. Takeichi O, Saito I, Tsurumachi T, Moro I, Saito T. Expression of inflammatory cytokine genes in vivo by human alveolar bone-derived polymorphonuclear leukocytes isolated from chronically inflamed sites of bone resorption. Calcif Tissue Int 1996;58:244–248.
125. Euler GJ, Miller GA, Hutter JW, D'Alesandro MM. Interleukin-6 in neutrophils from peripheral blood and inflammatory periradicular tissues. J Endod 1998;24:480–484.
126. Barkhordar RA, Hayashi C, Hussain MZ. Detection of interleukin-6 in human dental pulp and periapical lesions. Endod Dent Traumatol 1999;15:26–27.
127. Wang CY, Stashenko P. Kinetics of bone resorbing activity in developing periapical lesions. J Dent Res 1991;70:1362–1366.
128. Wang CY, Stashenko P. Characterization of bone resorbing activity in human periapical lesions. J Endod 1993;19:107–111.
129. Kakehashi S, Stanley HR, Fitzgerald RJ. The effects of surgical exposures of dental pulps in germ-free and conventional laboratory rats. Oral Surg 1965;20:340–344.
130. Wang CY, Stashenko P. The role of interleukin-1α in the pathogenesis of periapical bone destruction in a rat model system. Oral Microbiol Immunol 1993;8:50–56.
131. Seckinger P, Klein-Nulend J, Alander C, Thompson RC, Dayer JM, Raisz LG. Natural and recombinant human IL-1 receptor antagonist block the effects of IL-1 on bone resorption and prostaglandin production. J Immunol 1990;145:4181–4186.
132. Shimauchi H, Takayama S, Imai-Tanaka T, Okada H. Balance of interleukin-1 beta and interleukin-1 receptor antagonist in human periapical lesions. J Endod 1998;24:116–119.
133. Assuma R, Oates T, Cochran D, Amar S, Graves DT. IL-1 and TNF antagonists inhibit the inflammatory response and bone loss in experimental periodontitis. J Immunol 1998;160:403–409.
134. Chen C-P, Hertzberg M, Jiang Y, Graves DT. Interleukin-1 and tumor necrosis factor receptor signaling is not required for bacteria-induced osteoclastogenesis and bone loss but is essential for protecting the host from a mixed anaerobic infection. Am J Pathol 1999;155:2145–2152.
135. Graves DT, Chen C-P, Douville C, Jiang Y. Interleukin-1 receptor signaling rather than that of tumor necrosis factor is critical in protecting the host from the severe consequences of a polymicrobe anaerobic infection. Infect Immun 2000;68:4746–4751.
136. Furie MB, McHugh DD. Migration of neutrophils across endothelial monolayers is stimulated by treatment of the monolayers with interleukin-1 or tumor necrosis factor-alpha. J Immunol 1989;143:3309–3317.
137. Sample AK, Czuprynski CJ. Priming and stimulation of bovine neutrophils by recombinant human interleukin-1 alpha and tumor necrosis factor alpha. J Leukoc Biol 1991;49:107–115.
138. Cohen JS, Reader A, Fertel R, Beck M, Meyers WJ. A radioimmunoassay determination of the concentrations of prostaglandins E_2 and F_2 alpha in painful and asymptomatic human dental pulps. J Endod 1985;11:330–335.
139. McNicholas S, Torabinejad M, Blankenship J, Baklund L. The concentration of prostaglandin E_2 in human periradicular lesions. J Endod 1991;17:97–100.
140. Shimauchi H, Takayama S, Miki Y, Okada H. The change in periapical exudates prostaglandin E_2 levels during root canal treatment. J Endod 1997;23:755–758.
141. Lessard GM, Torabinejad M, Swope D. Arachidonic acid metabolism in canine tooth pulps and the effects of nonsteroidal anti-inflammatory drugs. J Endod 1986;12:146–149.
142. Okiji T, Morita I, Kobayashi C, Sunada I, Murota S. Arachidonic acid metabolism in normal and experimentally inflamed rat dental pulp. Arch Oral Biol 1987;32:723–727.
143. Okiji T, Morita I, Sunada I, Murota S. Involvement of arachidonic acid metabolites in increases in vascular permeability in experimental dental pulp inflammation in the rat. Arch Oral Biol 1989;34:523–528.
144. Stashenko P, Yu SM. Phenotypic characterization of inflammatory cells in induced rat periapical lesions. J Endod 1987;13:535–540.
145. Dewhirst FE, Ago JM, Stashenko P. Interleukin 1 interacts synergistically with forskolin and isobutylmethylxanthine in stimulating bone resorption in organ culture. Calcif Tissue Int 1989;47:1–7.
146. Oguntebi BR, Barker BF, Anderson DM, Sakamura J. The effect of indomethacin on experimental dental periapical lesions in rats. J Endod 1989;15:117–121.
147. Jeffcoat MK, Williams RC, Wechter WJ, Johnson HG, Kaplan ML, Gandrup JS, Goldhaber P. Flurbiprofen treatment of periodontal disease in beagles. J Periodont Res 1986;21:624–633.

148. Chyun YS, Raisz LG. Stimulation of bone formation by prostaglandin E2. Prostaglandins 1984;27:97–103.
149. Bo J, Sudmann E, Marton PF. Effect of indomethacin on fracture healing in rats. Acta Orthop Scand 1976;47:588–599.
150. Marks SC Jr, Miller SC. Local delivery of prostaglandin E_1 induces periodontal regeneration in adult dogs. J Periodont Res 1994;29:103–108.
151. Akira S. Functional roles of STAT family proteins: Lessons from knockout mice [review]. Stem Cells 1999;17:138–146.
152. Bonecchi R, Bianchi G, Bordignon PP, D'Ambrosio D, Lang R, Borsatti A, et al. Differential expression of chemokine receptors and chemotactic responsiveness of Th1 and Th2s. J Exp Med 1998;187:129–134.
153. Ho IC, Lo D, Glimcher LH. C-maf promotes T helper cell type 2 (Th2) and attenuates Th2 differentiation by both IL-4-dependent and -independent mechanisms. J Exp Med 1998;188:1859–1866.
154. Randolph DA, Huang G, Carruthers CJ, Bromley LE, Chaplin DD. The role of CCR7 in TH1 and TH2 cell localization and delivery of B cell help in vivo. Science 1999;286:2159–2162.
155. Seder RA, Gazzinelli R, Sher A, Paul WE. IL-12 acts directly on $CD4^+$ T cells to enhance priming for IFNγ production and diminishes IL-4 inhibition of such priming. Proc Natl Acad Sci U S A 1993;90:10188–10192.
156. Swain SL, Weinberg A, English M, Huston G. IL-4 directs the development of Th2 like helper effectors. J Immunol 1990;145:3796–3806
157. Gross A, Ben-Sasson SS, Paul WE. Anti-IL-4 diminishes in vivo priming for antigen-specific IL-4 production by T cells. J Immunol 1993;150:2112–2120.
158. McKenzie GJ, Emson CL, Bell SE, Anderson S, Fallon P, Zurawski G, et al. Impaired development of Th2 cells in IL-13-deficient mice. Immunity 1998;9:423–432.
159. Herrick CA, MacLeod H, Glusac E, Tigelaar RE, Bottomly K. Th2 responses induced by epicutaneous or inhalational protein exposure are differentially dependent on IL-4. J Clin Invest 2000;105:765–775.
160. Mosmann TR. Regulation of immune responses by T cells with different cytokine secretion phenotypes: Role of a new cytokine, cytokine synthesis inhibitory factor (IL-10) [review]. Int Arch Allergy Appl Immunol 1991;94:110–115.
161. Eastcott JW, Yamashita K, Taubman MA, Harada Y, Smith DJ. Adoptive transfer of cloned T helper cells ameliorates periodontal disease in nude rats. Oral Microbiol Immunol 1994;9:284–289.
162. Kawai T, Eisen-Lev R, Seki M, Eastcott JW, Wilson ME, Taubman MA. Requirement of B7 co-stimulation for Th1-mediated inflammatory bone resorption in experimental periodontal disease. J Immunol 2000;164:2102–2109.
163. Kawashima N, Stashenko P. Expression of bone resorptive and regulatory cytokines in infraosseus inflammation. Arch Oral Biol 1999;44:55–66.
164. Walker KF, Lappin DF, Takahashi K, Hope J, Macdonald DG, Kinane DF. Cytokine expression in periapical granulation tissue as assessed by immunohistochemistry. Eur J Oral Sci 2000;108:195–201.
165. Sasaki H, Hou L, Belani A, Wang CY, Uchiyama T, Muller R, Stashenko P. IL-10, but not IL-4, suppresses infection-stimulated bone resorption in vivo. J Immunol 2000;165:3626–3630.
166. Balto K, Sasaki H, Stashenko P. Interleukin-6 deficiency increases inflammatory bone destruction. Infect Immun 2001;69:744–750.
167. Watanabe K, Tanaka Y, Morimoto I, Yahata K, Zeki K, Fujihara T, et al. Interleukin-4 as a potent inhibitor of bone resorption. Biochem Biophys Res Comm 1990;172:1035–1041.
168. Kulkarni AB, Huh C, Becker D, Geiser A, Lyght M, Flanders KC, et al. Transforming growth factor β1 null mutation in mice causes excessive inflammatory response and early death. Proc Natl Acad Sci USA 1993;90:770–774.
169. Diebold RJ, Eis MJ, Yin M, Ormsby I, Bovin GP, Darrow BJ, et al. Early-onset multifocal inflammation in the transforming growth factor β1 null mouse is lymphocyte mediated. Proc Natl Acad Sci USA 1995;92:12215–12219.
170. Garrone P, Djossou O, Galizzi JP, Banchereau J. A recombinant extracellular domain of the human interleukin-4 receptor inhibits the biological effects of interleukin-4 on T and B lymphocytes. Eur J Immunol 1991;21:1365–1369.
171. Maliszewski CR, Sato TA, Davison B, Jacobs CA, Finkelman FD, Fanslow WC. In vivo biological effects of recombinant soluble interleukin-4 receptor. Proc Soc Exp Biol Med 1994;206:233–237.

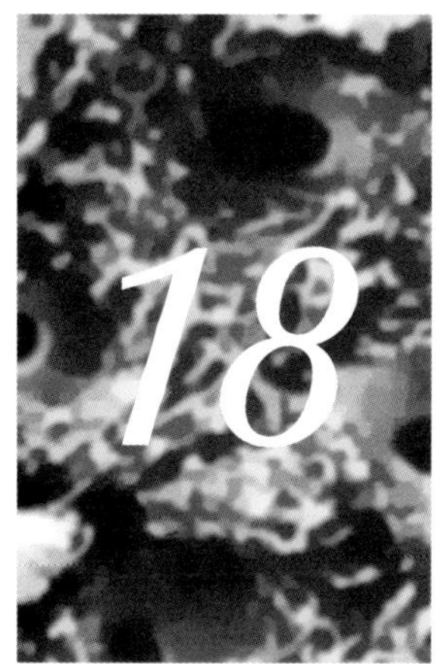

Interrelationship of Pulpal and Periodontal Diseases

R. Bruce Rutherford, DDS, PhD

A major theme of this book is the relationship between dental pulp and other tissues in health and disease. The complex relationship between diseases of the dental pulp and of the periodontium is evidenced in anthropologic specimens[1] and has long been recognized to be of potential pathologic significance.[2] Indeed, the presence of a periradicular radiolucency (apical periodontitis), as identified by radiographic evidence of bone loss surrounding the root apex, is often a clinician's first indication of pulpal pathosis. The relationship between pulpal disease and periradicular inflammation and tissue destruction is covered in detail in chapter 17. This chapter focuses on the interaction between the pulp and marginal periodontitis.

There is some evidence for claims that disease of the dental pulp, in addition to root perforations and fracture,[3] affects the health and healing capacity of the periodontium. Conversely, it is possible that disease of the periodontium can negatively affect the structure and function of the dental pulp. This chapter discusses the evidence for and against correlations between pulp and periodontal diseases and treatment. Clinical implications of such relationships coronal to the periradicular region, diagnostic approaches, and treatment options are discussed.

Classification of Pulpal and Periodontal Pathoses

Simon and colleagues[4] published a classification of pulp-periodontium relationships and treatment regimens[5,6] useful to both clinicians and investigators (Figs 18-1 and 18-2).[7-10] This classification scheme is based on the primary source of infection or inflammation. The principal distinction between primary periodontal lesions with secondary pulpal involvement and the primary pulpal lesion with secondary periodontal involvement is the order of events. Substantial evidence suggests that pulpal disease can contribute to periodontal disease; however, much more controversy surrounds the reverse situation. Evidence either supporting or refuting these relationships will be discussed below.

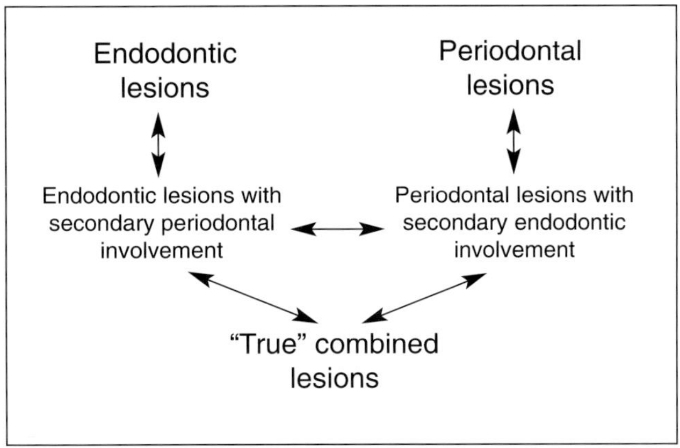

Fig 18-1 The clinical interrelationships of five classes of endodontic-periodontal lesions. (Reprinted from Simon et al[4] with permission.)

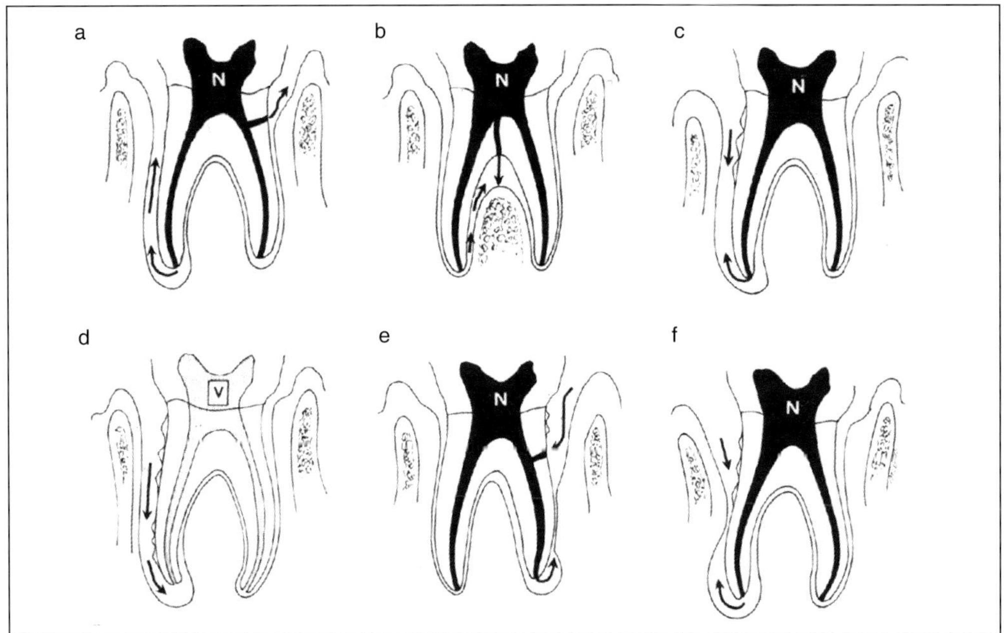

Fig 18-2 Schematic illustration depicting potential etiologic routes for development of endodontic-periodontal lesions. *(a)* Endodontic lesion. The pathway of communication is evident through the periodontal ligament from the apex or a lateral canal. *(b)* Communication through the apex or a lateral canal may cause bifurcation involvement. *(c)* Primary endodontic lesion with secondary periodontal involvement. The existing pathway as in *(a)* is shown, but with the passage of time periodontitis with calculus formation begins at the cervical area. *(d)* Periodontal lesion. The progression of periodontitis is toward the apex. Note the vital pulp (V). *(e)* Primary periodontal lesion with secondary endodontic involvement, showing the primary periodontal involvement at the cervical margin and the resultant pulpal necrosis once the lateral canal is exposed to the oral environment. *(f)* "True" combined lesion. The two separate lesions are heading to a coalescence, which forms the "true" combined lesion. N, necrotic pulp. (Reprinted from Simon et al[4] with permission.)

Anatomic relationships between the pulp and periodontium

The pulp connects to the periodontal ligament through the apical foramen (see chapter 17), lateral or accessory canals, and possibly through patent dentinal tubules in the presence or absence of cementum[11] (see chapters 4 and 19). The presence of lateral canals and their distribution in teeth have been demonstrated by a variety of methods. These techniques include microradiography (Fig 18-3),[12] pulp-chamber perfusion of

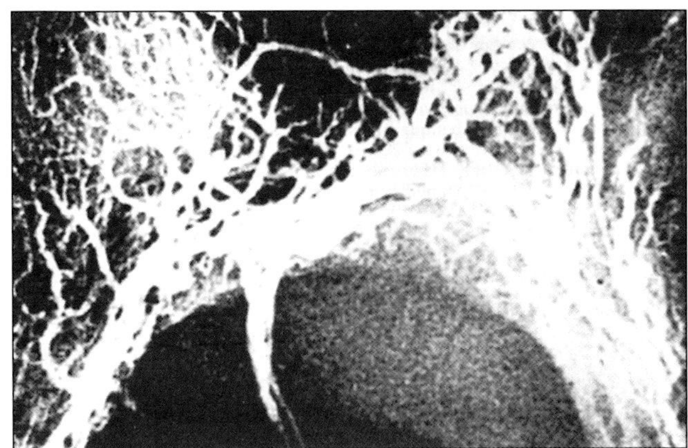

Fig 18-3 Microradiograph depicting the arrangement of blood vessels in the maxillary second molar of a 22-year-old male. Note the vascular bridge extending across the pulp chamber and connecting the root canal vessels. Aberrant vessels are entering the pulp chamber near the bifurcation of the roots. (Reprinted from Saunders[12] with permission.)

Fig 18-4 Histologic evaluation of combined pulpal-periodontal vasculature using india ink perfusion. (Reprinted from Kramer[14] with permission.)

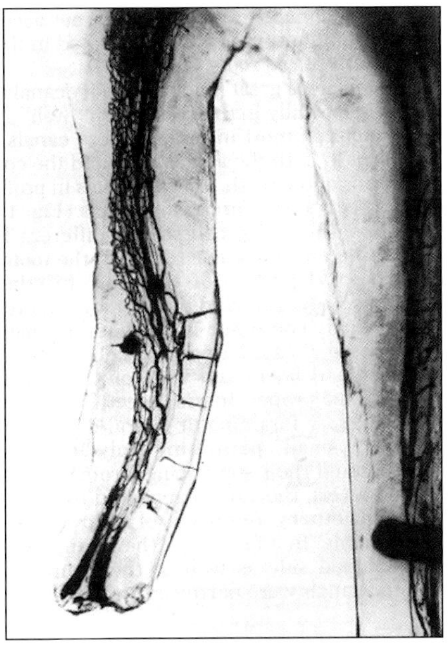

Fig 18-4a Buccal root of a maxillary first molar. Note six groups of blood vessels connecting the root canal with the periodontal ligament.

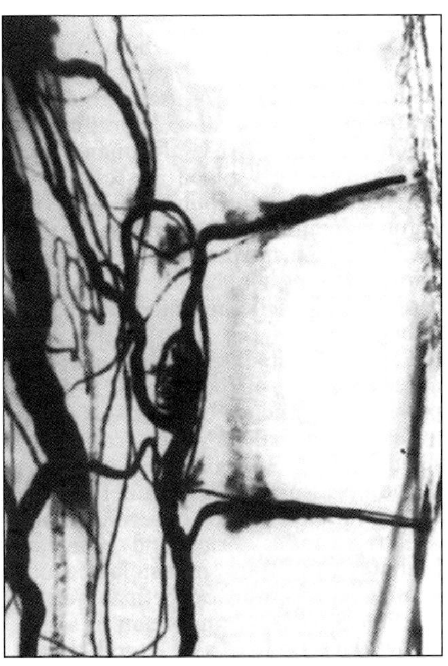

Fig 18-4b Higher magnification (×83) of Fig 18-4a showing that each canal connecting the pulp to the periodontium contains a pair of vessels with one vessel larger than the other. The smaller vessels resemble arteries and the larger vessels veins.

extracted teeth with india ink (Fig 18-4),[13] postoperative radiography of root canals filled by diffusion or pressure techniques (Fig 18-5), and conventional light microscopic examination (Fig 18-6).[15] These studies suggest that patent blood vessels course in lateral or accessory canals connecting the coronal and/or radicular pulp with the periodontal ligament. They appear to be distributed at any level of the root as well as on the floor of the pulp chamber.

Additional studies using histologic evaluation of serial sections indicate that most teeth contain

Fig 18-5 Post-endodontic treatment radiographs illustrating location and distribution of lateral canals as evidenced by presence of endodontic sealer. (Courtesy of Drs Karl Keiser, William Walker, William Schindler, and Kenneth Hargreaves.)

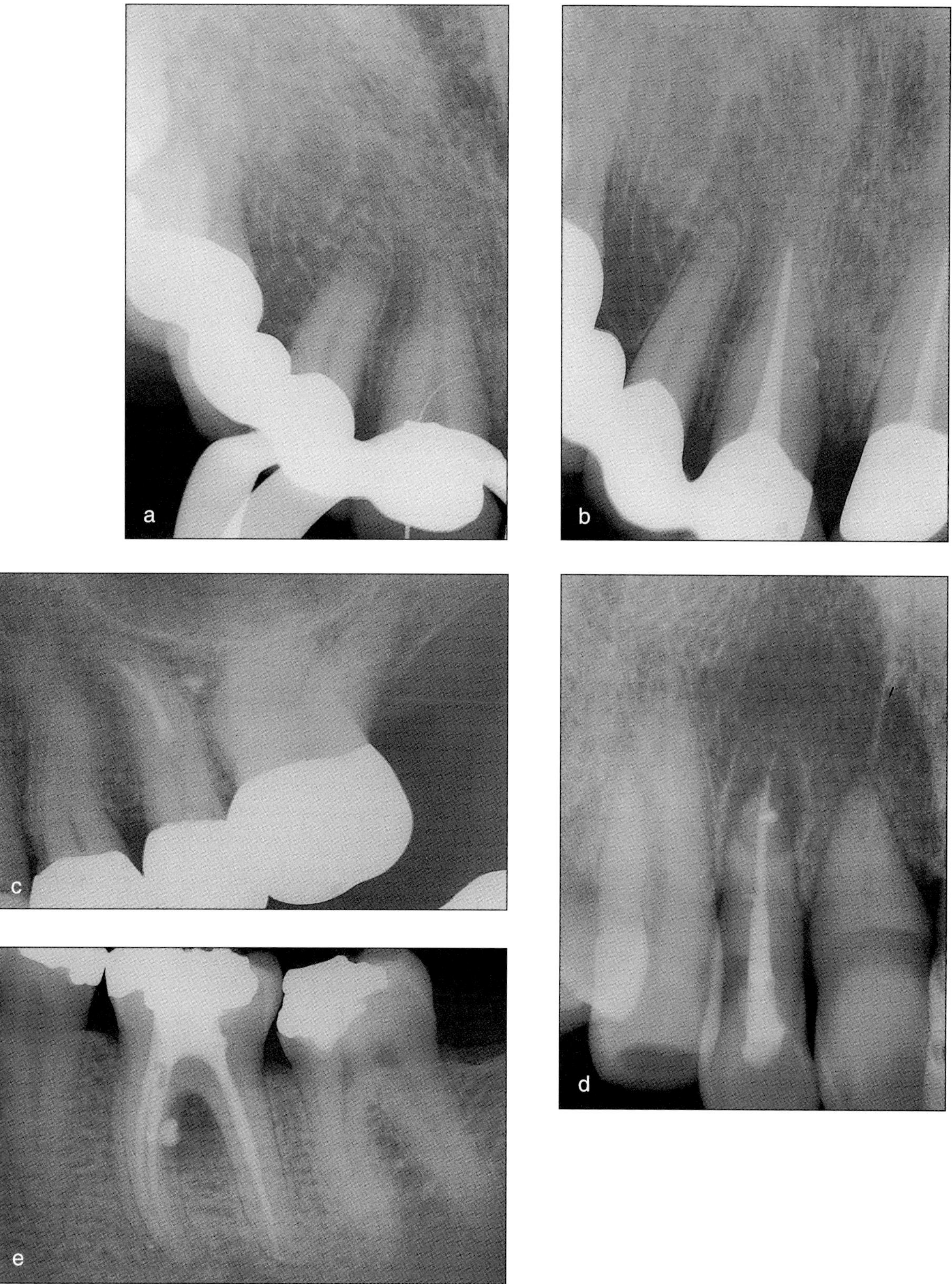

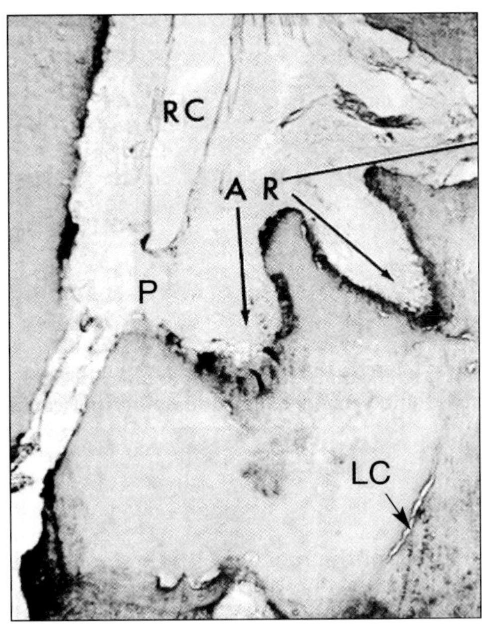

Fig 18-6 Composite section of a maxillary second premolar. Note the multiple apical ramifications (AR) of the pulp (P) in the apical portion of the root canal (RC). A lateral canal (LC) is present in the coronal portion of the apical third of the root. D, dentin (original magnification ×96). (Reprinted from Seltzer et al[16] with permission.)

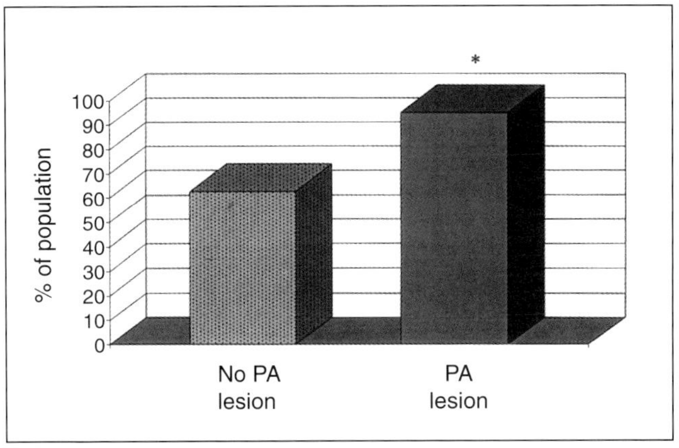

Fig 18-7 Incidence of furcation involvement, defined as > 3 mm horizontal depth, in mandibular molars with no periapical (PA) radiolucency (N = 223) compared to the incidence in mandibular molars with PA radiolucency (N = 41). $^{**}P < .05$. (Data from Jansson and Ehnevid.[20])

such pulp-periodontium communications.[15] In this study, not all canals appeared to be patent at the time of tooth extraction. In a few teeth, the foramina on the periodontal side as well as the lumina of the lateral canals were narrowed by cementum deposition. The distribution of lateral canals has been reported to be 17% in the apical third, 8.8% in the middle third, and 1.6% at the coronal portion of the root.[17] Substantial variation exists in the estimate of accessory canals in the area of the root furcation of multirooted teeth, with measured values ranging from 76%[18] to 28%.[19] These accessory canals may serve as pathways for bacteria in necrotic pulps to reach the furcal periodontium and contribute to periodontitis in this region (Fig 18-7).

The presence of patent accessory canals provides a potential pathway whereby disease processes, toxic substances, medicaments, or bacteria may spread between these two tissues at sites within the periodontium as well as the periradicular area. However, the apical foramen may be the more significant because total pulpal necrosis has been reported to occur only subsequent to bacterial invasion of all apical foramina of a given tooth.[21]

Fluid may flow through patent dentinal tubules (see chapter 4). Hence, in the absence of an intact enamel or cementum covering, the pulp may be considered exposed to the oral environment via the gingival sulcus or periodontal pocket. Experimental studies demonstrate that soluble material from bacterial plaque applied to dentin can cause pulpal inflammation.[22] The authors concluded that dentinal tubules may provide ready access between the periodontium and the pulp.

Noyes et al[23] report that 5% to 10% of human teeth display enamel-cemental dysjunction, exposing cervical dentinal tubules to the gingival sulcus. In addition, cementum may not always provide an impermeable covering for dentin. Studies indicate that cementum may be permeable in a number of conditions: young cementum is more permeable than old,[11] cemental defects may occur,[7] the cementum may be variably mineralized,[24] or it may be subject to resorption[11] (see chapter 19). In addition, dentinal tubules may be exposed in developmental anomalies such as lingual grooves, enamel projections, and other conditions.[5,9] Several other possible modes of pulp-periodontium communication should be considered, including neural reflex pathways, a common vasculature and lymphatic system, and root fracture (reviewed in Dongari and Lambrianidis[9]).

Effect of Pulpal Infection on Periodontal Disease

A causal relationship between root canal infection and periodontal disease requires *(1)* a patent route to the periodontium, *(2)* an infected root canal system, and *(3)* sufficient virulence of the pulpal bacteria to evoke marginal periodontitis. Unfortunately, there are no well-controlled prospective clinical studies demonstrating these three criteria. Instead, a causal relationship is often inferred from large-scale retrospective studies, from longitudinal studies, or from interventional preclinical studies. Although available data are not definitive, their quality appears to be sufficient to make inferences about whether pulpal infections serve as a risk factor for marginal periodontitis.[6]

Evidence in a variety of forms suggests that disease in the dental pulp alone can affect the health of the periodontium (Fig 18-8; see also Fig 18-2 [a–c]). Although the incidence of primary endodontic lesions that produce nonapical periodontal destruction has not been determined, it may be sufficiently often to confound epidemiologic studies estimating the prevalence of marginal periodontitis.[25]

Anthropologic data in early man reveal that pulpal exposure through occlusal attrition led to extensive angular alveolar defects apparently not related to marginal periodontitis.[1] These osseous defects were inferred to arise from pulpal disease with apical and/or lateral drainage into the periodontal ligament. Several case reports claim primary endodontic lesions manifesting as rapid nonapical periodontal destruction.[15,26–28] Some may manifest as a retrograde marginal periodontitis (reverse pocket) as drainage is established through the periodontium to the gingival sulcus (see Fig 18-2).[29] Such lesions have been induced experimentally in the teeth of cats, dogs, monkeys, and humans.[30–33] Seltzer and Bender[15] found granulomatous lesions associated with lateral and periradicular canals in extracted teeth.

The studies correlating endodontic infection or root canal therapy to periodontal disease utilized various techniques. Frequently the data came from retrospective analyses of data derived from human studies or experiments on animal models. In a series of retrospective studies on human patients referred to a periodontal clinic for treatment, Jansson and coworkers[34–39] concluded that loss of marginal periodontal attachment was directly correlated to the presence of endodontic infection. These studies demonstrated that teeth in patients prone to marginal periodontitis and with endodontic infections (periradicular radiolucencies) had deeper pockets, more attachment loss, and a higher frequency of angular (vertical) defects than teeth without radiographic evidence of endodontic infection (see Fig 18-7). Based on these findings, the authors concluded that pulpal infections serve as a risk factor in patients prone to periodontitis.

Prospective preclinical studies have also evaluated whether pulpal infection modifies the health of the marginal periodontium. For example, the effects of experimental root canal system infection on healing of surgically induced periodontal wounds was studied in monkeys.[41] A mixture of *Fusobacterium nucleatum*, *Streptococcus intermedius*, *Peptostreptococcus micros*, and *Porphyromonas gingivalis* was introduced into endodon-

Fig 18-8 Clinical example of a lesion of pulpal origin. (Reprinted from Wenckus et al[40] with permission.)

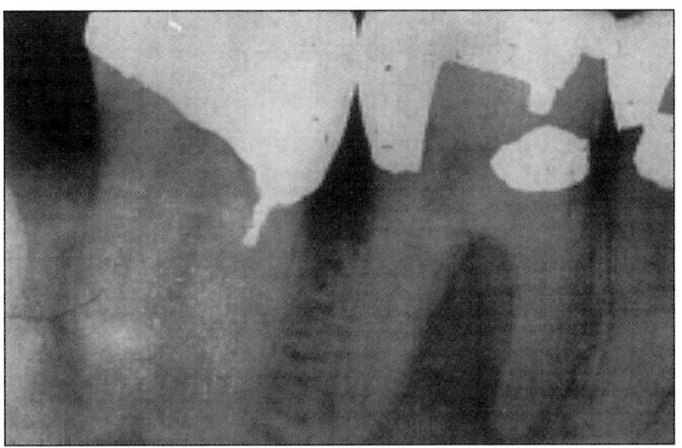

Fig 18-8a Preoperative radiograph illustrating a mandibular first molar with large periradicular radiolucency extending into the furcation.

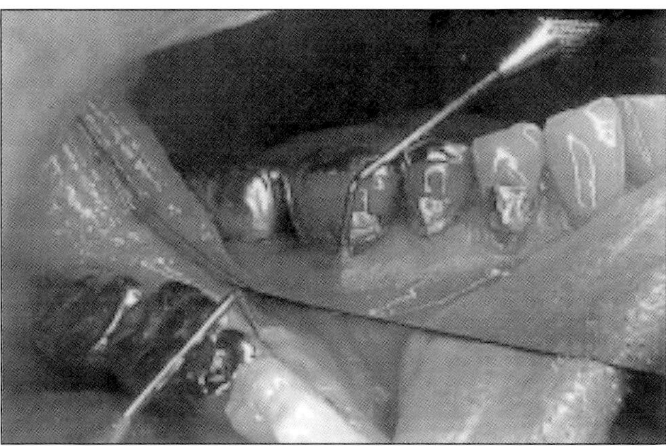

Fig 18-8b Note deep probing into the sinus tract that exited through the sulcus.

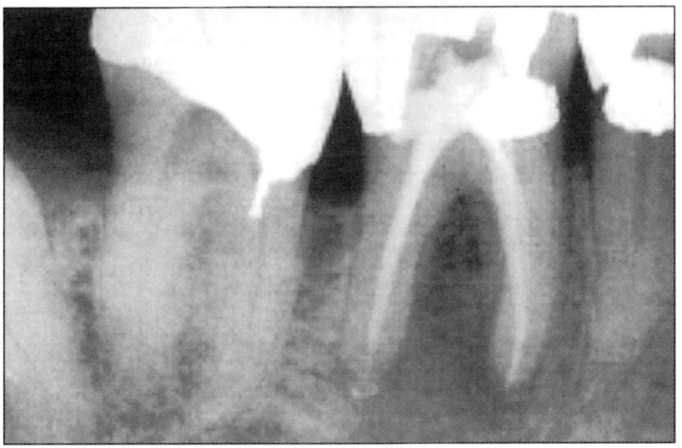

Fig 18-8c Nine-month postendodontic recall showing excellent, but incomplete, healing.

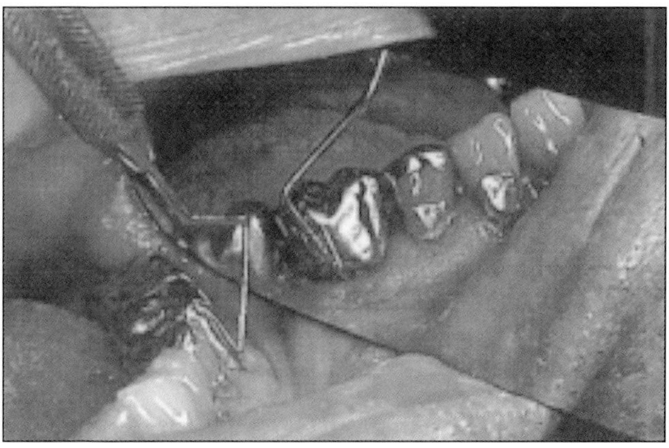

Fig 18-8d Nine-month recall showing no clinical probing into the sinus.

tically instrumented palatal roots of monkey premolars and molars. Cementum, ligament, and bone were then surgically removed from the palatal root, the root surface was acid etched, and healing observed. A greater fraction (20%) of the root was covered with epithelium in infected teeth when compared with noninfected teeth, whereas noninfected teeth had 10% more connective tissue covering the denuded root. Interestingly, the infections were more severe in the marginal region of the root, leading the authors to conclude that the cervical dentinal tubules were more patent than apical tubules, permitting a greater transport of bacteria or by-products (see also chapter 4).

However, not all investigators agree with the hypothesis that pulpal infections represent a risk factor for marginal periodontitis. For example, some investigators found no relationship between the physiologic status of the pulp (vital or nonvital) or periradicular radiologic anatomy and marginal periodontal attachment loss as assessed radiologically.[42] This study utilized patients from three separate populations in which the tooth with the periradicular pathosis was matched to a normal contralateral tooth. Others have contrasted the relatively high incidence of furcal accessory canals (28% to 76%) with the relatively poor evidence implicating them as a potential pathway for pathogens.[6] Finally, many authors contend that an intact cemental layer effectively prevents pulp-periodontium communication; this point is covered in more detail in chapter 19.

The extant data reveal that extensive pulpal infection spreading through patent lateral canals or dentinal tubules in the absence of an intact cemental layer may alter the periodontium. In such instances, periodontal treatment without root canal therapy is not sufficient. However, none of the reviewed clinical studies cited above completely answered the question of whether endodontic infections significantly affect periodontal health. More compelling evidence could be provided through prospective longitudinal studies.

Effect of Endodontic Treatment on Periodontal Healing

Information on the capacity of pulpal infections to influence periodontal healing after traumatic injury has been obtained from a series of experiments utilizing reimplanted teeth as a model.[43-48] These studies revealed that pulpal infections in reimplanted teeth may influence periodontal healing when the integrity of the cementum is breached by root resorption and dentinal tubules are exposed. Root resorption occurs in the presence of pulpal infection and absence of cementum, whereas cementum prevents root resorption associated with endodontic infection (see chapter 19). The presence of a root canal infection revealed radiograpically was also associated with diminished periodontal healing after scaling and root planing.[36] A later experiment using implanted monkey incisors demonstrated that root resorption was associated with experimentally infected pulp chambers only in the absence of cementum.[41] Although these studies do not provide definitive evidence of pulpal infection spreading to the periodontium, they do suggest the possibility that endodontic infection retards periodontal healing in the event of traumatic injury to the periodontium. These studies appear to reinforce the widely accepted clinical practice of filling root canals without altering the roots of reimplanted, fully formed, avulsed teeth. These studies, however, do not necessarily relate to plaque-associated (marginal) periodontitis.

Effect of Periodontal Lesions on Pulpal Pathosis

Although many clinicians and investigators have concluded that pulpal disease can affect periodontal health, there is less agreement that the converse is also true. Several studies have reported no association between the extent of periodontal tissue loss and markers of pulpal health. The histologic appearance of pulps in extracted human teeth from individuals exhibiting wide variation in the extent of periodontal destruction was all within normal limits.[49] Similar findings were reported by others also using histologic examination of extracted human teeth.[50,51] Other investigators using animal models have come to similar conclusions. In a rat model of induced periodontal disease, no pulpal disease was evident; however, the authors failed to document the presence of lateral canals or other means for pulp-periodontium communication.[52]

In contrast, Seltzer and Bender[15] interpret their data to be indicative of periodontal disease affecting pulpal physiology. The pulpal changes included pulpitis and necrosis. Other authors have reached similar conclusions.[21,53] Langeland and coworkers[21] reported that whereas pulpal changes were associated with periodontitis, pulpal necrosis was not evident in teeth without periradicular penetration by bacteria. For total necrosis, all periradicular foramina of a given tooth must have been infected. This study is weakened by the lack of a precise clinical description of the extent of the periodontitis and the lack of direct evidence of bacteria from the periodontium invading the pulp. Caution must attend interpretation of bacterial invasion of adjacent tissues from histologic sections because bacteria may be spread between tissues during preparation, eg, sectioning teeth prior to fixation.

However, a nonhuman primate study to determine the effect on pulpal health of periodontitis and scaling and plaque accumulation on exposed root dentin supports the existence of the primary periodontal lesion with pulpal involvement (see Fig 18-2 [e]).[54] Ligature-induced plaque-associated periodontitis was induced in six young-adult monkeys. Some of the animals received scaling and were then subjected to new plaque accumulation on the freshly exposed root dentin. Pulpal pathosis was associated with 57% of teeth subjected to experimental periodontitis while no pulpal changes were evident in control teeth (no induced plaque accumulation). However, the pulpal changes, tertiary dentin formation, and/or foci of inflammation were considered "mild," with only one necrotic pulp. The foci of pulpal inflammation occurred adjacent to areas of root resorption that could have exposed dentinal tubules. Scaling, root planing, and subsequent plaque accumulation had no additional effect on pulpal pathosis. Lateral canals were not identified. In another experimental study in rats, induction of periodontitis was associated with tertiary dentinogenesis[55] at the dentin-pulp junction adjacent to the periodontal lesion.[56] In this study, the single example of pulpitis and partial necrosis was associated with periradicular extension of the periodontitis.

The discrepant results among these studies probably reflect the different methodologies employed. Conclusions based on histologic examination of extracted teeth must be interpreted with caution. Some studies did not use age-matched teeth, did not examine the pulps of teeth without periodontal disease, did not collect sufficient numbers of subjects, or did not apply appropriate statistical analyses. The preponderance of evidence weighs against clinically relevant pulpal disease occurring because of marginal periodontitis that does not destroy periradicular tissue.

Diagnosis and Treatment

Effective diagnosis and treatment is aided by a biologically based and clinically relevant classification scheme such as that originally published by Simon and colleagues[4] (see Figs 18-1 and 18-2). This classification enables the tabulation of physical characteristics, clinical findings, treatments, and therapeutic considerations in relation to the several types of lesions associated with pulp and periodontal disease. This information is presented in Table 18-1 and is based on several recent reviews.[5,6,57] It is clear that the prognosis for most such lesions is good, with the success of periodontal care being the most difficult to predict. Careful diagnosis and a logical treatment plan conscientiously followed by thorough treatment regimens should lead to retention of most teeth with combined lesions (Figs 18-8 to 18-11).

Two of the major considerations in establishing these diagnoses are pulp vitality and the morphology of the periodontal defect. The clinician should realize that methods used to evaluate pulp vitality are susceptible to false-positive (ie, a positive response from a necrotic pulp) and false-negative (ie, a negative response from a vital pulp) results.[58,59] A recent study compared the cold test (ethyl chloride) to an electrical pulp test (Analytic Technolgy Pulp Tester [Analytic Technology, Redmond, WA]) to the gold standard (endodontic access and clinical verification of vitality) in 59 teeth of unknown pulpal status.[59] The probability of a negative test being a true necrotic pulp was similar for the cold and electrical tests (89% vs 88%). In addition, the probability of a positive test being a true vital pulp was similar for the cold and electrical tests (90% vs 84%). Overall, the cold test had slightly greater accuracy compared with the electrical test (86% vs 81%). However, the incidence of a false-posi-

Table 18-1 **Clinical classification system for diagnosis and treatment of lesions associated with pulpal and periodontal disease**

Diagnosis	Characteristics	Clinical findings	Treatment	Consideration
Endodontic lesion	Periapical bone loss Drainage through sulcus History/signs of extensive restorative treatment Gingival swelling Furcation bone loss	Pulp test negative Periodontal probing yields narrow, isolated pocket Evidence of inadequate root canal treatment Rapid onset	Endodontic treatment only	May be a risk factor in patient prone to periodontitis May spread through cervical tubules and main canal systems
Endodontic lesion with periodontal disease	Necrotic pulp Generalized periodontitis with plaque and calculus	Pulp test negative, evidence of inflammation/necrosis Generalized increase in pocket depth and attachment loss Radiographic evidence of pulp and periodontal disease	First: endodontic treatment, evaluate in 2 to 3 months Then: periodontal treatment	Avoid extensive root instrumentation during periodontal treatment that might remove cementum
Periodontal lesion	Deep pockets Extensive attachment loss No evidence of pulpal disease	History of disease progression/therapy Probing Pulp test positive	Periodontal therapy only	Be cautious of the reliability of pulp testing, especially in mutirooted teeth with severe periodontitis
Periodontal lesion with endodontic disease	Deep pockets Extensive attachment loss Increased pain Evidence of pulp disease	History of disease progression/therapy Probing Pulp test negative Pain Radiographic evidence	First: endodontic treatment, evaluate in 2 to 3 months Then: periodontal treatment	Weak evidence for this condition to occur
Combined lesion	Etiologic factors present for both conditions	Generalized periodontal destructon that connects to periapical lesion Test for root fracture Pulp test negative	Root canal therapy Periodontal therapy	Classic case is due to a fractured or perforated root

tive result may increase in cases of advanced periodontitis, with some studies reporting false-positive results as high as 52% in teeth with advanced periodontitis.[60] These authors suggest that in cases of severe periodontitis, the presence of vertical (deep narrow) pockets and furcal lesions should be considered predictors of pulpal necrosis in addition to cold or electrical test results. Moreover, the case of multirooted teeth adds another layer of complexity because some of the multiple root canal systems may be necrotic while the other systems remain vital.

The morphology of the periodontal lesion is another important diagnostic factor. In general, periodontitis is characterized by horizontal bone loss and is often generalized in the mouth with evident plaque and calculus formation. In contrast, the presence of a vertical bony lesion (deep narrow pocket) should lead the clinician to suspect an endodontic origin of the lesion, and the

Fig 18-9 Clinical example of a lesion of periodontal origin. (Reprinted from Wenckus et al[40] with permission.)

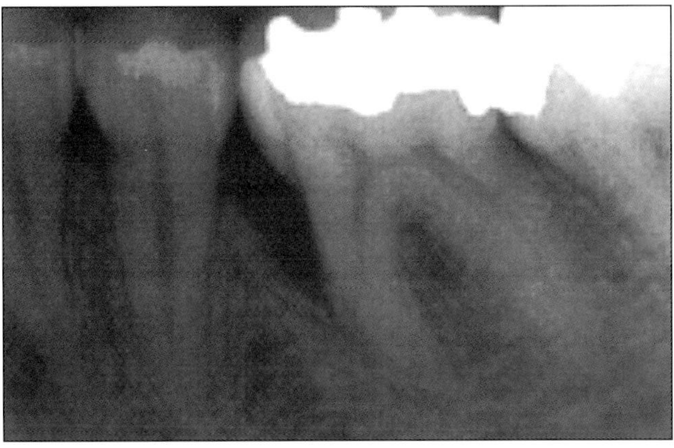

Fig 18-9a Preoperative radiograph illustrating a mandibular first molar with mesial radiolucency. Pulp testing revealed a vital pulp.

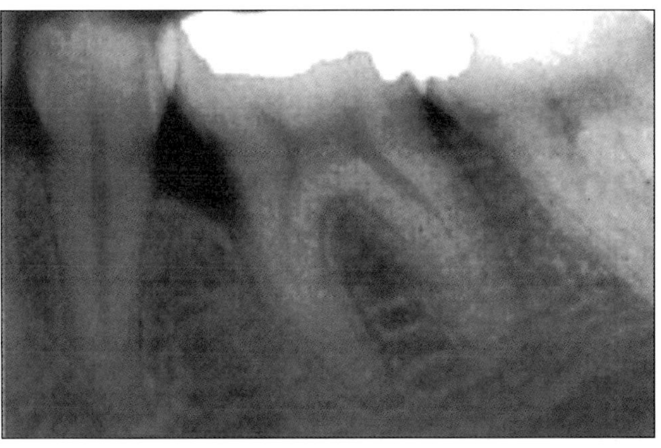

Fig 18-9b One-year recall after periodontal surgery and bone grafting reveals osseous healing. Pulp testing indicates continued pulpal vitality.

Fig 18-10 Clinical example of a combined lesion of primary pulpal and secondary periodontal origin. (Reprinted from Wenckus et al[40] with permission.)

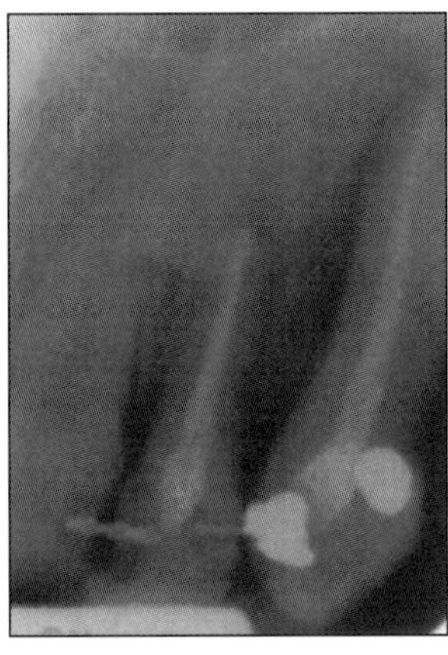

Fig 18-10a Preoperative radiograph illustrating a maxillary canine with a vertical periradicular radiolucency.

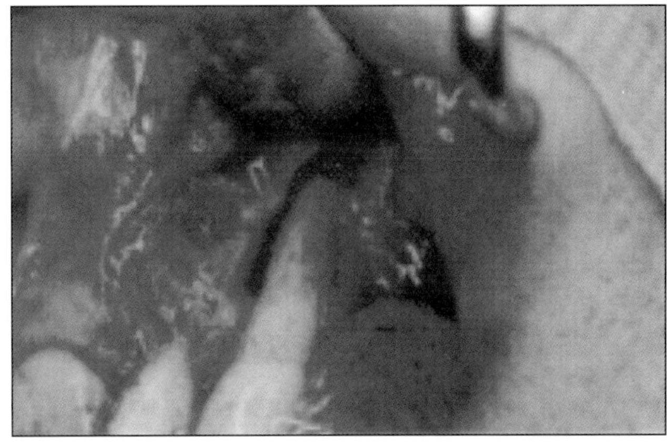

Fig 18-10b A complete dehiscence of the buccal cortical plate of bone was noted during periodontal surgery.

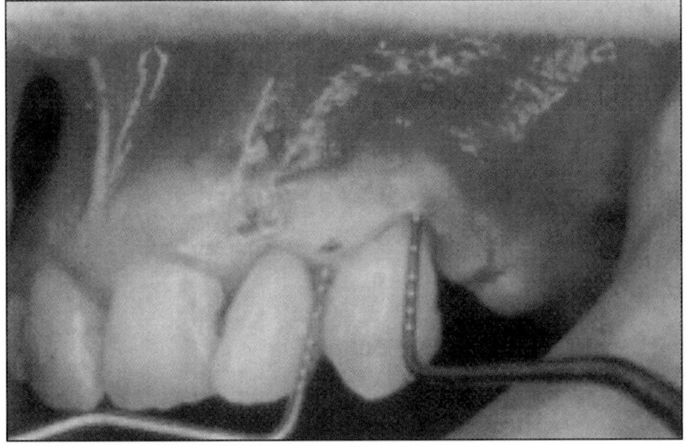

Fig 18-10c At the 4-months recall, the probing depths were only 3 mm.

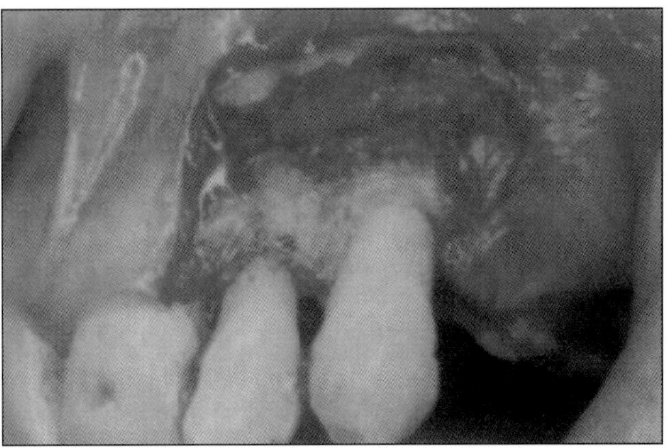

Fig 18-10d Upon re-entering the area, a complete regeneration of bone over the previous dehiscence was observed.

Fig 18-11 Clinical example of a combined lesion of concomitant pulpal and periodontal origin. (Reprinted from Wenckus et al[40] with permission.)

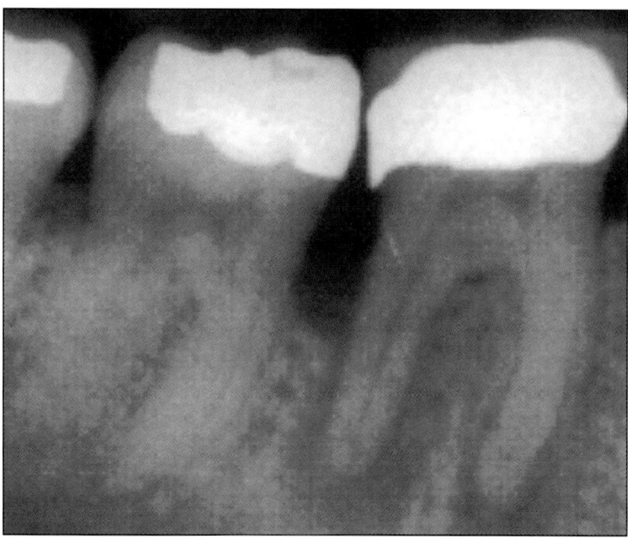

Fig 18-11a Preoperative radiograph illustrating a mandibular molar with a periradicular radiolucency.

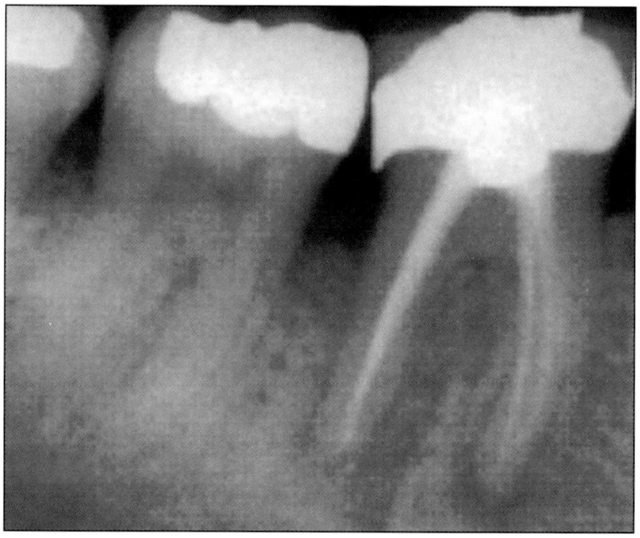

Fig 18-11b At 3 months after combined endodontic treatment and periodontal surgery with bone grafting, both the periradicular and gingival tissues appeared healthy.

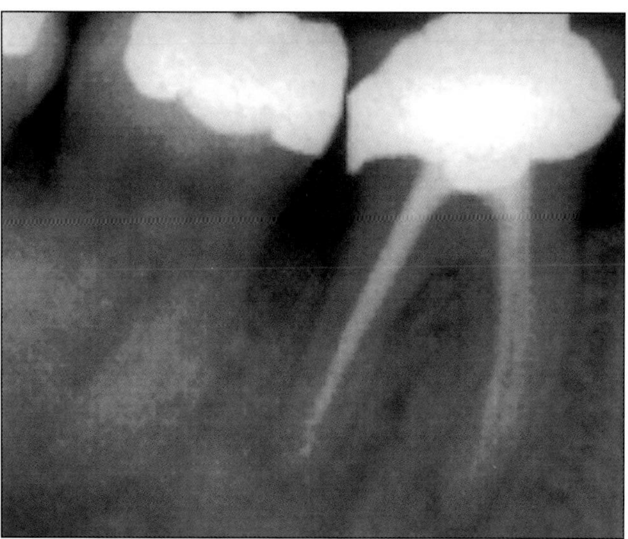

Fig 18-11c At 1 year, the periradicular healing was evident and the periodontal defect also appeared healed. The tooth probed within normal limits.

presence of a fractured root should be evaluated in these cases.

The treatment plan of a primary endodontic lesion with secondary periodontal lesion has been reviewed by several clinicians. In particular, investigators have noted the importance of completing the indicated endodontic treatment first and then re-evaluating the periodontal status 2 to 3 months following completion,[6,57] which allows sufficient time for initial healing events to present a more accurate picture of the status of periodontal tissue prior to developing the periodontal treatment plan. Moreover, given the high incidence of accessory canals in the furcal region or patent dentinal tubules in the cervical region, this treatment sequence also reduces the potential for pulpal bacteria or by-products to become risk factors for periodontitis. Given this consideration, some investigators have advocated the use of calcium hydroxide paste as an intracanal medicament for its known antimicrobial and proteolytic properties.[61]

References

1. Clarke NG. Periodontal defects of pupal origin: Evidence in early man. Am J Phys Anthropol 1990;82: 371-376.
2. Black GV. Amputation of the roots of teeth. In: Litch WF (ed). The American System of Dentistry. Philadelphia: Lea, 1887.
3. Frank AL. Resorption, perforations and fractures. Dent Clin North Am 1974;18:465-487.
4. Simon JHS, Glick DH, Frank AL. The relationship of endodontic-periodontic lesions. J Periodontol 1972;43: 202-208.
5. Belk CE, Gutmann JL. Perspectives, controversies and directives on pulpal-periodontal relationships. J Can Dent Assoc 1990;56:1013-1017.
6. Paul BF, Hutter JW. The endodontic-periodontal continuum revisited: New insights into etiology, diagnosis and treatment. J Am Dent Assoc 1997;128:1541-1548.
7. Hiatt WH. Pulpal periodontal disease. J Periodontol 1977;48:598-609.
8. Tal H. Differentiating between primary periodontal and endodontic lesions. Gen Dent 1984;32:433-435.
9. Dongari A, Lambrianidis T. Periodontally derived pulpal lesions. Endod Dent Traumatol 1988;4:49-54.
10. Rossman LE. Relationship between pulpal and periodontal diseases In: Genco RJ, Goldman HM, Cohen DW (eds). Contemporary Periodontics. St. Louis: Mosby, 1990.
11. Carranza FA. The periodontal pocket. In: Glickman's Clinical Periodontology, ed 6. Philadelphia: Saunders, 1984:201-226.
12. Saunders RL de CH. Microradiographic studies of periodontic and dental pulp vessels in monkey and man. In: Cosslett VE, Pattee HJ (eds). X-ray Microscopy and Microradiography. New York: Academic Press, 1957:561-571.
13. Kramer IRH. A technique for the injection of blood vessels in the dental pulp using extracted teeth. Anat Rec 1951;11:91.
14. Kramer IRH. Vascular architecture of human dental pulp. Arch Oral Biol 1960;2:177.
15. Seltzer S, Bender IB. The Dental Pulp: Biologic Considerations in Dental Procedures, ed 3. Philadelphia: Lippincott, 1984.
16. Seltzer S, Bender IB, Ziontz M. The interraelationship of pulp and periodontal disease. Oral Surg Oral Med Oral Pathol 1963;16:1474.
17. De Deus QD. Frequency, location, and direction of lateral, secondary and accessory canals. J Endod 1975;1:361.
18. Burch JG, Hulen S. A study of the presence of accessory formina and the topography of molar furcations. Oral Surg Oral Med Oral Pathol 1974;38:451-455.
19. Gutmann JL. Prevalence, location and patency of accessory canals in the furcation region of permanent molars. J Periodontol 1978;49:21-26.
20. Jansson L, Ehnevid H. The influence of endodontic infection on periodontal status in mandibular molars. J Periodontol 1998;68:1392-1396.
21. Langeland K, Rodrigues H, Dowden W. Periodontal diseases, bacteria and pulpal histopathology. Oral Surg Oral Med Oral Pathol 1974;37:257-270
22. Bergenholtz G, Lindhe J. Effect of soluble plaque factors on inflammatory reactions in the dental pulp. Scand J Dent Res 1975;83:153-158.
23. Noyes FB, Schour I, Noyes HJ. A Textbook of Dental Histology and Embryology, ed 5. Philadelphia: Lea & Febiger, 1998:113.
24. Linde J. Textbook of Clinical Periodontology. Copenhagen: Munksgaard, 1983:235-253.
25. Clark N, Hirsch R. Two critical confounding factors in periodontal epidemiology. Community Dent Health 1992;9:133-141.
26. Barkhordar RA, Stewart GG. The potential of periodontal pocket formation associated with untreated accessory root canals. Oral Surg Oral Med Oral Pathol 1990; 70:769-772.
27. Reeh ES, el Deeb M. Rapid furcation involvement associated with a devitalizing mandibular first molar. Oral Surg Oral Med Oral Pathol 1990;69:95-98.
28. Chang KM, Lin LM. Diagnosis of an advanced endodontic/periodontic lesion: Report of a case. Oral Surg Oral Med Oral Pathol Oral Radiol Endod 1997;84:79-81.
29. Simring M, Goldberg M. Pulpal pocket approach to retrograde periodontitis. J Periodontol 1964;35:22.
30. Moss SJ, Addelston H, Goldsmith ED. Histologic study of pulpal floor of deciduous molars. J Am Dent Assoc 1965;70:372-379.
31. Winter GB, Kramer IRH. Changes in periodontal membrane and bone following experimental pulpal injuries in deciduous molar teeth in kittens. Arch Oral Biol 1965;10:279.
32. Seltzer S, Bender IB, Nazimov H, Sinai I. Pulpitis-induced interradicular periodontal changes in experimental animals. J Periodontol 1967;38:124-129.
33. Winter GB, Kramer IRH. Changes in periodontal membrane, bone and permanent teeth following experimental pulpal injury in deciduous molar teeth of monkeys (*Macaca irus*). Arch Oral Biol 1972;17:1771-1779.
34. Jansson LE, Ehnevid H, Lindskog SF, Blomlof LB. Radiographic attachment in periodontitis-prone teeth with endodontic infection. J Periodontol 1993;64:947-953.
35. Jansson L, Ehnevid H, Lindskog S, Blomlof L. Relationship between periapical and periodontal status: A clinical retrospective study. J Clin Periodontol 1993;20: 117-123.

36. Ehnevid H, Jansson LE, Lindskog SF, Blomlof LB. Periodontal healing in relation to radiographic attachment and endodontic infection. J Periodontol 1993;64:1199-1204.
37. Ehnevid H, Jansson L, Lindskog S, Blomlof L. Periodontal healing in teeth with periapical lesions: A clinical retrospective study. J Clin Periodontol 1993;20:254-258.
38. Jansson L, Ehnevid H, Lindskog S, Blomlof L. The influence of endodontic infection on progression of marginal bone loss in periodontitis. J Clin Periodontol 1995;22:729-734.
39. Jansson L, Ehnevid H, Blomlof L, Weintraub A, Lindskog S. Endodontic pathogens in periodontal disease augmentation. J Clin Periodontol 1995;22:598-602.
40. Wenckus C, Gutmann J, Dorn S. Pulpal/periodontal relationships. Endodontics: Colleagues for Excellence 2001; Spring/Summer:2-3.
41. Ehnevid H, Jansson L, Lindskog S, Weintraub A, Blomlof L. Endodontic pathogens: Propagation of infection through patent dentinal tubules in traumatized monkey teeth. Endod Dent Traumatol 1995;11:229-234.
42. Miyashita H, Bergenholtz G, Grondahl K, Wennstrom JL. Impact of endodontic conditions on marginal bone loss. J Periodontol 1998;69:158-164.
43. Andreasen JO, Hjorting-Hansen E. Replantation of teeth. II. Histological study of 22 replanted anterior teeth in humans. Acta Odontol Scand 1966;24:287-306.
44. Andreasen JO, Hjorting-Hansen E. Replantation of teeth. I. Radiographic and clinical study of 110 human teeth replanted after accidental loss. Acta Odontol Scand 1966;24:263-346.
45. Andreasen JO. Analysis of pathogenesis and topography of replacement root resorption (ankylosis) after replantation of mature permanent incisors in monkeys. Swed Dent J 1980;231-240.
46. Andreasen JO. Relationship between surface and inflammatory resorption and changes in the pulp after replantation of permanent incisors in monkeys. J Endod 1981;7:294.
47. Andreasen JO, Kristerson L. The effect of limited drying or removal of the periodontal ligament: Periodontal healing after replantation of mature permanent incisors in monkeys. Acta Odontol Scand 1981;39:1-13.
48. Andreasen JO. Effect of extra-alveolar period and storage media upon periodontal and pulpal healing after replantation of mature permanent incisors in monkeys. Int J Oral Surg 1981;10:43.
49. Mazur B, Massler M. Influence of periodontal disease on the dental pulp. Oral Surg Oral Med Oral Pathol 1964;17:592.
50. Czarnecki RT, Schilder HA. Histological evaluation of the human pulp in teeth with varying degrees of periodontal disease. J Endod 1979;5:242-253.
51. Torabinejad M, Kiger RD. A histologic evaluation of dental pulp tissue of a patient with periodontal disease. Oral Surg Oral Med Oral Pathol 1985;59:198-200.
52. Hattler AB, Snyder DE, Listgarten M, Kemp W. The lack of pulpal pathosis in rice rats with the periodontal syndrome. Oral Surg Oral Med Oral Pathol 1979;44:939-948.
53. Mandi FA. Histological study of the pulp changes caused by periodontal disease. J Br Endod Soc 1972;6:80.
54. Bergenholtz G, Lindhe J. Effect of experimentally induced marginal periodontitis and periodontal scaling on the dental pulp. J Clin Periodontol 1978;5:59-73.
55. Smith AJ, Cassidy N, Perry H, Begue-Kirn C, Ruch JV, Lesot H. Reactionary dentinogenesis. Int J Dev Biol 1995;39:273-280.
56. Stahl SS. Pathogenesis of inflammatory lesions in pulp and periodontal tissues. Periodontics 1966;4:190.
57. Chapple I, Lumley P. The periodontal-endodontic interface. Dent Update 1999;26:331-334.
58. Hyman J, Cohen M. The predictive value of endodontic diagnostic tests. Oral Surg Oral Med Oral Pathol 1984;58:343-346.
59. Peterson K, Soderstrom C, Kiani-Araaraki M, Levy G. Evaluation of the ability of thermal and electrical tests to register pulp vitality. Endod Dent Traumatol 1999;19:127-131.
60. Hirsch R, Clarke N, Srikandi W. Pulpal pathosis and severe alveolar lesions: A clinical study. Endod Dent Traumatol 1989;5:48-54.
61. Solomon C, Chalfin H, Kellert M, Weseley P. The endodontic-peridontal lesion: A rational approach to treatment. J Am Dent Assoc 1995;126:473-479.

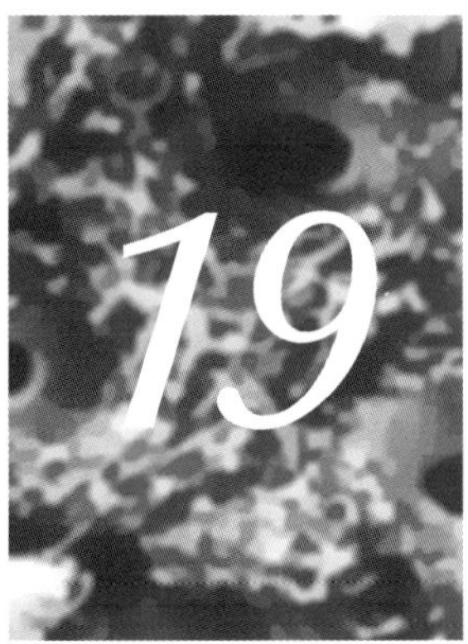

Root Resorption

Linda Levin, DDS, PhD
Martin Trope, BDS, DMD

Root resorption is a rare occurrence in permanent teeth. Unlike bone that undergoes resorption and apposition as part of a continual remodeling process, the roots of permanent teeth are not normally resorbed. Only resorption of primary teeth during exfoliation is considered physiologic.[1]

Mechanisms of Resorption

Even under conditions that would normally result in bone resorption, such as alterations in oxygen tension, hormonal fluctuations, locally produced chemical mediators, or electrical currents, the root is resistant to resorption on both its external and internal surfaces.[2] Although several hypotheses have been proposed, the exact mechanism by which the resorption process is inhibited is unknown. One hypothesis maintains that the remnants of the epithelial root sheath surround the root like a net and impart resistance to resorption and subsequent ankylosis.[3,4] This hypothesis, however, has not been supported.[5] A second hypothesis is based on the premise that the covering of cementum and predentin on dentin is essential in the resistance of the dental root to resorption. There is some support for this hypothesis in that it has long been noted that osteoclasts will not adhere to unmineralized matrix.[6] Osteoclasts will bind to extracellular proteins containing the agi-nine-glycine-aspartic acid (RGD) sequence of amino acids. These RGD peptides are bound to calcium salt crystals on mineralized surfaces and serve as osteoclast binding sites. Importantly, the most external aspect of cementum is covered by a layer of cementoblasts over a zone of nonmineralized cementoid, and therefore does not present a surface satisfactory for osteoclast binding. Internally the dentin is covered by predentin matrix, a similarly organic surface (Fig 19-1). Thus, the lack of RGD proteins in both cementum and predentin reduces osteoclast binding and confers resistance to resorption. Numerous studies lend support to this theory.[1,5,7-10] It has also been demonstrated in cases of extensive external root resorption that the circumpulpal dentin in close proximity to the predentin is spared even though most of the peripheral dentin may have been resorbed (Fig 19-2). Another prediction of this hypothesis is that damage to cementum or predentin increases the probability of osteoclast-induced resorption, which could occur in teeth damaged during avul-

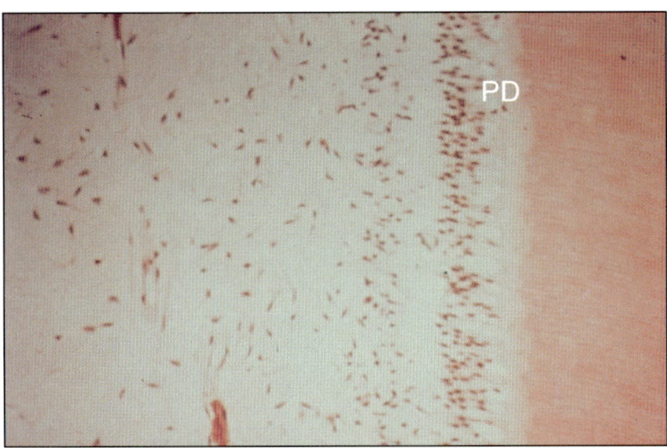

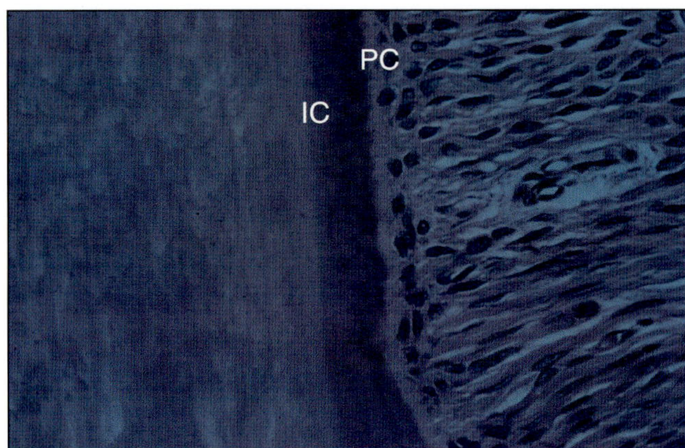

Fig 19-1 Histologic appearance of pulp, periodontal ligament, and adjacent dentin. The precementum (PC) and predentin (PD) have antiresorptive properties. If the intermediate cementum (IC) is penetrated, any pulpal toxins that may be present will cause periodontal inflammation with bone and root resorption (H&E stain, original magnification ×25).

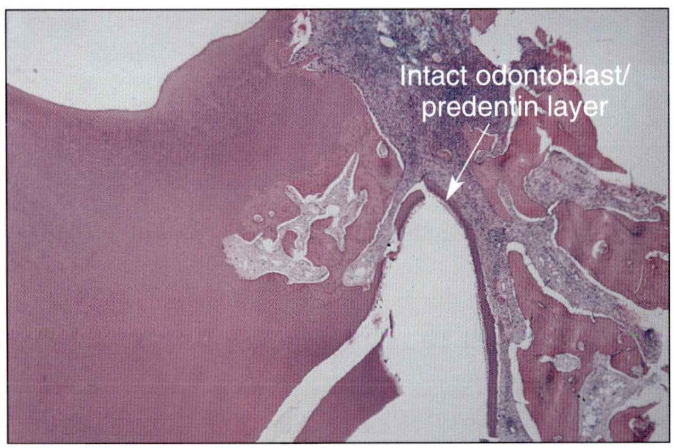

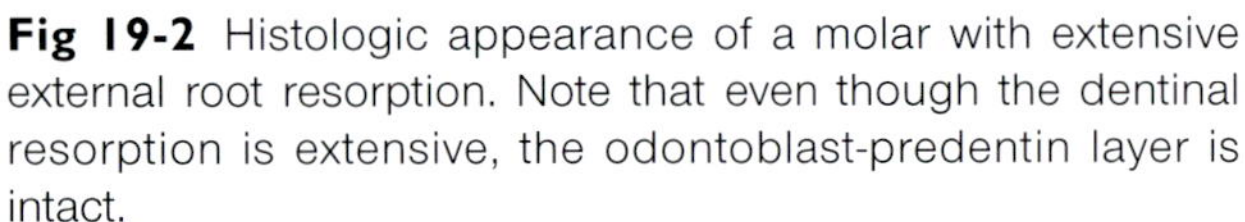

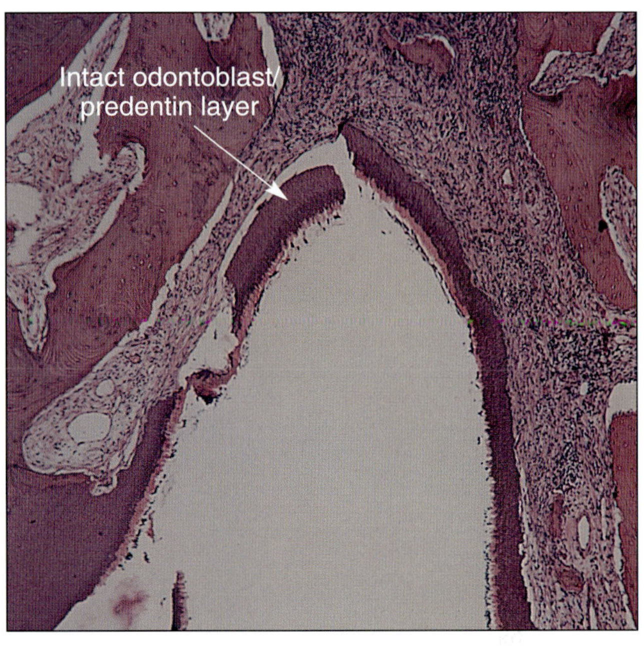

Fig 19-2 Histologic appearance of a molar with extensive external root resorption. Note that even though the dentinal resorption is extensive, the odontoblast-predentin layer is intact.

sions or other traumatic injuries. Although this hypothesis has both experimental support and clinical implications, other hypotheses have also been advanced.

Another hypothesis for the relative resistance of teeth to resorption maintains that intrinsic factors found in predentin and cementum act as inhibitors of resorptive cells. It is known, for example, that certain factors inhibit the resorptive process in bone. One such factor is osteoprotegerin (OPG), a novel member of the tumor necrosis factor (TNF) superfamily that has the ability to inhibit osteoclast-mediated bone loss. Osteoprotegerin acts as a "decoy receptor" by binding to the receptor activator of NF-κβ ligand (RANKL), which reduces its concentration and thereby inhibits the ability of RANKL to stimulate osteoclast production (osteoclastogenesis).[11] Whether cementoblasts produce OPG is not known; however, human gingival fibroblasts, human periodontal ligament cells, and human pulpal cells possess the ability.[12,13]

Finally, another hypothesis applicable to certain types of external root resorption involves the barrier formed by the highly calcified intermediate cementum (Fig 19-3).[5,14,15] The *intermediate cementum*, the innermost layer of cementum, creates a barrier between the dentinal tubules and the periodontal ligament.[16-18] Under normal circumstances, this barrier does not allow irritants such as bacterial by-products to pass from an infected pulp space to stimulate an inflammatory response in the adjacent periodontal ligament. However, if the intermediate cementum is lost or damaged, the inflammatory stimulators may diffuse from an infected pulp space into the periodontal ligament, setting up an inflammatory response and subsequent external inflammatory root resorption. It is clear that these different hypotheses are not mutually exclusive, and their relative contributions to various clinical conditions may also vary depending on the circumstances of each case.

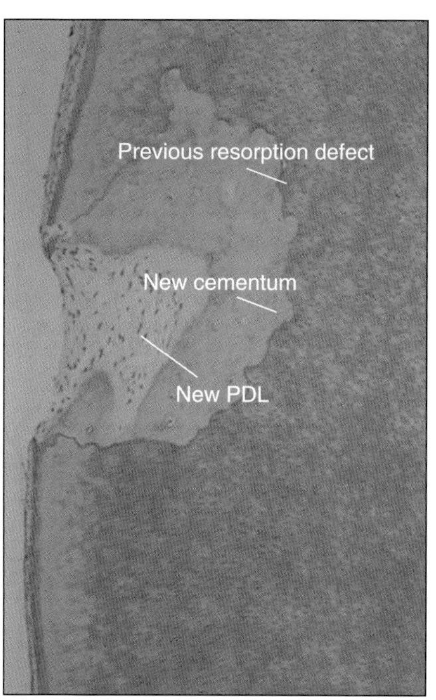

Fig 19-3 Histologic appearance of a localized area of root resorption that has healed with new cementum and periodontal ligament (PDL). The initial damage was caused by a mild localized luxation injury.

A variety of mediators such as hormones, integrins, transcription factors, and cytokines affect physiologic osteoclast function (see also chapter 17). The primary factors involved in pathologic root resorption are fewer, however, and are primarily or secondarily associated with the inflammatory response to infection. It is known that inflammatory mediators are potent stimulators of osteoclast/odontoclast function. Interleukin-1 (IL-1), IL-3, IL-11, leukemia inhibitory factor (LIF), ciliary neurotropic factor (CNTF), oncostatin M (OSM), TNF, granulocyte-macrophage colony-stimulating factor (GM-CSF), and c-kit ligand are known to stimulate osteoclast development and activity.[19] Colony stimulating factor 1 (CSF-1), in concert with TNF-related activation-induced cytokine (TRANCE), also called *receptor activator of NF-κB ligand* (RANKL), is critical for stromal cell mediation of osteoclast development (Fig 19-4).[20] IL-1 and TNF are potent stimulators of osteoclast ontogeny and function (see also chapters 15 and 17). IL-1 is produced by a variety of cells, including macrophages, marrow stromal cells, and odontoclasts, and has been shown to effect both an increase in osteoclast differentiation and activation of mature clastic cells.[21] Both TNF-α and TNF-β are likewise involved in dissolution of hard tissues by stimulating formation and proliferation of clastic cells.

Some of the mediators of inflammation-induced clastic function belong to the gp130 cytokine family that has been shown to play a key role in bone remodeling.[22] This family is a pleomorphic group that shares a common signal transducer (gp130) and includes cardiotrophin-1, OSM, CNTF, IL-6, IL-11, and LIF. Of these factors, IL-6 and IL-11 appear to have the most profound effect on hard tissue resorption, and IL-6 has been shown to stimulate osteoclastogenesis in the presence of IL-1 but not in the presence of anti-IL-1.[23] This effect is dependent on the expression of the IL-6 receptor on osteoblastic cells and occurs in a dose-dependent manner.[24] Interleukin-6 also appears to reverse the inhibitory effects of extracellular Ca^{2+} by reducing the ability of osteoclasts

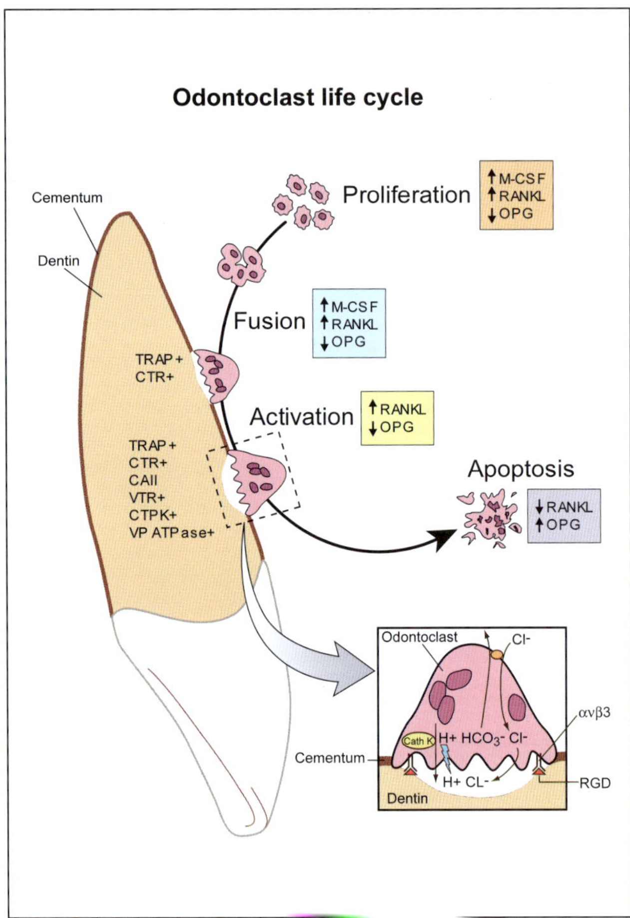

Fig 19-4 The odontoclast life cycle. Shaded boxes list molecules involved in osteoclast maturation, function, and demise. Tartrate-resistant acid phosphatase (TRAP), calcitonin receptors (CTRs), vitronectin receptors (VTRs), carbonic anhydrase II (CAII), cathepsin K (CTPK), and vacuolar proton V-H ATPase (VP ATPase) are molecular markers for the mature clastic phenotype. M-CSF, macrophage colony-stimulating factor.

to detect extracellular Ca^{2+} concentrations[25] and is expressed by cells of the stromal/osteoblastic lineage. IL-11 is an osteoblast-derived mediator that induces prostaglandin synthesis and thereby triggers differentiation of clastic cells. Cells of the osteoclast phenotype have been shown to express the IL-11 receptor gene that in turn seems to be related sequentially to expression of the calcitonin receptor gene, a recognized osteoclast differentiation marker.[26] Furthermore, gp130 signal induction by IL-11 appears to be necessary for IL-1–induced osteoclast formation.[22]

Due to the previously described inhibitory effects of organic precementum and predentin, an intact root is resistant to resorption even in the presence of inflammation. However, if an injury removes or alters the protective predentin or precementum, then inflammation in the pulp or periodontium will induce root resorption with multinucleated clastic cells similar to those seen in bone resorption.

The singular defining feature of the mature osteoclast is functional, namely the ability to resorb calcified tissues. Morphologically, the osteoclast is described as a multinucleated giant cell formed by the fusion of monocytic precursors.[1,27] Odontoclasts differ slightly from their bone-resorbing counterparts in that they are usually smaller, have fewer nuclei, and have very small (if any) sealing zones.[28] These cells nonetheless are thought to represent a variant of osteoclasts with morphologic differences reflecting the nature of the resorption substrate as well as the resorption kinetics of the cells.[29,30]

On a cellular level, osteoclasts are usually large with multiple nuclei. They possess a well-defined Golgi apparatus, numerous lysosomal vesicles, and high polarity.[31,32] A characteristic morphologic feature of the osteoclast is the ruffled border formed by membrane and cytoplasmic undulations and the sealing zone comprised of the ventral surface of the osteoclast membrane in contact with the targeted bone surface.[33] The mature osteoclast is further defined by a series of molecular markers, each representing genes integral to clastic function. These include transcripts coding for tartrate-resistant acid phosphatases (TRAPs), calcitonin receptors (CTRs), vitronectin receptors, carbonic anhydrase II, cathepsin K, and vacuolar proton V-H adenosine triphosphatase.[33]

A model for the process of root resorption can be depicted based on what is known about odontoclasts combined with data extrapolated from studies of osteoclasts (Fig 19-4). As previously mentioned, initiation of root resorption has two requirements: removal of the protective layer (predentin internally, precementum externally) of the root and the presence of a noxious stimulus that results in an inflammatory response adjacent to the damaged root surface. Given these conditions, the first step in root resorption is binding the clastic cell to its substrate. Various RGD-peptide–containing proteins (eg, osteopontin, bone sialoprotein, fibronectin, vitronectin) have been shown to be involved in osteoclast binding. Most notably, osteopontin has been shown to play an important role in regulating osteoclast recruitment and activation by binding to the osteoclast integrin receptor $\alpha_v\beta_3$. Osteopontin thus serves as a linker molecule, with one domain bound to calcium crystals in exposed dentin and another domain bound to the integrin protein ($\alpha_v\beta_3$) extending from the osteoclast's plasma membrane. Therefore, the binding of osteopontin to the $\alpha_v\beta_3$ integrin facilitates clastic cell adhesion and subsequent establishment of the clear zone or extracellular resorbing compartment. Specifically, the osteopontin-$\alpha_v\beta_3$ interaction with odontoclasts stimulates a second messenger pathway (ie, gelsolin association with phosphatidylinositol-3-hydroxyl kinase via a pp60src- and rhoA-dependent pathway) that mediates cytoskeletal rearrangement, ruffled border formation, and substrate adhesion.[34] Once the ruffled border has been formed, the odontoclast secretes an acidic solution containing proteolytic enzymes, specifically carbonic anhydrase and vacuolar type H^+ ATPase into the extracellular resorbing compartment to effect decalcification.[35]

Role of Dental Pulp in Resorption

Since the focus of this book is the dental pulp and its interaction with other tissues, those types of resorption in which the pulp plays a major role will be discussed in detail. However, it is important to discuss briefly additional common dental root resorptions because this knowledge allows the practitioner to accurately differentiate these resorption phenomena and supports correct diagnosis before treatment is rendered.

The pulp plays an essential role in two resorption types. The first type of resorption is *external* inflammatory root resorption. In external inflammatory root resorption, the necrotic infected pulp provides the stimulus for periodontal inflammation. If the situation arises where the cementum has been damaged and the intermediate cementum penetrated, as when the tooth undergoes a traumatic injury, the inflammatory stimulators in the pulp space are able to diffuse through the dentinal tubules and stimulate an inflammatory response over large areas of the periodontal ligament. Due again to the lack of cemental protection, the periodontal inflammation will result in root resorption as well as the expected bone resorption.

The second type of resorption in which pulpal tissue plays an important role is *internal* inflammatory root resorption. In internal inflammatory root resorption, the inflamed pulp is the tissue involved in resorbing the root structure. The pathogenesis of internal root resorption is not completely understood. It is thought that coronal necrotic infected pulp provides a stimulus for a pulpal inflammation in the more apical parts of the pulp. In rare cases where the inflamed pulp is adjacent to a root surface that has lost its precemental protection, internal root resorption will result. Thus, both the necrotic infected pulp and the inflamed pulp contribute to this type of root resorption.

External Root Resorption

External root resorption caused by an injury restricted to the external root surface

In this first example, an injury causes loss of the protective layer and serves as an inflammatory stimulus. This type of resorption is self-limiting. The injury is the cause of the attachment damage. The inflammatory mediators evoked by the mechanical damage stimulate the cellular inflam-

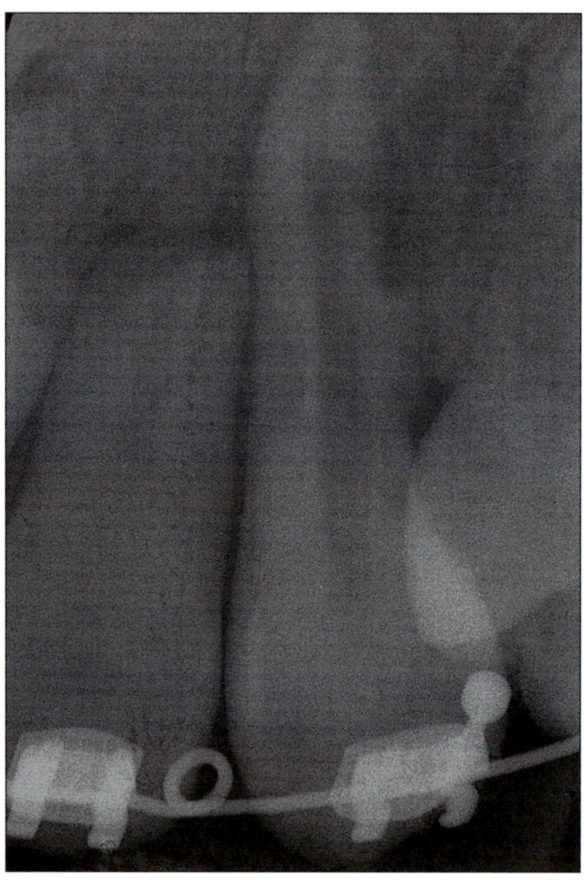

Fig 19-5 Active transient external inflammatory root resorption. Note the lucent areas on the root surface. Because the pulp is vital, a "wait-and-watch" strategy is followed.

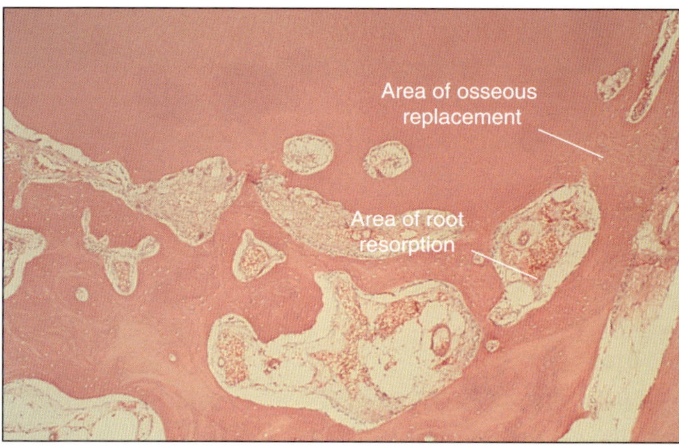

Fig 19-6 Histologic appearance of active osseous replacement. Without an intermediate periodontal ligament, bone attaches directly to the root. Areas of active root resorption are seen in the bone and root.

matory response. The healing response is dependent on the extent of the initial damage.

Localized injury: Healing with cementum

When the injury is localized (eg, after concussion or subluxation injury), mechanical damage to the cementum occurs, resulting in a local inflammatory response and a localized area of root resorption. If no further inflammatory stimulus is present, periodontal healing and root surface repair will occur within 14 days (see Fig 19-3).[1] The resorption is localized to the area of mechanical damage, and treatment is not required because it is free of symptoms and in most cases undetectable radiographically. However, in a minority of cases, small radiolucencies can be seen on the root surface if the radiograph is taken at a specific angle (Fig 19-5). It is important not to misinterpret these cases as progressive in nature. It is equally important to understand that the pulp is not involved in these cases. When no potential inflammatory stimulus can be identified (ie, when a positive sensitivity test indicates a vital pulp), no endodontic treatment should be performed. A "wait-and-see" attitude should be taken to allow spontaneous healing to take place.

Diffuse injury: Healing by osseous replacement

When the traumatic injury is severe (eg, intrusive luxation or avulsion with extended dry time), involving diffuse damage on more than 20% of the root surface, an abnormal attachment may occur after healing takes place.[36] The initial reaction is always inflammation in response to the severe mechanical damage of the traumatic and concomitant injuries to the root surface. After the initial inflammatory response, a diffuse area of root surface will be devoid of cementum. Cells in the vicinity of the denuded root compete to repopulate it, and often cells that are precursors of bone, rather than periodontal ligament cells, will move across from the socket wall and populate the damaged root. Bone comes into direct contact with the root, without the intermediate cementum serving as an attachment apparatus. This phenomenon is termed dentoalveolar ankylosis.[37] Bone resorbs and forms physiologically throughout life. Thus, the root is resorbed by the osteoclasts, but in the reforming stage, bone instead of dentin is laid down. In this way, the root is slowly replaced with bone, a process called *osseous replacement* (Fig 19-6). The trauma produces mechanical debris that elicits an initial inflammatory response that may be reversed. However, the subsequent ankylosis and osseous replacement cannot be reversed and can be considered a physiologic process because bone resorbs and reforms throughout life. In these traumatic cases, however, the resorptive phase includes the root (Fig 19-7).

Treatment strategies are directed at avoiding or minimizing the initial inflammatory response. Five specific strategies should be considered[38]: *(1)* prevention of the initial injury should be emphasized by counseling or advocating use of mouthguards for athletic endeavors; *(2)* treatment should minimize additional damage after the initial injury; *(3)* pharmacologic interventions that inhibit the initial inflammatory response should be considered; *(4)* the possibility of stimulating cemental (rather than osseous) healing should be considered; and *(5)* interventions that reduce the rate of osseous replacement, when inevitable, should be considered. Space precludes a more thorough review of these current areas of therapy and research; the interested reader is encouraged to seek reviews on this aspect of care.[38]

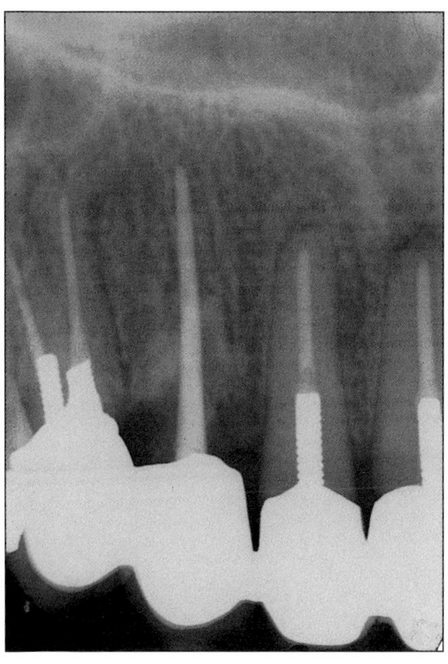

Fig 19-7 Radiographic appearance of osseous replacement. A mottled appearance of bone replacing root is visible. Radiolucencies in the adjacent bone are not apparent.

External root resorption caused by an injury to the external root surface with an inflammatory component

There are three general types of inflammatory stimuli that cause external root resorption: pressure, pulp space infection, and sulcular infection.

Pressure

Pressure both damages the cementum and provides a continuous stimulus for the resorbing cells. The most common example of this type of pressure resorption is root resorption due to excessive forces of orthodontic tooth movement. Other examples are resorption from impacted teeth and tumors.

Pressure resorption has been assumed to be external in nature, but this is not necessarily true. In orthodontics, for example, the process takes place at the apex of the tooth near the cementodentinal junction. Since the force affects the apical root, either the cementum or predentin may be damaged. Because the predentin may

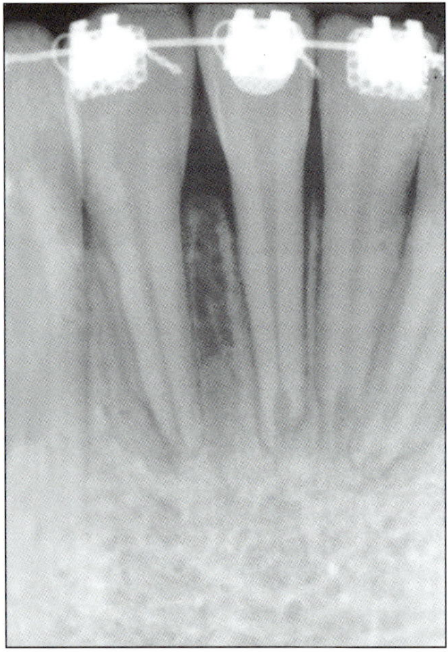

Fig 19-8 Root resorption during active orthodontic tooth movement. Mandibular central incisors show apical external and internal resorption.

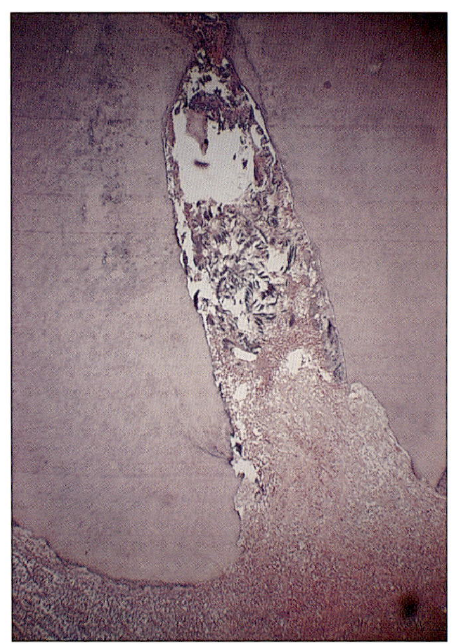

Fig 19-9 Histologic appearance of apical resorption due to an infected root canal. Chronic inflammation is present apically. Resorption of the external and internal aspects of the root can be seen.

be affected also, it is not unusual to see radiographic evidence of internal apical resorption in the active stage of the process (Fig 19-8). In 1997, Bender and colleagues labeled this type of resorption *periapical replacement resorption* (PARR) and offered a hypothetical explanation for it, suggesting that pulpal neuropeptides may be involved in PARR in both vital and endodontically treated incisors.[39] Their review of 43 cases indicated that endodontically treated incisors show a statistically significant reduced frequency and severity of apical resorption versus untreated teeth. However, it is unlikely that endodontic treatment will completely reverse active resorption due to pressure. Only removal of the pressure will stop the resorption.

Pulp space infection

Pulp space infection represents the second general type of inflammatory stimuli that can cause external root resorption. Pulp space infection can lead to external root resorption in either the apical or lateral regions of the root. The classic example of pulp space infections causing apical external root resorption is apical periodontitis with apical root resorption.

The etiology for this form of apical external root resorption is pulpal necrosis. The pulp of the tooth may become necrotic for many reasons, but the predominant cause is a bacterial challenge through caries (see chapter 12). When the pulp defenses are overcome, the pulp becomes necrotic and infected, with subsequent diffusion of bacteria and by-products into the surrounding periodontium. In most routine cases, the root surface is protected by its intact cementum, and communication will be primarily through the apical foramina or occasionally through accessory canals.

Invariably the periodontal inflammation is accompanied by slight resorption of the root at the cementodentinal junction. This resorption in usually not apparent radiographically but is routinely seen upon histologic evaluation (Fig 19-9). It is not obvious why the apex of the root is not as well protected from the resorbing factors produced during the inflammatory response as the other areas of the root. A simple explanation might be that inflammation is confined to a small area at the apex of the root so that the concentration of resorbing factors is so high that the resistance of the root to resorption is overcome. Another speculation is that the junction of the cementum and dentin (CDJ) at the apical foramen provides an extremely thin protective layer compared with the other areas of the root.[40] It is also possible that the cementum and dentin could fail to meet in a certain percentage of the cases, as with the cementoenamel junction (CEJ). Thus the mineralized tissue would be exposed, permitting attachment of the clastic resorbing cells to RGD-containing peptides such as osteopontin. There are no clinical manifestations because apical root resorption is asymptomatic. Symptoms that might lead to its diagnosis are associated with periapical inflammation and not root resorption per se.

The radiographic appearance, as described above, is not detectable in most cases, but when apparent, the radiolucencies are evident at the root tip and adjacent bone. Irregular shortening, stumping, or thinning of the root tip is sometimes seen (Fig 19-10). The histologic appearance of a periapical lesion may be either granulomic or cystic.[41,42] On the root surface, resorption of the cementum and dentin results in a scalloped appearance of the root end (see Fig 19-9). Attempts at repair are often seen in the presence of the resorption lacunae, resulting in resorptive and mineralization processes observed adjacent to each other.[2]

The treatment protocol for external root resorption with apical periodontitis should be directed at removing the stimulus for the underlying inflammatory process, ie, the bacteria in the root canal system.[43,44] If a thorough disinfection protocol is followed, an extremely high success rate can be expected.[45,46] At present, the treatment protocol of choice is complete debridement of the root canal systems with sodium hypochlorite irrigation at the first visit. A creamy mix of calcium hydroxide is then introduced with a lentulo instrument. After the intracanal medicament has been in place for at least 7 days,

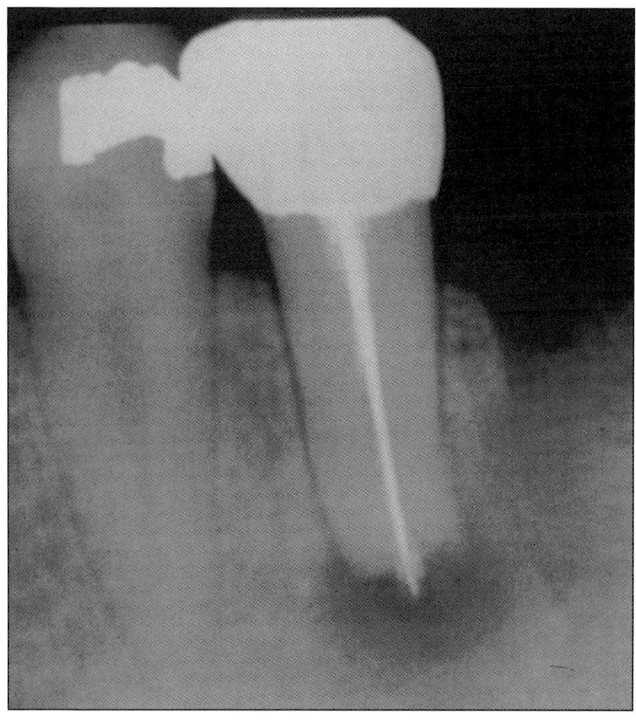

Fig 19-10 Tooth with external apical resorption due to apical periodontitis. The pulp of the tooth is necrotic and infected.

the root canal systems are obturated at the second visit. Recent research indicates that the canal may be obturated after the first visit if larger than currently accepted instrumentation is used.[47] When extensive resorption is present apically, the clinician should account for canal-altering pathologic processes when establishing a working length for canal debridement. Attempts should be made to instrument the full length of the remaining canal while creating a dentin shelf to serve as a stop for the gutta-percha obturation. Apical closure techniques with long-term calcium hydroxide treatment or short-term barriers (eg, mineral trioxide aggregate, collagen plugs) may also be used to ensure a better prognosis for nonsurgical endodontic therapy.[48] If nonsurgical therapy has been unsuccessful in arresting the resorption, apical surgery should be attempted, provided sufficient crown-root ratio will be present after the surgery.

The second type of external root resorption due to pulp space infection is lateral external inflammatory resorption. Lateral periodontitis

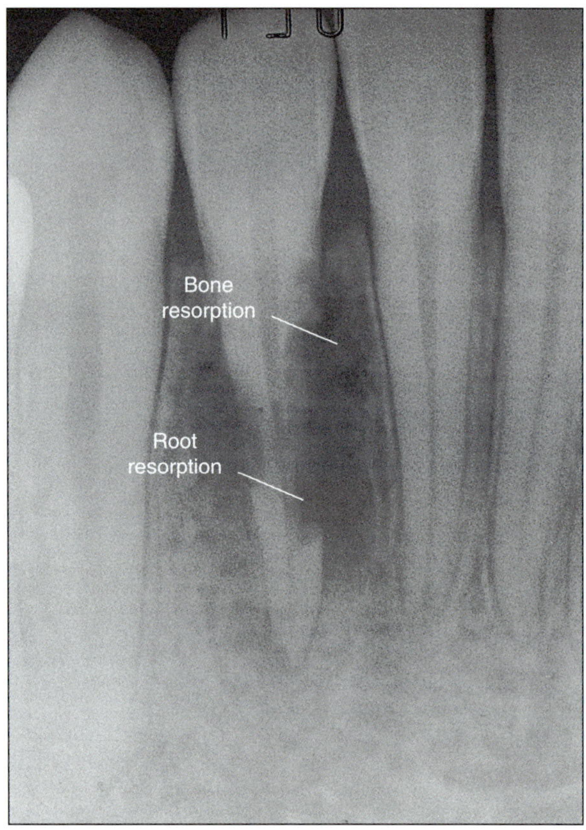

Fig 19-11 Radiographic appearance of external inflammatory resorption due to pulpal infection. Note the radiolucencies in the root and adjacent bone.

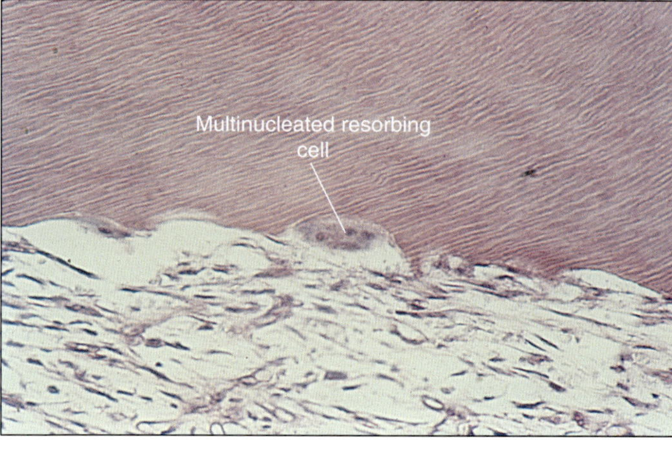

Fig 19-12 Histologic appearance of inflammatory resorption revealing chronically inflamed tissue in relation to the resorbed root surface. Multinucleated giant cells are present in the areas of active resorption on the root surface.

with external root resorption may result when the root loses its cemental protection (Fig 19-11). For pulp space infection to develop, the pulp must first become necrotic. Necrosis occurs after a serious injury in which displacement of the tooth results in severing of the apical blood vessels. In mature teeth, pulp cannot regenerate, and the necrotic pulp will usually become infected by 3 weeks. For details on the typical bacterial contents of a traumatized necrotic pulp, see chapter 12.[49] Because a serious injury is required for pulp necrosis, the protective cemental covering of the root is usually damaged or lost, as well. As described in chapter 4, studies have shown that the loss of the cementum layer leads to a large increase in permeability. Bacterial toxins are free to pass through the dentinal tubules and stimulate an inflammatory response in the corresponding periodontal ligament.[50] The result is resorption of the root and bone. The periodontal infiltrate consists of granulation tissue with lymphocytes, plasma cells, and polymorphonuclear leukocytes. Multinucleated giant cells may bind to exposed RGD peptides and resorb the denuded root surface. This process continues until the stimulus (pulp space bacteria) is removed (Fig 19-12).[51] Radiographically, the resorption is observed as progressive radiolucent areas of the root and adjacent bone (see Fig 19-11).

The treatment protocol for external root resorption due to sulcular inflammation is to first recognize the attachment damage due to the traumatic injury and minimize the subsequent inflammation. The clinician should ideally evaluate pulp space infection 7 to 10 days after the injury.[52,53] Disinfection of the root canal systems removes the stimulus to the periradicular inflammation and the resorption will stop.[1] In most cases, a new attachment will form, but if a large area of root is affected, osseous replacement may result by the mechanism already described.

The two major treatment principles are prevention of pulp space infection and elimination of any bacteria present in the pulp space. An effective way to prevent pulp space infection is, of course, to maintain the vitality of the pulp. If the pulp stays vital, the canal will be free of bacteria and thus this type of external inflammatory root resorption will not occur. In severe injuries where vitality has been lost it is possible under some circumstances to promote revascularization of the pulp. Such revascularization is possible in young teeth with incompletely formed apices if replaced in their original position within 60 minutes of the injury.[54] If the tooth has been avulsed, soaking it in doxycycline for 5 minutes before replantation has been shown to double the revascularization rate.[54] However, even under the best conditions, revascularization will occur only about 50% of the time, which poses a diagnostic dilemma. If the pulp revascularizes, external root resorption will not occur and the root will continue to develop and strengthen. However, if the pulp becomes necrotic and infected, the subsequent external inflammatory root resorption that develops could result in the loss of the tooth in a very short time. At present, the diagnostic tools available cannot detect a vital pulp in this situation for approximately 6 months following successful revascularization. This period of time is obviously unacceptable because by that time the teeth that have not revascularized would be lost to the resorption process. Recently, however, the laser Doppler flowmeter has been shown to be an excellent diagnostic tool for the detection of revascularization in immature teeth. This device appears to accurately detect the presence of vital tissue in the pulp space by 4 weeks after the traumatic injury.

A second major treatment principle is the elimination of any bacteria present in the pulp space. Revascularization cannot occur in teeth with closed apices. These teeth must be endodontically treated before the ischemically necrosed pulp becomes infected, ie, within 7 to 10 days of the injury.[52,53] From a theoretical point of view, timely treatment of these teeth may be considered equivalent to the treatment of teeth with vital pulp. Therefore, endodontic treatment may be completed in one visit. However, efficient treatment is extremely difficult so soon after a serious traumatic injury; therefore, it is beneficial to start the endodontic treatment with chemomechanical preparation, after which an intracanal dressing of creamy calcium hydroxide is placed.[53] The practitioner can then obturate the canal at his or her convenience when periodontal healing of the injury is complete, approximately 1 month after the instrumentation visit. There appears to be no need for long-term calcium hydroxide treatment in cases where endodontic treatment is started within 10 days of the injury. The calcium hydroxide can be applied in a compliant patient for up to 6 months to ensure periodontal health prior to root canal filling with gutta-percha.

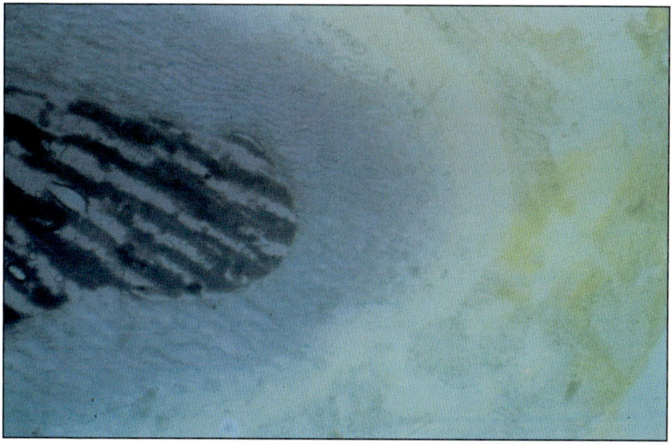

Fig 19-13 Cross section of root filled with calcium hydroxide. The pH indicator shows that the canal and surrounding dentin are basic compared with the surrounding tissue, which is slightly acidic.

When root canal treatment is initiated later than 10 days after the accident or when active external inflammatory resorption is observed, the preferred antibacterial protocol consists of chemomechanical preparation followed by long-term dressing with densely packed calcium hydroxide, which creates an alkaline pH in the surrounding dentinal tubules (Fig 19-13), kills

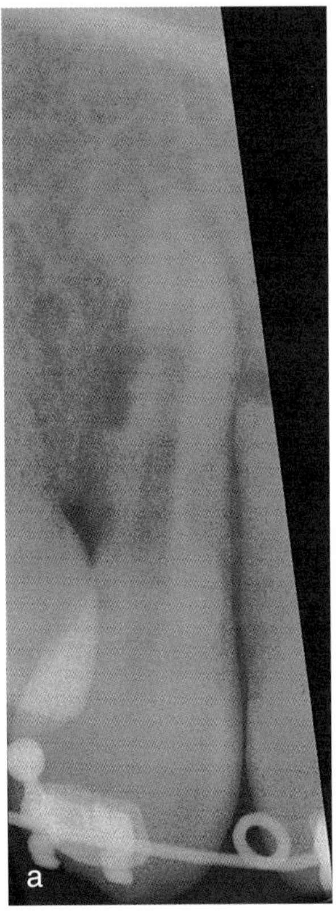

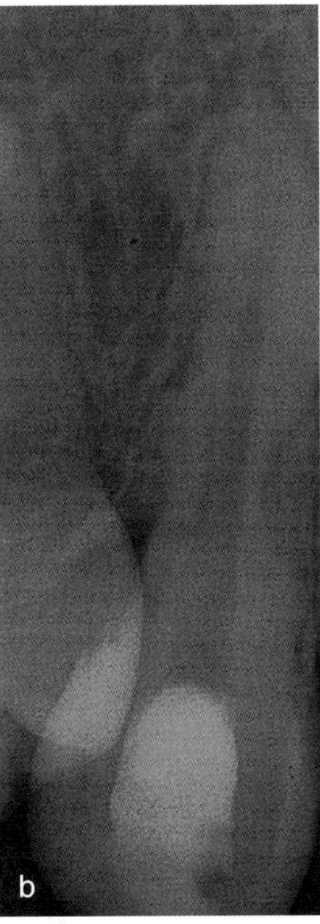

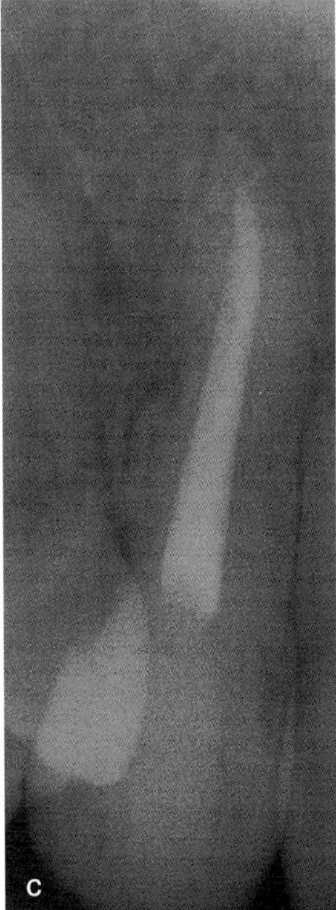

Fig 19-14 Tooth treated for external inflammatory resorption with long-term calcium hydroxide medication. *(a)* At the start of treatment, radiolucencies are present in the root and adjacent bone, indicating active resorption. *(b)* At the 9-month follow-up, the lucencies have disappeared on the adjacent bone and a lamina dura has re-formed, indicating that the process has stopped. *(c)* The canal is obturated with gutta-percha and sealer.

bacteria, and neutralizes endotoxin, a potent inflammatory stimulator.[53]

The patient's first visit consists of thorough chemomechanical instrumentation of the root canal systems and placement of a creamy mix of calcium hydroxide, an intracanal antibacterial agent, using a lentulo instrument. The patient is then seen in approximately 1 month, at which time the canal systems are filled with a dense mix of calcium hydroxide. Once filled, the canals appear radiographically to be calcified, for the radiodensity of calcium hydroxide in the canal is usually similar to the surrounding dentin. Radiographs are then taken at 3-month intervals. At each visit, the tooth is tested for symptoms of periodontitis. In addition to tracking the resorptive process, the presence or absence of the calcium hydroxide (ie, calcium hydroxide washout) is assessed. Because the root surface is so radiodense as to make the assessment of healing difficult, healing of the adjacent bone is also assessed. If the adjacent bone has healed, the resorptive process can be presumed to have stopped in the root as well, and the canal systems may be obturated with gutta-percha (Fig 19-14). If the practioner believes that additional healing before obturation would be beneficial, then the need for replacing the calcium hydroxide in the canal should be assessed. If the canal still appears radiographically to be calcified, there is no need to replace the calcium hydroxide. If on the other hand the canal has regained its radiolucent appearance, then the calcium hydroxide should be repacked and reassessed in another 3 months.

Sulcular inflammation

Sulcular inflammation represents the third general type of inflammatory stimulus that can cause

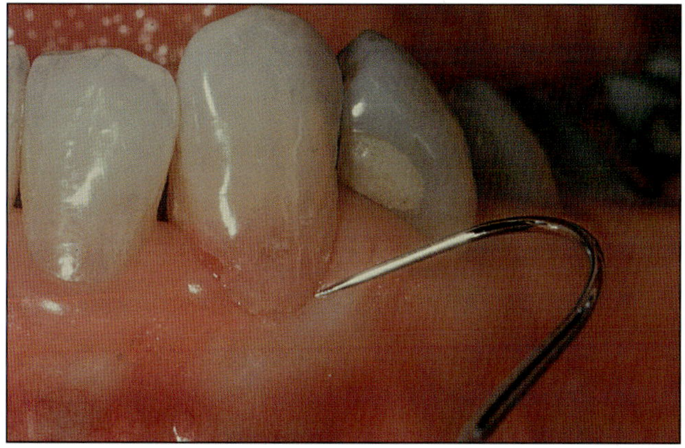

Fig 19-15a A "pink spot" of external inflammatory resorption. The granulomatous tissue has spread coronally and undermined the enamel, causing the pink color in the crown. (Courtesy of Dr Henry Rankow.)

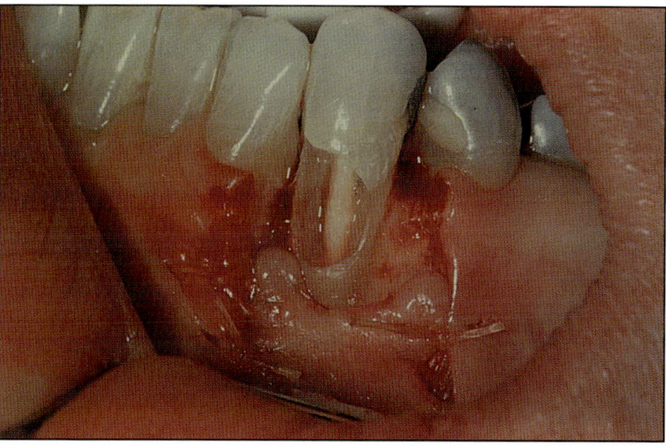

Fig 19-15b Careful removal of the granulomatous tissue shows the canal to be almost entirely encircled but not penetrated by the resorptive defect. (Courtesy of Dr Henry Rankow.)

external root resorption. This progressive external root resorption of inflammatory origin occurs immediately below the epithelial attachment of the tooth, usually but not exclusively at the cervical area of the tooth. Because of this location, it has been referred to as *subepithelial inflammatory root resorption*. Although it is often called *cervical root resorption*, the periodontal attachment of teeth is not always at the cervical margin; the same process can occur more apically on the root surface. In fact, the anatomic connotation of "cervical" root resorption has led to confusion and misdiagnosis of this condition, inspiring attempts to rename this type of external resorption.[55,56]

The pathogenesis of cervical root resorption is not fully understood.[51] However, because its histologic appearance and progressive nature are identical to other forms of progressive inflammatory root resorption, it seems logical that the pathogenesis would be the same (ie, an unprotected or altered root surface attracting resorbing cells and an inflammatory response maintained by infection). Causes of root damage immediately below the epithelial attachment of the root include orthodontic tooth movement, trauma, nonvital bleaching, and other less definable factors. It is important to realize that the pulp plays no role in subepithelial inflammatory root resorption and is usually normal in these cases.[51] Because the source of stimulation (infection) is not the pulp, it has been postulated that bacteria in the sulcus of the tooth stimulate and sustain an inflammatory response in the periodontium at the attachment level of the root.[51]

Subepithelial inflammatory root resorption is asymptomatic and is usually detected only through routine radiographs. Occasionally, symptoms of pulpitis will develop if the resorption is extensive. When the resorption is long-standing, granulation tissue may be seen to undermine the enamel of the crown of the tooth, resulting in a pinkish appearance. This "pink spot" has traditionally been used to describe the pathognomonic clinical picture of internal root resorption, leading to the misdiagnosis and treatment of many cases of subepithelial inflammatory root resorption as internal root resorption (Fig 19-15).

The radiographic appearance of subepithelial inflammatory root resorption can be quite variable. If the resorptive process occurs mesially or distally on the root surface, small radiolucent openings into the root are common. The radiolucency expands coronally and apically in the dentin and reaches, but usually does not perforate, the root canal (Fig 19-16). If the resorptive pro-

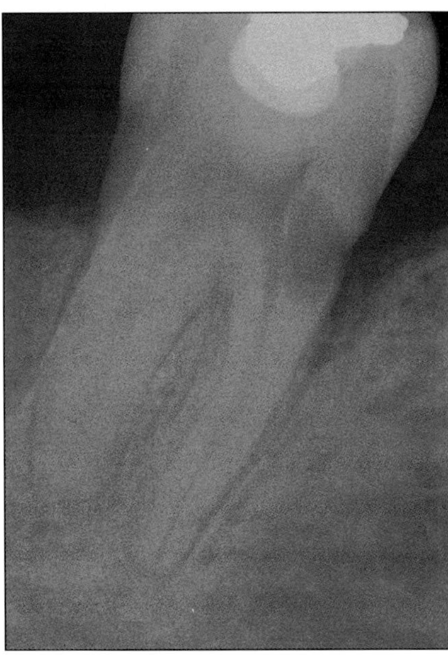

Fig 19-16 Radiographic appearance of external subepithelial root resorption. The resorptive defect on the mesial side of the molar shows a small opening into the root. The apical and coronal expansion reaches but does not penetrate the pulp canal. Note the adjacent bone resorption.

cess is buccal or palatolingual, the radiographic picture is dependent on the extent to which the resorptive process has spread in the dentin. It is seen as a radiolucency at the attachment level or as mottled if it has spread coronally or apically to any considerable degree. Because the pulp is not involved, its outline can usually be distinguished through the resorptive defect (Fig 19-17).

Space limitations preclude a complete review of the treatment strategies for subepithelial inflammatory root resorption. Fortunately, recent reviews discuss strategies for treating this form of external root resorption.[57]

Internal Root Resorption

Internal root resorption is rare in permanent teeth. When it does occur, it is characterized by an oval-shaped enlargement of the root canal space.[58] External resorption, which is much more common, is often misdiagnosed as internal resorption.

Etiology of internal root resorption

Internal root resorption is marked by resorption of the internal aspect of the root via multinucleated giant cells adjacent to granulation tissue in the pulp (Fig 19-18). Chronic inflammatory tissue is common in the pulp, but only rarely does it result in the conditions necessary for recruitment and activation of the clastic cells that mediate resorption. There are different hypotheses on the origin of the pulpal granulation tissue involved in internal resorption. The first and most widely accepted hypothesis is that infected coronal pulp tissue leads to the formation of adjacent apical granulation pulp tissue (see also chapter 10). A second hypothesis proposes that the granulation tissue is of nonpulpal origin, possibly originating from cells circulating in the vascular compartment or from cells originating in the periodontium. It has been shown that communication between the coronal necrotic tissue and the vital pulp is through appropriately oriented dentinal tubules (see Fig 19-18).[59] One investigation reported that resorption of the dentin is frequently associated with deposition of hard tissue resembling bone or cementum, not dentin.[54] The investigators postulate that the resorbing tissue is not of pulpal origin but is actually "metaplastic" tissue derived from the pulpal invasion of macrophage-like cells circulating in the vascular compartment. Still others have proposed that the pulp tissue is replaced by periodontium-like connective tissue when internal resorption is present.[60] These hypotheses are not mutually exclusive, and it is possible that all contribute to the formation of granulation tissue in pulp in various clinical cases.

In addition to the presence of granulation tissue in pulp, internal root resorption takes place only when the odontoblastic layer and predentin are lost or altered.[51] Causes of predentin loss adjacent to granulation tissue are not obvious, but trauma has been frequently suggested,[2,61] perhaps even as an initiating factor in internal resorption.[59]

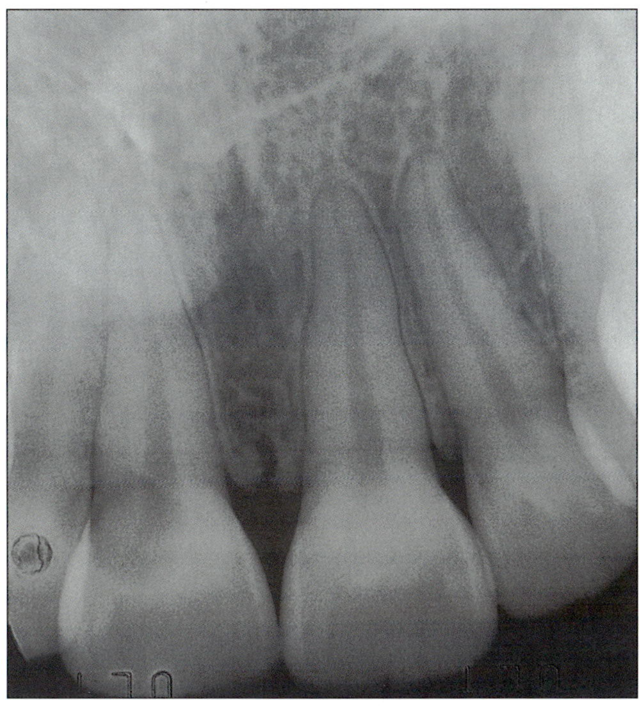

Fig 19-17a Radiographic appearance of a maxillary incisor with external resorption extending coronally. Note the outline of the root canal through the resorptive radiolucency.

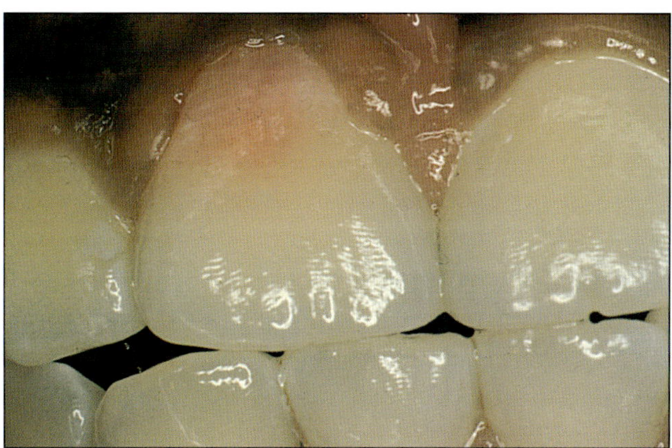

Fig 19-17b The clinical appearance shows a pink spot close to the gingival margin on the labial surface of the tooth.

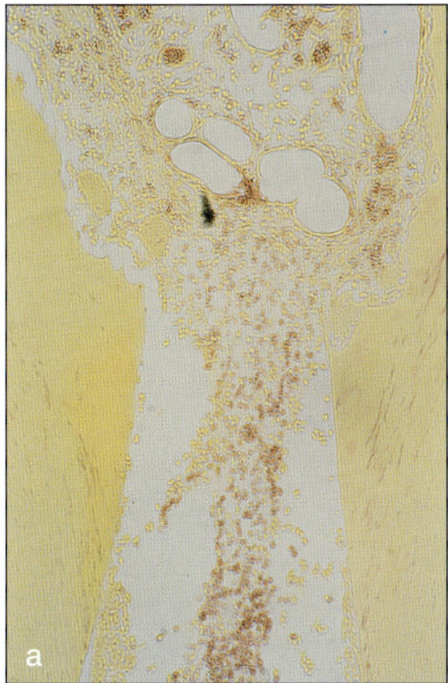

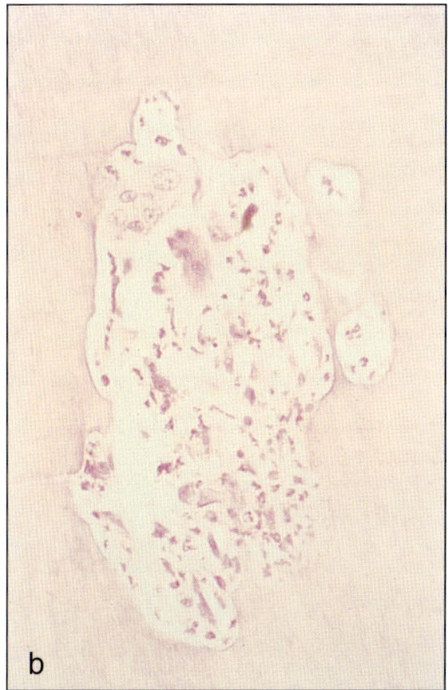

Fig 19-18 Histologic section of internal root resorption stained with Brown and Brenn. *(a)* Bacteria are seen in the dentinal tubules communicating between the necrotic coronal segment and the apical granulation tissue and resorbing cells. *(b)* Apical dentin is resorbed. (Courtesy of Dr Leif Tronstad.)

Traumatic episodes are divided into two types: transient and progressive, the latter of which requires continuous stimulation by infection. Another possible cause of predentin loss may be extreme heat produced by cutting on dentin without an adequate water spray (see also chapters 15 and 16).The heat presumably destroys the predentin layer, predisposing the tooth to internal resorption if the coronal aspect of the pulp subsequently becomes infected. Under these conditions, bacterial products could initiate typical inflammation in conjunction with resorbing giant cells in the vital pulp adjacent to the denuded root surface. In support of this possible scenario, internal root resorption has been produced experimentally by the application of diathermy.[62]

Clinical manifestations of internal root resorption

Internal root resorption is usually asymptomatic and is first recognized clinically through routine radiographs. Pain may be a presenting symptom if perforation of the crown occurs and the granulation tissue is exposed to oral fluids. For internal resorption to be active, at least part of the pulp must be vital so that a positive response to pulp sensitivity testing is possible. It should be remembered that the coronal portion of the pulp is often necrotic, whereas the apical pulp, which includes the internal resorptive defect, may remain vital. Therefore, a negative sensitivity test result does not rule out active internal resorption. It is also possible that the pulp becomes nonvital after a period of active resorption, giving a negative sensitivity test, radiographic signs of internal resorption, and radiographic signs of apical inflammation. Traditionally, the pink tooth, due to the granulation tissue in the coronal dentin undermining the crown enamel, has been thought to be pathognomonic of internal root resorption (Fig 19-19). However, as described above, a pink tooth can also be a feature of subepithelial external inflammatory root resorption, which must be ruled out before a diagnosis of internal root resorption is made.

Radiographic appearance of internal root resorption

The usual radiographic presentation of internal root resorption is a fairly uniform radiolucent enlargement of the pulp canal (Fig 19-20). Because the resorption is initiated in the root canal, the resorptive defect includes some part of the root canal space. Therefore, the original outline of the root canal is distorted. Only on rare occasions, when the internal resorptive defect penetrates the root and impacts the periodontal ligament, does the adjacent bone show radiographic changes.

Histologic appearance of internal root resorption

Like that of other inflammatory resorptive defects, the histologic presentation of internal resorption is granulation tissue with multinucleated giant cells (see Fig 19-18). An area of necrotic pulp is found coronal to the granulation tissue. Dentinal tubules containing microorganisms and communicating between the necrotic zone and the granulation tissue can sometimes be seen (see Fig 19-18).[10,51,52,59,63,64] Unlike external root resorption, the adjacent bone is not affected by internal root resorption.

Treatment of internal root resorption

Treatment of internal root resorption is conceptually very easy. Because the resorptive defect is the result of the inflamed pulp and the blood supply to the tissue is through the apical foramina, endodontic treatment that effectively removes the blood supply to the resorbing cells is the treatment approach. After adequate anesthesia is obtained, the canal apical to the internal defect is explored and a working length short of the radiographic apex is used. The apical canal is thoroughly instrumented to ensure that the blood supply to the tissue resorbing the root is cut off. Upon completion of the root canal instrumentation, paper points should be able to

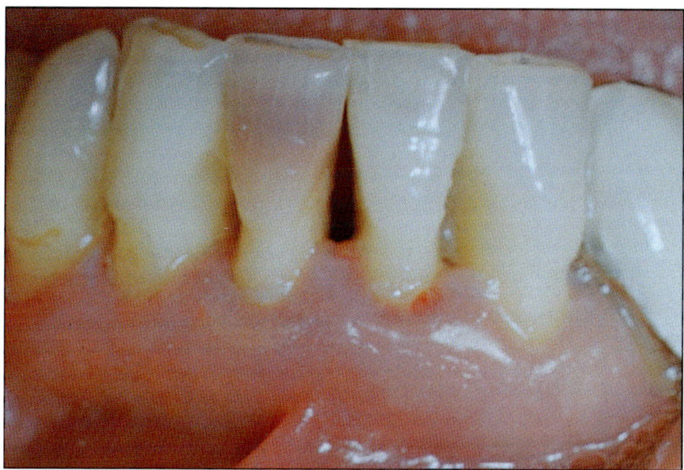

Fig 19-19 Pink spot on a mandibular central incisor indicating internal root resorption. The pink discoloration is due to the undermining of the enamel by the granulomatous tissue. Because the pink spot is so far from the periodontal attachment level, this example is unlikely to be external in nature.

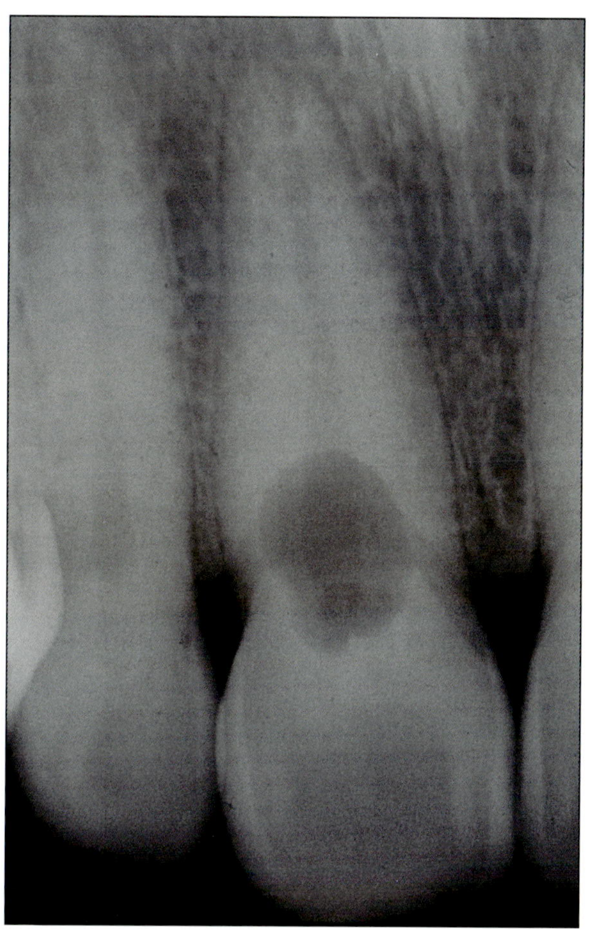

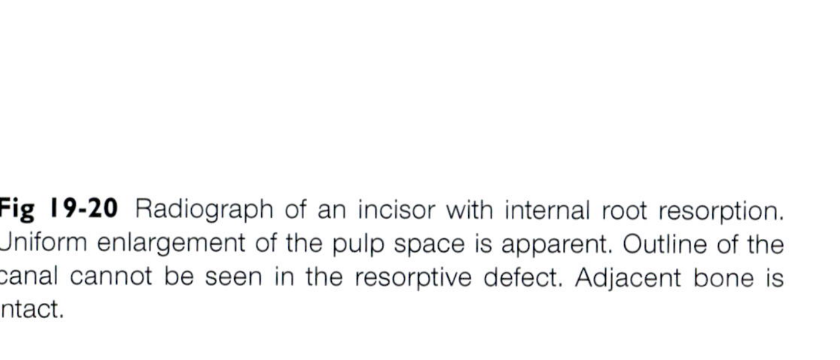

Fig 19-20 Radiograph of an incisor with internal root resorption. Uniform enlargement of the pulp space is apparent. Outline of the canal cannot be seen in the resorptive defect. Adjacent bone is intact.

maintain a blood-free, dry canal. Calcium hydroxide is administered into the canal to facilitate removal of the tissue in the irregular defect at the next visit, when the tooth and defect are filled with softened gutta-percha. In rare cases involving extremely large internal resorptive defects in the apical part of the canal, it may be possible to surgically remove the defective root and place an endodontic implant in order to maintain stability of the tooth. However, with modern dental techniques this treatment alternative should be weighed against the advantages of implant dentistry.

Summary: Diagnostic Features of External vs Internal Root Resorption

It is often very difficult to distinguish external from internal root resorption, so misdiagnosis and incorrect treatment can result. What follows is a list of typical diagnostic features of each resorptive type. Box 19-1 provides an overview of the key elements of these diagnostic features and may serve as a quick reference in clinical practice.

Box 19-1 Summary of typical diagnostic features of root resorption

- External inflammatory root resorption due to pulp infection
  - Apical external root resorption
  - Negative pulp sensitivity test, with or without a history of trauma
- Lateral external root resorption
  - History of trauma
  - Negative pulp sensitivity test
  - Lesion moves on angled X rays
  - Root canal visualized radiographically overlying the defect
  - Bony radiolucency apparent
- Subepithelial external inflammation due to sulcular infection
  - History of trauma (often forgotten or not appreciated by the patient)
  - Positive pulp sensitivity test
  - Lesion located at the attachment level of the tooth
  - Lesion moves on angled X rays
  - Root canal outline is undistorted and can be visualized radiographically
  - Crestal bony defect associated with the lesion
  - Pink spot possible
- Internal root resorption
  - History of trauma, crown preparation, or pulpotomy
  - Positive pulp sensitivity test likely
  - May occur at any location along the root canal (not only at attachment level)
  - Lesion stays associated with the root canal on angled X rays
  - Radiolucency contained in the root without an adjacent bony defect
  - Pink spot possible

Radiographic features

A change of X-ray angle should give a fairly good indication of whether a resorptive defect is internal or external. A lesion of internal origin appears close to the canal whatever the angle of the X ray (Figs 19-21 and 19-22). On the other hand, a defect on the external aspect of the root moves away from the canal as the angle changes (Figs 19-21 and 19-23). In addition, it is usually possible to distinguish whether the external root defect is buccal or palatolingual by using the buccal object rule. In internal resorption, the outline of the root canal is usually distorted and the root canal and the radiolucent resorptive defect appear contiguous (see Figs 19-20 to 19-22). When the defect is external, the root canal outline appears normal and can usually be seen "running through" the radiolucent defect (see Figs 19-17 and 19-23).

It is important to realize that external inflammatory root resorption is always accompanied by resorption of the bone in addition to the root (see Figs 19-11 and 19-16). Therefore, radiolucencies are apparent in the root as well as the adjacent bone. Internal root resorption does not involve the bone; as a rule, the radiolucency is confined to the root (see Figs 19-20 and 19-21). On rare occasions, if the internal defect perforates the root, the adjacent bone is resorbed and appears radiolucent on the radiograph.

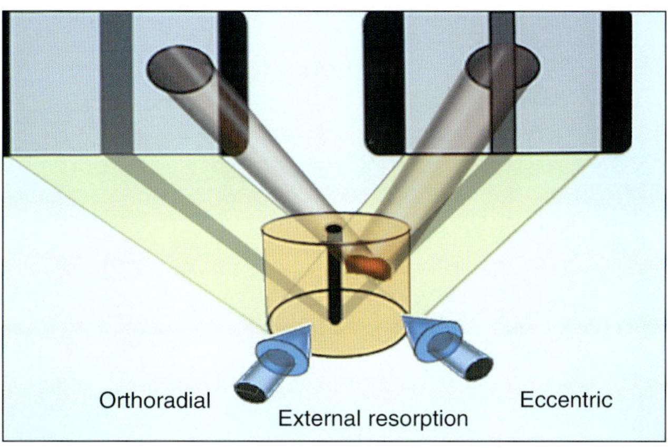

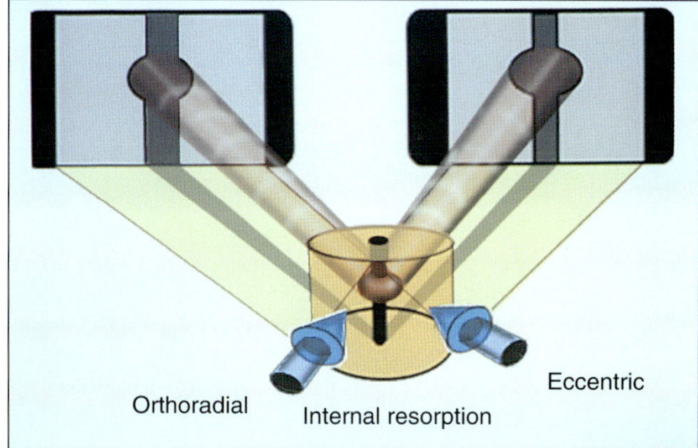

Fig 19-21 Diagrammatic representation of the difference between internal and external root resorption when the X-ray angle is changed. (Courtesy of Dr Claudia Barthel.)

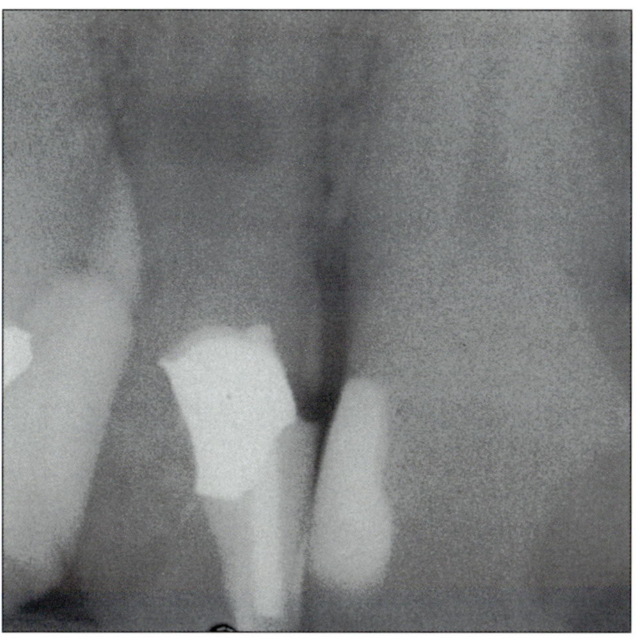

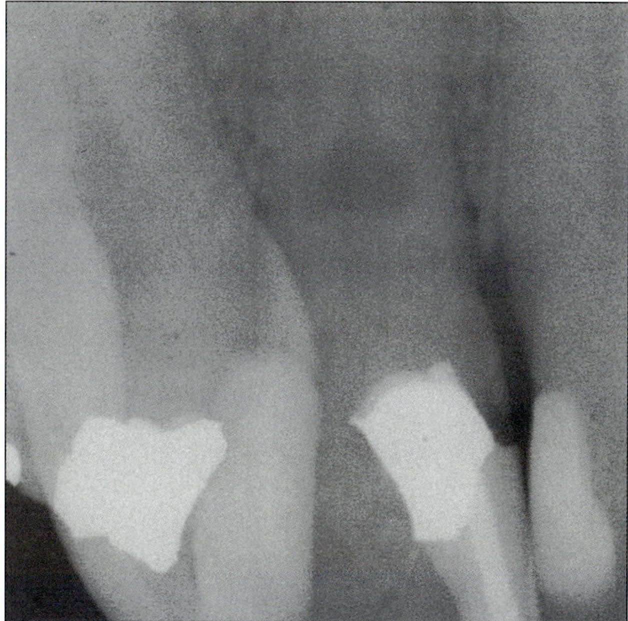

Fig 19-22 Internal resorption. Radiographs from two different horizontal projections depict the lesion within the confines of the root canal in both views.

Vitality testing

External inflammatory resorption on the apical and lateral aspects of the root involves an infected pulp space, indicated by a negative response to sensitivity tests. On the other hand, because subepithelial external root resorption does not involve the pulp (the bacteria are thought to originate in the sulcus of the tooth), this type of resorption is often associated with a normal response to sensitivity testing. Internal root resorption usually occurs in teeth with vital pulps and elicits a positive response to sensitivity testing. However, teeth that exhibit internal root resorption sometimes register a negative response to sensitivity testing, often in cases where the

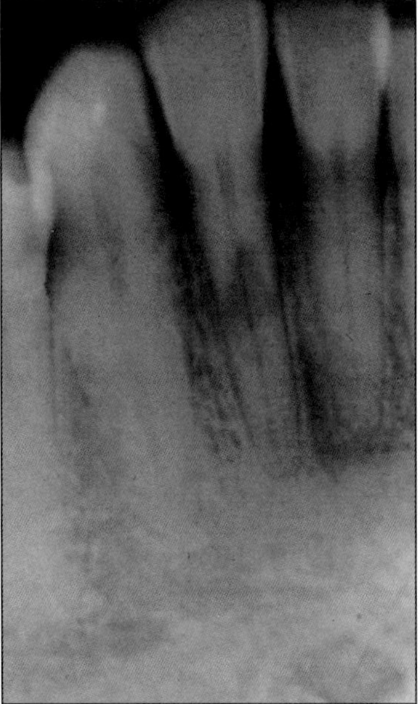
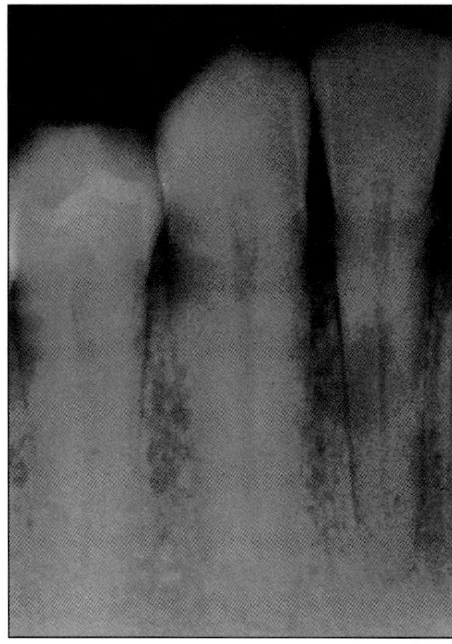

Fig 19-23 External resorption. Radiographs from two different horizontal projections depict movement of the lesion to outside the confines of the root canal.

coronal pulp is removed or necrotic and the active resorbing cells are more apical in the canal. In addition, the pulp may become necrotic after active resorption has taken place.

Pink spot

Because the pulp is nonvital in either apical or lateral external root resorption, the granulation tissue that produces a pink spot is not present in such cases. However, a pink spot caused by granulation tissue undermining enamel is a possible sign of both subepithelial external (see Fig 19-15) and internal root resorption (see Fig 19-19).

Common misdiagnoses

The majority of misdiagnoses of resorptive defects are made in distinguishing subepithelial external and internal root resorption. A diagnosis should always be confirmed while treatment is proceeding. When root canal therapy is the treatment of choice for an apparent internal root resorption, bleeding within the canal should cease quickly after pulp extirpation if the blood supply to the granulation tissue is the apical blood vessels. But if bleeding continues during treatment, particularly if it is still present at the second visit, the source of the blood supply is external and treatment for external resorption should be carried out. Also, upon obturation in cases of internal resorption, it should be possible to fill the entire canal from within. Failure to fill the canal suggests an external lesion. Finally, if the blood supply of an internal resorption defect is removed upon pulp extirpation, any continuation of the resorptive process on recall radiographs should alert the dentist to the possibility that an external resorptive defect was misdiagnosed.

Systemic Causes of Root Resorption

The roots of teeth show a remarkable resistance to detectable resorption, even with systemic diseases that can cause significant bone resorption (see also chapter 21). With hyperparathyroidism osteitis deformans (Paget disease), for example, radiographically apparent bone resorption is not accompanied by resorption of the roots.[65] However, hormonal disturbances and genetic factors have been shown sometimes to cause resorption of the root.[66] Renal dystrophy results in an increased oxylate concentration in the blood and precipitation in the hard tissues, which can cause root resorption.[8,55,67,68] Genetic linkage is implicated because external root resorption of no apparent cause has been found in members of the same family.[67] As our knowledge and test procedures advance, resorption presently diagnosed as idiopathic will in the future probably be increasingly found to be of systemic or genetic origin.

References

1. Hammarstrom L, Lindskog S. General morphologic aspects of resorption of teeth and alveolar bone. Int Endod J 1985;18:93-108.
2. Seltzer S. Endodontology. Philadelphia: Lea and Febiger, 1988.
3. Orban B. The epithelial network in the periodontal membrane. J Am Dent Assoc 1952;44:632.
4. Loe H, Waerhaug J. Experimental replantation of teeth in dogs and monkeys. Arch Oral Biol 1961;3:176.
5. Andreasen JO. Review of root resorption systems and models: Etiology of root resorption and the homeostatic mechanisms of the periodontal ligament. In: Davidovitch Z (ed). The Biologic Mechanisms of Tooth Eruption and Resorption. Birmingham, AL: EB-SCOP Media, 1989.
6. Nakamura I, Takahashi N, Sasaki T, Jimi E, Kurokawa T, Suda T. Chemical and physical properties of the extracellular matrix are required for the actin ring formation in osteoclasts. J Bone Miner Res 1996;11:1873-1879.
7. Karring T, Nyman S, Lindhe J. Healing following implantation of periodontitis affected roots into bone tissue. J Clin Periodontol 1980;7:96-105.
8. Polson AM, Caton JM. Factors influencing periodontal repair and regeneration. J Periodontol 1982;53:617-625.
9. Stenvik A, Mjor IA. Pulp and dentin reaction to experimental tooth intrusion: A histologic study of the initial changes. Am J Orthod 1970;57:370-385.
10. Wedenberg C. Evidence for a dentin-derived inhibitor of macrophage spreading. Scan J Dent Res 1987;95: 381-388.
11. Kong YY, Yoshida H, Sarosi I, Tan HL, Timms E, Capparelli C, et al. OPGL is a key regulator of osteoclastogenesis, lymphocyte development and lymph-node organogenesis. Nature 1999;397:315-323.
12. Wada N, Maeda H, Tanabe K, Tsuda E, Yano K, Nakamuta H, Akamine A. Periodontal ligament cells secrete the factor that inhibits osteoclastic differentiation and function: The factor is osteoprotegerin/ osteoclastogenesis inhibitory factor. J Periodontal Res 2001;36:56-63.
13. Sakata M, Shiba H, Komatsuzawa H, Fujita T, Ohta K, Sugai M, et al. Expression of osteoprotegerin (osteoclastogenesis inhibitory factor) in cultures of human dental mesenchymal cells and epithelial cells. J Bone Miner Res 1999;14:1486-1492.
14. Hopewell-Smith A. The process of osteolysis and odontolysis or so-called "absorption" of calcified tissues: A new original investigation. Dent Cosmos 1903;72:323.
15. Selvig KA, Zander HA. Chemical analysis and microradiography of cementum and dentin from periodontically diseased human teeth. J Periodontol 1962;33:103.
16. Saygin NE, Giannobile WV, Somerman MJ. Molecular and cell biology of cementum [review]. Periodontol 2000;24:73-98.
17. Andreasen JO. Relationship between surface and inflammatory resorption and changes in the pulp after replantation of permanent incisorss in monkeys. J Endod 1981;7:294-301.
18. Andreasen JO. The effect of pulp extirpation or root canal treatment upon periodontal healing after replantation of permanent incisors in monkeys. J Endod 1981;7:245-252.
19. Manolagas SC. Birth and death of bone cells: Basic regulatory mechanisms and implications for the pathogenesis and treatment of osteoporosis. Endocr Rev 2000;21; 115-137.
20. Reddy SV, Roodman GD. Control of osteoclast differentiation. Crit Rev Eukaryotic Gene Expression 1998;8: 1-17.
21. Okamura T, Shimokawa H, Takagi Y, Ono H, Sasaki S. Detection of collagenase mRNA in odontoclasts of bovine root-resorbing tissue by in situ hybridization. Calcif Tiss Int 1993;52:325-330.
22. Heyman D, Rousselle A. Gp130 cytokine family and bone cells. Cytokine 2000;12:1455-1468.
23. Kulihara N, Bertolini D, Suda T, Akiyama Y, Roodman GD. IL-6 stimulates osteoclast-like multinucleated cell formation in long term human marrow cultures by inducing IL-1 release. J Immunol 1990;144:4226-4230.
24. Udagawa N, Takahashi N, Katagiri T, Tamura T, Wada S, Findlay DM, et al. Interleukin (IL-6) induction of osteoclast differentiation depends on IL-6 receptors expressed on osteoblastic cells but not on osteoclastic progenitors. J Exp Med 1995;182:1461-1468.

25. Adebanjo OA, Moonga BS, Yamate T, Sun L, Minkin C, Abe E, Zaidi M. Mode of action of interleukin-6 on mature osteoclasts: Novel interactions with extracellular Ca^{2+} sensing in the regulation of osteoclastic bone resorption. J Cell Biol 1996;142:1349–1356.
26. Goldring SR, Gorn AH, Yamin M, Krane SM, Wang JT. Characterization of the structural and functional properties of cloned calcitonin receptor cDNAs. Horm Metab Res 1993;25:477–480.
27. Suda T, Udagawa N, Takahasi N. Cells of bone: Osteoclast generation. In: Bilezikian JP, Raisz LG, Rodan GA (eds). Principles of Bone Biology. San Diego: Academic, 1996:87–102.
28. Lindskog S, Blomlof L, Hammarstrom L. Repair of periodontal tissues in vivo and vitro. J Clin Periodontol 1983;10:188–205.
29. Nilsen R. Microfilaments in cells associated with induced heterotopic bone formation in guinea pigs: An immunofluorescence and ultrastructural study. Acta Pathol Microbiol Scand 1980;88:129–134.
30. Pierce AM. Cellular Mechanisms in Bone and Tooth Resorption [dissertation]. Stockholm: Karolinska Institute, 1988.
31. Aubin JE. Osteoclast adhesion and resorption: The role of podosomes. J Bone Miner Res 1992:7:365–368.
32. Vaananen K. Osteoclast function: Biology and mechanisms. In: Bilezikian JP, Raisz LG, Rodan GA (eds). Principles of Bone Biology. San Diego: Academic, 1996: 103–113.
33. Aubin JE, Bonnelye E. Osteoprotegerin and its ligand: A new paradigm for regulation of osteoclastogenesis and bone resorption. Osteoporos Int 2000;11:905–913.
34. Giachelli CM, Steitz S. Osteopontin: A versatile regulator of inflammation and biomineralization. Matrix Biol 2000;19:615–622.
35. Bartkiewicz M, Hernando N, Reddy SV, Roodman DG, Baron R. Characterization of the osteoclast vacuolar H+-ATPase B-subunit. Gene 1995;160:157–164.
36. Lindskog S, Pierce AM, Blomlof L, Hammarstrom L. The role of the necrotic periodontal membrane in cementum resorption and ankylosis. Endod Dent Traumatol 1985;1:96–101.
37. Hammarstrom L, Pierce A, Blomlof L, Feiglin B, Lindskog S. Tooth avulsion and replantation: A review. Endod Dent Traumatol 1986;2:1–8.
38. Trope M. Luxation injuries and external root resorption: Etiology, treatment and prognosis. CDA J 2000;11: 860.
39. Bender IB, Byers MR, Mori K. Periapical replacement resorption of permanent, vital, endodontically treated incisors after orthodontic movement: Report of two cases. J Endod 1997;23:768–773.
40. Kuttler Y. Microscopic investigation of root apexes. J Am Dent Assoc 1955;50:544.
41. Bhaskar SN. Periapical lesions: Types, incidence, and clinical features. Oral Surg Oral Med Oral Pathol 1966; 21:657–671.
42. Lalonde ER, Luebke RG. The frequency and distribution of periapical cysts and granulomas: An evaluation of 800 specimens. Oral Surg Oral Med Oral Pathol 1968; 25:861–868.
43. Dalton C, Phillips C, Pettiette M, Trope M. Bacterial reduction with nickel titanium rotary instruments. J Endod 1998;24:763–777.
44. Shuping GB, Orstavik D, Sigurdsson A, Trope M. Reduction of intracanal bacteria using nickel-titanium rotary instrumentation and various medicaments. J Endod 2000;26:751–755.
45. Byström A, Happonen R, Sjögren U, Sundqvist G. Healing of periapical lesions of pulpless teeth after endodontic treatment with controlled asepsis. Endod Dent Traumatol 1987;3:58–63.
46. Sjögren U, Figdor D, Persson S, Sundqvist G. Influence of infection at the time of root filling on the outcome of endodontic treatment of teeth with apical periodontitis. Int Endod J 1997;30:297–306.
47. Card S, Trope M, Sigurdsson A, Orstravik D. The effectiveness of increased apical enlargement in reducing intracanal bacteria. J Endod (in press).
48. Kerekes K, Heide S, Jacobsen I. Follow-up examination of endodontic treatment in traumatized juvenile incisors. J Endod 1980;6:744–748.
49. Bergenholtz G. Micro-organisms from necrotic pulp of traumatized teeth. Odont Rev 1974;25:347–358.
50. Andreasen JO. Periodontal healing after replantation of traumatically avulsed human teeth: Assessment by mobility testing and radiography. Acta Odontol Scand 1975;33:325.
51. Tronstad L. Root resorption: Etiology, terminology and clinical manifestations. Endod Dent Traumatol 1988;4: 241–252.
52. Trope M, Yesilsoy C, Koren L, Moshonov J, Friedman S. Effect of different endodontic treatment protocols on periodontal repair and root resorption of replanted dog teeth. J Endod 1992;18:492–496.
53. Trope M, Moshonov J, Nissan R, Buxt P, Yesilsoy C. Short-versus long-term $Ca(OH)_2$ treatment of established inflammatory root resorption in replanted dog teeth. Endod Dent Traumatol 1995;11:124–128.
54. Cvek M, Cleaton-Jones P, Austin J, Lownie J, Kling M, Fatti P. Effect of topical application of doxycycline on pulp revascularization and periodontal healing in reimplanted monkey incisors. Endod Dent Traumatol 1990;6: 170–176.
55. Frank AL, Bakland LK. Nonendodontic therapy for supraosseous extracanal invasive resorption. J Endod 1987;13: 348–355.

56. Trope M. Root resorption of dental and traumatic origin: Classification based on etiology. Pract Periodontics Aesthet Dent 1998;10:515–522.
57. Trope M. Subattachment inflammatory root resorption: Treatment strategies. Pract Periodontics Aesthet Dent 1998;10:1005–1010.
58. Andreasen JO, Andreasen FM. Textbook and Color Atlas of Traumatic Injuries to the Teeth, ed 3. Copenhagen and St. Louis: Munksgaard and Mosby, 1994.
59. Wedenberg C, Lindskog S. Experimental internal resorption in monkey teeth. Endod Dent Traumatol 1985;1:221–227.
60. Stanley HR. Diseases of the dental pulp. In: Tieck RW (ed). Oral Pathology. New York: McGraw Hill, 1965.
61. Wedenberg C, Zetterqvist L. Internal resorption in human teeth: A histological, scanning electron microscope and enzyme histo-chemical study. J Endod 1987;13:255–259.
62. Gottlieb B, Orban B. Veränderungen in Periodontium nach chirurgischer Diathermie. ZJ Stomatol 1930;28:1208.
63. Tronstad L, Andreasen JO, Hasselgren G, Kristerson L, Riis I. pH changes in dental tissues after root canal filling with calcium hydroxide. J Endod 1980;7:17–21.
64. Silverman S Jr, Ware WH, Gillooly C Jr. Dental aspects of hyperparathyroidism. Oral Surg Oral Med Oral Pathol 1968;26:184–189.
65. Smith BJ, Eveson JW. Paget's disease of bone with particular reference to dentistry. J Oral Pathol 1981;10:223–247.
66. Sharawy AM, Mills PB, Gibbons RJ. Multiple ankylosis occurring in rat teeth. Oral Surg 1968;26:856–860.
67. Gold SI, Hasselgren G. Peripheral inflammatory root resorption: A review of the literature with case reports. J Clin Periodontol 1992;19:523–534.
68. Moskow BS. Periodontal manifestations of hyperoxaluria and oxalosis. J Periodontol 1989;60:271–278.

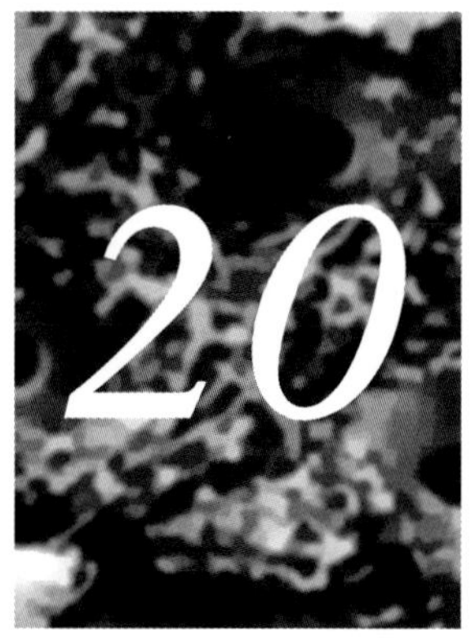

Differential Diagnosis of Odontalgia

Samuel Seltzer, DDS
Kenneth M. Hargreaves, DDS, PhD

Epidemiologic studies indicate that toothaches represent the most prevalent form of orofacial pain, with about 12% to 14% of the population reporting a history of a toothache over a 6-month period.[1-3] Although these studies indicate that dental pain is the most commonly reported form of orofacial pain, it should be recognized that this symptom could be caused by painful disorders of either odontogenic or nonodontogenic origin. Thus, pain management begins with developing an accurate differential diagnosis of dental pain. This is a critical first step in pain management since effective treatment is directed at removing or controlling the underlying condition (see chapter 9).

Understanding the basic science of pain mechanisms and the therapeutics of pain management is a major theme in pulpal biology. Accordingly, this text includes detailed reviews on common etiologic factors (chapter 12), inflammatory responses in pulpal (chapters 5, 10, and 11) and periradicular tissue (chapter 17), the neuroanatomy and neurophysiology of dental pulp (chapter 7), pain mechanisms in pulpal tissue and the brain (chapter 8), and strategies for pain management (chapter 9). This chapter contributes to that foundation of knowledge by focusing on the differential diagnosis of odontogenic and nonodontogenic dental pain.

The last decade has seen an explosion in the area of pain research, leading to the development of new theories, diagnostic tests, and treatment strategies. Major references on this topic are available to the interested reader.[4-6] However, the primary purpose of this chapter is not to provide a broad overview of this topic, but instead to focus on strategies for developing a differential diagnosis of odontogenic and nonodontogenic dental pain. Other sources should be reviewed for an extensive discussion of etiology, diagnosis, and management of various nonodontogenic pain disorders.[6-19]

Common Features of Odontogenic and Nonodontogenic Dental Pain

Fortunately, the large majority of patients reporting dental pain have symptoms that are caused by odontogenic pain mechanisms (see chapters

Box 20-1 Common features of odontogenic dental pain

- Presence of etiologic factors for an odontogenic origin of pain (eg, caries, leakage of restorations, trauma, fracture)
- Ability to reproduce chief complaint during examination
- Pain reduction by local anesthetic injection
- Unilateral pain
- Pain qualities: Dull, aching, throbbing
- Localized pain*
- Sensitivity to temperature*
- Sensitivity to percussion, digital pressure*

*Diagnosis-specific.

Box 20-2 Selected features of nonodontogenic dental pain

- No apparent etiologic factors for odontogenic pain (eg, no caries, leaky restorations, trauma, fracture)
- No consistent relief of pain by local anesthetic injection
- Bilateral pain or multiple painful teeth
- Chronic pain that is not responsive to dental treatment
- Pain qualities: Burning, electric shooting, stabbing, dull ache*
- Pain that occurs with a headache*
- Increased pain associated with palpation of trigger points or muscles*
- Increased pain associated with emotional stress, physical exercise, head position, etc*

*Diagnosis-specific.

7 and 8). Examples of pathoses producing odontogenic pain include reversible pulpitis, irreversible pulpitis, acute apical periodontitis, and acute apical abscess.[19,20] However, the clinician will certainly encounter those patients reporting dental pain that is actually caused by a nonodontogenic etiology. Therefore, it is necessary to be diligent in developing a differential diagnosis for all patients.[14-18]

Common features associated with pain of odontogenic origin are listed in Box 20-1.[12,15-21] Although this list provides a useful summary of characteristic features of odontogenic pain, the skilled clinician will realize that not all cases present with exactly the same findings. Indeed, pain of pulpal origin is often characterized by difficulty in localizing the source of pain. In contrast, pain originating from acutely inflamed periradicular tissue is generally much easier for the patient to localize. Thus, "common" features do not imply ubiquitous features, and several of those clinical findings listed in Box 20-1 are specific to certain diagnoses. For example, discriminant analysis of 74 orofacial pain patients indicates that pain due to pulpal pathosis is significantly associated with thermal allodynia (ie, temperature sensitivity; odds ratio of 9.0 versus apical periodontitis; $P < .001$), whereas pain due to apical periodontitis is significantly associated with mechanical allodynia (ie, digital or percussion sensitivity; odds ratio of 6.9 versus pulpitis; $P < .01$).[18]

The absence of common features should prompt the clinician to expand the differential diagnosis to consider other possibilities. For example, local anesthetic injections can be used as a diagnostic test to provide an approximate localization of the source of the pain. If pain persists even in the presence of an effective local anesthetic injection, then the clinician should consider the possibility of either a nonodontogenic etiology of the pain or that the pain was referred from a tooth that was not located in the field of anesthesia.[7-9,20] From this perspective, the clinician should consider all local anesthetic injections as a diagnostic procedure in pain patients and evaluate whether they reduce patient pain reports. Although this test is very useful, potential false positive results can occur. In one such case, intraoral local anesthetic injections reduced dental pain in a patient with an epidermoid cyst in the brain stem (S. Milam, personal communication, 2001). Thus, the local anesthetic test must be considered in the context of the other findings of each case (see Box 20-1). The local anesthetic test provides only an approximate localization since multiple teeth are anesthetized even when injections are given by intraosseous or intraligamentary routes.[22,23] Similarly, if a clinician cannot reproduce the patient's chief complaint (eg, lingering pain to cold stimulus in a patient reporting thermal sensitivity), then alternative origins of the pain should be considered, including even teeth previously provided with nonsurgical root canal treatment.[21]

A summary of features of nonodontogenic dental pain is provided in Box 20-2.[7-16] Once again, the skilled clinician will recognize that these features are not pathognomonic, but instead are markers that should raise the index of suspicion for pain of a nonodontogenic origin. For example, maxillary sinusitis is characterized as a dull, aching pain sensation that is perceived to involve multiple maxillary posterior teeth.[8,9] In contrast, trigeminal neuralgia is often characterized as producing sharp, stabbing, often electric shock-like pains that may involve one or more teeth.[9] Note that both of these disorders represent nonodontogenic dental pain, but that the perceptual pain qualities and the localization may be different for each diagnosis.

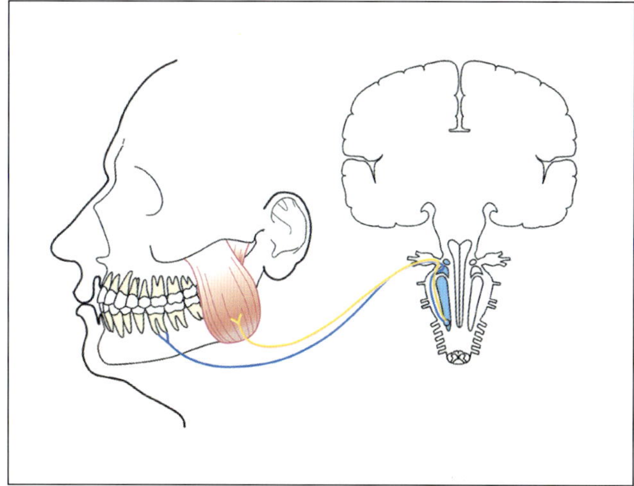

Fig 20-1 Schematic drawing illustrating convergence of afferent fibers from dental pulp onto the same projection neuron in the trigeminal nuclear complex that receives afferent input from other craniofacial tissues (in this example, the masseter muscle). (Reprinted from Hargreaves and Keiser[24] with permission.)

Mechanisms of Nonodontogenic Dental Pain

There are three primary mechanisms that cause pain of a nonodontogenic origin to be perceived as a toothache. The first and probably most common mechanism is *referred pain*. Although several mechanisms for referred pain have been proposed (see chapter 8), a commonly accepted hypothesis is convergence (Fig 20-1). The convergence hypothesis proposes that certain afferent sensory neurons have peripheral terminals that innervate different tissues, yet their central terminals converge onto the same second-order projection neuron located in the trigeminal nuclear complex. This hypothesis is supported by strong experimental data that indicate that afferent neurons from multiple peripheral tissues indeed have central terminals that converge onto the same trigeminal projection neuron, which receives sensory input from dental pulpal neurons (see Fig 8-17).[25] In fact, it has been estimated that about 50% of all pulpal neurons converge with other neurons onto the same trigeminal projection neurons.[26]

The hypothesis of convergence has important clinical implications because it explains how the "site" of pain perception can be different from the "origin" of nociceptor activation. In the example illustrated in Fig 20-1, the tooth is perceived as the "site" of pain perception but the origin of nociceptor activation is actually the masseter muscle. This example provides a rationale for using an intraoral local anesthetic injection, which would not be expected to reduce the patient's pain perception in this scenario, as a diagnostic tool. Conversely, in this example, palpation of trigger points located in the masseter muscle would be expected to increase pain perception. Referred pain is thought to contribute to the sensation of nonodontogenic dental pain in many patients, including those with temporomandibular dysfunction (TMD), fibromyalgia, trigeminal neuralgia, cardiac pain, and neurovascular disorders (eg, migraine or cluster headaches; see Fig 8-8).

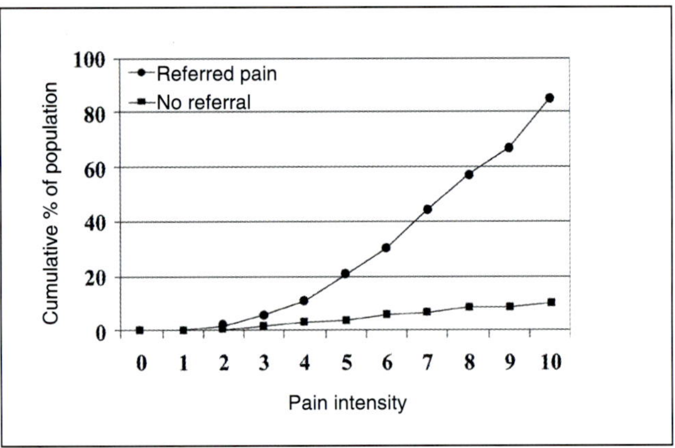

Fig 20-2 Relationship of pain referral to pain intensity in 400 patients reporting odontogenic pain (posterior teeth only). Pain intensity was measured on a 0 to 10 integer scale; 0 = no pain, 10 = extreme pain. Referred pain was determined by how patients marked areas of pain perception on a mannequin. (Modified from Falace et al[28] with permission.)

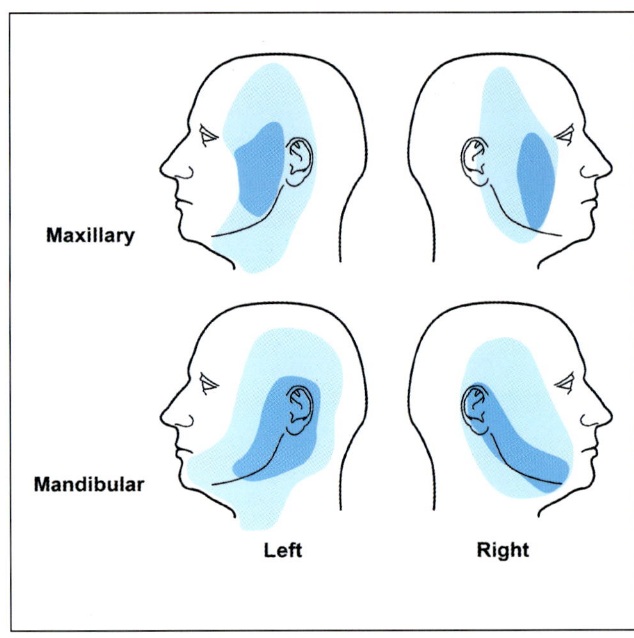

Fig 20-3 The extraoral referral patterns of pain originating from maxillary and mandibular right (n = 27, n = 31) and left (n = 38, n = 47) first molars. The dark blue shading indicates the most frequent areas of pain referral; the light blue shading indicates less frequent areas of referral. Note that the referred pain does not generally cross the midline. (Modified from Falace et al[28] with permission.)

However, pain also can originate from pulpal nociceptors and be referred to other craniofacial structures such as the preauricular region.[27] This was diagrammatically represented in Fig 8-18, in which a patient with irreversible pulpitis had pain that was referred to a large portion of the mandibular and maxillary divisions of the trigeminal nerve. Other studies have demonstrated that more intense pain has a greater probability of referral to other regions. For example, a study of 400 patients with odontogenic pain indicated that its intensity, but not its duration or quality, is significantly associated with pain referral to other craniofacial structures (Fig 20-2).[28] In this study, about 90% of all patients reporting moderate to severe odontogenic pain (5 or more on a 0 to 10 scale) also reported pain referred to nearby craniofacial regions. Thus, as pain intensity increases, there is an increasing likelihood of patients reporting a history of referred pain. The most common areas of extraoral pain referred from first molar odontogenic pain are shown in Fig 20-3.[28] In summary, it is important to realize that craniofacial pain can originate from other tissues and be referred to teeth, and, conversely, that pain may originate from pulpal nociceptors and be referred to other craniofacial tissues.

The second general mechanism of nonodontogenic dental pain is a *systemic disorder* that interacts with pulpal or periradicular tissue. In these cases, the systemic disorder serves as an etiologic factor for pain that originates from pulpal or periradicular nociceptors but is not derived from dental pathoses; thus dental treatment may prove ineffective in reducing pain. In most of these cases, appropriate clinical care would include recognition of the systemic etiology of the pain report and referral for medical evaluation or treatment. Examples include herpes zoster, malignant neoplasia, diabetes, sickle cell anemia, and developmental disorders. For example, patients with sickle cell anemia may report dental pain that signals an impending sickling crisis rather than an indication of a local, dental pathosis.[29,30] The effect of systemic disorders on dental pulp is covered later in this chapter and reviewed extensively in chapter 21.

The third general mechanism of nonodontogenic dental pain is caused by higher brain functions that are commonly classified as *psychosocial* or *behavioral factors*. Psychosocial, behavioral, cultural, and environmental factors have two major levels of impact on pain.[9,31,32] First, they can influence a patient's interpretation and report of pain. For example, one study reporting on cultural differences in pain language found that 82% of Mandarin-speaking Chinese reported tooth-drilling preparations as producing a "sourish" sensation, whereas only 8% of English-speaking Americans used this term.[33] In another example, environmental factors were found to influence pain reports. In this study, female subjects reported significantly greater anxiety and lower thresholds for electric pulpal stimulation when tested in a dental operatory as compared to a research laboratory setting.[34] These studies illustrate the fact that the skilled clinician must interpret the patient's pain report with consideration given to psychosocial and cultural factors. Moreover, clinicians should appreciate the fact that their own psychosocial and cultural factors may influence how they interpret a patient's pain report.

Under certain conditions, psychosocial, behavioral, or other factors may have a second impact on pain. Under these pathologic circumstances, these factors may contribute to the perception of chronic craniofacial or dental pain. Examples include somatoform pain disorders and Munchausen syndrome. Although uncommon, these conditions may contribute to the (fortunately) rare case in which a patient presents after receiving multiple endodontic procedures to treat a recurring pain complaint.

Types of Nonodontogenic Dental Pain

There are several classification schemes for categorizing orofacial pain. Four of the more common approaches include those described in the following publications: *(1)* Bell's classic text,[7] *(2)* a monograph by the American Academy of Orofacial Pain[35] (with input from the International Headache Society), *(3)* a report by the International Association for the Study of Pain,[36] and *(4)* the Research Diagnostic Criteria advanced by Dworkin and colleagues.[37] Although these diagnostic schemes share many similarities, they are not identical, and they have not all been validated in large-scale, multicenter studies. Because the goal of this chapter is to provide a useful overview of those pain disorders that contribute to dental pain of nonodontogenic origin and to provide sufficient information for clinicians to develop a differential diagnostic list, a generalized classification of nonodontogenic pain disorders will be presented here. The ultimate diagnosis and clinical management of these nonodontogenic dental pain disorders should be considered within the context of a team of pain clinicians for each patient with nonodontogenic pain.

Nonodontogenic dental pain of musculoskeletal origin

Myofascial pain: Temporomandibular dysfunction

Etiology This classification is an umbrella term for several chronic pain disorders involving masticatory and proximate muscles and the temporomandibular joint (TMJ).[36-39] Pain of myofascial origin can result in nonodontogenic dental pain. Classic studies by Travell and Simons have shown that several muscles including the masseter, temporal, and digastric muscles can refer pain to teeth.[38]

The etiologic basis for these chronic pain conditions is unknown.[40] Studies have been conducted in twins to determine the relative contribution of genetic (ie, anatomic or physiologic) versus environmental (ie, learned) factors. Evaluation of 494 monozygotic and dizygotic twins determined the relative genetic contribution to TMD pain by measuring the heritability of craniofacial pain, clenching, grinding, and joint sounds.[41] Interestingly, there was no difference between monozygotic and dizygotic twins for any of the outcome measures; therefore, this study found no significant genetic contribution to these measures of orofacial pain or disorder. Instead, the authors concluded that environmental factors unique to each twin appear to exert a major influence on the presentation of pain, joint sounds, and clenching and grinding habits. Another study using 335 pairs of twins also has reported little to no heritability for self-report of any joint pain.[42] Additional studies have indicated that there was no significant genetic influence on the dolorimetric measurement of pressure pain thresholds in 609 female-female twins.[43] Taken together, these preliminary studies are consistent with the hypothesis that environmental factors play a major role in the development of these disorders and that genetic factors may not be as important. The replication and extension of these findings will undoubtedly be an important focus of future research in chronic pain patients.

Differential diagnosis Myofascial pain is often described as a deep, dull, aching pain of diffuse localization. A diagnosis of nonodontogenic dental pain evoked by muscle pain, rather than one of odontogenic pain, often is found when: *(1)* pain is not restricted to a tooth (ie, diffuse pain, see Fig 8-18), *(2)* pain is exacerbated by palpation of trigger points (myofascial pain) or muscles, *(3)* pain is unrelieved by a diagnostic intraoral local anesthetic block, *(4)* there is restriction of jaw opening or pain upon opening the jaw (masseter or medial pterygoid pain), and *(5)* pain is not altered by intraoral thermal stimuli (eg, normal thermal responsiveness).[7,9,39,44] In one study of 312 patients, pain duration was significantly longer in TMD patients (mean, 13.4 ± 17 months) than in odontogenic pain patients (mean, 3.7 ± 3.8 months), but the high standard deviation suggests that this measure has low specificity.[44] There is no difference in electric pulpal testing thresholds between patients with myofascial pain and control subjects.[45]

The muscles that typically contribute to nonodontogenic dental pain (and the teeth to which the pain is referred) are the superior belly of the masseter (maxillary posterior teeth), the inferior belly of the masseter (mandibular posterior teeth), anterior digastric (mandibular anterior teeth), and temporal (maxillary anterior or posterior teeth) muscles.[7,38,46,47] An overview of techniques for palpating these muscles is presented in Figs 20-4 to 20-9.

Several investigators have reported on the propensity of these musculoskeletal disorders to evoke nonodontogenic dental pain.[7,38,44,47,48] In a series of 230 cases of patients with a diagnosis of TMD, 85% reported referred pain after firm palpation of muscles or trigger points.[47] A total of more than 1,000 sites of referred pain were recorded in this study; common regions of palpation-induced referred pain were to the cheek (21% of all referred pain reports), ear (14.6%), forehead (14.5%), and teeth (11.6%).[47] Figure 20-10 presents the distribution of muscles that, when palpated in these patients, refer pain to teeth.[47] There are four main points to be concluded from Fig 20-10. First, molars are the teeth that most frequently receive referred pain from muscle or trigger-point palpation. Second, the masseter muscle is the most common muscle referring nonodontogenic dental pain to teeth. Third, the total frequency for pain referred to maxillary and mandibular teeth is about the same. Fourth, palpation of four sites (masseter, lateral pterygoid, temporalis, and TMJ) produced a total of 132 reports of pain referred to teeth. In contrast, palpation of seven additional sites (medial pterygoid, coronoid process, trapez-

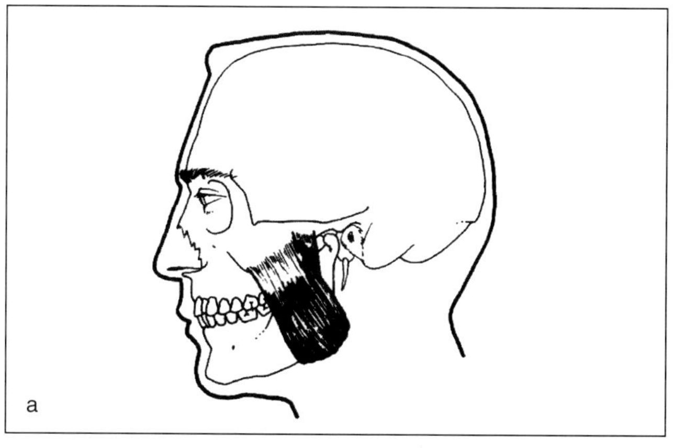

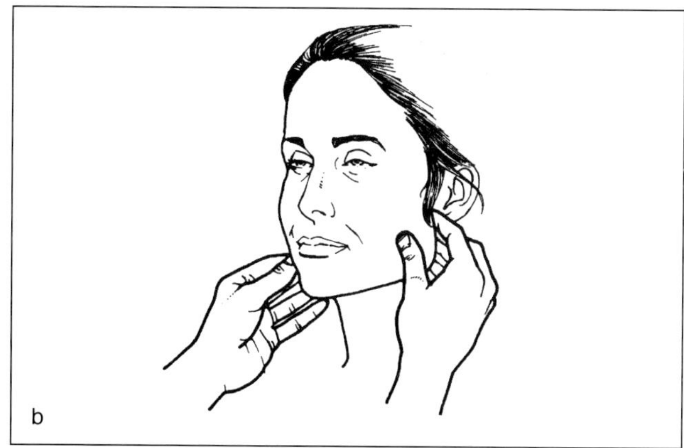

Fig 20-4 *(a)* Masseter muscle. *(b)* Palpation of masseters. (Illustrations by Robert Minor, DDS.)

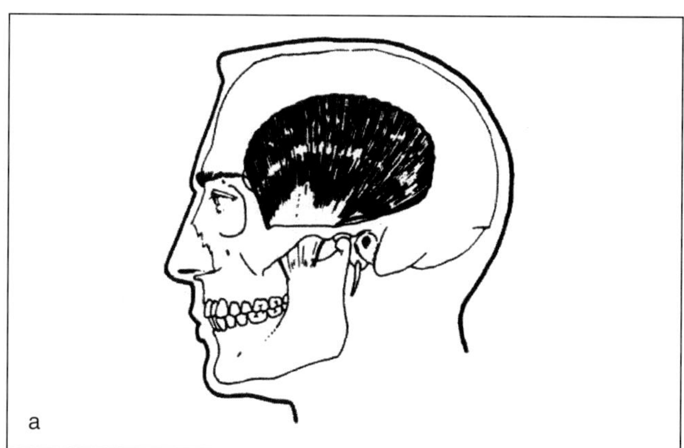

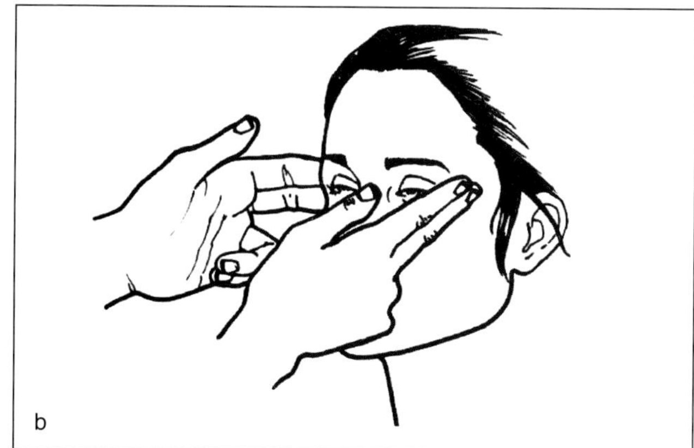

Fig 20-5 *(a)* Temporal muscles. *(b)* Palpation of temporal muscles. (Illustrations by Robert Minor, DDS.)

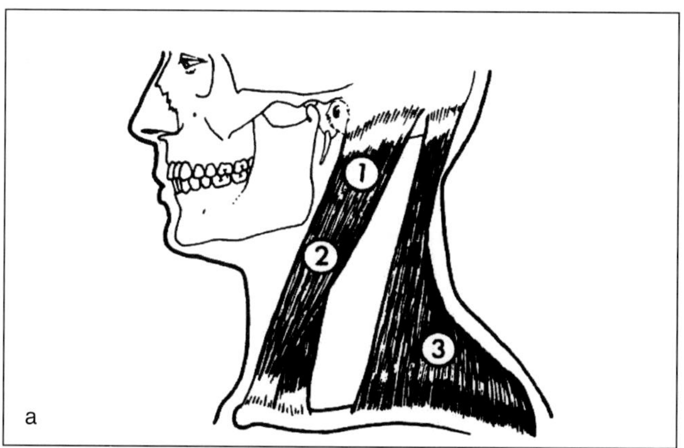

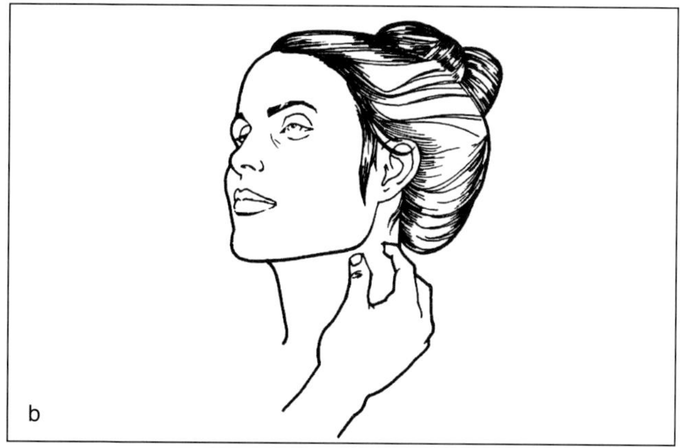

Fig 20-6 *(a)* Sternocleidomastoid (1,2) and trapezius muscles (3). Areas 1 and 2 should be palpated first, then area 3. *(b)* Palpation of sternocleidomastoid muscles (area 2). (Illustrations by Robert Minor, DDS.)

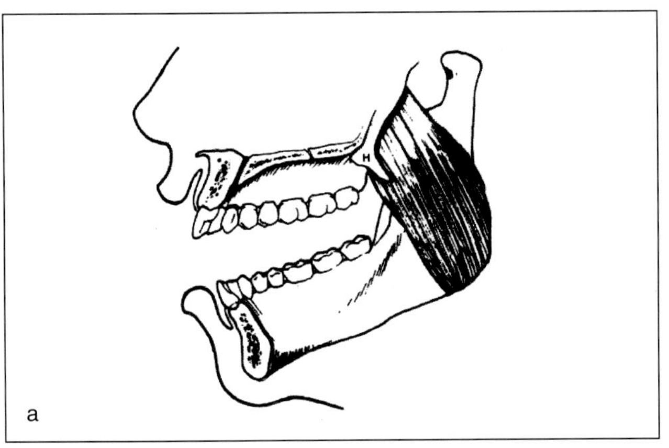

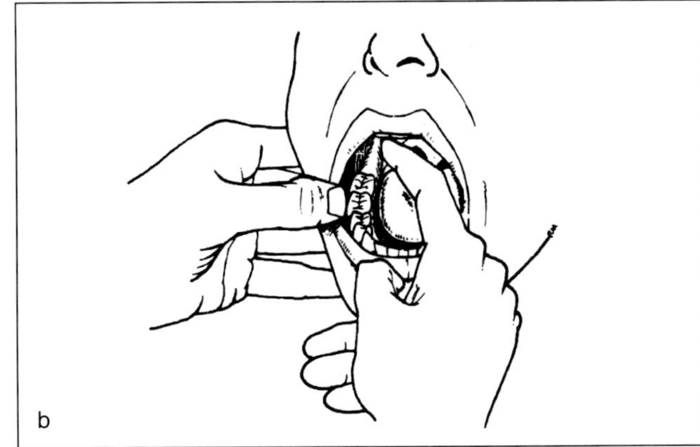

Fig 20-7 *(a)* Digastric muscles. *(b)* Palpation of anterior belly of digastric muscle. (Illustrations by Robert Minor, DDS.)

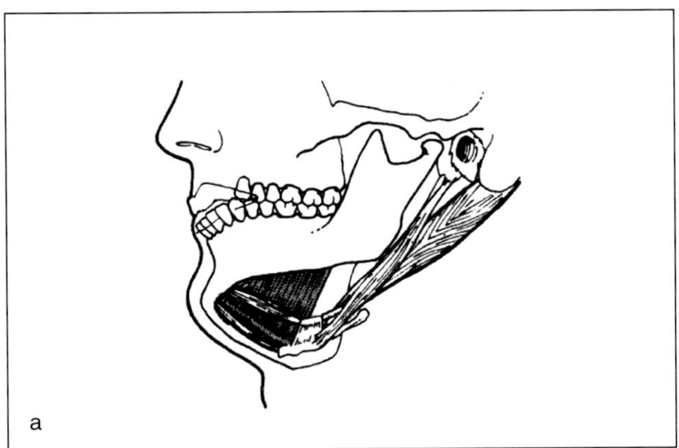

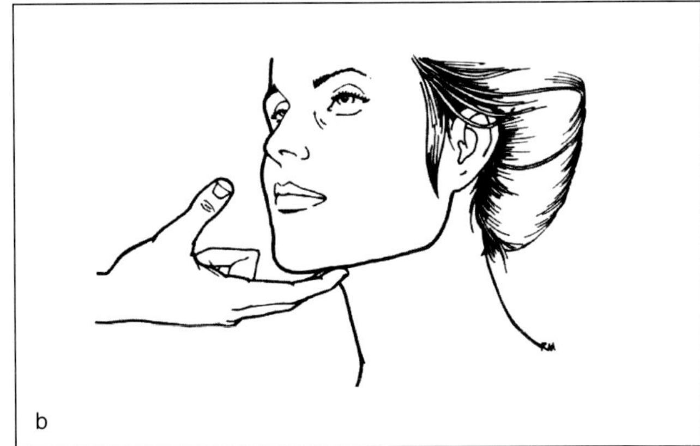

Fig 20-8 *(a)* Medial pterygoid muscle. *(b)* Palpation of medial pterygoid muscle. (Illustrations by Robert Minor, DDS.)

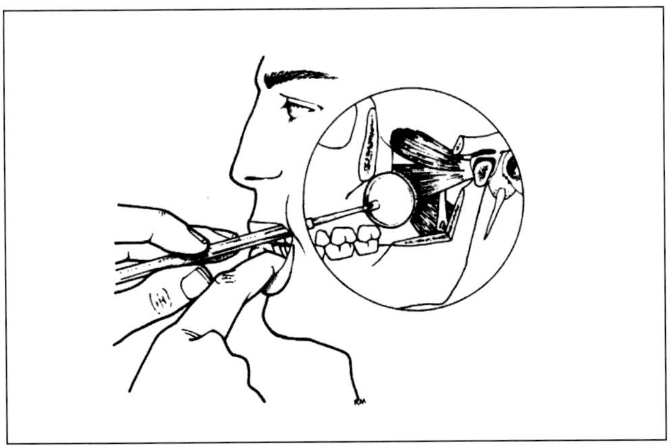

Fig 20-9 Test of origin of lateral pterygoid muscles using a mouth mirror. (Illustration by Robert Minor, DDS.)

ius, splenius capitus, sternocleidomastoid, anterior digastric, and posterior digastric) produced a total of only 9 reports of pain referred to teeth.[47] Thus, palpation of the masseter, lateral pterygoid, and temporal muscles, as well as the TMJ, should be considered first when evaluating the potential for a myofascial origin of nonodontogenic dental pain.

Treatment Several treatment modalities have been evaluated for these patients. A partial list includes identification and elimination of contributory factors, mild analgesics, spray and stretch therapy, massage, splints, biofeedback, and deep heat. The specific combination of treatments depends upon the diagnosis and treatment philosophy of the clinician.[7,38]

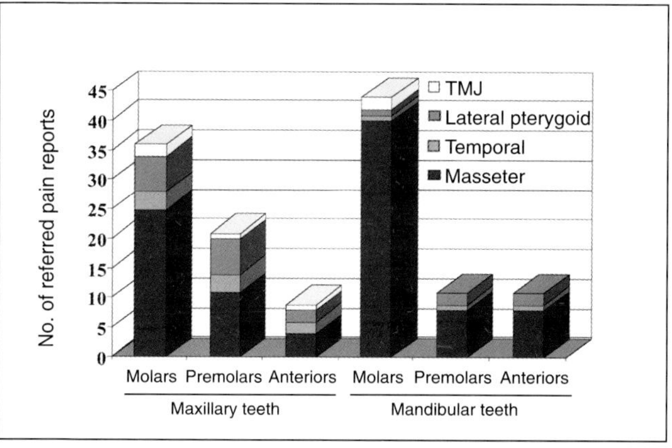

Fig 20-10 Frequency distribution of nonodontogenic dental pain referred to teeth after palpation of selected muscles in a group of 230 patients with TMD. Firm pressure was applied for 5 seconds to selected sites, and the patients were instructed to report on palpation-induced referred pain during stimulation. Muscles were palpated by applying sustained firm pressure while sliding the fingers along the length of the muscle. The entire body of the masseter muscle was palpated. The temporal muscle was palpated superior to the zygomatic arch. The lateral pterygoid was palpated by applying the fifth digit along the buccal alveolar ridge just apical to the maxillary molars. The lateral pole and posterior aspect of the TMJ were palpated with the mouth open. (Data from Wright.[47])

Nonodontogenic dental pain of neuropathic origin

Trigeminal neuralgia

Etiology The etiology of trigeminal neuralgia (also known as *tic douloureux*) is unclear; however, vascular compression of the trigeminal nerve is a common hypothesis that has gained considerable credibility with the demonstration that compression of either the sciatic or trigeminal (infraorbital) nerves in rats produces models of neuropathic pain.[49,50]

Differential diagnosis The differential diagnosis between nonodontogenic dental pain evoked by trigeminal neuralgia and odontogenic pain often includes pain quality and duration (eg, patients with trigeminal neuralgia will often report severe, shooting, electric-like pain that lasts only a few seconds).[5,7,10] A trigger point is often found in patients with trigeminal neuralgia; a gentle touch may be all that is required to evoke a paroxysmal attack. Other distinguishing features include pain not always restricted to a tooth, pain unrelieved by a diagnostic intraoral local anesthetic block (unless the trigger point is in the field of anesthesia), and pain not altered by intraoral thermal stimuli.[5,7,9] The frequency of involvement in the trigeminal divisions is mandibular > maxillary >> ophthalmic.[5,7,10,11] The pain is often severe; patients have reported the pain as being the most intense they have ever experienced and may be able to trace the pain along the distribution of the nerve.[9]

A proposed diagnosis related to trigeminal neuralgia is pretrigeminal neuralgia.[10,51-53] This is thought to be an early form of trigeminal neuralgia. It is characterized as a sinus pain or nonodontogenic dental pain and does not present with the classic paroxysmal pain. The pain is often aching in quality and the duration is minutes to several hours. These patients may subsequently develop trigeminal neuralgia.[52,53]

Patients with trigeminal or pretrigeminal neuralgia may report a nonodontogenic dental pain. In one series of 41 patients with trigeminal neuralgia and 19 with pretrigeminal neuralgia, a total of 61% reported an initial dental pain.[10] In another series of cases, a total of 29% of 24 patients reporting on symptoms during pretrigeminal neuralgia reported dental pain.[53]

Patients with trigeminal neuralgia may receive endodontic treatment for their dental pain.[54-56] Additional case reports also provide examples of the opposite diagnostic problem: patients with odontogenic dental pain being diagnosed as having trigeminal neuralgia.[57] In both types of misdiagnosis, the lack of response to treatment was a key factor in prompting reassessment of the differential diagnosis.

Treatment Several treatment modalities have been evaluated for patients with trigeminal neuralgia, including carbamazepine, gabapentin, baclofen, phenytoin, and valproic acid.[10,53,56,58] Local anesthetic injections into the area of the trigger point often relieve pain. In a series of 24 cases, intraoral administration of capsaicin to mucosa resulted in complete or partial relief of pain in approximately 63% of the patients.[59] Surgical procedures such as percutaneous rhizotomy or nerve decompression are considered in refractory cases.[5,7]

Atypical odontalgia

Etiology The etiology of atypical odontalgia (phantom toothache, deafferentation pain) is unknown, but is often associated with trauma or inflammation in the region.[39,60-63] For this reason, it has been proposed to be a type of deafferentation pain, although vascular hypotheses also have been advanced.[61,64,65] The possibility of a psychosocial etiology has been supported in some studies,[65] but not others.[63,64,66-68] Prior studies conducted in animals have shown that trigeminal deafferentation produces central plasticity in the trigeminal nuclear complex in the brain stem (see Fig 8-15).[69] In addition, there may be a sympathetic component to the pain.[67] Although no large-scale clinical trials have been conducted, atypical odontalgia has been estimated to be 10 times more prevalent than trigeminal neuralgia and may include up to 3% of patients receiving pulpal extirpation procedures.[39,70]

Differential diagnosis The following characteristics of nonodontogenic dental pain evoked by atypical odontalgia can be used to differentiate it from odontogenic pain: diffuse pain; pain not always restricted to a tooth (eg, the area may be edentulous); pain that is almost always continuous; a pain quality often described as a dull, aching, throbbing, or burning sensation; pain that may or may not be relieved by a diagnostic intraoral local anesthetic block; pain that often lasts more than 4 months; and pain not altered by intraoral thermal stimuli.[7,9,11,62,67,68,71,72]

Patients with atypical odontalgia often report a history of trauma or ineffective dental treatment in the area.[61] In a study of 42 patients with atypical odontalgia, 86% of the patient population was female and 78% reported maxillary pain; out of 119 reported areas of pain, the most common were the molar (59%), premolar (27%), and canine (4%) regions.[64,68] The pain may change in location over time; some studies have reported pain shifting location in up to 82% of the subjects.[67,71] Thermography has been proposed as a diagnostic test, and although the differences in facial thermal asymmetry between control subjects and patients with atypical odontalgia are statistically significant, they are not large in magnitude (18%).[73]

Patients with atypical odontalgia may receive multiple endodontic treatments or extractions for their dental pain.[64,71,72,74,75] In many of these cases, the lack of response to treatment was a key factor in prompting reassessment of the differential diagnosis.[39] In one case report, the lack of an effect of a local anesthetic injection on reducing the intensity of pain was a significant finding that prompted consideration of nonodontogenic dental pain.[75]

Treatment Management of patients with atypical odontalgia is difficult and patients may receive repeated (but ineffective) dental treatment directed at removing their symptoms. Interventions have included tricyclic antidepressants, capsaicin, sympathetic block (eg, stellate block), and systemic lidocaine or lidocaine patch.[9,12,58,60,63,64,67,72,76] In one study on 50 patients, a 5-minute application of a lidocaine 2.5% and prilocaine 2.5% cream produced a mean 60% ± 29% pain reduction; a 4-week trial of 0.025% capsaicin produced no effect in 11 patients and an average 58% ± 25% pain reduction in 19 patients.[67] The finding that peripheral interventions may reduce chronic pain is potentially important not only from a patient management perspective, but also because it suggests that a persistent peripheral input at the site of injury may contribute to central sensitization (see chapter 8).[77,78]

Glossopharyngeal neuralgia

Etiology The etiology of glossopharyngeal neuralgia is unknown, but may involve vascular compression of the ninth cranial nerve.[9,11] Accordingly, some investigators have suggested that glossopharyngeal neuralgia and trigeminal neuralgia have similar etiologies (ie, vascular compression) involving different cranial nerves. Glossopharyngeal neuralgia appears to be about one tenth as prevalent as trigeminal neuralgia.[11,79]

Differential diagnosis Glossopharyngeal neuralgia is similar to trigeminal neuralgia in that both disorders are episodic; however, the pain associated with glossopharyngeal neuralgia is generally not as intense. Moreover, patients with glossopharyngeal neuralgia do not commonly report pain referred to teeth.

The differential diagnosis between nonodontogenic dental pain evoked by glossopharyngeal neuralgia and odontogenic pain often includes pain quality and duration (the former involves severe shock-like pain that lasts only a few seconds).[7,9,10,58] The pain is often elicited by swallowing; however, it may also be elicited by chewing or talking. The distribution of pain includes the posterior mandible, oropharynx, tonsillar fossa, and ear.[9,79] Other distinguishing features include pain unrelieved by a diagnostic intraoral local anesthetic block (unless the trigger point is in the field of anesthesia), and pain not altered by intraoral thermal stimuli.[7,9,59]

Treatment Treatments reported for glossopharyngeal neuralgia include gabapentin, phenytoin, and carbamazepine.[58,79] Resistant cases have been treated with surgical decompression.[79]

Neuralgia-inducing cavitational osteomyelitis/osteonecrosis

Etiology Ratner et al and Roberts et al advanced the hypothesis that certain forms of chronic orofacial pain are caused by cavitational defects in the mandible or maxilla, a condition called neuralgia-inducing cavitational osteomyelitis (or osteonecrosis) (NICO).[80-82] A proposed etiology is chronic inflammation or necrosis from bacterial osteomyelitis or vascular pathosis following tooth extraction.[80,81,83] However, this proposed disorder is controversial, is not supported by scientific evidence, and the defining characteristics have changed over time.[64,84-89] A comprehensive monograph on pain published in 2001 did not describe NICO.[5]

Bone cavities have indeed been observed in some patients with chronic orofacial pain.[80,81,83] However, it has been suggested that these cavities are a normal anatomic structure because they also have been found in cadavers of patients who had not reported pain and they are not necessarily found in patients with atypical facial pain.[83,89] A recent tomographic study using technetium-99 labeling of bone regions found higher uptake in patients with idiopathic jaw pain, but concluded that this technique is unable to serve as a diagnostic test for pain disorders because of low sensitivity and specificity.[90] Other investigators have challenged the use of this diagnostic term and the implication that it is involved in pain.[86-88]

Differential diagnosis According to Ratner et al, the diagnosis of NICO is based on tenderness upon palpation over an edentulous region of alveolar bone over an extraction site, lack of radiographic findings, and rapid pain reduction with local anesthetic infiltration.[80,81] Reported treatments include surgical debridement of the bone cavities and antibiotic treatment.

NICO-like nonodontogenic dental pain has been reported. For example, a cavitational bone defect has been reported in an endodontic patient. The case report ascribed the pain to a cavitational bone defect containing necrotic cells, although the bone defect was separated from the involved teeth by normal-appearing bone.[91]

Nonodontogenic dental pain of neurovascular origin

Migraine

Etiology Migraine is one of the most common forms of pain of neurovascular origin in the trigeminal system.[7,9,11] Although the etiology is unknown, a neurovascular hypothesis postulating vasodilation of cephalic and cerebral arteries with activation of sensitized perivascular nociceptors has experimental support.[92,93] Genetic factors are involved and serve as risk factors for developing migraine.[94] Migraine with aura, known as *classic migraine*, is a risk factor for stroke and justifies medical referral.[95] Migraine without aura is termed *common migraine*. Migraines may be evoked by stress, dietary factors, altered sleep patterns, or menstruation.[11]

Differential diagnosis Nonodontogenic dental pain evoked by migraine can be differentiated from odontogenic pain in that the former often is characterized by pain not restricted to a tooth (ie, diffuse pain); a unilateral dull, throbbing pain quality; pain unrelieved by a diagnostic intraoral local anesthetic block; and pain not altered by intraoral thermal stimuli.[11,96] The diagnosis is often made by a temporal relationship in which the dental pain subsides as the headache symptoms are reduced. Physical activity (eg, walking a flight of stairs) often increases pain intensity. Migraines are often associated with nausea, emesis, affective changes in mood, and sensitivity to light or sound.[11] Migraine occurs more frequently in females, particularly in those younger than 50 years.[96]

In one case report, a 35-year-old woman reported dental pain in a mandibular canine.[97] The pain persisted after extraction of the tooth. Subsequent examination revealed that the pain was associated with nausea and sensitivity to loud sounds. The patient denied experiencing an aura during the attacks. Treatment with anti-migraine drugs and cessation of oral contraceptives reduced the migraine episodes.

Treatment Migraine treatment is of two types: prophylactic drugs and abortive drugs.[96] Migraine patients have been treated successfully with sumatriptan and other serotoninergic agents that block the $5HT_1$ or $5HT_3$ serotoninergic receptors.[93,98,99] Clinical trials have also demonstrated efficacy for gabapentin and injection of botulinum toxin in the reduction of migraine pain.[100,101] Ergotamine has been largely replaced by these alternatives because they have a lower incidence of adverse effects.

Cluster headache

Etiology The etiology of cluster headache (Sluder neuralgia) is unknown, but has been hypothesized to be caused by episodic vasodilation activating perivascular nociceptors. The term *cluster* denotes the observation that these pain episodes often last about 6 to 8 weeks and then are followed by a relatively long pain-free period. Although less common than migraines, cluster headaches are often considered to produce more intense pain.[11,79,96]

Differential diagnosis Nonodontogenic dental pain evoked by cluster headache is distinct from odontogenic pain in that it is often characterized by pain not restricted to a tooth (ie, pain includes retro-orbital and sinus regions), pain exacerbated by drugs or occuring during sleep, pain unrelieved by a diagnostic intraoral local anesthetic block, and pain not altered by intraoral thermal stimuli.[7,11,102] Cluster headaches can be triggered by drugs such as alcohol and cocaine.[11,102] The pain is generally described as hot, stabbing, and paroxysmal in nature. The pain attacks often occur at the same time of day (especially 4:00 AM to 10:00 AM), and often last 30 to 180 minutes.[96] The attack may be associated with rhinorrhea, nasal congestion, and lacrimation from the involved eye.[11] Cluster headaches occur most often in male patients (male-female ratio, 6:1) in the range of 30 to 50 years of age. The pain distribution is often located in the maxillary posterior teeth, sinus, and retro-orbital regions. A related condition is chronic paroxysmal hemicrania. This disorder has similar pain characteristics, is completely responsive to indomethacin, and is observed mostly in females.[96]

Cluster headaches often evoke nonodontogenic dental pain. In one study, 43% of subjects with cluster headache were initially treated by a dentist.[103] However, a relatively uncommon variant of cluster headache (migrainous neuralgia) is associated with a nonodontogenic dental pain without the headache component.[9] A case report described three patients with nonodontogenic dental pain due to cocaine-induced cluster headaches.[102] One patient described unilateral maxillary pain in the premolar region that lasted for 30 to 120 minutes after cocaine use. Another patient reported continued nonodontogenic dental pain in the maxillary molar region. The pain persisted after endodontic treatment and subsequent extraction; only later did the patient report that the pain started about 1 to 2 hours after cocaine ingestion. The third patient also reported nonodontogenic dental pain in the maxillary premolar region after consumption of cocaine.

Treatment Patients with cluster headache are treated with oxygen therapy, sumatriptan, prednisone, gabapentin, and calcium channel blockers.[96,104,105] Ergotamine has been largely replaced by these alternatives because of the lower incidence of adverse effects.

Temporal arteritis (giant cell arteritis) and carotidynia represent relatively rare neurovascular conditions that may lead to a misdiagnosis.[9,11,96] Because of their relatively rare occurrence and comparatively few published studies, as well as space considerations, the interested reader is encouraged to seek cited references.

Nonodontogenic dental pain due to inflammatory conditions

Sinusitis

Etiology The two major forms of sinusitis are those due to bacterial infection and the more common form due to allergies. The etiology for the nonodontogenic pain includes both referred pain mechanisms and an acute neuritis of dental nerves leaving the apical foramina and coursing through the floor of the sinus.

Differential diagnosis Unlike odontogenic pain, nonodontogenic dental pain evoked by sinusitis is often characterized by pain not restricted to a single tooth (ie, pain may include malar and maxillary alveolus regions), pain that may be partially relieved by a diagnostic intraoral local anesthetic block, pain that increases after percussion, and occasional thermal sensitivity to cold.[7,9,11,96] Patients may report a sense of pressure or fullness in the infraorbital region over the involved sinus. A particularly distinguishing characteristic is the presentation of multiple maxillary posterior teeth having percussion sensitivity with a positive response to pulpal vitality testing. The intranasal application of a 4% lidocaine spray is considered diagnostic if the pain is reduced.[96] Alternatively, a swab soaked with 5% lidocaine can be placed in the middle meatus for 30 seconds for evaluation of pain reduction.[8]

Bacteria-induced sinusitis pain is characterized as a severe, throbbing, stabbing pain with a sense of pressure. More than 70% of cases are caused by *Streptococcus pneumoniae* and *Haemophilus influenzae*.[106] In cases of moderate to severe sinusitis, a positive "head-dip" test is observed (ie, pain increases when patient lays down or places head below the knees), and patients may report a purulent nasal discharge. Placing a fiberoptic probe against the palate in a darkened operatory reveals transmitted light through a normal sinus and greatly reduced light when transmitted through an antrum filled with fluid.[84] Radiographic imaging of the sinuses, particularly a Waters view, may reveal fluid accumulation.

Allergy-induced sinusitis tends to be seasonal in colder climates but can occur at any time in temperate climates. The pain is often characterized as a chronic dull ache in the maxillary posterior region with a positive percussion test of molars or premolars. Interestingly, patients also may report an "itching" sensation in the maxillary teeth.

Case reports of patients with nonodontogenic dental pain due to sinusitis indicate a diffuse throbbing, aching pain.[107] The lack of complete response to endodontic treatment prompted expansion of the differential diagnosis.

Treatment Bacterial sinusitis is often treated with β-lactamase-resistant antibiotics such as amoxicillin with clavulanic acid or trimethoprim-sulfamethoxazole.[106] Allergic sinusitis is often treated with antihistamines or decongestants.

Pain in the maxillary sinuses as well as in the maxillary and mandibular teeth also can be triggered by reduced atmospheric pressure. Several case reports have described odontogenic and nonodontogenic dental pain in patients during or after airplane flights or scuba diving.[108-110] It has been recommended that dental treatment, including root canal obturations, be completed more than 24 hours prior to exposure to reduced atmospheric pressure.[109]

There are several additional inflammatory conditions that may lead to a misdiagnosis. These include pain referred from another tooth (see chapter 8), impacted third molars,[111] eruption sequestra of bone,[112] otitis media, and foreign bodies impacted into periodontal tissues during mastication[113] or retained under surgical tissue flaps.[114] The correct diagnosis requires careful history taking, clinical examination, and interpretation of findings.

Nonodontogenic dental pain due to systemic disorders

Several systemic disorders can lead to nonodontogenic dental pain. Chapter 21 provides an extensive review of their etiology and their pathophysiologic effects on dental pulp. Therefore, this section will simply provide an overview of these disorders from the perspective of developing a differential diagnosis of nonodontogenic dental pain.

A classic example of a systemic disorder producing nonodontogenic dental pain is cardiac pain.[51,115-117] In about 10% of cases, cardiac pain is referred to the left posterior mandible or to the inferior border of the mandible.[118] These case reports relate that in some patients the nonodontogenic dental pain is the only symptom; whereas in other patients it occurs together with substernal pain or pressure. The nonodontogenic dental pain is not altered by local anesthetic injection, but nitroglycerin may be effective in reducing pain.[9]

Herpes zoster has been reported to produce nonodontogenic dental pain preceding the eruption of vesicles. These case reports are mixed, with some reporting pulpalgia-like symptoms and others reporting necrosis with the presence of periradicular lesions.[119-122]

Patients with sickle cell anemia may present with nonodontogenic dental pain.[29,30] In a 12-month study, 68% of 51 patients with sickle cell anemia reported dental pain with no evident dental pathosis; in contrast, no differences were observed in patients with the sickle cell trait compared to controls.[123,124]

Several studies have reported on various neoplastic diseases associated with nonodontogenic dental pain. Although rare, these reports describe dental pain as an initial or severe symptom in patients with glioblastoma multiforme[125]; metastases from breast, lungs, or prostate[126-128]; osteoblastoma[129]; carcinoma[130,131]; sarcoma[131]; non-Hodgkin lymphoma[132,133]; and Burkitt lymphoma.[134] Key findings that prompted consideration of a nonodontogenic origin of the dental pain included subsequent paresthesia or anesthesia, positive responses to pulpal testing, failure of dental treatment, diffuse or spreading nature of pain, unusual-appearing radiographic lesions (eg, diffuse borders involving multiple teeth or "moth-eaten" trabecular pattern), and lack of etiologic factors.[125,126,129,130,132,133] In one series of 763 patients with nonspecific jaw pain, 1.2% of the population had pain that was caused by metastases located in the mandible.[127]

Patients with multiple sclerosis (MS) may present with nonodontogenic dental pain. In one case, toothache was the initial presenting symptom in a patient with MS (S. Milam, personal communication, 2001). Later, the emergence of electric shock-like pain, as well as the lack of evidence of dental pathoses, contributed to expansion of the differential diagnosis and prompted evaluation for MS. MS is typically diagnosed in young female patients.

A pulpal pain correlated with the menstrual cycle has been reported by some authors.[14] Although pulpal levels of estrogen receptors are low to nondetectable, it is interesting to note that progesterone receptors have been detected in dental pulp.[135] Additional studies are required to determine the prevalence, mechanisms, and differential diagnostic evaluation of this form of odontalgia.

Nonodontogenic dental pain of psychogenic origin

Etiology It is likely that in the past far too many patients have been classified as having pain of a psychogenic origin when, in fact, no psychosocial or behavioral etiology was confirmed. Instead, the assignment was often based on a diagnosis of exclusion. This situation has been described as being unjustifiable, with the suggestion that these patients are more accurately classified as having idiopathic pain disorder.[96]

Patients who have pain that is caused by psychogenic mechanisms are appropriately placed in this category. The term *somatoform pain disorder* is used to describe a cognitive perception of pain that has no demonstrable physical basis.[136-138] Four proposed subtypes include somatic delusions, somatization disorder, depression, and conversion.[11,96,139,140]

Differential diagnosis Patients with somatoform pain disorders may report pain from multiple teeth that often shifts in location, pain of long duration (chronic pain), pain that does not respond to appropriate treatment, pain that crosses anatomic distribution of peripheral nerves, pain that frequently changes in character, pain with no identifiable etiology, and pain that may or may not be reduced with a diagnostic local anesthetic block.[7,96,141]

Treatment Treatment requires the expertise of a psychologist or psychiatrist with experience in dealing with somatoform pain disorders.

Conclusions

It has been stated that clinicians who treat pain patients should remember the classic tale of the blind men describing the elephant.[142] In this tale, each blind man described the elephant as a completely different animal, depending on whether he was touching the trunk, ears, or legs. Similarly, clinicians tend to interpret the symptoms and results of the clinical examination of pain patients based on their own focus of training. Clinicians should consider the whole animal when assessing patient reports of dental pain. As seen in the examples given in this chapter, many painful disorders can result in nonodontogenic dental pain. Accordingly, prior to focusing on the planned dental treatment, clinicians should carefully consider the clinical findings and the differential diagnosis.

To ensure appropriate diagnosis of patients reporting dental pain, clinicians should follow these guidelines:

1. Be diligent in establishing a differential diagnosis.
2. Reproduce the patient's chief complaint.
3. Determine the etiology of the dental pain. Is the pain of dental origin?
4. Consider all local anesthetic injections as diagnostic. Evaluate patient response.
5. Monitor treatment outcome.
6. Know your regional pain team (eg, pain dentists, neurologists, psychologists, radiologists, and otolaryngologists), and consult with them when necessary.

Effective pain control is a hallmark of clinical excellence, and this starts with active consideration of the differential diagnosis of odontogenic and nonodontogenic dental pain.

References

1. Locker D, Grushka M. Prevalence of oral and facial pain and discomfort: Preliminary results of a mail survey. Community Dent Oral Epidemiol 1987;15:169–172.
2. Lipton J, Ship J, Larach-Robinson D. Estimated prevalence and distribution of reported orofacial pain in the United States. J Am Dent Assoc 1993;124:115–121.
3. Riley J, Gilbert G. Orofacial pain symptoms: An interaction between age and sex. Pain 2001;90:245–56.
4. Wall P, Melzack R (eds). Textbook of Pain, ed 4. Edinburgh, NY: Churchill Livingstone, 1999.
5. Loeser J, Bonica J. Bonica's Management of Pain, ed 3. Philadelphia: Lippincott Williams & Wilkins, 2001.
6. Lund J, Lavigne G, Dubner R, Sessle B. Orofacial Pain: From Basic Science to Clinical Management. Chicago: Quintessence, 2001.
7. Okeson J. Bell's Orofacial Pain, ed 5. Chicago: Quintessence, 1995.
8. Schwartz S, Cohen S. The difficult differential diagnosis. Dent Clin North Am 1992;36:279–292.
9. Okeson J, Falace D. Nonodontogenic toothache. Dent Clin North Am 1997;41:367–93.
10. Merrill R, Graff-Redford S. Trigeminal neuralgia: How to rule out the wrong treatment. J Am Dent Assoc 1992; 123:63–68.
11. Pertes R, Heir G. Chronic orofacial pain: A practical approach to differential diagnosis. Dent Clin North Am 1991;35:123–140.
12. Byers M, Burgess J. Pain of dental and intraoral origin. In: Loeser J, Bonica J. Bonica's Management of Pain, ed 3. Philadelphia: Lippincott Williams & Wilkins, 2001: 909–924.
13. Graff-Radford S. Regional myofascial pain syndrome and headache: Principles of diagnosis and management. Curr Pain Headache Rep 2001;5:376–381.
14. Seltzer S, Toglia J. Nondental conditions that cause head and neck pain. In: Seltzer S. Pain Control in Dentistry. Philadelphia: Lippincott Williams & Wilkins, 1978: 78–104.
15. Bender IB. Pulpal pain diagnosis: A review. J Endod 2000;26:175–179.
16. Bender IB. Reversible and irreversible painful pulpitides: Diagnosis and treatment. Aust Endod J 2000;26: 10–14.
17. Seltzer S, Boston D. Hypersensitivity and pain induced by operative procedures and the "cracked tooth syndrome." Gen Dent 1997;45:148–159.
18. Klausen B, Helbo M, Dabelsteen E. A differential diagnostic approach to the symptomatology of acute dental pain. Oral Surg Oral Med Oral Pathol 1985;59: 297–301.
19. Holland GR. Management of dental pain. In: Lund J, Lavigne G, Dubner R, Sessle B (eds). Orofacial Pain: From Basic Science to Clinical Management. Chicago: Quintessence, 2001:211–220.
20. Schmidt J, Wong M. The anesthetic test: A diagnostic aid for referred pain. Gen Dent 1994;42:338–340.
21. Keir D, Walker W, Schindler W, Dazey S. Thermally induced pulpalgia in endodontically treated teeth. J Endod 1990;17:38–40.
22. Replogle K, Reader A, Nist R, Beck M, Weaver J, Meyers W. Anesthetic efficacy of the intraosseous injection of 2% lidocaine (1:100,000 epinephrine) and 3% mepivacaine in mandibular first molars. Oral Surg Oral Med Oral Pathol Oral Radiol Endod 1997;83:30–37.
23. Kim S. Ligamental injection: A physiological explanation of its efficacy. J Endod 1986;12:486–491.
24. Hargreaves K, Keiser K. Development of new pain management strategies. J Dent Educ 2002;66:113–121.
25. Sessle BJ, Hu JW, Amano N, Zhong G. Convergence of cutaneous, tooth pulp, visceral, neck and muscle afferents onto nociceptive and non-nociceptive neurones in trigeminal subnucleus caudalis (medullary dorsal horn) and its implications for referred pain. Pain 1986; 27:219–235.
26. Sessle BJ. Recent developments in pain research: Central mechanisms of orofacial pain and its control. J Endod 1986;12:435–444.
27. Wright E, Gullickson D. Dental pulpalgia contributing to bilateral preauricular pain and tinnitus. J Orofac Pain 1996;10:166–168.
28. Falace D, Reid K, Rayens M. The influence of deep (odontogenic) pain intesity, quality and duration on the incidence and characteristics of referred orofacial pain. J Orofac Pain 1996;10:232–239.

29. Cox G. A study of oral pain experience in sickle cell patients. Oral Surg Oral Med Oral Pathol 1984;58: 39–41.
30. May O. Dental management of sickle cell patients. Gen Dent 1991;39:182–183.
31. Chapman CR, Turner J. Psychological aspects of pain. In: Loeser J, Bonica J. Bonica's Management of Pain, ed 3. Philadelphia: Lippincott Williams & Wilkins, 2001: 180–190.
32. LaResche L. Gender, cultural and environmental aspects of pain. In: Loeser J, Bonica J. Bonica's Management of Pain, ed 3. Philadelphia: Lippincott Williams & Wilkins, 2001:191–195.
33. Moore R, Brodsgaard I, Miller M. Consensus analysis: Reliability, validity and informant accuracy in use of American and Mandarin Chinese pain descriptors. Ann Behav Med 1997;19:295–300.
34. Dworkin S, Chen A. Pain in clinical and laboratory contexts. J Dent Res 1982;61:772–774.
35. Okeson J. Orofacial Pain. Guidelines for Assessment, Diagnosis, Management. Chicago: Quintessence, 1996.
36. Merskey H, Bogduk N (eds). Classification of Chronic Pain: Descriptions of Chronic Pain Syndromes and Definitions of Pain Terms, ed 2. Seattle: IASP Press, 1994.
37. Dworkin S, LaResche L. Research diagnostic criteria for temporomandibular disorders: Review, criteria, examinations, and specifications. J Craniomandib Disord 1992;6:301–355.
38. Travell J, Simons D. Myofascial Pain and Dysfunction. Baltimore: Williams & Wilkins, 1983.
39. Klausner J. Epidemiology of chronic pain: Diagnostic usefulness in patient care. J Am Dent Assoc 1994;125: 1604–1611.
40. Hargreaves K. The promise and pitfalls of polymorphisms and pain. J Orofac Pain 2001;15:89–90.
41. Michalowicz B, Pihlstrom B, Hodges J, Bouchard T. No heritability of temporomandibular joint signs and symptoms. J Dent Res 2000;79:1573–1578.
42. Charles S, Gatz M, Pederson N, Dahlberg L. Genetic and behavioral risk factors for self-reported joint pain among a population-based sample of Swedish twins. Health Psychol 1999;18:644–654.
43. MacGregor A, Griffiths G, Baker J, Spector T. Determinants of pressure pain threshold in adult twins: Evidence that shared environmental influences predominate. Pain 1997;73:253–257.
44. Gerke D, Richards L, Goss A. A multivariate study of patients with temporomandibular joint disorder, atypical facial pain, and dental pain. J Prosthet Dent 1992; 68:528–532.
45. Xie Q, Hampf G. Sensibility threshold in patients with masticatory muscle pain. Acta Odontol Scand 1994;52: 33–35.
46. Fricton J, Kroening R, Haley D, Siegert R. Myofascial pain syndrome of the head and neck: A review of clinical characteristics of 164 patients. Oral Surg Oral Med Oral Pathol 1985;60:615–623.
47. Wright E. Referred craniofacial pain patterns in patients with temporomandibular disorder. J Am Dent Assoc 2000;131:1307–1315.
48. Reeh E, elDeeb M. Referred pain of muscular origin resembling endodontic involvement. Case report. Oral Surg Oral Med Oral Pathol 1991;71:223–227.
49. Bennett G, Xie Y. A peripheral neuropathy in rat that produces disorders of pain sensation like those seen in man. Pain 1988;33:87–107.
50. Idanpaan-Heikkila J, Gulbaud G. Pharmacologic studies in a rat model of trigeminal neuropathic pain: Baclofen, but not carbamazepine, morphine or tricyclic antidepressants attenuates the allodynia-like behaviour. Pain 1999;79:281–290.
51. Drinnan A. Differential diagnosis of orofacial pain. Dent Clin North Am 1987;31:627–635.
52. Fromm G. Trigeminal neuralgias and related disorders. Neurol Clin 1989;7:305–323.
53. Fromm G, Graff-Radford S, Terrence C, Sweet W. Pretrigeminal neuralgia. Neurology 1990;40:1493–1495.
54. Goddard G. Case report of trigeminal neuralgia presenting as odontalgia. Cranio 1992;10:245–247.
55. Francica F, Brickman J, LoMonaco C, Lin L. Trigeminal neuralgia and endodontically treated teeth. J Endod 1988;14:360–362.
56. Law A, Lilly J. Trigeminal neuralgia mimicking odontogenic pain. A report of two cases. Oral Surg Oral Med Oral Pathol Oral Radiol Endod 1995;80:96–100.
57. Donlon W. Odontalgia mimicking trigeminal neuralgia. Anesth Prog 1989;36:98–100.
58. Loeser J. Cranial neuralgias. In: Loeser J, Bonica J. Bonica's Management of Pain, ed 3. Philadelphia: Lippincott Williams & Wilkins, 2001:855–866.
59. Epstein J, Marcoe J. Topical application of capsaicin for treatment of oral neuropathic pain and trigeminal neuralgia. Oral Surg Oral Med Oral Pathol 1994;77: 135–140.
60. Marbach J. Phantom tooth pain. J Endod 1978;4: 360–372.
61. Marbach J. Orofacial phantom pain: Theory and phenomenology. J Am Dent Assoc 1996;127:221–229.
62. Rees R, Harris M. Atypical odontalgia. Br J Maxillofac Surg 1979;16:212–218.
63. Graff-Radford S, Solberg W. Is atypical odontalgia a psychological problem? Oral Surg Oral Med Oral Pathol 1993;75:579–582.
64. Solberg W, Graff-Radford S. Orodental considerations in facial pain. Semin Neurol 1988;8:318–323.

65. Marbach J. Is phantom tooth pain a deafferentation (neuropathic) syndrome? Part II: Psychosocial considerations. Oral Surg Oral Med Oral Pathol 1993;75: 225–232.
66. Schnurr R, Brooke R. Atypical odontalgia. Update and comment on long-term follow-up. Oral Surg Oral Med Oral Pathol 1992;73:445–448.
67. Vickers E, Cousins M, Walker S, Chisholm D. Analysis of 50 patients with atypical odontalgia: A preliminary report on pharmacological procedures for diagnosis and treatment. Oral Surg Oral Med Oral Pathol Oral Radiol Endod 1998;85:24–32.
68. Graff-Redford S, Solberg W. Atypical odontalgia. J Craniomandib Disord 1992;6:260–265.
69. Kwan C, Hu J, Sessle BJ. Effects of tooth pulp deafferentation on brainstem neurons of the rat trigeminal subnucleus oralis. Somatosens Mot Res 1993;10: 115–131.
70. Marbach J, Hulbrock J, Hohn C, Segal A. Incidence of phantom tooth pain: An atypical facial neuralgia. Oral Surg Oral Med Oral Pathol 1982;53:190–193.
71. Lilly J, Law A. Atypical odontalgia misdiagnosed as odontogenic pain: A case report and discussion of treatment. J Endod 1997;23:337–339.
72. Battrum D, Gutmann J. Phantom tooth pain: A diagnosis of exclusion. Int Endod J 1996;29:190–194.
73. Gratt B, Sickles E, Graff-Radford S, Solberg W. Electronic thermography in the diagnosis of atypical odontalgia: A pilot study. Oral Surg Oral Med Oral Pathol 1989;68: 472–481.
74. Reik L. Atypical odontalgia: A localized form of atypical facial pain. Headache 1984;24:222–224.
75. Kreisberg M. Atypical odontalgia: Differential diagnosis and treatment. J Am Dent Assoc 1982;104:852–854.
76. Bates R. Atypical odontalgia: Phantom tooth pain. Oral Surg Oral Med Oral Pathol 1991;72:479–483.
77. Ren K, Dubner R. Focus article: Central nervous system plasticity and persistent pain. J Orofac Pain 1999;13: 155–163.
78. Woda A. Mechanisms of neuropathic pain. In: Lund J, Lavigne G, Dubner R, Sessle B (eds). Orofacial Pain: From Basic Science to Clinical Management. Chicago: Quintessence, 2001:67–78.
79. Lazar M, Greenlee R, Naarden A. Facial pain of neurologic origin mimicking oral pathologic conditions: Some current concepts and treatment. J Am Dent Assoc 1980;100:884–888.
80. Ratner E, Person P, Kleinman D, Shklar G, Socransky S. Jawbone cavities and trigeminal facial neuralgias. Oral Surg Oral Med Oral Pathol 1979;48:3–20.
81. Ratner E, Langer B, Evins M. Alveolar cavitational osteopathosis. Manifestations of an infectious process and its implication in the causation of chronic pain. J Periodontol 1986;57:593–603.
82. Roberts A, Person P, Chandran N, Hori J. Further observations of dental parameters of trigeminal and atypical facial neuralgias. Oral Surg Oral Med Oral Pathol 1984;58:121–129.
83. Bouquot J, McMahon R. Neuropathic pain in maxillofacial osteonecrosis. J Oral Maxillofac Surg 2000;58: 1003–1020.
84. Eversoll L, Chase P. Nonodontogenic orofacial pain and endodontics: Pain disorders involving the jaws that simulate odontalgia. In: Cohen S, Burns R (eds). Pathways of the Pulp, ed 8. St. Louis: Mosby, 2002:77–89.
85. Zuniga J. Challenging the neuralgia-inducing cavitational osteonecrosis concept. J Oral Maxillofac Surg 2000;58:1021–1028.
86. Woda A, Pionchon P. A unified concept of idiopathic orofacial pain: Pathophysiologic procedures. J Orofac Pain 2000;14:196–212.
87. Donlon W. Long-term effects of jawbone curretage on the pain of facial neuralgia. Discussion. J Oral Maxillofac Surg 1995;53:397–398.
88. Sciubba J. Long-term effects of jawbone curretage on the pain of facial neuralgia. Discussion. J Oral Maxillofac Surg 1995;53:398–399.
89. Loeser J. Tic douloureux and atypical facial pain. RCDC Symposium. J Can Dent Assoc 1985;51:917–923.
90. DeNucci D, Chen C, Sobiski C, Meehan S. The use of SPECT bone scans to evaluate patients with idiopathic jaw pain. Oral Surg Oral Med Oral Pathol Oral Radiol Endod 2000;90:750–757.
91. Segall R, del Rio C. Cavitational bone defect: A diagnostic challenge. J Endod 1991;17:396–400.
92. Moskowitz M, Henrikson B, Markowitz S. Intra- and extravascular nociceptive mechanisms and the pathogenesis of head pain. In: Olsen J, Edvinsson L (eds). Basic Mechanisms of Headache. Amsterdam: Elsevier, 1988:429–435.
93. Spierings E. Mechanism of migraine and action of antimigraine medications. Med Clin North Am 2001;85: 943–958.
94. Erdal M, Herken H, Yilmaz M, Bayazit Y. Association of the T102C polymorphism of 5-HT2A receptor gene with aura in migraine. J Neurol Sci 2001;188:99–101.
95. Hering-Hanit R, Friedman Z, Schlesinger I, Ellis M. Evidence for activation of the coagulation system in migraine with aura. Cephalalgia 2001;21:137–139.
96. Graff-Radford S. Headache problems that can present as toothache. Dent Clin North Am 1991;35:155–170.
97. Namazi M. Presentation of migraine as odontalgia. Headache 2001;41:420–421.
98. Wolf H. Preclinical and clinical pharmacology of the 5-HT3 receptor antagonists. Scand J Rheumatol Suppl 2000;113:37–45.
99. Deleu D, Hanssens Y. Current and emerging second-generation triptans in acute migraine therapy: A comparative review. J Clin Pharm 2000;40:687–700.

100. Magnus L. Nonepileptic uses of gabapentin. Epilepsia 1999;40(suppl 6):S66–S72.
101. Gobel H, Heinze A, Heinze-Kuhn K, Jost W. Evidence-based medicine: Botulinium toxin A in migraine and tension-type headache. J Neurol 2001;248(suppl 1):34–38.
102. Penarrocha M, Bagan J, Penarrocha M, Silvestre F. Cluster headache and cocaine use. Oral Surg Oral Med Oral Pathol Oral Radiol Endod 2000;90:271–274.
103. Bittar G, Graff-Radford S. Retrospective study of patients with cluster headaches. Oral Surg Oral Med Oral Pathol 1992;73:519–522 .
104. Tay B, Ngan Kee W, Chung D. Gabapentin for the treatment and prophylaxis of cluster headache. Reg Anesth Pain Med 2001;26:373–375.
105. Salvesen R. Cluster headache. Curr Treat Options Neurol 1999;1:441–449.
106. Fagnan L. Acute sinusitis: A cost-effective approach to diagnosis and treatment. Am Fam Physician 1998;58: 1795–1802.
107. Chen Y, Tseng C, Chao W, Harn W, Chung S. Toothache with a multifactorial etiology: A case report. Endod Dent Traumatol 1997;13:245–247.
108. Kieser J, Holborow D. The prevention and management of oral barotraumas. N Z Dent J 1997;93:114–116.
109. Kollmann N. Incidence and possible causes of dental pain during simulated high altitude flights. J Endod 1993:19:154–159.
110. Goethe W, Laban C, Beter H. Barodontalgia and barotrauma in the human teeth: Findings in navy divers, frogmen, and submariners of the Federal Republic of Germany. Mil Med 1989;54:491–495.
111. Punwutikorn J, Waikakul A, Ochareon P. Symptoms of unerupted third molars. Oral Surg Oral Med Oral Pathol Oral Radiol Endod 1999;87:305–310.
112. Schuler J, Camm J, Houston G. Bilateral eruption sequestra: Report of case. ASDC J Dent Child 1992;59:70–72.
113. Gallin D. "The clam syndrome" dental pain of unusual etiology. N Y State Dent J 1991;57:41.
114. Ludlow M, Brenneise C, Haft T. Chronic pain associated with a foreign body left under the soft tissue flap during periapical surgery. J Endod 1994;20:48–50.
115. Batchelder B, Krutchkoff D, Amara J. Mandibular pain as the initial and sole clinical manifestation of coronary insufficiency: Report of a case. J Am Dent Assoc 1987; 115:710–712.
116. Natkin E, Harrington G, Mandel M. Anginal pain referred to the teeth. Oral Surg Oral Med Oral Pathol 1975;40: 678–680.
117. Graham L, Schinbeckler G. Orofacial pain of cardiac origin. J Am Dent Assoc 1982;104:47–52.
118. Sandler N, Ziccardi V, Ochs M. Differential diagnosis of jaw pain in the elderly. J Am Dent Assoc 1995;126: 1263–1270.
119. Lopes A, de Souza Filho F, Jorge Junior J, de Almeida O. Herpes zoster infection as a differential diagnosis of acute pulpitis. J Endod 1998;24:143–144.
120. Goon W, Jacobsen P. Prodromal odontalgia and multiple devitalized teeth caused by a herpes zoster infection of the trigeminal nerve: Report of a case. JAMA 1988;166: 500–504.
121. Gregory WB, Brook LE, Penmick EC. Herpes zoster associated with pulpless teeth. J Endod 1975;1:32–38.
122. Rauckhorst AJ, Baumgartner C. Zebra XIX. Part 2. Oral herpes zoster. J Endod 2000;26:469–471.
123. O'Rourke C, Mitropoulos C. Orofacial pain in patients with sickle cell disease. Br Dent J 1990;169:130–132.
124. O'Rourke C, Hawley G. Sickle cell disorder and orofacial pain in Jamaican patients. Br Dent J 1998;185:90–92.
125. Cohen S, Baumgartner C, Carpenter W. Oral prodromal signs of a central nervous system malignant neoplasm—Glioblastoma multiforme. Report of a case. J Am Dent Assoc 1986;112:643–645.
126. Glaser C, Lang S, Pruckmayer W, Millesi W, Rasse M, Marosi C, Leitha T. Clinical manifestations and diagnostic approach to metastatic cancer of the mandible. Int J Oral Maxillofac Surg 1997;26:365–368.
127. Pruckmayer M, Glaser C, Marosi C, Leitha T. Mandibular pain as the leading clinical symptom for metastatic disease: Nine cases and review of the literature. Ann Oncol 1998;9:559–564.
128. Selden H, Manhoff D, Hatges N, Michel R. Metastatic carcinoma to the mandible that mimicked pulpal/periradicular disease. J Endod 1998;24:267–270.
129. Ribera M. Osteoblastoma in the anterior maxilla mimicking periapical pathosis of odontogenic origin. J Endod 1996;22:142–146.
130. Miyaguchi M, Sakai S. Spontaneous pain in patients with maxillary sinus carcinoma in relation to T-classification and direction of tumor spread. J Laryngol Otol 1992; 106:804–806.
131. Saxby P, Soutar D. Intra-oral tumors presenting after dental extraction. Br Dent J 1989;166:337–338.
132. Bavitz J, Paterson D, Sorensen S. Non-Hodgkin's lymphoma disguised as odontogenic pain. J Am Dent Assoc 1992;123:99–100.
133. Kant S. Pain referred to teeth as the sole discomfort in undiagnosed mediastinal lymphoma: Report of a case. J Am Dent Assoc 1989;118:587–588.
134. Alaluusua S, Donner U, Rapola J. Nonendemic Burkitt's lymphoma with jaw involvement: Case report. Pediatr Dent 1987;9:158–162.
135. Whitaker S, Singh B, Weller R, Bath K, Loushine R. Sex hormone receptor status of the dental pulp and lesions of pulpal origin. Oral Surg Oral Med Oral Pathol Oral Radiol Endod 1999;87:233–237.
136. Frances A, Pincus H, First M. Diagnostic and Statistical Manual of Mental Disorders. Washington, DC: American Psychiatric Associaton, 1994:458–462.
137. Bjil P. Psychogenic pain in dentistry. Compendium 1995; 16:46–54.

138. Dworkin S, Burgess J. Orofacial pain of psychogenic origin: Current concepts and classification. J Am Dent Assoc 1987;115:565–571.

139. Fordyce W, Steger J. Chronic pain. In: Pormerteau D, Brady J (eds). Behavior Medicine: Theory and Practice. Baltimore: William & Wilkins, 1979:125.

140. Hathaway K. Psychiatric and somatoform pain disorders: The least common diagnosis. In: Fricton JR, Kroenning RJ, Hathaway KM (eds). TMJ and Craniofacial Pain: Diagnosis and Management. St Louis: Ishiyaku EuroAmerica, 1988:149–158.

141. Ide M. The differential diagnosis of sensitive teeth. Dent Update 1998;25:462–466.

142. Hargreaves KM. The elephant. J Orofac Pain 1999;13:77.

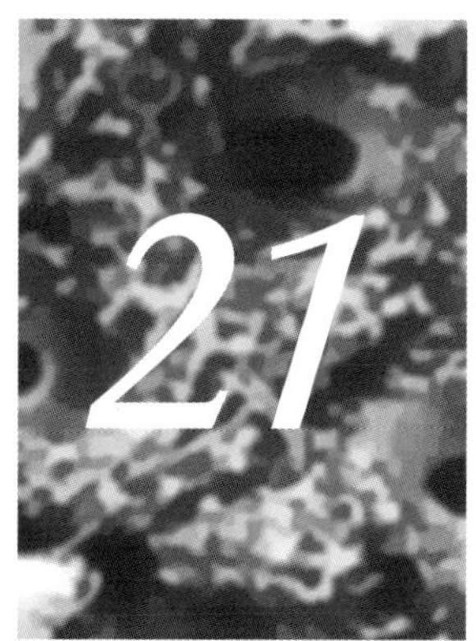

The Dental Pulp in Systemic Disorders

I. B. Bender, DDS
Kenneth M. Hargreaves, DDS, PhD

A major theme of this textbook is the interrelationship between dental pulp and other tissues in health and disease. This relationship is truly bidirectional in that the pulp has the potential to affect systemic health (eg, the potential bacteremia associated with infective endocarditis[1-4]) and systemic disorders have the potential to affect dental pulp.[5-9] Indeed, the effect of systemic disorders on the dental pulp is so strong that it has been suggested that dental pulp "biopsies" be used to diagnose certain systemic diseases.[10-12]

This chapter focuses on selected systemic disorders and their effect on the dental pulp. Related issues are discussed in chapters 2, 17, and 20. The focus and scope of this chapter preclude an extensive discussion of the effect of systemic disorders on teeth, periodontal structures, and bone; the interested reader is encouraged to seek other reviews on these important topics.[5,13-15] Other sources should be reviewed to provide background information on the pathogeneses and nonpulpal features of these systemic disorders.[16,17]

Systemic Viral Infections and the Dental Pulp

Human immunodeficiency virus (HIV)

Infection by HIV is a well-recognized worldwide epidemic that can lead to the development of acquired immunodeficiency syndrome (AIDS). Several studies have reported on the dental pathoses associated with HIV infection. Children who are perinatally infected with HIV and who have low CD4 cell counts (a marker for the helper T subclass of lymphocytes) have higher caries rates and fewer remaining teeth than do children with higher CD4 cell counts.[18,19] The increased incidence of tooth loss may be due in part to an enhanced sensitivity to bacterial lipopolysaccharide that is observed in monocytes collected from HIV-infected patients. The exposure of lipopolysaccharide to monocytes from HIV-infected patients produces significantly greater release of pro-inflammatory cytokines (eg, interleukin-1β, interleukin-6, tumor necrosis factor α) than does exposure to monocytes from

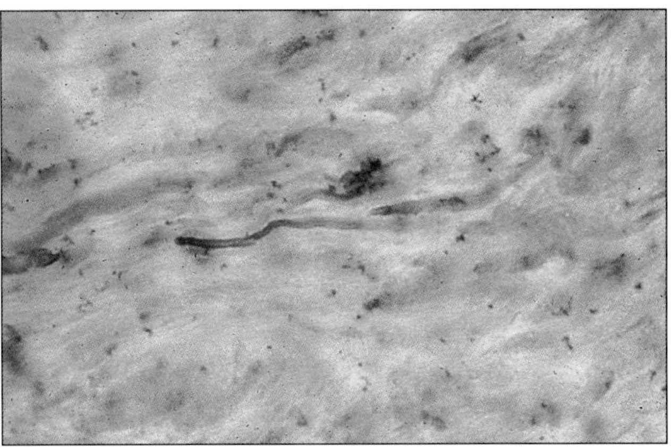

Fig 21-1 Evaluation of the presence of HIV in human dental pulp using in situ hybridization histochemistry. Dental pulp tissue from an HIV-positive patient was fixed, sectioned, and incubated with one of two biotinylated oligonucleotide probes complementary to a region of messenger RNA specific to HIV. Sections were incubated, washed, and developed. A positive signal is visible as a dark spot in the figure. (Reprinted from Glick et al[22] with permission.)

control patients; this excessive release of cytokines may lead to increased incidences of periodontitis and tooth loss in patients with HIV.[20,21]

HIV has been found in dental pulp[22] and in periradicular lesions of pulpal origin[23]; this finding has clinical implications in reinforcing universal precautions (Fig 21-1).

The reduced specific immune response observed in patients with low CD4 cell counts does not appear to be associated with an increase in endodontic complications after root canal treatment (see chapter 17).[24,25]

Herpesvirus infections

Herpes infection has been proposed to be a potential etiologic factor of pulpal necrosis and should be considered in the differential diagnosis of odontalgia (see chapter 20). Two forms of herpes simplex virus (HSV-1 and HSV-2) have been implicated in clinical viral infections. HSV-1 is associated with trigeminal infections, including herpes labialis and herpetic stomatitis.

The pathophysiology of herpes viral infections is known to involve sensory nerves and their peripheral termini. Therefore, it has been suggested that the clinical presentation may include multiple unilateral necrotic dental pulps, and this should alert the clinician to a possible herpesvirus etiology. However, in one study, HSV was not detected (using polymerase chain reaction) in 11 pulps with a diagnosis of irreversible pulpitis or in an additional 17 teeth with necrotic pulps.[26]

Herpes zoster (shingles) is caused by neuronal infection of the varicella zoster virus, which also causes chicken pox in children. Herpes zoster can occur more frequently in immunocompromised patients (eg, patients with lymphoma, Hodgkin disease, lymphatic leukemia, or AIDS) or the elderly. The activation of herpesvirus in the trigeminal nerve is characterized by a prodromal period of severe pain, usually lasting 2 to 3 days, followed by the classic vesicular eruption along the nerve pathway of the involved dermatome area, an area of the skin or mucosa supplied by an afferent nerve fiber. These vesicles subsequently rupture, and can lead to scarring, postherpetic neuralgia, and paresthesia.

This type of pain is very severe and continuous and, if intraoral, may be reported to involve several teeth. The prodromal pain may create a diagnostic problem, because it can mimic acute odontalgia.[27-30] Viral eruption patterns may include peripheral nerve endings in the pulp and periodontal ligament, leading to pain and possibly to pulpal necrosis[29,31-34] or internal resorption.[28] Surveys indicate that fewer than 2% of all herpes zoster cases involve the mandibular or maxillary divisions of the trigeminal nerve,[35] and only a few case reports involving teeth have been published. Involved teeth may show signs of acute pulpitis or present as necrotic with apical periodontitis (Fig 21-2). A common feature of these case reports is the presence of stress in the patient's life prior to the outbreak (loss of job, holiday season, etc).[27,29,33,34]

Fig 21-2 Periradicular radiograph of a patient 5 months after a herpes zoster outbreak. Note the periradicular radiolucencies of the maxillary left canine and first and second premolar. (Reprinted from Goon and Jacobsen[34] with permission.)

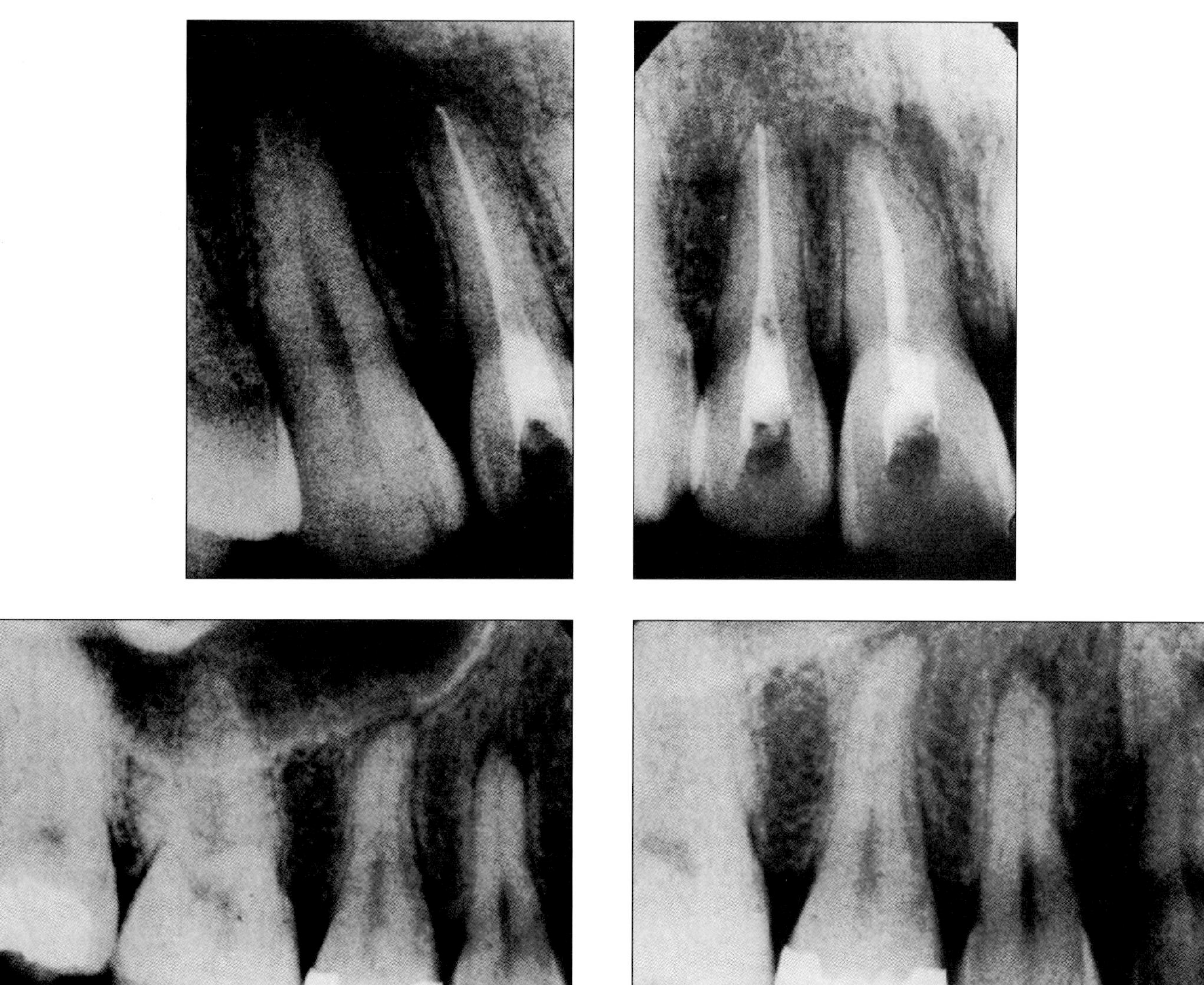

Rubella (German measles)

Rubella infections and their effects on the dental pulp may begin in the first trimester of pregnancy when the mother contracts rubella, causing cytopathic effects in the ameloblasts of primary teeth in the developing embryo. The ensuing enamel defect in the affected tooth leaves a telltale pathognomonic clinical sign of rubella[36,37] (Fig 21-3). With vaccination of the mother, the disease is now rare in many countries.

Other exanthematous disorders, eg, measles or chicken pox, may cause enamel defects of a linear type in permanent teeth (Fig 21-4) because these diseases occur after birth. Because enamel is continuously elaborated during tooth development, it is possible to estimate the age at which the fever occurred by the location of the linear defect on the enamel surface of the tooth. Thus, the enamel presents a clinical clue as to when the systemic disorder occurred.

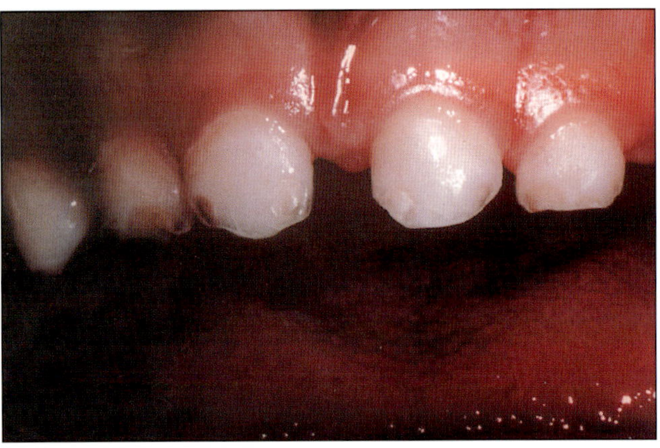

Fig 21-3 Patient with rubella. Note the discoloration of the maxillary anterior teeth.

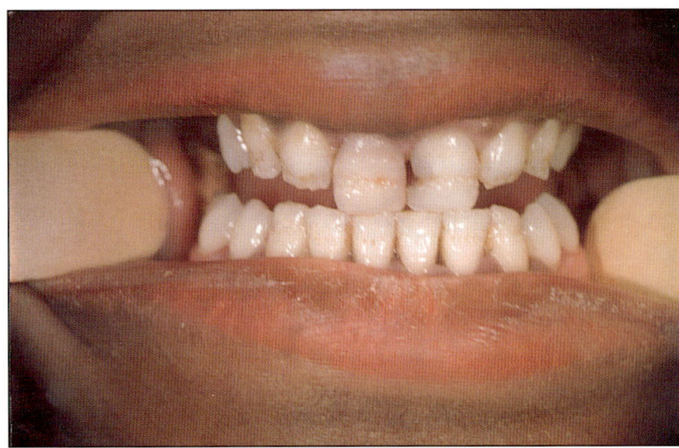

Fig 21-4 Enamel hypoplasia. Note the linear defect in enamel formation that may occur from any of the exanthematous fevers (eg, rubella, measles, or chicken pox). The position of the linear defect depends on the age of morphodifferentiation of the different permanent teeth at the time of the infection.

Paget disease (osteitis deformans)

Paget disease is a chronic, progressive bone disease characterized by active bone turnover.[38,39] Although it has an unknown etiology, it is included in this section of the chapter because the measles virus of the paramyxovirus family is implicated as the causative agent of this disorder[40,41] and electron microscopy of involved bone is consistent with viral infection.[16,40,42,43] Moreover, virus-infected bone cells collected from patients with Paget disease have been shown to generate bone resorptive factors, including interleukin-6, a resorptive cytokine.[44-46] A candidate gene on chromosome 18q may also serve as a risk factor for Paget disease.[39] Paget disease is found in about 3% of patients older than 40 years of age and in 11% of patients older than 90 years of age.

Paget disease is often detected through a routine dental radiographic examination because of the pathognomonic "cotton wool" appearance of the bone.[47] The exuberant metabolic increase in osteoclastic and osteoblastic activity, high blood serum alkaline phosphatase, and increase in urinary hydroxyproline excretion are important pathogenic features in this disease, leading to a disorganized bone breakdown, bone deformity, bone pain, fracture, and osteomyelitis.

Studies have shown that 93% of patients with Paget disease who have bone changes in the maxilla or mandible also have dental problems. In contrast, only 10% of Paget patients who have bone changes in other distant body parts or changes restricted to the skull (excluding the mandible and maxilla) have dental problems.[48] The appearance of bony changes in the maxilla or mandible is associated with a higher incidence of cardiac disease.[48]

Most posterior teeth in patients in the sclerotic phase of Paget disease manifest a hyperplasia of the cementum. A large amount of cementum is deposited in the apical two thirds of the roots, giving the tooth the appearance of a baseball bat (Fig 21-5). The cementum of the root appears to be fused at times with the adjacent sclerotic bone[49] (Fig 21-6); there is no evidence of periodontal ligament space. Teeth may be abnormally firm when hypercementosis is present.[50] Hypercementosis of roots may occur without the presence of bone sclerosis in either jaw. The presence of root hypercementosis in dentate patients older than 40 years is pathognomonic for Paget disease.

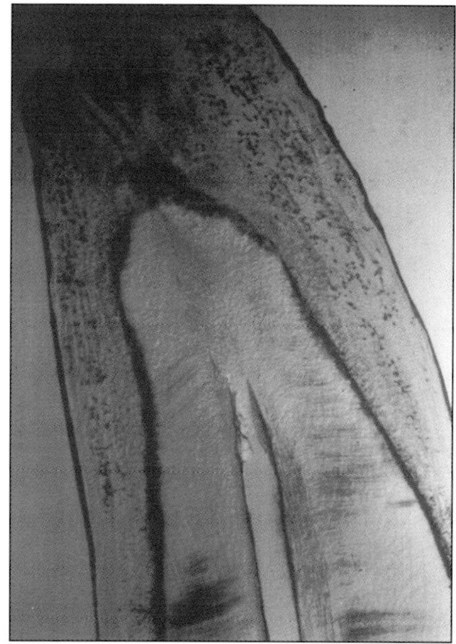

Fig 21-5 Ground section of a maxillary second premolar showing the extensive hypercementosis associated with Paget disease.

Fig 21-6 Characteristic intraoral radiographic features of Paget disease. Note the variable appearance of canal space, periodontal ligament space, and lamina dura. (Reprinted from Barnett and Elfenbein[49] with permission.)

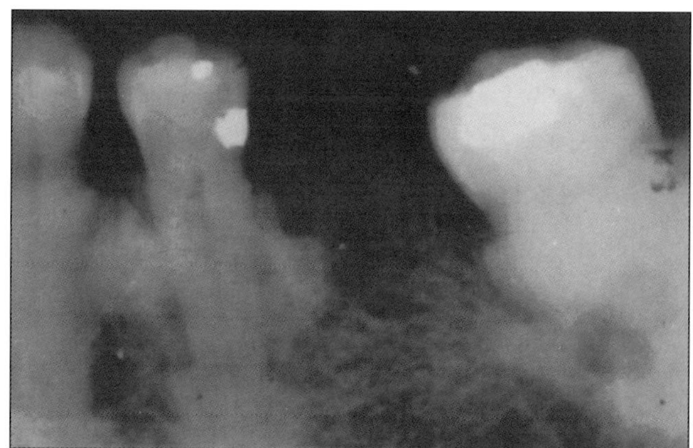

Fig 21-6a Areas of radiolucency.

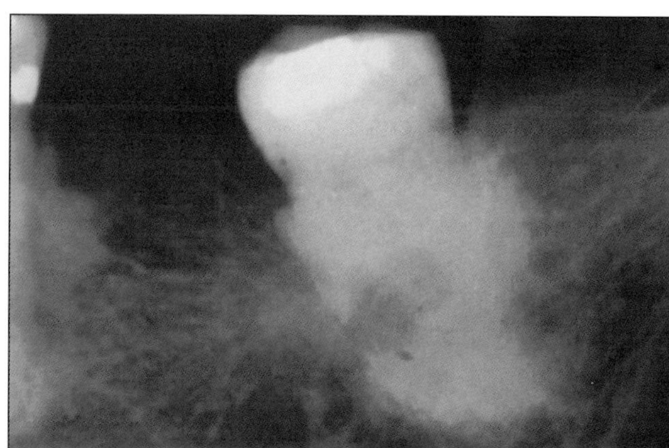

Fig 21-6b Isolated sclerosis.

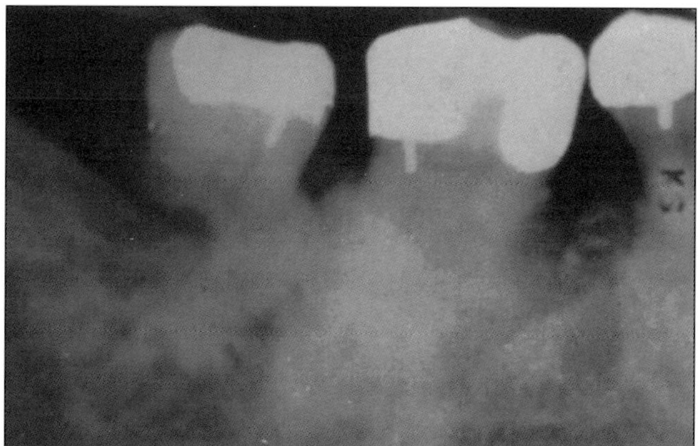

Fig 21-6c Isolated sclerosis and distal root resorption of the maxillary second molar.

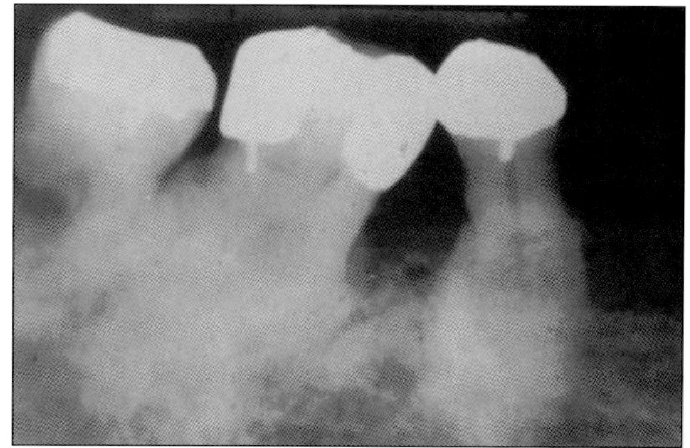

Fig 21-6d Isolated sclerosis and hypercementosis of the second premolar.

Table 21-1 Dental findings in 50 cases of hereditary vitamin D–resistant rickets*

Observation	No. of cases	%
Large pulps	30	60
Pulp horns (DEJ)	25	50
Enamel hypoplasia	14	28
Radiolucent band	7	14
Thin enamel	27	54
Periapical rarefactions	23	46
Sinus tracts	18	36
Lamina dura absent	9	18
Globular dentin	14	100

*Data from Bender and Naidorf.[5]

At other times, most likely during the lytic phase, the periodontal ligament space is wider because of the loss of the lamina dura. Absence of alveolar lamina dura in Paget disease is restricted to certain groups of teeth and never affects all teeth, as occurs in primary or secondary hyperparathyroidism. Additional changes during the lytic phase include root resorption associated with loosening of teeth.[49] Root resorption may be present in some teeth and hypercementosis in others, just as both resorption and formation of hard tissue may be found in bone.

Paget disease also affects the dental pulp. The strongest evidence is a radiographic appearance of pulpal obliteration.[51] There are relatively few published histologic studies.[52,53] In one case report on a mandibular third molar, there were signs of internal resorption of dentin; direct apposition of cellular hard tissue partially occluded the coronal pulp. This pulpal tissue, too, had the mosaic pattern that was present in the bone and cementum. The radicular region of the pulp displayed dystrophic calcification.[52,53]

In the endodontic treatment of pagetic teeth, it is sometimes difficult to establish the location of the terminal apical ending. This objective is essential to preventing periradicular irritation that may lead to osteomyelitis, a frequent complication in teeth affected by Paget disease. Under these circumstances, it may be prudent to use an apex locator to establish the canal length.

Genetic and Developmental Disorders and the Dental Pulp

The molecular basis of several of the following developmental disorders is reviewed in chapter 2.

Hypophosphatemic rickets

Hypophosphatemic rickets (hereditary vitamin D-resistant rickets) is a genetic disorder that is inherited as an X-linked dominant trait and therefore is often more severe in male patients.[16,54] It is characterized by hypophosphatemia, reduced intestinal absorption of calcium, and osteomalacia (ie, rickets) that do not respond to vitamin D therapy. In type I hypophosphatemic rickets, circulating levels of vitamin D3 are reduced; in the second form of this disorder (type II), cellular response to vitamin D is reduced, possibly because of a reduced expression of its receptor.

Many clinical features have been noted,[16] including several found in the dental pulp and oral tissues. The major clinical findings include frontal bossing of the skull, bowing of the legs, short stature, enlarged wrists and ankles, a waddling gait, and alopecia totalis. The primary laboratory finding is hypophosphatemia, although increased urinary phosphate excretion and increased serum levels of alkaline phosphatase may also be observed.

Both pathognomonic radiographic signs and periradicular lesions that are resistant to endodontic therapy are found in patients with this disorder.[5] The dental features are summarized in Table 21-1. The critical sign in this disease is the radiographic finding of pulp horns that extend to the dentinoenamel junction (DEJ) in all teeth, both primary and permanent. This sign can be viewed on a single intraoral radiograph and is looked on as a pathognomonic sign in this disease (Fig 21-7). Under normal conditions, the pulp horns are confined within the coronal dentin of the tooth and do not extend to the inner enamel surface or DEJ (Fig 21-8).[5]

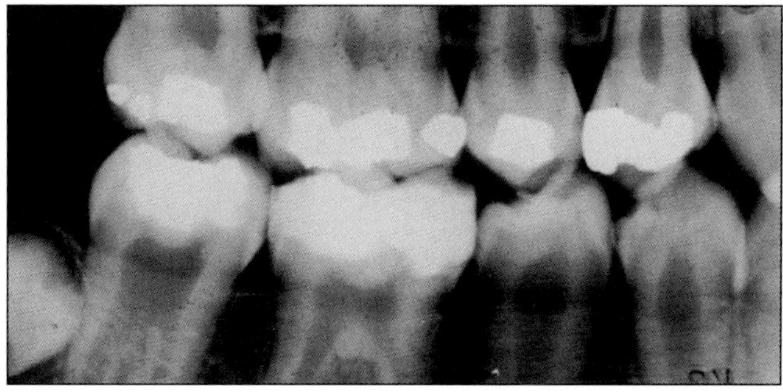

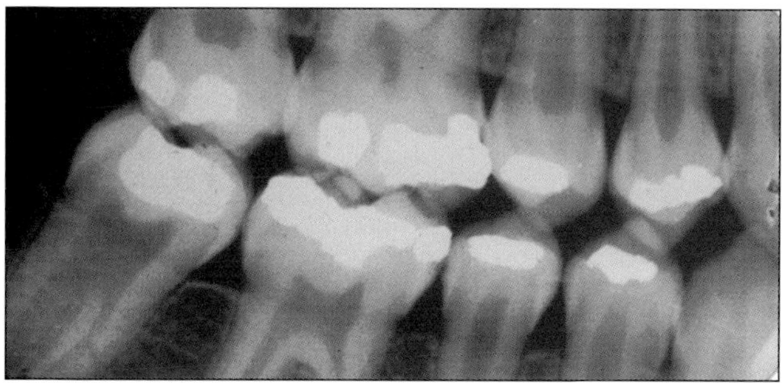

Fig 21-7 Bitewing radiographs of a patient with vitamin D–resistant rickets. Note the enlarged pulp chambers, large root canal systems, and pulp horns that extend to the DEJ. (Reprinted from Bender and Naidorf[5] with permission.)

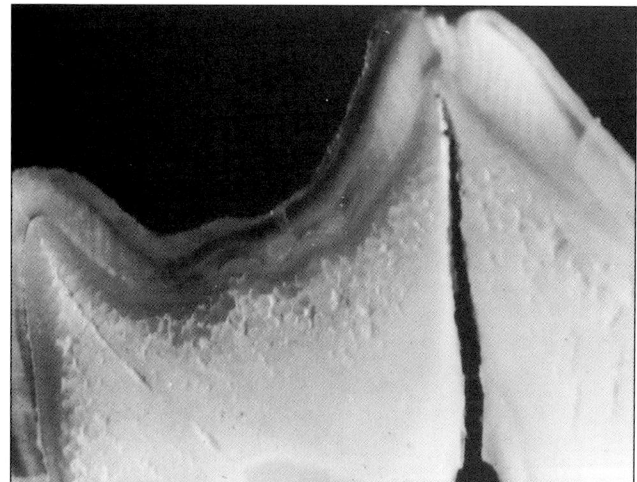

Fig 21-8 Ground section of a premolar from a patient with vitamin D–resistant rickets showing the extension of the pulp horn to the dentinoenamel junction. Note also the appearance of hypoplastic enamel and interglobular dentin. (Courtesy of Dr C. J. Witkop.)

The severity of the clinical and radiographic dental lesions is influenced by the patient's age, the type of teeth (prenatal or postnatal odontogenesis), and whether the patient was undergoing therapy prior to the time of examination. During odontogenesis, large daily doses of calcitriol or vitamin D can cause complete obliteration of the large pulp chambers.[55] Patients often exhibit a delay in apical maturation or closure, particularly in the permanent teeth. The different type of dental changes observed in individual patients may be attributed to the existence of different clinical forms of this disease and the presence or absence of associated hypophosphatemia.[56]

In radiographs of normal teeth, the enamel is distinctly more radiopaque than dentin. However, the enamel of teeth in patients with hereditary vitamin D-resistant rickets appears to be only slightly more radiopaque than the dentin (see Fig 21-7). This difference may be attributed to the presence of thin enamel in approximately 54% of patients affected by hereditary vitamin D-resistant rickets (see Table 21-1). The thin enamel is caused by a hypocalcification that is characterized by a deficiency in quantity of mineral per unit of volume. This finding is supported by studies showing that vitamin D deficiency causes a reduction in tooth mass and absolute weight of the deposited mineral.[57]

Dental radiographic changes most often observed in patients with hereditary vitamin D-resistant rickets include radiographic manifesta-

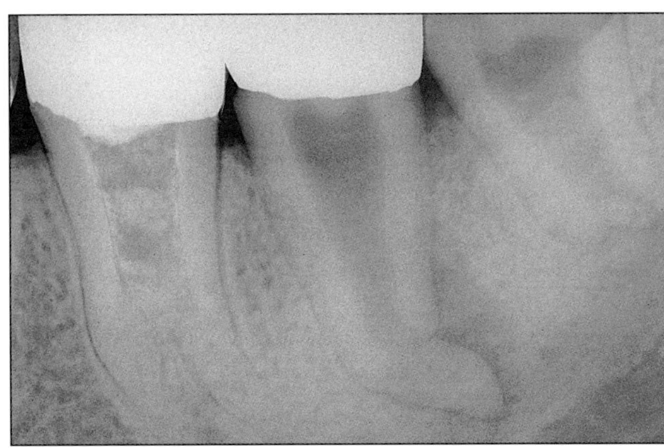

Fig 21-9 Preoperative radiograph of a taurodontic mandibular right second molar. Note the relatively large pulp chamber and shortened roots with distal caries. (Reprinted from Hayashi[67] with permission.)

tions of enlarged pulp chambers, wide root canals, and pulp horns extending to the DEJ. Another, less frequently observed, radiographic sign is a radiolucent band that surrounds the region of the entire DEJ in both primary and permanent teeth.[58,59] This radiolucent band is caused by the larger zones of poorly calcified interglobular dentin at the periphery of the DEJ.[60]

A conspicuous and frequent oral clinical feature of hereditary vitamin D-resistant rickets is the presence of draining sinus tracts and swellings with periradicular abscesses. This is attributed to pulpal necrosis caused by a rapid entry of bacteria and their toxins through the poorly mineralized enamel and dentin.[61] The incidence of the clinical lesions has been estimated to be 36% (see Table 21-1).[5] The pulpal-periradicular abscesses do not appear to be the result of caries.[61]

The reason for the dental complications of pulpal necrosis and subsequent periradicular lesions becomes apparent when histologic and ground sections of the teeth are examined (see Fig 21-8). The pulp horn defect that extends to the DEJ appears as a tubular cleft covered only by a thin layer of hypoplastic enamel. The subsequent attrition of the enamel allows bacterial entry into the dentinal tubules and pulp.[8,61,62] Longitudinal studies on these patients indicate that there is a continuous progression of periradicular disease that develops in affected teeth.[5,6]

Taurodontism

Taurodontism is a developmental disturbance of teeth that results in abnormally large pulp chambers. This is accompanied by a morphologic change in tooth structure in which the crown of the tooth is larger and the roots are shorter than the typical form.[56,63-65] Taurodontism occurs most frequently in molars and may be unilateral or bilateral in its expression. Patients with chromosomal aneuploides, particularly additional X chromosomes, have a higher incidence of taurodontic teeth.[63,66]

Radiographs of teeth affected by taurodontism reveal much longer pulp chambers and shortened root canal systems[67] (Fig 21-9). This may resemble the presentation of teeth affected by hereditary vitamin D-resistant rickets, except that the critical sign, pulp horns that extend to the DEJ, is not evident. Endodontic treatment of taurodonts must take into account the larger pulp chambers, the greater difficulty in locating canal orifices, and the potential for additional root canal systems (eg, five canals in mandibular molars).[67,68]

Dens in dente (dens invaginatis) and dens evaginatus

There are several examples of developmental disorders of morphodifferentiation of teeth. Dens in dente (dens invaginatus) and dens evaginatus, two of the more common disorders of morphodifferentiation that have pulpal implications, are reviewed in this section. The reader is encouraged to review oral pathology textbooks for a complete discussion of other disorders of morphodifferentiation (eg, gemination, fusion, concrescence, and dilacerations).[13-15]

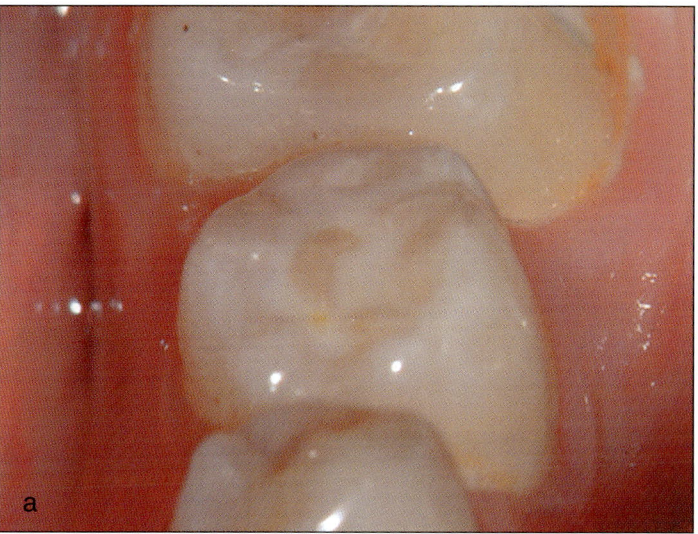
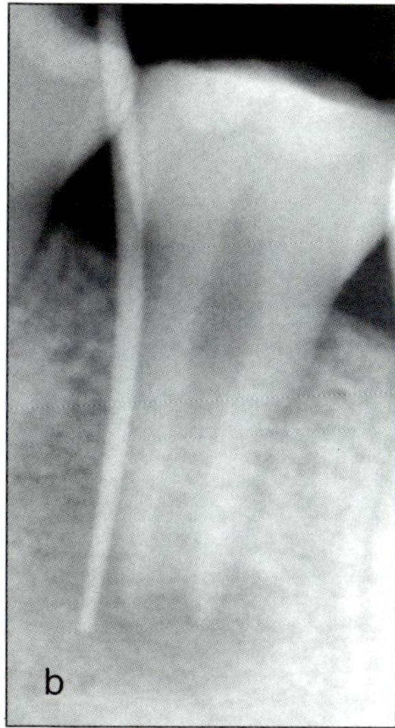
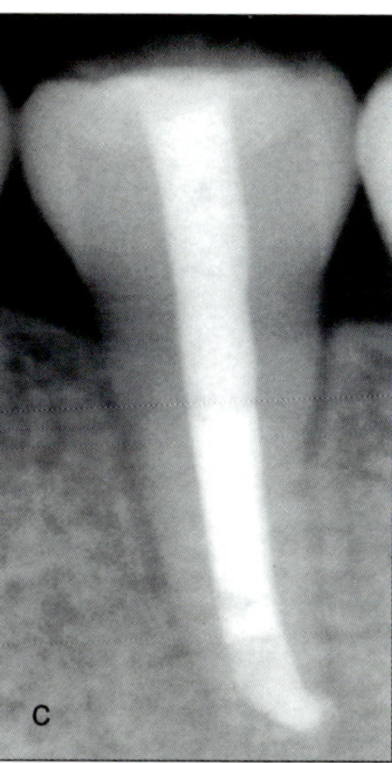

Fig 21-10 Clinical and radiographic views of dens evaginatus in an 11-year-old boy. *(a)* Clinical view of external anatomy. *(b)* Preoperative radiograph. Note the extensive periradicular radiolucency, complex root canal systems, and immature apex. The sinus tract is traced with a gutta-percha cone. *(c)* Postoperative view illustrating the use of Collatape (Sulzer Dental, Carlsbad, CA) and mineral trioxide aggregate (MTA) as an internal barrier and final obturation with thermoplasticized gutta-percha. (Courtesy of Drs Neil Begley and William Schindler.)

Dens in dente is a developmental disorder in which a portion of the crown undergoes an invagination prior to calcification. This is thought to involve an infolding of the dental papilla during development and may occur because of altered tissue pressures, trauma, infection, or localized discrepancies in cellular hyperplasia (eg, apically directed proliferation of ameloblasts). Dens in dente is characterized by a deep infolding of enamel and dentin and often involves maxillary lateral incisors.[69] Teeth affected by dens in dente are classified into three types: type 1 is an enamel-lined relatively minor defect; type 2 is an enamel-lined blind sac that invades the root; and type 3 invades the root and has a secondary foramen. The prevalence has been reported to be between 0.04% and 10%.[15]

There are several points of clinical significance in the dens in dente tooth. First, there is an increased risk of bacteria-induced pulpal necrosis, and prophylactic placement of sealants may be indicated.[69,70] Second, nonsurgical root canal treatment is difficult because the anatomic complexity makes both tissue debridement and complete obturation extremely challenging. Suggested treatment approaches include the use of ultrasonic files, calcium hydroxide dressings, and obturation with a thermoplasticized gutta-percha technique.

Dens evaginatus is a localized outgrowth of ameloblasts that appears clinically as a globule of enamel and may be reminiscent of an accessory cusp. This outgrowth contains enamel, dentin, and pulp. It typically occurs on premolars or molars. The prevalence is higher among Asians (about 15%) than among Caucasians.[15] The clinical significance of this disorder is that the relatively narrow shelf of enamel, once penetrated, often leads to pulpal exposure.

A clinical example of a dens evaginatus is presented in Fig 21-10. An 11-year-old boy presented with bilateral dens evaginatus of the first premolars. The mandibular left premolar was necrotic

Fig 21-11 Periradicular radiographs of a patient with type I dentinogenesis imperfecta.

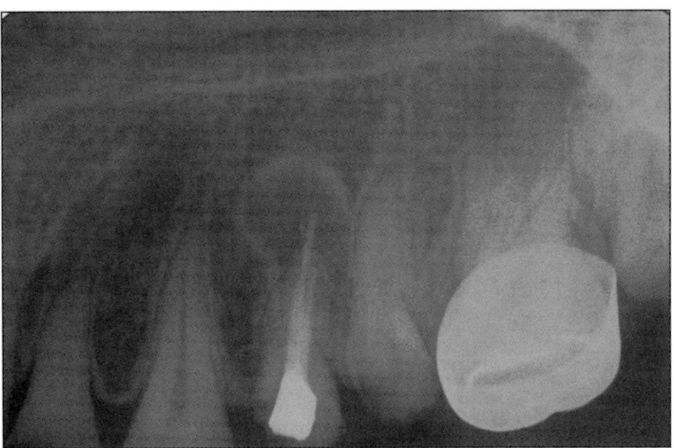

Fig 21-11a Preoperative radiograph. Note the reduced size of the pulp chamber, canal orifices, and canal systems in the first premolar, as well as the over-extended gutta-percha and apical periodontitis.

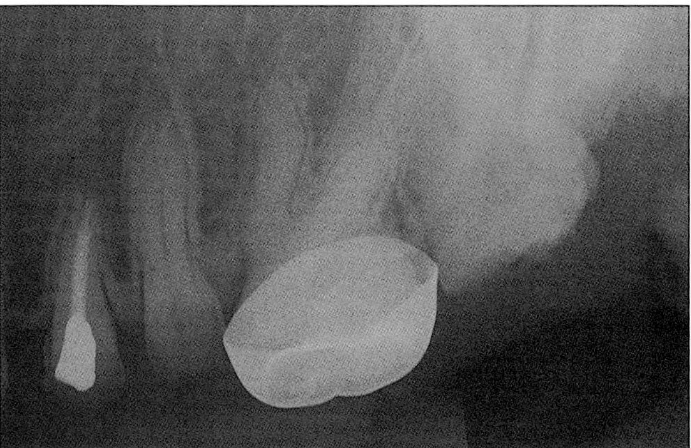

Fig 21-11b One-year follow-up after root-end resection and MTA retrofill of the first premolar.

and exhibited suppurative apical periodontitis. The root canal system was chemomechanically debrided and then treated with calcium hydroxide for 3 months with replacements every 4 to 6 weeks. An artificial barrier of absorbable collagen membrane (Collatape) and MTA (ProRoot MTA [Tulsa Dental, Tulsa, OK]) was placed, and the tooth was obturated with thermoplasticized gutta-percha.

Dentinogenesis imperfecta

Dentinogenesis imperfecta is an autosomal-dominant hereditary developmental disorder characterized by an altered expression of dentin matrix proteins. The most common of dental genetic diseases, it is found in about 1:6,000 individuals.[71-74] The three major types of dentinogenesis imperfecta are type I, associated with osteogenesis imperfecta; type II, dentin matrix only, also known as *hereditary opalescent dentin*; and type III, which is characterized by frequent pulpal exposures, large pulp chambers, and a "shell" tooth appearance.[71-75] The disorder can be expressed in either the primary or the permanent dentition.

The clinical presentation of dentinogenesis imperfecta includes amber to bluish-green teeth, crowns with severe attrition, and root canal chambers that become radiographically obliterated because of overproduction of dentin (Fig 21-11). In early stages of dentinogenesis imperfecta, the appearance may resemble the large pulp chambers found in hereditary vitamin D–resistant rickets or taurodontism, but the differential diagnosis is apparent on clinical examination because all teeth with dentinogenesis imperfecta manifest the amber to bluish-green color and radiographically obliterated pulp spaces.

Nonsurgical root canal treatment of teeth with dentinogenesis imperfecta is difficult because of obliteration of the pulp system, including mineralization of the pulp chamber, canal orifices, and systems.[76] Surgical root canal treatment of these teeth is also problematic because it is difficult to identify canal systems even after root resection.[76]

Amelogenesis imperfecta

Amelogenesis imperfecta comprises a large group of developmental disorders that results in impaired enamel formation.[63,73,77,78] It is estimated to occur in 1:14,000 patients and may arise from multiple etiologies because its inheritance pattern has been suggested to be autosomal dominant, autosomal recessive, or X-linked.[77]

In one study of nine unrelated families, about 20% of the patients with amelogenesis imperfecta were found to have increased pulpal calcifications as well as the expected disturbances in enamel formation.[77] Endodontic treatment considerations in these patients relate in part to the long-term prognosis of these teeth and the restorative difficulties.[79-81]

Gaucher disease

Gaucher disease (glucocerebroside lipidosis) is a genetic recessive disorder characterized by an accumulation of glucocerebrosides in the reticuloendothelial cells of the body. The accumulation of glucocerebrosides results from the deletion or reduced activity of the enzyme acid β-glucosidase in macrophages and an accumulation of lipids in these cells. Three different types of Gaucher disease have been described, characterized in part by age of onset.[16] Type 1 Gaucher disease is the most common form and is found in adults. It is the most prevalent genetic disease of Ashkenazi Jews.

Because dental radiographic examinations are usually performed more frequently than any other radiographic examination, some occult systemic disorders can be detected from dental radiographs in the absence of clinical symptoms.[5,6,82-85] This is the case for Gaucher disease. In Gaucher disease, radiographic bone changes manifest generalized osteopenia, including loss of trabecular structure, cortical thinning, and an Erlenmeyer flask-like appearance of the distal head of the femur (looked on as a pathognomonic sign for Gaucher disease).

Gaucher disease can manifest radiographic bone changes in the body of the mandible and in the region of the first molar and premolar (Fig 21-12). Cases with 13- and 60-year follow-ups have been published.[6] This radiographic bone lesion was a consistent finding in 11 patients with type 1 Gaucher disease.[86-93] Comparative radiographs taken over a 60-year time span show that lesions enlarge and temporary bone regeneration occurs after tooth extraction in proximity to the lesion or following a fracture of the long bone or curettage of the lesion in the mandible.[6] However, this healing is subsequently followed by the reformation of the lytic bony changes.

In skeletal surveys, the jaws, and particularly the mandible, are often ignored. Yet, all 11 cases described in Table 21-2 show most of the aforementioned radiographic changes in the molar and premolar region of the mandible. This finding indicates that the observed changes are not of local origin. This region normally contains hematopoietic marrow. The mandible also manifests increased osteolysis and osteosclerosis. Twelve to 15 years after the onset of Gaucher disease, the myeloid packing of glucocerebroside in the apical region of the first molar and second premolar region can become so great that it causes a slow, uniform, apical resorption of those teeth without producing the complications of pulpal necrosis (see Fig 21-12). Electric pulp testing in the reported cases gave positive responses.[94]

Accumulation of Gaucher cells causes a scalloped appearance in the endosteal bone region. Both the mandible and maxilla manifest an osteoporotic pattern similar to that found in patients with hemoglobinopathies (Figs 21-12 and 21-13).

Another dental pathogenetic disorder that has been observed in patients with Gaucher disease is periapical replacement resorption[93] (see Fig 21-12). This is commonly found in the first molar and premolar region of the mandible, bilaterally. Biopsy and autopsy evidence discloses that periapical cementum is replaced with Gaucher cells and fibrous tissue.[87,89] Systemic periapical replacement resorption also occurs in Paget disease.[95]

Fig 21-12 Radiographic presentation of Gaucher disease. (Reprinted from Bender and Bender[6] with permission.)

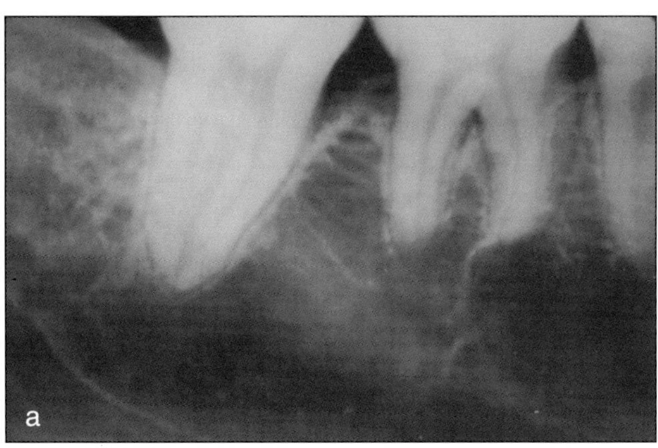

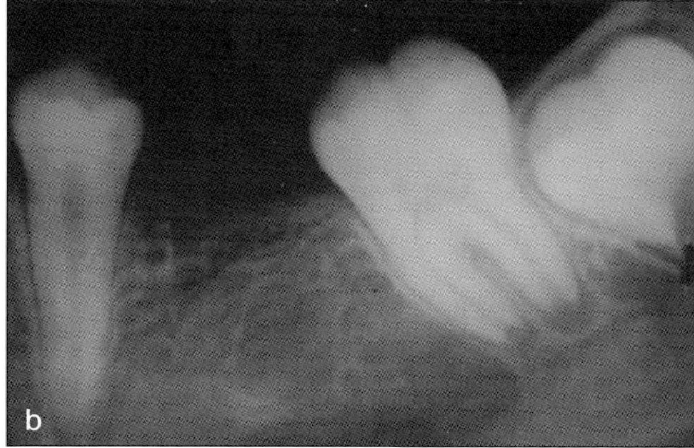

Figs 21-12a and 21-12b Uniform bilateral periapical radiolucency of the mandibular second premolars and first molars.

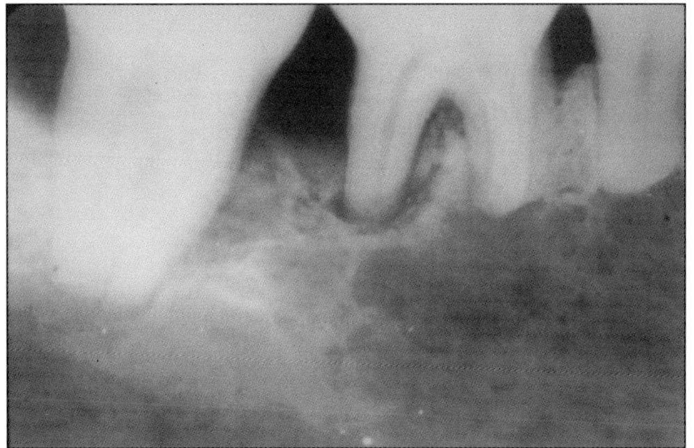

Fig 21-12c Twenty-year follow-up revealing evidence of periapical root resorption on the second premolar and first molar. The resorption only occurs in the apical portion of the roots.

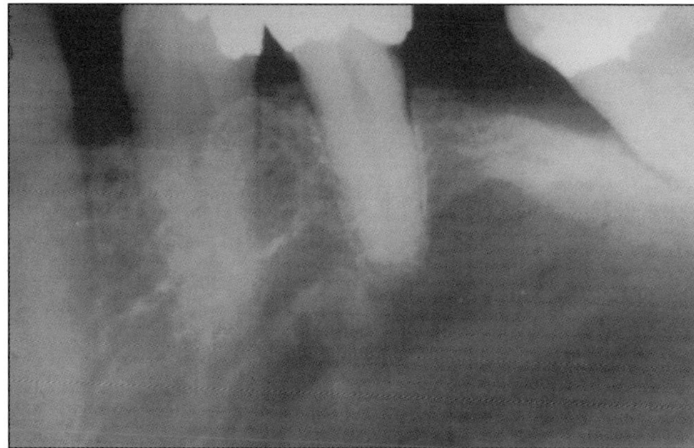

Fig 21-12d Twenty-year follow-up of the contralateral side reveals less periapical root resorption.

Table 21-2 Dental observations in 11 cases of Gaucher disease (type 1)*

Mandibular radiolucency	Maxillary radiolucency	Osteopenia	Sclerotic changes	Biopsy	Hemorrhagic diathesis	Radiologic root resorption
+	+	+	–	–	–	+
+	+	+	–	–	–	–
+	–	+	–	+	+	+
+	0	+	–	+	+	–
+	+	+	–	–	+	–
+	0	+	+	0	–	–
+	0	+	+	0	–	+
+	0	+	–	0	+	+
+	0	+	–	+a	+a	–
+	+	+	+	+	0	+b
+	0	+	0	+	0	0

*+, Present; –, absent; 0, not mentioned; +a, autopsy; +b, histologic resorption.

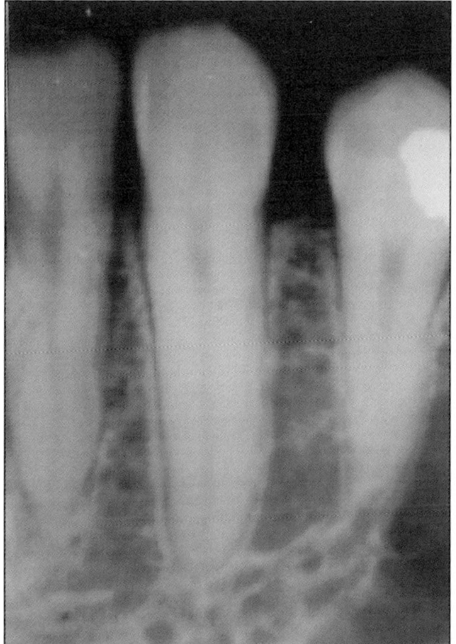

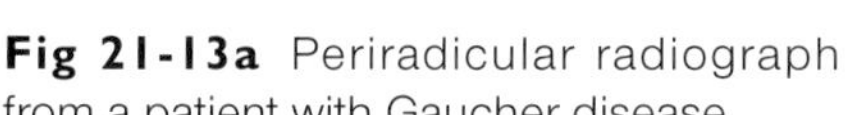

Fig 21-13a Periradicular radiograph from a patient with Gaucher disease.

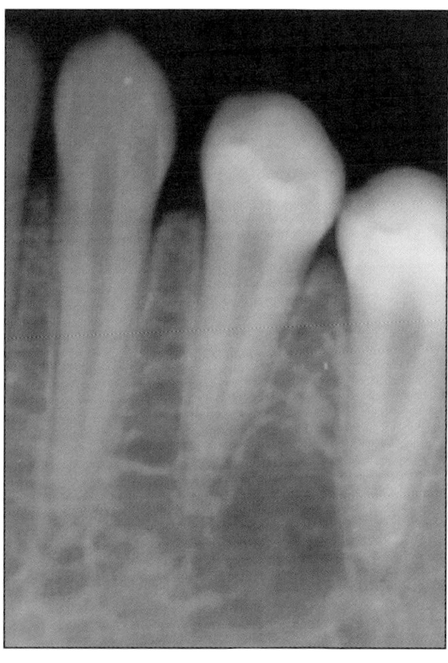

Fig 21-13b Periradicular radiograph from a patient with sickle cell anemia.

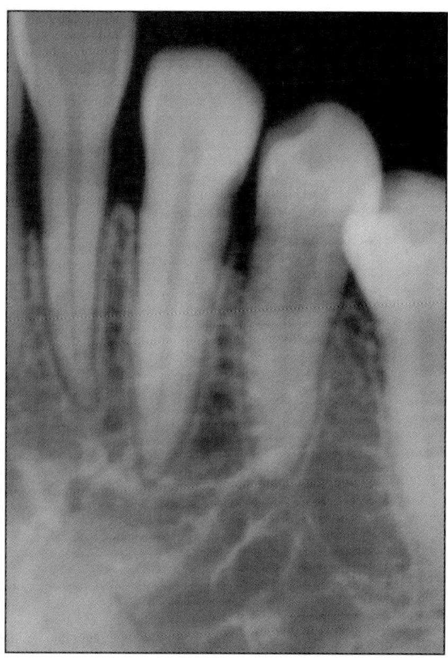

Fig 21-13c Periradicular radiograph from a patient with thalassemia.

Hemoglobinopathies

Hemoglobinopathies are a group of hereditary blood disorders. The two most common examples of the many autosomal gene mutation disorders are sickle cell anemia and thalassemia.

Sickle cell anemia

Sickle cell anemia (SCA) is the most common familial hereditary hematologic disorder in patients of African descent. Patients with SCA are homozygous for the mutant gene and patients with sickle cell trait are heterozygous for this gene. The mutation is a single codon substitution that leads to the inclusion of a valine amino acid in the β globin protein instead of glutamate. Approximately 8% to 12% of the African-American population of the United Stated carries the sickle cell trait (heterozygous). Sickle cell trait is usually less severe than SCA. However, it is important from a genetic counseling perspective.[16,96]

The distorted red sickle cell of SCA patients is relatively hydrophobic and cannot bend as the cell attempts to move through the capillaries. This causes a vaso-occlusion, an associated anemia, pallor, and tissue deterioration (eg, retinopathy, nephropathy, leg ulcers, and osteomyelitis of long bones and mandible). Patients with SCA have enlarged spleens or splenomegaly; this is attributed to the short life span (14 to 17 days) of the sickle cell. The complication of vaso-occlusion in SCA and the associated tissue hypoxia lead to the common pain crises known as *sickling crises*; these involve pain in the abdomen, joints, muscle, and bones.[97]

The most common oral complication of SCA in the facial skeleton is in the mandible, a frequent site of osteomyelitis in patients with SCA (Fig 21-13b). The disease occurs 200 times more often in the mandibles of patients with SCA than in the unaffected population. An estimated 28% of patients with SCA have had an osteomyelitis episode.[98]

Patients with sickle cell disorder may report odontalgia even in the absence of any evident dental pathosis.[99] In one study of 51 patients with sickle cell disorder and 51 matched controls, 67% of the sickle cell patients reported odontalgia in the prior year.[100] In half of these sickle cell patients, there was no evident dental pathosis. In contrast, none of the control subjects reported odontalgia in teeth without evident pathosis.[100]

However, other studies have reported a lower incidence of odontalgia. In a study with an 8-year follow-up, only 9% of patients with SCA (2 of 22) complained of intermittent toothache during sickling crises.[9] Histologic examination of a dental pulp from a patient with SCA revealed dilated blood vessels that were filled with microthrombi comprising sickle cells. The difference in pain that was reported in these studies may be related in part to the patients who were included because patients with SCA have a significantly higher incidence of reported odontalgia than do patients with sickle cell trait.[101]

Both localized and generalized pathoses have led to pulpal necrosis and treatment challenges in sickle cell patients.[83,102-109] Localized impairment of pulpal vasculature is associated with asymptomatic pulpal necrosis.[83,102] In one study, 22 homozygous patients with SCA (aged 12 to 37 years) were examined, and endodontic treatment was performed without anesthesia.[102] Five of the 22 patients (23%) had asymptomatic radiolucencies, and one patient had five different periradicular radiolucencies. A 4-year radiographic follow-up found good-to-complete radiographic healing.

Pulpal necrosis can also occur because of generalized vascular pathoses in sickle cell patients. In one report, a unilateral infarct of the mandible during a sickle cell crisis produced a generalized necrosis of mandibular premolars and molars.[103]

When pulpal pathoses occur in patients with SCA, it is prudent to consider endodontics rather than exodontics. The complication of vaso-occlusion following surgery could lead to osteomyelitis or infarction of the mandible.[83,100,103-106]

Thalassemia

Thalassemia is one of the most common genetic hemoglobinopathies and consists of a group of heterogenous blood disorders characterized by an inherited defect in the synthesis of at least one globin protein (β, α, γ, or δ globin) leading to a disorder in erythropoiesis.[16] The β-thalassemia form is the result of reduced synthesis of β globin; heterozygotes are carriers with mild-to-moderate anemia (eg, thalassemia minor), whereas homozygotes express the classic phenotype (eg, thalassemia major).

Thalassemia major (also known as *Cooley anemia*) is characterized by a severe microcytic hypochromic anemia with red cell counts of 1 million red cells/mm^3 of blood. Stained peripheral blood smears show numerous abnormal red blood cells, including immature cells, stippled cells, and target cells. Splenohepatomegaly and hyperactivity of the bone marrow cause bone radiolucency in long bones and the mandible. There is a shift toward the primitive cell forms, including erythroblasts and stem cells.[16]

Oral manifestations of β-thalassemia major include an enlarged maxilla, spacing of the anterior teeth, and an associated overjet, which result in poor occlusion. The hairbrush-like appearance on skull radiographs appears more pronounced in thalassemia major, although this finding is not pathognomonic.[106,107] The marked trabeculation and stepladder effect are illustrated in Fig 21-13c. Clinical features such as vaso-occlusive pain crisis, mandibular osteomyelitis, anesthesia of the mental nerve, and pulpal necrosis[108-110] have been reported in patients with hemoglobinopathies.

Several treatment interventions for thalassemia patients are in development. Dilazep (Tocris, Ellisville, MO) has been used in patients with β-thalassemia with significant increases in hemoglobin levels; however, one patient in this clinical trial exhibited substantial bleeding after a tooth extraction.[111] Another approach to treating patients with homozygous hemoglobinopathies, especially thalassemia major, is bone marrow transplantation for patients younger than 16 years of age.[112]

Fig 21-14 Periradicular radiographs of a patient with an autoimmune disorder directed against a membrane protein on neutrophils. The patient's circulating immunoglobulin A binds to a surface protein on neutrophils and blocks their chemotaxis and oxidative burst.

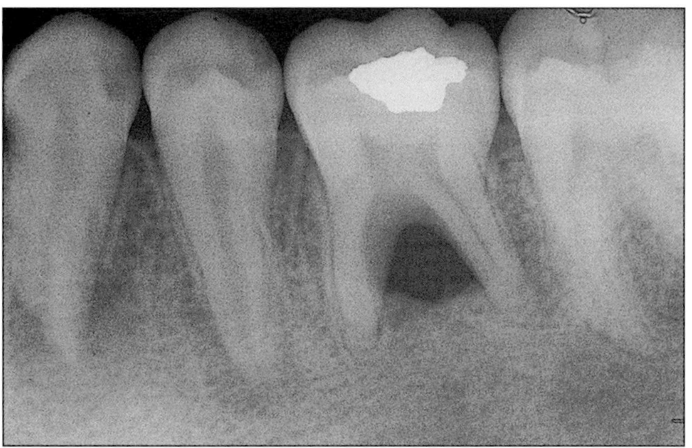

Fig 21-14a Extensive periradicular radiolucencies despite the absence of etiologic factors (caries, extensive restorations, advanced periodontitis, etc).

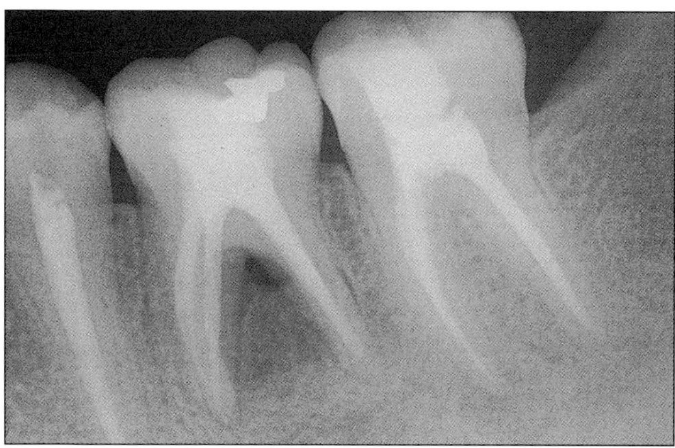

Fig 21-14b One-year follow-up revealing partial healing.

Genetic disorders of the immune system

Several genetic immunodeficiencies have profound dental implications. These include disorders of nonspecific immunity (eg, chronic granulomatous disease, cyclic neutropenia, Papillon-Lefèvre syndrome, Chédiak-Higashi syndrome, and leukocyte adhesion deficiencies) and disorders of specific immunity (eg, DiGeorge syndrome [thymic aplasia resulting in a decrease or absence of T cells], hypogammaglobulinemias, and selective immunoglobulin A and immunoglobulin G deficiencies). The implications of these disorders for pulpal and periradicular pathoses are reviewed in chapters 11 and 17.

One example of the effect of an immune disorder on pulpal tissue is presented here (Fig 12-14). The patient presented in severe pain. Multiple teeth were diagnosed as being necrotic and revealed apical periodontitis. The patient reported taking prednisone, gamma interferon, clindamycin, and ciprofloxacin. The medical history revealed a familial immunoglobulin A gammopathy in which circulating immunoglobulin A bound to a 62kd protein expressed on neutrophil membranes. Incubation of the patient's immunoglobulin A with either normal neutrophils or the patient's own neutrophils reduced chemotaxis by 80% and inhibited neutrophil responsiveness to test stimuli (eg, phorbol esters).[113]

The patient presented with extensive facial nodules (because of recurrent staphylococcal infections) and intermittent neutropenia. Clinical examination failed to reveal any potential etiologic factors for pulpal necrosis (ie, no caries, fractured teeth, history of trauma, periodontitis, or leaking restorations). Because etiologic factors were not evident, it is possible that pulpal necrosis occurred because of hematogenous infection from orofacial abscesses (anachoresis was not considered because there was no evidence of pre-existing pulpal inflammation).

Other developmental disorders affecting the dental pulp

A number of other developmental disorders have been shown to manifest themselves in the dental pulpal tissue. They are grouped together in this section merely because of their relatively low frequency of expression or because of the relative lack of studies describing their impact on dental pulp physiology.

Fabry disease is a rare X-linked disorder of lipid metabolism characterized by accumulation of trihexoside ceramide in blood vessels. It results from reduced activity of the lysosomal enzyme α-galactosidase A.[16] Clinical findings include characteristic skin lesions, renal failure, and cardiac complications. Histologic findings of dental pulp are characterized by trihexoside ceramide in the blood vessels.[11]

Lowe syndrome is a rare X-linked recessive disorder characterized by mental retardation, cataracts, and rickets. It is caused by a defect in glucosaminoglycogen metabolism.[114] Dental findings include large pulp chambers and altered dentinal formation.[115]

Niemann-Pick disease (sphingomyelin lipidosis) is a collection of four types of disorders of lipid metabolism, specifically affecting sphingomyelinase. It is characterized by severe neurologic disturbances, including mental retardation.[116] Reticuloendothelial cells are characterized as "foam cells" because of altered lipid levels and have been described in dental pulp.

Oxalosis (hyperoxaluria) is a rare autosomal-recessive disorder characterized by oxalate deposits in the kidney (leading to renal failure) and other tissues.[16] Dental findings include slate-gray teeth, odontalgia, pulpal calcifications of oxalate crystals, and root resorption.[117,118] The root resorption may be sufficiently extensive to necessitate tooth extraction.[119]

Endocrine Disorders and the Dental Pulp

Diabetes mellitus

Diabetes mellitus is a common metabolic disorder affecting more than 15 million persons in the United States.[120] The diabetic is not more vulnerable to bacterial infections, but there is a greater probability that infections that do develop will be more serious.[121,122] This susceptibility is due, in part, to a generalized circulatory disorder that results in inadequate blood supply to regions of injury.[16,123]

There are two major forms of diabetes mellitus. Type 1 diabetes mellitus is associated with a defect or an absence of the insulin-producing beta cells of the pancreas.[16] In this type, originally known as *insulin-dependent diabetes mellitus*, the patient needs exogenous insulin for survival. Type 2 diabetes mellitus, which occurs because of an impaired function of the beta cells or resistance to insulin effects, is the more common type.[16] Type 2 was previously referred to as *non-insulin-dependent diabetes mellitus*. The onset of type 2 occurs in midlife or later, whereas type 1 can begin during childhood or in the teenage years.

An important consideration in both type 1 and type 2 diabetes mellitus is the vascular system. The blood vessels are compromised by the continuous accumulation of atheromatous deposits in the intimal tissues of the blood vessel lumens. In addition, blood vessels, particularly capillaries, develop a thickened basement membrane that impairs leukocyte responses, and there is a decrease in the killing activity of polymorphonuclear neutrophil leukocytes.[121-125] The degree of vascular thickening is correlated to the duration of the disease.

Oral manifestations of infections occur more readily and more severely in type 1 than in type 2 diabetes. This may be influenced by age, duration of the disease, and the degree of metabolic control. Xerostomia, enlargement of the parotid glands, and an altered taste sensation can be observed.[120,126-128] There is also an increase in incidence of caries and periodontitis. Patients with either type 1 or type 2 diabetes mellitus, particularly those with poor insulin control, often have an increased risk of oral infections and periodontitis.[120,126-129]

Detailed human pulp studies in patients with diabetes mellitus do not exist, although two reports are found in the literature. One study described the pulpal histology in noncarious teeth extracted from seven diabetic patients with long-term disease of 15 to 24 years' duration and compared the findings to pulps from 13 control subjects.[130] The ages varied from 23 to 39 years, suggesting that these patients may have had type 1 diabetes mellitus. The pulpal tissues from the diabetic patients were characterized by the presence of large-vessel and small-vessel angiopathies and a thickened basement membrane. Many of the samples from diabetic patients contained numerous sickle-shaped calcifications that occluded vessels. Although this was a small study sample, the results suggest that late-stage diabetics experience both vascular changes and calcifications in the dental pulp.

A second study reported on histologic changes in dental pulps from 21 diabetic patients and 20 matched controls.[131] Extensive amorphous calcifications were observed in the pulps from the diabetics. However, no vascular changes were found in the dental pulps of the diabetic patients, although changes were evident in gingival biopsies. Because the patients' durations of illness were not stated in this study, it is possible that diabetes-related vascular changes in the pulp take longer to occur than do similar changes in gingival tissue.

Patients with diabetes have larger or more prevalent periradicular lesions of endodontic origin. A clinical and radiographic survey compared 94 patients with diabetes of long duration and 86 patients with diabetes of short duration to 86 individuals without diabetes (aged 20 to 70 years); there was a greater prevalence of periradicular lesions in patients with type 1 diabetes.[132] In particular, those with long-duration diabetes exhibited teeth with periradicular lesions more frequently than did the other groups. In addition, women with long-duration diabetes exhibited more endodontically treated teeth with periradicular lesions than did women with short-duration diabetes and women without diabetes.[133] This appears to be a generalized feature of diabetes; even rats with short-term streptozotocin-induced diabetes have significantly larger periradicular lesions of endodontic origin than do control animals.[134]

Diabetes-related odontalgia has been reported.[14,135,136] Unexplained odontalgia may be a clue to unrecognized diabetes mellitus, and, because diabetes leads to circulatory impairment with ischemia, pulpal necrosis may occur occasionally. For example, a 32-year-old white woman complained of a mild, constant, bilateral odontalgia (Bender, unpublished observations). Her medical history at the time of dental examination was noncontributory. The oral and radiographic examinations revealed low caries frequency and a few shallow restorations. There were no periradicular areas of rarefaction. She was instructed to see her physician and to return in 1 month.

She returned in 6 weeks, reporting that she still had unilateral pain and that her physician had diagnosed her with diabetes mellitus and prescribed insulin therapy. The patient was radiographically re-examined, and seven teeth with periradicular radiolucencies were noted. These teeth did not respond originally to the electric pulp tester. The teeth responded favorably to endodontic treatment. It is apparent that the patient was suffering from unrecognized diabetes mellitus.

Glucocorticoids

Cortisol, a naturally occurring glucocorticoid of the adrenocortex, has numerous effects on connective tissue, including dental pulp. Excessive cortisol production causes Cushing syndrome, while a deficiency produces Addison disease. An increase in production of cortisol by the adrenal gland may be caused by an adrenal adenoma or pituitary tumor (via release of corticotropin). Prolonged use of exogenous glucocorticoids can also produce effects similar to Cushing syndrome, including a rounded, plethoric face and trunk obesity.[16]

The chronic administration of high doses of glucocorticoids has numerous effects on the connective tissue of the dental pulp. This is observed

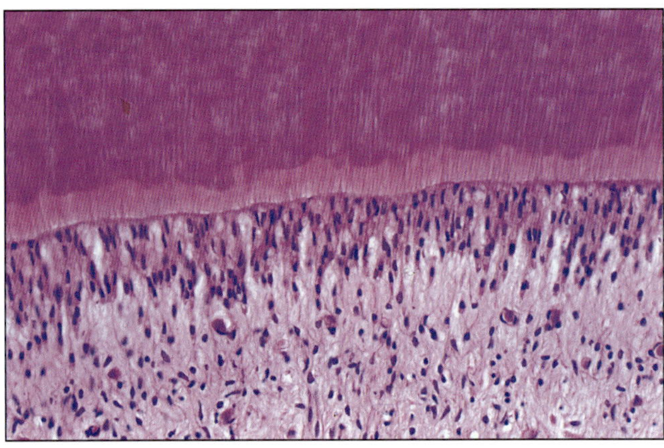

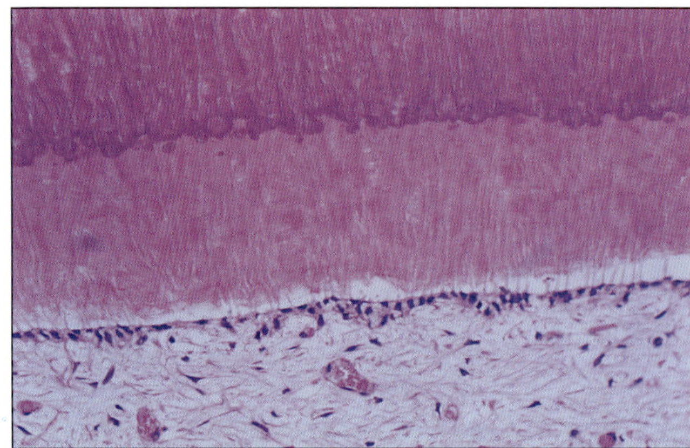

Fig 21-15 Comparison of predentin thickness in teeth collected from a healthy patient *(left)* and a patient who was chronically treated with glucocorticoids, suffering from renal failure, and undergoing dialysis *(right)*. The predentin is about four times wider in the former than it is in the latter (H&E stain). (Reprinted from Wysocki et al[140] with permission.)

particularly in patients with end-stage renal disease, who are often treated chronically with steroids.[137-140] Periradicular radiographic examination of these patients often reveals narrowing of the dental pulp chamber or complete pulpal obliteration. One study evaluated pulpal changes in 42 patients with renal disease who received prolonged glucocorticoid treatment and were followed for at least 2 years.[138] Radiographic examination revealed that 50% of these patients exhibited narrowing of the pulp chamber. Subset analysis revealed that this effect occurred more frequently in the group undergoing renal transplant (74%) than in the group undergoing hemodialysis (33%) or the group receiving immunosuppressive therapy (29%).[137,138] The earliest recording of pulpal narrowing was 10 months after renal transplantation.

Steroid-induced pulpal narrowing is the result of deposition of mineralized tissue in the pulp chamber. In a postmortem study of five patients who had been treated by renal transplantation, histologic examination of the dental pulp revealed a widened predentin zone, four times its normal width.[137] Similar results have been noted by other investigators examining pulp from patients undergoing hemodialysis (Fig 21-15).[140,141]

Rats undergoing long-term treatment with cortisone also exhibit excessive formation of a mineralized tissue in the dental pulp chamber.[139,142] The greatest dentinal deposition appeared to occur on the roof of the pulp chamber, suggesting that the pattern of dentinal deposition in the glucocorticoid-treated patient is different from that of the normal aging process.[143]

Cancer

There are relatively few reports of malignancies in dental pulp. In reviewing the dental literature published over a 100-year span (1870 to 1970), Stanley[7] reported fewer than 20 case reports of pulpal cancers.

However, several more recent case reports have described leukemic cellular infiltrates in dental pulp or periapical tissue.[7,144-147] Acute leukemias are characterized by malignant transformation of hematopoetic stem cells that often rapidly proliferate to replace bone marrow cells. The two major

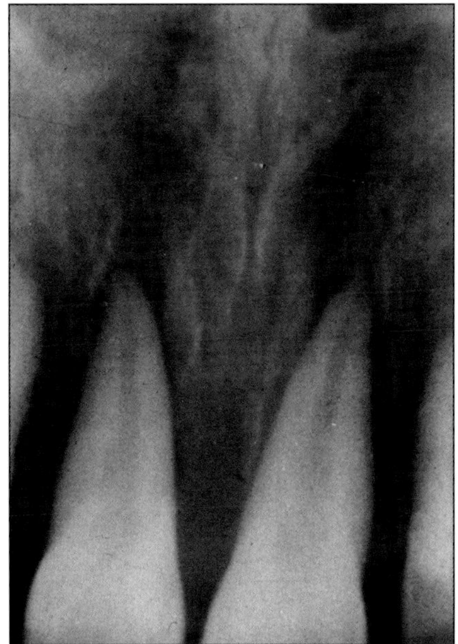
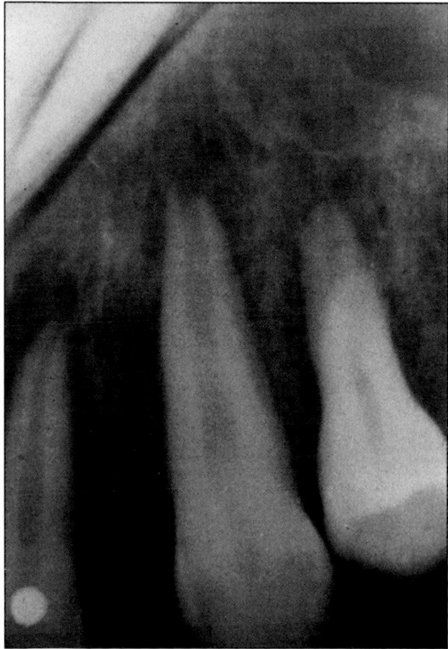

Fig 21-16 Periradicular radiographs of a 13-year-old patient with acute monocytic leukemia. Note the uniform widening of the periodontal ligament space.

classes of acute leukemia are acute lymphoblastic leukemia and acute myelogenous leukemia. Both types have been reported in dental pulp or periradicular tissue.[144-147]

Case reports have indicated that clinical findings include percussion sensitivity,[147] periradicular radiolucencies,[145-147] gingival swelling, odontalgia,[145,148] and a numb chin.[147] Other studies have noted that patients with acute myelogenous leukemia are five times more likely to have periodontal infections and two times more likely to have mucosal infections than they are to have periradicular pathoses.[149] Figure 21-16 shows radiographs from a patient with acute lymphocytic leukemia, revealing uniform widening of the periodontal ligament space.

Lymphomas are characterized as a malignant clonal proliferation of lymphoid cells in tissues comprising the immune system (eg, lymph nodes, spleen, bone marrow, gastrointestinal tract). The two major classes of lymphoma are Hodgkin disease and non-Hodgkin lymphoma.[16] Non-Hodgkin lymphoma is more prevalent than Hodgkin disease; about 50,000 new cases are diagnosed in the United States each year.

One form of non-Hodgkin lymphoma, Burkitt lymphoma, is more prevalent in central Africa than in the United States, and the Epstein-Barr virus is thought to be an etiologic agent. It may present as an enlargement of the jaws in children. Burkett lymphoma has been reported in dental pulp, where it completely replaced all pulpal cells.[7] Other case reports have noted that clinical findings of orofacial lymphomas include odontalgia,[150,151] tooth mobility,[151] periradicular radiolucencies,[151-153] jaw swelling,[7,151,154] numb lip,[155] and generalized osteolytic lesions.[151]

Many other forms of neoplasia have not been reported in dental pulp but must be considered in the differential diagnosis of periradicular lesions that are visible on radiographs. A partial list of primary and metastatic disorders includes carcinoma, adenocarcinoma, osteogenic sarcoma, multiple myeloma, sarcoma, and ameloblastoma.[7,13-17,152,156-161] Mandibular pain not related to a dental pathosis has been noted as an important symptom of the presence of metastatic neoplasia.[150-152,156-159]

Conclusion

A major theme of this textbook is the interrelationship between dental pulp and other tissues in health and disease. Although most of the chapters in this book have focused on the dental pulp and its effects on other tissues, chapters 20 and 21 have focused on the effect that systemic disorders have on dental pulp and patients' symptoms. Space limitations preclude a general review of the pathophysiology of these disorders or an extensive review of their effects on other orofacial tissues; the clinician is encouraged to seek other sources for this information.[13-17,96,161]

One of the most challenging steps in providing dental care to patients is establishing the differential diagnosis. In evaluating the patient's symptoms and the results of the clinical examination, the clinician should develop a differential diagnosis that considers both local and systemic pathoses. The lack of evident local etiologic factors (eg, caries or leaking restoration) or the presence of unusual findings (eg, numb lip or vital tooth with periradicular radiolucency) should prompt rapid and effective review of possible contributing systemic disorders.

References

1. Baumgartner JC, Heggers JP, Harrison JW. The incidence of bacteremias related to endodontic procedures 1. Nonsurgical endodontics. J Endod 1976;2:135–140.
2. Bender IB, Seltzer S, Yermish M. The incidence of bacteremia in endodontic manipulation. Oral Surg 1960; 13:353.
3. Bender IB, Barkan MJ. Dental bacteremia and its relationship to bacterial endocarditis: Preventive measures. Compend Contin Educ Dent 1989;10:472–483.
4. Debelian GJ, Olsen I, Tronstad L. Bacteremia in conjunction with endodontic therapy. Endod Traumatol 1995;11:142–149.
5. Bender IB, Naidorf I. Dental observations in vitamin D-resistant rickets with special reference to periapical lesions. J Endod 1985;11:514–520.
6. Bender IB Bender AL. Dental observations in Gaucher's disease: Review of literature and two case reports with 13- and 60-year follow-ups. Oral Surg Oral Med Oral Pathol 1996;82:650–659.
7. Stanley HR. The effect of systemic diseases on the human pulp. Oral Surg Oral Med Oral Pathol 1972;33: 606–648.
8. Seow W, Needleman H, Holm I. Effect of familial hypophosphatemic rickets on dental development: A controlled longitudinal study. Pediatr Dent 1995;17: 346–350.
9. Witkop CJ. Manifestations of genetic diseases in the human pulp. In: Siskin M (ed). The Biology of the Human Dental Pulp. St Louis: Mosby, 1973:215–257.
10. Stewart R. Dental pulp biopsy in the diagnosis of neurological disorders in childhood. J Hosp Dent Pract 1970;4:13–17.
11. Desnick S, Witkop C, Krivit W, Thies J, Desnick R. Fabry's disease (ceremide trihexosidase deficiency): Diagnostic confirmation by analysis of dental pulp. Arch Oral Biol 1972;17:1473–1479.
12. Carlo J, Willis J, McGarry P, Duncan M. Examination of dental pulp to diagnose infantile neuroaxonal dystrophy. Arch Neurol 1982;39:422–423.
13. Langlais R, Miller C. Color Atlas of Common Oral Diseases, ed 2. Philadelphia: Lippincott, 1998.
14. Lynch M. Burket's Oral Medicine: Diagnosis and Treatment, ed 9. Philadelphia: Lippincott, 1998.
15. Neville B, Damm D, Allen C, Bouquot J. Oral and Maxillofacial Pathology. Philadelphia: Saunders, 1995.
16. Beers M, Berkow R. The Merck Manual of Diagnosis and Therapy, ed 17. Whitehouse Station, NJ: Merck, 1995.
17. Jones JH, Mason D. Oral Manifestations of Systemic Disease. London: Bailliere Tindall, 1990.
18. Hicks M, Flats C, Carter A, Cron S, Rossmann S, Simon C, et al. Dental caries in HIV-infected children: A longitudinal study. Pediatr Dent 2000;22:359–364.
19. Ramos-Gomez F, Petu A, Hilton J, Canchola A, Wra D, Greenspan J. Oral manifestations and dental status in paediatric HIV infection. Int J Paediatr Dent 2000;10: 3–11.
20. Baqui A, Jabra-Rizx M, Kelley J, Zhang M, Falkler W, Meiller T. Enhanced interleukin 1β, interleukin 6, and tumor necrosis a production by LPS stimulated human monocytes isolated from HIV+ patients. Immunopharmacol Immunotoxicol 2000;22:401–422.
21. Baqui A, Meiler T, Jabra-Rizk M, Zhang M, Kelley J, Falkler W. Enhanced interleukin 1β, interleukin 6, and tumor necrosis factor α in gingival crevicular fluid from periodontal pockets of patients infected with human immunodeficiency virus 1. Oral Microbiol Immunol 2000;15:67–73.
22. Glick M, Trope M, Bagasra O, Pliskin M. Human immunodeficiency virus infection of fibroblasts in dental pulp of seropositive patients. Oral Surg Oral Med Oral Pathol Oral Radiol Endod 1991;71:733–736.

23. Elkins D, Torabinejad M, Schmidt R, Rossi J, Kettering J. Polymerase chain reaction detection of human immunodeficiency virus DNA in human periradicular lesions. J Endod 1994;20:386–388.
24. Cooper H. Root canal treatment in patients with HIV infection. Int Endod J 1993;26:369–371.
25. Glick M, Abel S, Muzyka B, DeLorenzo M. Dental complications after treating patients with AIDS. J Am Dent Assoc 1994;126:296–301.
26. Heling I, Morag-Hezroni M, Marwa E, Hochman N, Zakay-Rones Z, Morag A. Is herpes simplex virus associated with pulp/periapical inflammation? Oral Surg Oral Med Oral Pathol Oral Radiol Endod 2001;91: 359–361.
27. Rauckhorst AJ, Baumgartner C. Zebra XIX. 2. J Endod 2000;26:469–471.
28. Solomon CS, Coffiner MO, Chalfm [AU: Please confirm author's name]FIE. Herpes zoster revisited: Implicated in root resorption. J Endod 1986;12:210–213.
29. Gregory WB, Brook LE, Pennick EC. Herpes zoster associated with pulpless teeth. J Endod 1975;1:32–38.
30. Schwartz O, Kvorming SH. Tooth exfoliation, osteonecrosis of the jaw and neuralgia following herpes zoster of the trigeminal nerve. Int J Oral Surg 1982; 11:364–371.
31. Barakat H, Latronica R, Loiselle R. Herpes zoster simulating odontalgia. Rev Dent Liban 1960;19:80.
32. Heiman J. Odontalgia resulting from prodromal herpes zoster. J Mich Dent Assoc 1972;54:102–105.
33. Sigurdsson A, Jacoway J. Herpes zoster infection presenting as an acute pulpitis. Oral Surg Oral Med Oral Pathol Oral Radiol Endod 1995;80:92–95.
34. Goon W, Jacobsen P. Prodromal odontalgia and multiple devitalized teeth caused by a herpes zoster infection of the trigeminal nerve: Report of a case. J Am Dent Assoc 1988;166:500–504.
35. Ragozzino M, Melton L, Kurland L. Population-based study of herpes zoster and its sequelae. Medicine 1982; 61:310–316.
36. Guggenheimer J, Nowak A, Michaels R. Dental manifestations of the rubella syndrome. Oral Surg 1971;32: 30–37.
37. Hall R. Prevalence of developmental defects of tooth enamel (DDE) in a pediatric hospital department of dentistry population. Adv Dent Res 1989;3:114–119.
38. Theriault R, Hortobagyi G. The evolving role of bisphosphonates. Semin Oncol 2001;28:284–290.
39. Noor M, Shoback D. Paget's disease of bone: Diagnosis and treatment update. Curr Rheumatol Rep 2000;2: 67–73.
40. Rebel A, Malkani K, Basle MF, Bregeon C. Osteoclast ultrastructure in Paget's disease. Calcif Tissue Res 1976; 22:187–199.
41. Niedermeyer H, Arnold W, Neubert W, Sedlmeier R. Persistent measles virus infection as a possible cause of osteosclerosis: State of the art. Ear Nose Throat J 2000; 79:552–558.
42. Mills BG, Singer FR. Nuclear inclusions in Paget's disease of bone. Science 1976;194:201–202.
43. Mirra JM. Pathogenesis of Paget's disease based on viral etiology. Clin Orthop Related Res 1987;217:162–170.
44. Mills BG, Frausto A, Singer FR, Ohsaki Y, DeMulder A, Roodman GD. Multinucleated cells formed in vitro from Paget's bone marrow express viral antigens. Bone 1994;15:443–448.
45. Ischimi Y, Miyaura C, Jin CH. IL-6 is produced by osteoblasts and induces bone resorption. J Immunol 1990; 145:3297–3303.
46. Manolagas SC, Jilka RL. Bone marrow, cytokines, and bone remodeling. N Engl J Med 1995;332:305–311.
47. Carter LC. Paget's disease: Important features for the general practitioner. Compend Contin Educ Dent 1990;11:662–669.
48. Wheeler T, Alberts M, Dolan T, McGorray S. Dental, visual, auditory and olfactory complications of Paget's disease of bone. J Am Geriatr Soc 1995;43:1384–1391.
49. Barnett F, Elfenbein L. Paget's disease of the mandible: A review and report of a case. Endod Dent Traumatol 1985;1:39–42.
50. Smith SJ, Eveson JW. Paget's disease of bone with particular reference to dentistry. J Oral Pathol 1982;10: 233–247.
51. Wood NK, Goaz PW. Differential Diagnosis of Oral Lesions, ed 2. St Louis: Mosby, 1980:598–60l.
52. Aldred MJ, Cooke BED. Paget's disease of bone with involvement of the dental pulp. J Oral Pathol 1989;18: 184–185.
53. Lucas RB. The jaws and teeth in Paget's disease of bone. J Clin Pathol 1955;8:195–200.
54. Rosenberg LE. Inborn errors of metabolism. In: Duncan GD (ed). Duncan's Diseases of Metabolism. Philadelphia: Saunders 1974:53.
55. Chesney RW, Maxess RB, Rose P, Hamstra AJ, DeLuca HF, Breed AIL. Long-term influence of calcitriol (1-25 dihydroxy vitamin D) and supplemental phosphate in x-linked phosphatemic rickets. Pediatrics 1983;71: 559–567.
56. Witkop K. Manifestations of genetic diseases in the human pulp. Oral Surg Oral Med Oral Pathol Oral Radiol Endod 1971;22:278–316.
57. Shusterman S, Fellers FX The prevalence of enamel defects in childhood nephrotic syndrome. ASDC J Dent Child 1969;36:435–440.
58. Via W. "Spontaneous" degeneration of the dental pulp associated with phosphate diabetes. Oral Surg 1967; 24:623–628.
59. Ainley JE. Manifestations of familial hypophosphatenuria. J Endod 1978;4:26–28.

60. Shellis R. Structural organization of calcospherites in normal and rachitic human dentine. Arch Oral Biol 1983;28:85-95.

61. Murayama T, Iwatsubo R, Shigehisa A, Atsuo A, Ichijiro M. Familial hypophosphatemic vitamin D-resistant rickets: Dental findings and histologic findings of teeth. Oral Surg Oral Med Oral Pathol Oral Radiol Endod 2000;90:310-316.

62. Hillmann G, Geurtsen W. Pathohistology of undecalcified primary teeth in vitamin D-resistant rickets. Oral Surg Oral Med Oral Pathol 1996;82:218-224.

63. Witkop CJ Jr, Keenan K, Cervenka J, Jaspers M. Taurodontism: An anomaly of teeth reflecting disruptive homeostasis. Am J Med Genet Suppl 1988;4:85-97.

64. Jaspers M. Taurodontism in the Down syndrome. Oral Surg Oral Med Oral Pathol Oral Radiol Endod 1981;51:632-636.

65. Hata S, Fujita Y, Mayanagi H. The dentofacial manifestations of XXXXY syndrome: A case report. Int J Paediatr Dent 2001;11:138-142.

66. Varrela J, Alvesalo L. Taurodontism in 47,XXY males: An effect of the extra X chromosome on root development. J Dent Res 1988;67:501-502.

67. Hayashi Y. Endodontic treatment in taurodontism. J Endod 1994;20:357-358.

68. Yeh S, Hsu T. Endodontic treatment in taurodontism with Klinefelter's syndrome: A case report. Oral Surg Oral Med Oral Pathol Oral Radiol Endod 1999;88:612-615.

69. Hulsmann M. Dens invaginatus: Aetiology, classification, prevalence, diagnosis, and treatment considerations. Int Endod J 1997;30:79-90.

70. De Sousa SM, Bramante CM. Dens invaginatus: Treatment choices. Endod Dent Traumatol 1998;14:152-158.

71. Sapir S, Shapira J. Dentinogenesis imperfecta: An early treatment strategy. Am Acad Pediatr Dent 2001;23:232-237.

72. Patel P. Soundbites. Nat Genet 2001;27:129-130.

73. Witkop C. Amelogenesis imperfecta, dentinogenesis imperfecta and dentin dysplasia revisited. Problems in classification. J Oral Pathol 1989;17:547-553.

74. MacDougall M, Jeffords L, Gu T, Knight C, Frei G, Reus B, et al. Genetic linkage of the dentinogenesis imperfecta type III locus to chromosome 4q. J Dent Res 1999;78:1277-1282.

75. Shields E, Bixler D, El-Kafrawy A. A proposed classification for heritable human dentin defects with a description of a new entity. Arch Oral Biol 1973;18:543-553.

76. Pettiette M, Wright T, Trope M. Dentinogenesis imperfecta: Endodontic implications. Oral Surg Oral Med Oral Pathol Oral Radiol Endod 1998;86:733-737.

77. Collins M, Mauriello S, Tyndall D, Wright J. Dental anomalies associated with amelogenesis imperfecta: A radiographic assessment. Oral Surg Oral Med Oral Pathol Oral Radiol Endod 1999;88:258-264.

78. Paine M, Zhu D, Luo W, Bringas P, Goldberg M, White S, et al. Enamel biomineralization defects result from alterations to amelogenin self-assembly. J Struct Biol 2000;132:191-200.

79. Hulsmann M. Root canal treatment as a treatment modality for temporary tooth retention in adolescent patients. J Clin Pediatr Dent 1997;22:109-115.

80. Bouvier D, Duprez J, Bois D. Rehabilitation of young patients with amelogenesis imperfecta: A report of two cases. ASDC J Dent Child 1996;63:443-447.

81. Williams W, Becker L. Amelogenesis imperfecta: Functional and esthetic restoration of a severely compromised dentition. Quintessence Int 2000;31:397-403.

82. Bender IB. Dental observations in Gaucher's disease. J Dent Res 1938;11:359-360.

83. Smith HH, McDonald DK, Miller RI. Dental management of patients with sickle cells disorders. J Am Dent Assoc 1987;114:85-87.

84. Soderholm G, Lysell L, Svensson A. Changes in the jaws in chronic renal insufficiency and haemodialysis. Report of a case. J Clin Periodontol 1974;1:36-42.

85. Smith NHH. Albers-Schonberg disease (osteopetrosis). Oral Surg 1966;22:699-710.

86. Tassman GC, Bender IB. Gaucher's disease. J Am Dent Assoc 1940;27:1268.

87. Browne WO. Oral pigmentation and root resorption in Gaucher disease. J Oral Surg 1977;25:153-155.

88. Goldman HM. Gaucher's disease. Compend Contin Educ Dent 1988;9:42-43.

89. Heasman PA. Mandibular lesions in Gaucher disease. Oral Surg Oral Med Oral Pathol 1991;72:506.

90. Michanowicz AE, Michanowicz JP, Stine GM. Gaucher's disease. Oral Surg 1967;23:36-42.

91. Moch WS. Gaucher's disease with mandibular bone lesions. Oral Surg 1953;6:1250.

92. Sela J, Polliak A, Ulmansky M. Involvement of the mandible in Gaucher's disease: Report of a case with post-mortem findings. Br J Oral Surg 1972;9:246-250.

93. Weigler JM, Seldin R, Minkowitz S. Gaucher's disease involving the mandible: Report of a case. J Oral Surg 1967;25:158-163.

94. Bender IB. Dental observations in Gaucher's disease. A twenty-year follow-up. Oral Surg 1957;12:546-561.

95. Bender IB, Byers M, Mori K. Periapical replacement resorption of permanent, vital, endodontically treated incisors after orthodontic movement: Report of two cases. J Endod 1997;23:768-773.

96. Kumar V, Cotran R, Robbins S. Basic Pathology, ed 6. Philadelphia: Saunders, 1997.

97. King KE, Ness PM. Treating anemia. Hematol Oncol Clin North Am 1996;10:1305-1320.

98. Lawrenz DR. Sickle cell disease: A review and update of current therapy. J Oral Maxillofac Surg 1999;57:171-178.

99. Cox G. A study of oral pain experience in sickle cell patients. Oral Surg Oral Med Oral Pathol 1984;58:39–41.
100. May O. Dental management of sickle cell patients. Gen Dent 1991;39:182–183.
101. O'Rourke C, Mitropoulos C. Orofacial pain in patients with sickle cell disease. Br Dent J 1990;169:130–132.
102. Andrews CH, England MC, Kemp WC. Sickle cell anemia: An etiological factor in pulpal necrosis. J Endod 1983;9:249–252.
103. Bishop K, Briggs P, Kelleher M. Sickle cell disease: A diagnostic dilemma. Int Endod J 1995;28:297–302.
104. Shroyer JV III, Law D, Abreo F, Unhold CP. Osteomyelitis of the mandible as a result of sickle cell disease. Report and literature review. Oral Surg Oral Med Oral Pathol 1991;72:25–28.
105. Olaitan A, Amuda J, Adekeye E. Osteomyelitis of the mandible in sickle cell disease. Br J Oral Maxillofac Surg 1997;35:190–192.
106. Mourshed F, Tuckson CR. A study of the radiographic features of the jaws in sickle-cell anemia. Oral Surg 1974;37:812–819.
107. Ziccardi VB, Ferreti A, Schneider W. Management of sickle cell/thalassemia patient with severe odontogenic infection. NY State Dent J 1996;62:28–32.
108. Kelleher M, Bishop K, Briggs P. Oral complications associated with sickle cell anemia: A review and case report. Oral Surg Oral Med Oral Pathol Oral Radiol Endod 1996;82:225–228.
109. Duggal M, Bedi R, Kinsey S, Williams S. The dental management of children with sickle cell disease and β-thalassemia: A review. Int J Paediatr Dent 1996;6:227–234.
110. Bender IB. Pulpal pain diagnosis—A review. J Endod 2000;26:175–179.
111. Opartkiattikul N, Sukpanichnant S, Funahara Y, Sumiyoshi A, Wanachiwanawin W, Tatsumi N, et al. Cross-over placebo control trial of dilazep in β-thalassemia/hemoglobin E patients. SE Asian J Trop Med Public Health 1999;30:307–310.
112. Lucarelli G. Galimberti M, Polchi P, Angelucci E, Baronciani D, Giardini C, et al. Bone marrow transplantation in patients with thalassemia. N Engl J Med 1990; 322: 417–421.
113. Moy J, Nelson R, Richards K, Hostetter M. Identification of an IgA inhibitor of neutrophil chemotaxis and its membrane target for the metabolic burst. Immunology 1990;69:257–263.
114. Monnier N, Satre V, Lerouge E, Berthoin F, Lunardi J. OCRL1 mutation analysis in French Lowe's syndrome patients: Implications for molecular diagnosis strategy and genetic counseling. Hum Mutat 2000;16:157–165.
115. Harrison M, Odell E, Sheehy E. Dental findings in Lowe's syndrome. Pediatr Dent 1999;21:425–428.
116. Kolodny E. Niemann-Pick disease. Curr Opin Hematol 2000;7:48–52.
117. Boyce B, Prime S, Halls D, Johnson E, Critchlow H, McDonald D, et al. Does osteomalacia contribute to the development of oral complications of oxalosis? Oral Surg Oral Med Oral Pathol 1986;61:272–277.
118. Moskow B. Periodontal manifestations of hyperoxaluria and oxalosis. J Periodontol 1989;60:271–278.
119. Rahima M, DiMauro M. Primary hyperoxaluria in a pediatric dental patient: A case report. Pediatr Dent 1992;14:260–262.
120. Mealey B. Impact of advances in diabetes care on dental treatment of the diabetic patient. Compend Contin Educ Dent 1998;19:41–50.
121. Tennenberg S, Finkenauer R, Dwivedi A. Absence of lipopolysaccharide-induced inhibition of neutrophil apoptosis in patients with diabetes. Arch Surg 1999; 134:1229–1233.
122. Mealey B. Diabetes and periodontal diseases. J Periodontol 1999;70:935–49.
123. Bell GW, Large DM, Barclay SC. Oral health care in diabetes mellitus. Dent Update 199;26:322–330.
124. Witko-Sarsat V, Rieu P, Descamps-Latsha B, Halbwachs-Mercarelli L. Neutrophils: Molecules, functions and pathophysiological aspects. Lab Invest 2000;80:617–653.
125. Liles W, Klebanoff S. Regulation of apoptosis in neutrophils—Fast track to death? J Immunol 1995;155:3289–3291.
126. Rees T. The diabetic dental patient. Dent Clin North Am 1994;38:447–463.
127. Sandberg G, Sundberg H, Fjellstrom C, Wikblad K. Type 2 diabetes and oral health. A comparison between diabetic and non-diabetic subjects. Diabetes Res Clin Pract 2000;50:27–34.
128. Vernillo A. Diabetes mellitus: Relevance to dental treatment. Oral Surg Oral Med Oral Pathol Oral Radiol Endod 2001;91:263–270.
129. Ueta E, Osaki T, Yonda K, Yamamoto T. Prevalence of diabetes mellitus in odontogenic infections and oral candidiasis: An analysis of neutrophil suppression. J Oral Pathol Med 1993;22:168–174.
130. Russell B. The dental pulp in diabetes mellitus. Acta Pathol Microbiol Scand 1967;70:319–320.
131. Bissada NF. Sharawy AM. Histologic study of gingival and pulpal vascular changes in human diabetics. Egypt Dent J 1970;283–296.
132. Falk H, Hugoson A, Thorstensson H. Number of teeth, prevalence of caries and periapical lesions in insulin-dependent diabetics. Scand J Dent Res 1989;97:198–206.
133. Tenuvuo J, Alanen P, Larjava H, Virkari J, Lehtonen O-P. Oral health of patients with insulin-dependent diabetes mellitus. Scand J Dent Res 1986;94:338–346.
134. Kohsaka T, Kumazawa M, Yamasaki M, Nakamura H. Periapical lesions in rats with streptozotocin-induced diabetes. J Endod 1996;22:418–421.

135. Bender IB, Seltzer S. Special report: Dental procedures of interest to the physician in the management of patients with cardiovascular disease. Am Heart J 1963; 66:679.
136. Seltzer S, Bender IB. The Dental Pulp. Philadelphia: Lippincott, 1984:369.
137. Nässtrӧm K. Dentin formation after corticosteroid treatment. A clinical study and an experimental study on rats. Swed Dent J 1996;115(suppl):1–45.
138. Nässtrӧm K, Forsberg B, Petersson A, Westesson PL. Narrowing of the dental pulp chamber in patients with renal diseases. Oral Surg Oral Med Oral Pathol 1985;54: 242–246.
139. Nässtrӧm K, Moller B, Petersson A. Effect on human teeth of renal transplantation: A postmortem study. Scand J Dent Res 1993;101:202–209.
140. Wysocki GP, Valey TD, Ulan RA. Predentin changes in patients with chronic renal failure. Oral Surg Oral Med Oral Pathol 1983;56:167–173.
141. Ganibegovic M. Dental radiographic changes in chronic renal disease. Med Arh 2000;54:115–118.
142. Anneroth G, Bloom G. Structural changes in the incisors of cortisone-treated rats. J Dent Res 1966;45: 229–235.
143. Symons A, Symons DJ. Pulpal obliteration related to long-term glucocorticosteroid medication. Spec Care Dent 1994;14:103–107.
144. Maygarden S, Askin F, Burkes E, McMillan C, Sanders J. Isolated extramedullary relapse of acute myelogenous leukemia in a tooth. Mod Pathol 1989;2:59–62.
145. Peterson D, Gerad H, Williams L. An unusual instance of leukemic infiltrate. Diagnosis and management of periapical tooth involvement. Cancer 1983;51:1716–1719.
146. Morgan L. Infiltrate of chronic lymphocytic leukemia appearing as a periapical radiolucent lesion. J Endod 1995;21:475–478.
147. Hiraki A, Nakamura S, Abe K, Takensohita Y, Horinouchi Y, Shinohara M, et al. Numb chin syndrome as an initial symptom of acute lymphocytic leukemia: Report of three cases. Oral Surg Oral Med Oral Pathol 1997;83: 555–561.
148. Kanas R, Jensen J, DeBoom G. Painful, nonhealing tooth extraction socket. J Am Dent Assoc 1986;113:441–442.
149. Peterson D, Overholser C. Increased morbidity associated with oral infection in patients with acute nonlymphocytic leukemia. Oral Surg Oral Med Oral Pathol 1981;51:390–393.
150. Kant S. Pain referred to teeth as the sole discomfort in undiagnosed mediastinal lymphoma: Report of a case. J Am Dent Assoc 1989;118:587–588.
151. Svoboda W, Aaron G, Albano E. North American Burkitt's lymphoma presenting with intraoral symptoms. Pediatr Dent 1991;13:52–58.
152. Wannfors K, Hammarstrom L. Periapical lesions of mandibular bone: Difficulties in early diagnostics. Oral Surg Oral Med Oral Pathol 1990;70:483–489.
153. Heng C, Heng J. Implications of malignant lymphoma on a periapical mandibular lesion. Gen Dent 1995;43: 454–458.
154. Tsui S, Wong M, Lam W. Burkitt's lymphoma presenting as mandibular swelling—Report of a case and review of publications. Br J Oral Maxillofac Surg 2000;38:8–11.
155. Landesberg R, Yee H, Datikashvili M, Ahmed A. Unilateral mandibular lip anesthesia as the sole presenting symptom of Burkitt's lymphoma: Case report and review of the literature. J Oral Maxillofac Surg 2001;59: 322–326.
156. Pruckmayer M, Glaser C, Marosi C, Leitha T. Mandibular pain as the leading clinical symptom for metastatic disease: Nine cases and review of the literature. Ann Oncol 1998;9:559–564.
157. Glaser C, Lang S, Pruckmatyer M, Millesi W, Rasse M, Marosi C, et al. Clinical manifestations and diagnostic approach to metastatic cancer of the mandible. Int J Oral Maxillofac Surg 1997;26:365–368.
158. Boyczuk E, Solomon M, Gold B. Unremitting pain to the mandible secondary to metastatic breast cancer: A case report. Compend Contin Educ Dent 1991;12:104–110.
159. Selden H, Mannhoff D, Hatges N, Michel R. Metastatic carcinoma to the mandible that mimicked pulpal/periodontal disease. J Endod 1998;24:267–270.
160. Todd H, Langeland K. Pulpal destruction of neoplastic etiology. J Endod 1987;13:299–301.
161. White S, Pharoah M. Oral Radiology. Principles and Interpretation, ed 4. St Louis: Mosby, 2000.

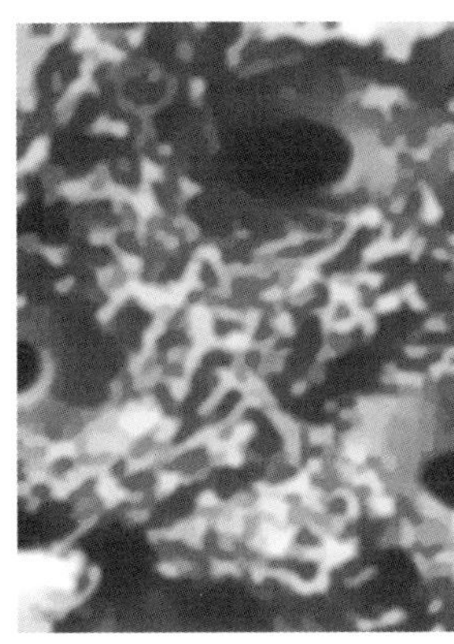

Index

Page references followed by "f" indicate figures, "t" indicate tables

R

S

T

U

V

W

Z